SECOND EDITION

Psychosocial Nursing Care Along the Cancer Continuum

Edited by
Rose Mary Carroll-Johnson, RN, MN
Linda M. Gorman, RN, MN, APRN, BC, OCN®, CHPN
Nancy Jo Bush, RN, MN, MA, AOCN®

D1231426

Oncology Nursing Society
Pittsburgh, Pennsylvania

ONS Publishing Division
Publisher: Leonard Mafrica, MBA, CAE
Director, Commercial Publishing: Barbara Sigler, RN, MNEd
Technical Editor: Angela Klimaszewski, MSN, RN
Production Manager: Lisa M. George, BA
Staff Editor: Lori Wilson, BA
Copy Editor: Amy Nicoletti, BA
Graphic Designer: Dany Sjoen

Psychosocial Nursing Care Along the Cancer Continuum (Second Edition)

Library of Congress Control Number: 2005936605

ISBN 1-890504-57-2

Publisher's Note

This book is published by the Oncology Nursing Society (ONS). ONS neither represents nor guarantees that the practices described herein will, if followed, ensure safe and effective patient care. The recommendations contained in this book reflect ONS's judgment regarding the state of general knowledge and practice in the field as of the date of publication. The recommendations may not be appropriate for use in all circumstances. Those who use this book should make their own determinations regarding specific safe and appropriate patient-care practices, taking into account the personnel, equipment, and practices available at the hospital or other facility at which they are located. The editors and publisher cannot be held responsible for any liability incurred as a consequence from the use or application of any of the contents of this book. Figures and tables are used as examples only. They are not meant to be all-inclusive, nor do they represent endorsement of any particular institution by ONS. Mention of specific products and opinions related to those products do not indicate or imply endorsement by ONS.

ONS publications are originally published in English. Permission has been granted by the ONS Board of Directors for foreign translation. (Individual tables and figures that are reprinted or adapted require additional permission from the original source.) However, because translations from English may not always be accurate or precise, ONS disclaims any responsibility for inaccuracies in words or meaning that may occur as a result of the translation. Readers relying on precise information should check the original English version.

Printed in the United States of America

Oncology Nursing Society
Integrity • Innovation • Stewardship • Advocacy • Excellence • Inclusiveness

To Sally Galbraith Thomas, RN, PhD, whose lessons regarding psychosocial nursing are as true today as when she mentored me 25 years ago.

Rose Mary Carroll-Johnson, RN, MN

To my dad, Henry Vodicka, who always believed in me and encouraged me to pursue my dreams. His death from lung cancer heightened my awareness of the impact of this disease and inspired me to continue working to educate others about it.

Linda M. Gorman, RN, MN, APRN, BC, OCN®, CHPN

For my son Derek, the miracle in my life. His courage and spirit have taught me the true meaning of coping and survivorship. Inspiration comes in many forms; mine is a product of his love.

Nancy Jo Bush, RN, MN, MA, AOCN®

Contributors

Editors

Rose Mary Carroll-Johnson, RN, MN
Editor, *Oncology Nursing Forum*
Valencia, California
Chapter 3. Life's Meaning and Cancer

Nancy Jo Bush, RN, MN, MA, AOCN®
Oncology Nurse Practitioner
Lecturer/Assistant Clinical Professor
School of Nursing
University of California, Los Angeles
Los Angeles, California
Chapter 4. Coping and Adaptation
Chapter 13. Anxiety and the Cancer Experience
*Chapter 35. Stress Management for Oncology Nurses:
    Finding a Healing Balance*

Linda M. Gorman, RN, MN, APRN, BC, OCN®,
    CHPN
Palliative Care/Hospice Clinical Nurse
    Specialist
Cedars-Sinai Medical Center
Los Angeles, California
*Chapter 1. The Psychosocial Impact of Cancer on the
    Individual, Family, and Society*
Chapter 16. Denial
Chapter 22. Powerlessness
Chapter 27. The Close of Life

Authors

Angela V. Albright, RN, APRN, BC, PhD
Associate Dean
College of Health and Human Services
California State University, Dominguez Hills
Carson, California
Chapter 15. Depression and Suicide

Paula J. Anastasia, RN, MN, AOCN®, OCN®
Gynecology-Oncology Clinical Nurse Specialist
Cedars-Sinai Medical Center
Los Angeles, California
*Chapter 5. Gender and Age Differences in the
    Psychological Response to Cancer*
Chapter 20. Altered Sexuality

Roberta H. Baron, RN, MSN, AOCN®
Clinical Nurse Specialist
Breast Surgical Oncology
Memorial Sloan-Kettering Cancer Center
New York, New York
*Chapter 30. Genetic Susceptibility Testing: Issues and
    Psychosocial Implications*

Susan Bauer-Wu, DNSc, RN
Director
Phyllis F. Cantor Center
Dana-Farber Cancer Institute
Instructor of Medicine
Harvard Medical School
Boston, Massachusetts
*Chapter 28. Psychoneuroimmunology: The Mind-
    Body Connection*

Libby Bowers, RN, MSN, CHPN, CCRN
Assistant Clinical Professor and Lecturer
School of Nursing
University of California, Los Angeles
Palliative Care Nurse Practitioner
Los Angeles, California
*Chapter 33. Ethical Issues Along the Cancer
    Continuum*

Deborah A. Boyle, RN, MSN, AOCN®, FAAN
Practice Outcomes Nurse Specialist
Project Leader, Gero-oncology and Survivorship
    Nursing Studies Program
Banner Good Samaritan Medical Center
Phoenix, Arizona
Chapter 2. Survivorship

Katherine Brown-Saltzman, RN, MA
Executive Director, Healthcare Ethics Center
University of California, Los Angeles Medical
    Center
Assistant Clinical Professor
School of Nursing
University of California, Los Angeles
Los Angeles, California
Chapter 18. Transforming the Grief Experience

Carol Campbell-Norris, BA, MS
Marriage and Family Therapist
Bereavement Counselor
Hospice of the Comforter
Altamonte Springs, Florida
Chapter 17. Body Image Disturbance

Peggy Compton, RN, PhD
Associate Professor
School of Nursing
University of California, Los Angeles
Los Angeles, California
Chapter 34. Substance Abuse

Phyllis Gorney Cooper, RN, MN
Community Health Consultant and Educator
Editor, *Nursing Forum*
COOPER CONSULTING
El Segundo, California
*Chapter 8. The Influence of Hope on the Psychosocial
    Experience*
Chapter 19. Guilt

Carol P. Curtiss, RN, MSN
Clinical Nurse Specialist Consultant
Curtiss Consulting
Greenfield, Massachusetts
*Chapter 9. The Psychosocial Impact of the Pain
    Experience*

Sheila M. Ferrall, RN, MS, AOCN®
Oncology Clinical Nurse Specialist
H. Lee Moffitt Cancer Center & Research
    Institute
Tampa, Florida
Chapter 36. Caring for the Family Caregiver

Betty R. Ferrell, PhD, FAAN
Research Scientist
City of Hope National Medical Center
Nursing Research and Education
Duarte, California
Chapter 10. Suffering

Margaret I. Fitch, RN, MScN, PhD
Head, Oncology Nursing and Supportive Care
Director, Psychosocial and Behavioral Research
    Unit
Toronto Sunnybrook Regional Cancer Centre
Toronto, Canada
*Chapter 25. Programmatic Approaches to Psychosocial
    Support*

Diane M. Fletcher, MA, RN, OCN®
Chief Executive Officer
Southwest Georgia Cancer Coalition
Albany, Georgia
*Chapter 32. Complementary and Alternative Medicine:
    Moving Toward Integrative Cancer Care*

Judi Johnson, PhD, RN, FAAN
Nurse Consultant
HealthQuest
Minneapolis, Minnesota
*Appendix. Psychosocial Support Programs and
    Resources for People Surviving Cancer and Their
    Families*

Catherine H. Kelley, RN, MSN
Manager, Clinical Scientists
Centocor, Inc.
Horsham, Pennsylvania
*Chapter 31. Psychosocial Aspects of Hematopoietic Stem
    Cell Transplantation*

Paula Klemm, DNSc, RN, OCN®
Associate Professor
School of Nursing
University of Delaware
Newark, Delaware
*Chapter 26. Technologic Advances: Psychosocial
    Implications for Patient Care*

Angela D. Klimaszewski, RN, MSN
Nurse Consultant
ADK Communications
Canton, New York
*Chapter 29. Psychosocial Aspects of Experimental
    Therapy: Clinical Trials*

Robin M. Lally, PhD(c), RN, MS, AOCN®, CNS
Clinical Nurse Specialist
Jane Brattain Breast Center
Park Nicollet Health Services
Minneapolis, Minnesota
Appendix. Psychosocial Support Programs and Resources for People Surviving Cancer and Their Families

Dale G. Larson, PhD
Professor
Department of Counseling Psychology
Santa Clara University
Santa Clara, California
Chapter 35. Stress Management for Oncology Nurses: Finding a Healing Balance

Esther Muscari, RN, MSN, APRN, BC
Director, Oncology
The Cancer Center at Henrico Doctor's Hospital
Richmond, Virginia
Chapter 12. Cognitive Impairment in Cancer
Chapter 21. Delirium and Dementia

Kathryn E. Pearson, RN, CNS, MN, AOCN®
Oncology Clinical Nurse Specialist
St. Jude Medical Center
Fullerton, California
Chapter 23. Interpersonal and Therapeutic Skills Inherent in Oncology Nursing

Janice E. Post-White, PhD, RN, FAAN
Research Consultant in Complementary and Alternative Medicine
Adjunct Associate Professor
School of Nursing
University of Minnesota
Minneapolis, Minnesota
Chapter 28. Psychoneuroimmunology: The Mind-Body Connection

Judith A. Shell, PhD, LMFT, RN, AOCN®
Medical Family Therapist
Marriage and Family Therapist
Osceola Cancer Center
Kissimmee, Florida
Chapter 17. Body Image Disturbance

Mady C. Stovall, RN, MSN, ONP, OCN®
Oncology Nurse Practitioner
University of California, Los Angeles
Los Angeles, California
Chapter 11. Cancer-Related Fatigue

Virginia Sun, MSN, RN
Senior Research Specialist
Departments of Medical Oncology and Nursing Research and Education
City of Hope National Medical Center
Duarte, California
Chapter 10. Suffering

Elizabeth Johnston Taylor, PhD, RN
Associate Professor
School of Nursing
Loma Linda University
Loma Linda, California
Chapter 7. Spirituality and Spiritual Nurture in Cancer Care

Sharon M. Valente, RN, APRN, BC, PhD, FAAN
Assistant Chief
Nursing Research and Evaluation
Veterans Administration Greater Los Angeles Healthcare System
Los Angeles, California
Chapter 15. Depression and Suicide

Sharon Van Fleet, MS, APRN, BC
Clinical Nurse Specialist
H. Lee Moffitt Cancer Center & Research Institute
Tampa, Florida
Chapter 24. Crisis Intervention

Ashby C. Watson, APRN, BC, OCN®
Psychosocial Oncology Clinical Nurse Specialist
Virginia Commonwealth University Medical Center
Richmond, Virginia
Chapter 14. Anger and Cancer

DeLois P. Weekes, RN, BS, MS, DNSc
President and Chief Executive Officer
Lester L. Cox College of Nursing and Health Sciences
Springfield, Missouri
Chapter 6. Cultural Influences on the Psychosocial Experience

Mercedes K. Young, RN, MSN, ONP
Oncology Nurse Practitioner
Norris Comprehensive Cancer Center and Hospital
University of Southern California
Los Angeles, California
Chapter 11. Cancer-Related Fatigue

Table of Contents

Section IV. Psychosocial Interventions   383

Appendix   611

Index   649

Preface

Seven years have passed since we wrote the Preface to the first edition of this book. We are seven years older and wiser, we have passed seven more anniversaries of the heart, our children are now young adults, we have lost parents, our health and the health of those we love has been hard won, and America has lived through 9/11, another Iraq war, and the worst natural disaster ever to hit our shores. What has not changed is the inevitability of the presence of cancer in our personal and professional lives. Perhaps because of the added burdens in our daily lives, the need to confront and intervene with the psychological ravages of cancer has become even more a priority for healthcare professionals.

Over the last seven years, some advances in the treatment of cancer have been made. Some cancers appear less frequently, but others continue to present our patients and their families with increasingly complicated challenges. Many new drugs and treatments are available to us now, but with them come the inevitable side effects and potential long-term problems. Many more of our fellow Americans are without healthcare coverage, and those who have coverage fight the eroding of their benefits with each passing month. The personal crisis that is cancer can tax even the strongest copers beyond the limits of their endurance. The need for psychological and emotional support for everyone concerned—patients, family members, healthcare providers—has grown and will continue to grow.

This book is intended to help nurses and other related healthcare providers to understand and be able to intervene with the psychosocial turmoil faced by those diagnosed with cancer. This second edition attempts to improve on the quality work done by our contributors in the first edition in a number of critical ways. First and foremost, the content has been updated with the addition of new source material and identification of knowledge generated in the seven years since the first edition was published. Some chapters have been reconfigured to better reflect the nature of our current practice, and some topics only touched on seven years ago get full treatment in this edition. The presence and importance of technology, specifically the Internet, is acknowledged, and a comprehensive list of resources for patients and families is provided. From a professional point of view, we have sought to incorporate principles of evidence-based practice into the chapters to further highlight what we know and what continues to require further examination. We acknowledge changes in practice such as collaborative practice and the shift to nurse practitioners in many settings. Still, at the center of it all is a patient struggling to understand what is happening and why—a patient who continues to deal daily with the fear and sadness a diagnosis of cancer inevitably brings. And still it usually falls to a nurse to guide, educate, console, support, and encourage those patients. Despite new advances and new treatments, we can be assured that some things will never change, and oncology nurses will remain first responders for individuals caught up in the personal disaster that is cancer.

As we edited this second edition, we became yet again aware of the interconnectedness of the content. Books are neatly divided into chapters of discrete information, but as you use the book you will come to see, as we did, that the human psyche and its emotions are multifaceted and connected on many different levels. Reading individual chapters will help to enlighten you with respect to a particular topic, but it also will point you in the direction of two or three other chapters, each relevant to the problem you originally looked up. Take the time to consider that you likely will find the information you need in a number of places. It is not so much duplication of content as it is a testament to the holistic nature of the mind and body. This can be reassuring in some sense. The number of interventions becomes greater and our chance of success in helping our patients and their families to cope multiplies exponentially the more directions you can take to deal with a problem. The importance of this aspect of our nursing care cannot be underestimated, and it is our sincere wish that this book can help you in those endeavors.

Special thanks to the authors of chapters in the first edition. Their work laid the foundation for this second edition. We are grateful to colleagues, new and old, for their work to update the content and make it as useful as it can be. Barbara Sigler and her staff at the Oncology Nursing Society were helpful and gracious at each step. A book like this is truly a partnership, and we had the best of help from every corner. Finally, thanks to our families for their support, love, and pride in our work and our accomplishments and for believing that all those book meetings were worth the sacrifice on their parts. We are blessed with all that we have been given.

SECTION I

The Psychosocial Impact of Cancer on the Individual, Family, and Society

CHAPTER 1

The Psychosocial Impact of Cancer on the Individual, Family, and Society

LINDA M. GORMAN, RN, MN, APRN, BC, OCN®, CHPN

We are not ourselves when nature, being oppressed, commands the mind to suffer with the body.
—William Shakespeare

It is now known that psychosocial issues affect patients in all stages of cancer. Emotional response can influence both morbidity and mortality (Holland, 2002). The increased emphasis on psychosocial oncology in recent years has led to more research, education, and training programs as more professionals appreciate the importance of this aspect of care. Psychosocial care of patients is needed in all phases of the cancer experience. Holland (2003) identified three factors contributing to psychological adaptation: (a) type of cancer, (b) personal coping skills, and (c) society's prevailing attitudes toward cancer.

Diagnosis

The anxiety and uncertainty of a cancer diagnosis can create extreme disruption in the life of almost any individual. A cancer diagnosis can create a threat to one's general sense of security and orderliness in life. Although the vast majority of cancers are treatable, many people retain deep-seated fears that any cancer represents pain, suffering, and death. Holland (2002) noted that no disease has sustained as strong of a negative stigma as cancer. These fears can contribute to a person's reaction to a new cancer diagnosis. Whatever the type of cancer, people are faced with ongoing uncertainty about their future as they deal with the potential for an unpredictable course (Dankert et al., 2003). A cancer diagnosis leads to a complex set of issues, including dealing with physical symptoms from the disease and treatment, facing the existential dimension of the illness, and seeking a comforting philosophical, spiritual, or religious belief structure or values that give meaning to life and death (Holland, 2002).

Awareness

Prior to the diagnosis, the individual may be aware of body changes that could indicate cancer (e.g., a lump, abnormal bleeding). Nail (2001) called this the Recognition Phase. This awareness creates a state of hyperalertness that eventually leads to action in most people. How quickly this action occurs depends on many variables, including past experience with cancer in oneself or one's family. An experience with cancer may encourage some to seek quick medical attention. The experience of others may cause them to avoid medical attention because they are fearful of what the symptoms could mean. Pain or discomfort created by the symptoms tends to motivate people to seek medical attention (Mood, 1996). Other factors may contribute to delays, such as feeling uncomfortable around healthcare providers, financial considerations, fear of dependency, and fear of disfigurement. Fear of cancer treatment may contribute to an individual's acknowledgment of symptoms. Family members with similar values may inadvertently promote the same delaying behaviors that the patient is using. Lack of knowledge about symptoms also may cause a delay.

Receiving the Cancer Diagnosis

In the United States, adherence to the ethical principle of autonomy has resulted in physicians directly telling patients about the diagnosis of cancer. The principle of autonomy dictates that the individual has the right to determine his or her own course of action with a self-determined plan (Beauchamp & Childress, 2001). In the healthcare field, this means one has the right to know and participate in all healthcare decisions. The original 1847 Code of Ethics of the American Medical Association (cited in Katz, 1984) noted that a physician's duty is to avoid all things that could discourage or depress the spirit. This philosophy contributed to physicians receiving limited education in medical school about how to deliver bad news (Girgis & Sanson-Fisher, 1995). In 1961, 90% of surveyed physicians preferred not to directly tell patients about a cancer diagnosis (Oken, 1961). In 1977, more than 90% of physicians favored sharing such information with patients (Novack, Plumer, & Smith, 1978). This dramatic change in practice reflected the social changes of the 1960s and 1970s that resulted in an emphasis on openness. Access to oncology specialists who had experience in sharing bad news became widely available during that time. The development of research protocols emphasizing informed consent was another factor (Holland, 2002).

At times, families still ask that patients not be told about the diagnosis. This creates ethical dilemmas for healthcare providers about obtaining informed consent for treatment from their patients. Being pressured to use words like "growth" for the cancer or "special medicine" for chemotherapy makes providing care to these patients more difficult. Dunn, Patterson, and Butow (1993) noted that not being open about the diagnosis still leads to patients suspecting it and thinking that the cancer must be so horrible that even physicians or nurses will not acknowledge it. Avoiding the use of the word "cancer" reinforces the fear associated with the word (Holland, 2002, 2003).

If physicians do not tell patients the diagnosis, a risk always exists that someone will inadvertently share the information with the patient, causing the patient to greatly distrust the healthcare team and family. Dunn et al. (1993) identified the tendency of healthcare professionals and family members to avoid patients who have not been told the truth because of the fear of misspeaking. Openness about the diagnosis and prognosis enables patients to think more realistically about their condition and participate actively in treatment planning. Most individuals are able to adjust to the diagnosis over time (Dunn et al.). It is important to note that autonomy is not practiced worldwide. Patients and families from other cultures may be unprepared to receive the diagnosis directly. Healthcare professionals need to address the family's fears about sharing the news and offer suggestions for assisting the patient. Creating a balance between providing some information without alienating the patient and family can be difficult.

How one receives news of a cancer diagnosis is an important factor in how one responds (Dias, Chabner, Lynch, & Penson, 2003; Rabow & McPhee, 1999; Tulsky, 1998). Figure 1-1 lists some helpful guidelines for sharing the news of a cancer diagnosis. Healthcare professionals, including oncology nurses, need to develop skills in presenting information accurately yet gently, thus maintaining hope regardless of the prognosis. Although nurses may not deliver the initial diagnosis, they often are in a position to reinforce information, provide support, and consult with physicians about sharing the news. Schofield et al. (2003) reported that patients experience less anxiety associated

---

Figure 1-1. Guidelines for Giving a Cancer Diagnosis

- Provide privacy and adequate time to share the information and provide support.
- Ask the patient how much he or she wants to know.
- Encourage the patient to bring a family member to the meeting.
- Consider taping the meeting or providing a written summary of the information.
- Monitor for signs of emotional distress and respond as needed.
- Give the information gradually rather than starting with the diagnosis.
- Listen to the patient's and family's concerns.
- Assess their understanding of what has been shared throughout the process.
- Develop an alliance with the patient about the treatment plan.
- If needed, ensure that professional interpreters are available.
- If the prognosis is very poor, avoid giving a definite time frame.
- Reinforce information given on subsequent visits and when the patient and family see other healthcare professionals.
- Provide resources for follow-up support.

Note. Based on information from Buckman, 1992; Fried et al., 2003; Girgis & Sanson-Fisher, 1995; Tulsky, 1998.

---

with the following communication style of how news is given: The physician prepares the patient ahead of time for a possible cancer diagnosis, provides written information, and openly discusses life expectancy and severity of the cancer; the patient has someone with him or her when information is given; questions are addressed on the same day as the initial discussion; and the patient is involved in treatment decisions.

The Patient's Response to the Diagnosis

Whether a person anticipates the diagnosis, his or her initial response usually is disbelief, numbness, and anxiety. Receiving a cancer diagnosis is associated with a peak of negative mood and distress for many (Nail, 2001). Waves of intense emotions similar to a grief reaction with periods of calmness are common. Generally, following the initial days after receiving the diagnosis, most individuals are able to develop a constructive plan of action. Healthcare professionals must remember that no matter how compassionate and skilled the person is in giving the bad news, patients still may experience extreme emotional reactions (Shell & Kirsch, 2001).

To integrate the idea of having cancer into one's psyche, the patient may feel the need to identify the cause. Asking "why me?" may be part of this process. Seeking information about the type of cancer and its treatment can give the person some sense of control. Information seeking is a more common coping mechanism in the early stages of the disease, when the diagnosis is new and the patient is dealing with a variety of new healthcare professionals (Nail, 2001).

Some individuals initially respond with denial. They cannot allow themselves to think about what will happen if the treatment does not work or how this will affect the family. Denial is a protective mechanism from this tremendous threat. It is a common initial reaction to the overwhelming threat but generally decreases over time. Some individuals are able to forestall any emotional reaction to the news as they research the disease, consider treatment options, and interview physicians. This allows patients to remain more focused on the decision making. However, an emotional reaction can surface at any time.

In a landmark study, Weisman and Worden (1976–1977) examined 120 patients in the first 100 days after receiving a cancer diagnosis and described the extreme distress commonly experienced in hearing the news. Intermittent periods of anxiety and depression were common. Some of the factors they found that contributed to poor overall psychosocial adaptation included having more physical symptoms, perceiving the physician as being less helpful, having a psychiatric history, and having a pessimistic view of the world. The most significant variables were a perceived lack of a personal support system, having a more advanced illness, and viewing the physician as being unsupportive. Lampic, Thurfjell, Bergh, Carlsson, and Sjoden (2003) found that patients with a new diagnosis of breast cancer attributed significantly more importance to closer and more positive relationships with people in their lives.

As the patients return to their normal routine, some of the initial intense reactions tend to decrease, with intermittent periods of increased intensity. Everyone needs to view life as existentially meaningful, and cancer undermines this effort (Northouse & Northouse, 1996). Weisman and Worden (1976–1977) found that within three months of the diagnosis, most individuals began examining and reviewing their lives, as well as looking for meaning in what was happening to them. This period of intense existential analysis can be difficult and painful for patients and their families. Patients may challenge long-held beliefs and values of the family and search for new areas of meaningfulness that family members do not share.

Family Reactions

When cancer enters an individual's life, it also enters the lives of family members and close friends. Research clearly indicates that cancer enters the emotional, social, physical, and spiritual well-being of patients and their family members (Northouse, 2005). It presents a major crisis for them as well as the patient (Glajchen, 2004). Walking the illness journey with a loved one can contribute to many reactions, including feelings of loss of control, disrupted family organization, and altered relationships (Shell & Kirsch, 2001). They also noted that the initial uncertainty contributes to many extremes in reactions. The initial response is similar to the patient's: extreme distress and disruption. A sense of vulnerability and awareness of the inability to protect a loved one can lead to an intense sense of helplessness. Because family members and patients often share common beliefs, the reactions of family members may parallel those of patients (Lederberg, 1998). Denial or blaming others for the diagnosis may occur in close family members as well. Family members may experience vulnerability with the realization that this could happen to themselves.

Seeing a loved one vulnerable and fearful can create much distress, especially if this is a big change from the patient's normal personality. Family members often face many role changes at the time of the cancer diagnosis. Disruptions in schedules and taking on new roles of caregiving, meal preparation, and other family duties may put a strain on some family members. Role changes can contribute to communication problems if one is not sure of the usual routines or schedules. The financial demands of treatment options can create concerns about the need to continue working. The strain of feeling continuously "on duty" to provide physical and emotional support, on top of dealing with their own fears, adds to the pressures of family members. They also may need to conceal their own feelings and fears of what will be expected of them in the future if the disease progresses.

Some family members may assume the role of cheerleader to remain upbeat and encourage the patient to remain optimistic. This role can become very draining. It can lead to resentment if one's own needs are not being recognized or met. Resentment can occur regarding the stress and inconvenience imposed on the family, as well as past behaviors that they attribute to causing the cancer (e.g., smoking, high-stress lifestyle) (Mood, 1996). Some members may take on additional roles, such as assisting with research and treatment decisions, if the patient is paralyzed by anxiety or is too ill to participate.

Family members play a key role in the support system of most patients. How to provide support to patients and best meet their needs may require a period of trial and error. For example, patients may want to be more independent, whereas family members may feel the need to be protective, leading to resentment and increased stress on both sides. A lack of communication can lead to feeling that one's needs are going unrecognized and feelings of being smothered or isolated from family life.

Spouses often feel devastated because they have not considered what life together with illness would involve (Shell & Kirsch, 2001). A cancer diagnosis can bring couples closer or can distance them as more stress is added to the relationship (Glajchen, 2004).

Life Span Considerations

The response of family members to the diagnosis of a childhood cancer often is profound shock and disruption. Parents particularly are overwhelmed with the realization of their child's vulnerability to this disease. Parents may experience high levels of anxiety as they try to protect their child from any distress. In addition to the emotional distress, family members must face the disease-related demands that affect the entire family. These can include financial demands, transportation to multiple medical visits, supporting other family members, and conducting research related to the disease (Kristjanson & Ashcroft, 1994).

A child's response to a cancer diagnosis in a family member depends on the child's developmental and cognitive level, as well as on how the parent responds (Northouse, Cracchiolo-Caraway, & Appel, 1991). During the time of family disruption caused by the diagnosis, the child may exhibit behavioral and adjustment problems (e.g., problems with school attendance, sleep, aggression) in response to his or her anxiety. Children need to become more adaptive to change at these times (King, 2003). Children must receive information about what is happening, but it must be at a level that they can comprehend.

Cancer is increasingly more likely to occur as one ages (Jemal et al., 2005). Thus, older adults are more at risk. The strain on an older couple, especially when one is already frail, can be overwhelming. This can create an added burden for the patient with cancer who wants to protect the other spouse. Financial demands as well as limited support systems and problems with caregiving are other concerns.

Cancer Treatment

As the diagnostic phase is completed and treatment decisions are made, the patient and family face new experiences that will affect them psychosocially. These include hospitalization, surgery, insertion of a central line, starting chemotherapy or other treatments, and frequent doctor visits. An urgency often exists to begin treatment, and no matter how much education the patient receives, he or she still may feel unprepared to enter this unfamiliar world. Each type of treatment creates its own psychosocial impact.

Surgery

Surgery is the oldest form of cancer treatment (Jacobsen, Roth, & Holland, 1998). Surgery alone as a cancer treatment may not be associated with the same negative view as other treatments that are more closely aligned to cancer. Patients are more familiar with surgery than other types of cancer treatments because surgery is routinely performed for noncancerous conditions with positive outcomes. It is viewed as a way to eliminate the cancer from one's body. However, mastectomies, genital surgeries, head and neck surgeries, and colostomies generally are associated with more distress because of the obvious changes in appearance and body function (Jacobsen et al.). For the individual who receives the news of the cancer diagnosis postoperatively, pain and weakness from the surgery will add to the distress and depression created by the new diagnosis. Borneman et al. (2003) found that caregivers for patients undergoing palliative surgery experienced more intense psychological distress.

Chemotherapy

The public often views chemotherapy negatively. This may be based on irrational fears, misperceptions, and inaccurate or outdated information (Knobf, 1998). Most individuals have preconceived ideas about chemotherapy and its side effects. While still reeling from the diagnosis, starting chemotherapy can intensify the sense of vulnerability to one's already weakened coping reserves. The protective equipment worn by staff members who administer chemotherapy may add to this fear. However, chemotherapy is an active treatment that can give patients a sense of strength as they hope for a cure. Many patients are under the impression that chemotherapy must be given through IV to be effective. However, many new oral agents with lower side effect profiles are now available and can increase survival (Bedell, 2003).

Nausea and vomiting from chemotherapy tend to be major concerns for patients. Education about the medications available to control these symptoms can address these concerns. Alopecia has the emotional impact of being a constant reminder of the diagnosis, forcing patients to immediately integrate the diagnosis into their lives. It is a visible reminder to the world that a person has cancer, impeding the opportunity to keep the diagnosis private (Freedman, 1994). Fatigue and risk for infection also contribute to psychosocial distress.

Chemotherapy forces the patient and family to adhere to schedules of medical appointments or hospitalizations and to reallocate family roles because the patient usually cannot meet obligations because of fatigue or other side effects. Seeing the patient in a vulnerable state while coping with the effects of chemotherapy may increase the distress on family members who must watch their loved one suffer. Fatigue and irritability experienced by the patient and family can increase the negative impact on the family system.

Radiation Therapy

People are taught to fear and avoid radiation. However, the patient then is told that radiation is a treatment for the cancer. This dichotomy can create deep-seated anxieties related to the cancer treatment (Greenberg, 1998). Radiation presents many unknowns to the patient. Meeting a new physician and treatment team in the radiation therapy department and lying alone on a table with a large machine overhead can create a sense of isolation and anxiety. Fears about being burned and having visible skin tattoos may contribute to one's distress and create self-consciousness. Patients may have heard myths concerning the side effects of this therapy and need extensive education about what to expect. Patients with many side effects from the radiation treatment experience more negative emotions and intrusive negative thoughts about the cancer while receiving radiation therapy than patients with fewer side effects (Walker, Nail, Larsen, Magill, & Schwartz, 1996). This emphasizes the need for ongoing education and assessment of the effects of treatment.

The Patient's and Family's Response to Cancer Treatment

As the patient continues to receive chemotherapy, radiation therapy, or other treatments (e.g., stem cell transplants, immunotherapy), the patient and family hope for and seek a return to the former routines of their daily lives. Weeks and months of disruption and emotional upheaval throughout the treatment process can create a yearning for normalcy. Hilton (1996) found that families of patients with early-stage breast cancer achieved normalcy by viewing the cancer as "temporary" (with a focus on the belief that it would be cured); de-emphasizing the illness by keeping busy or adding distractions to their daily lives; maintaining flexibility in roles; and de-emphasizing or minimizing the demands and changes brought on by the treatment. The patient's and family's ability to return to usual patterns of activities is a way to put the cancer behind them. Congruency between family members in regard to their beliefs about the cancer also was important. This congruency made supporting each other easier for family members. Hilton found that the negative perceptions that patients or families retained about the cancer or its treatment affected their ability to enhance normalization. The ability to view the cancer as a temporary, short-term problem was extremely important in this process. Patients and families also face burdens of shortened hospital stays with patients returning home with more care needs (Holland, 2003) and the need for more involved home care and monitoring (Rawl et al., 2002). Family members are therefore likely to take on the role of caregiver (Given et al., 2004).

Nursing's Role

Patients who are receiving a new diagnosis, starting treatment, and continuing treatment are part of the daily practice of most oncology nurses. These patients and their families are facing one of the biggest crises of their lives. The oncology nurse's role must incorporate an awareness of the tremendous psychosocial implications that exist. Northouse and Northouse (1996) delineated the important interpersonal roles of oncology nurses as imparting information, communicating hope, and dealing with the many emotions that are part of the patient's cancer experience. They viewed the major issues confronting patients as maintaining a sense of control, obtaining information, searching for meaning, and disclosing feelings.

Nurses play an important role in assisting patients in all of these areas. Although nurses are not able to control the disease, they still can provide support in controlling patients' responses to the illness and education about the disease and its treatment. Education will provide patients with the control necessary to deal with side effects and will help them to make the best decisions. Providing education enhances emotional support and fosters development of a trusting relationship with patients. Helping patients to confront intense and confusing emotions is a key role for nurses and is an important component of the nurse/patient relationship.

Recurrence

Because of the unpredictable nature of cancer, many individuals facing a diagnosis and initial treatment eventually must face recurrence. Recurrence is defined as the return of the disease after an initial course of treatment with a disease-free period. The disease may recur at the same site, recur near the site, or metastasize to a distant site. The threat of recurrence is one of the reasons why cancer is such a feared disease. Long-term survivors continue to experience distress over fear of recurrence (Gill et al., 2004). Although recurrence does not necessarily lead to terminal illness, it certainly increases its likelihood (Mahon, 1991). Pasacreta, Minarik, and Nield-Anderson (2001) noted that recurrence is a period characterized by increased pessimism, renewed preoccupation with death, and disenchantment with the medical system. Frost et al. (2000) found that recurrence was associated with increased uncertainty and symptom distress as well as less hope. It also means returning to active treatment, which can bring back memories of past suffering (Glajchen, 1999). At this time, patients not only face the realization that treatment has failed and cure may be unattainable, but they must prepare themselves, as well as loved ones, for the possibility of death. Dankert et al. (2003) reported that recurrence is one of the main fears of people with cancer. Patients may face multiple recurrences during their lifetimes; therefore, psychological response to recurrence remains a common concern for patients, families, and healthcare professionals (Vickberg, 2001).

Psychosocial Response to Recurrence

Fear of recurrence continues after the initial diagnosis (Ferrell, Grant, Funk, Otis-Green, & Garcia, 1998; Vickberg, 2001). If the cancer returns, it is a distinctly different emotional event from the initial cancer diagnosis (Mahon, 1991). Although recurrence entails different stressors and the need for different interventions, research has not conclusively indicated that it is necessarily more stressful. Mahon, Cella, and Donovan (1990) noted that the majority of patients in their study found recurrence to be more upsetting than the initial diagnosis and that they were less hopeful than they were at the time of the initial diagnosis. Sarna et al. (2005) found that women with lung cancer had more distress over fears of recurrence and metastasis. Conversely, Munkres, Oberst, and Hughes (1992) found no significant differences in mood scores between patients with an initial cancer diagnosis and those with recurrence. Schulz et al. (1995) reported similar results; however, financial problems, less social support, and lower levels of optimism were associated with more psychological distress. Weisman and Worden (1986) found that the degree of psychological distress at the time of recurrence depended on the degree of symptomatology from the recurrence. Thirty percent of their sample actually reported less distress with the recurrence. This group was less surprised by the recurrence and had not let themselves believe they were cured. In fact, for some, recurrence was a relief from the distressing uncertainty with which they had been living as they waited for the disease to return (Holland, 1998). For these patients, the uncertainty can be more distressing than the actual return of disease.

Psychosocial problems that emerged from the initial diagnosis and treatment will resurface in recurrence (Holland, 1998). For example, a patient who initially responded to the diagnosis with severe anxiety or serious depression could be expected to respond to news of recurrence in a similar way. This demonstrates the need to obtain a thorough psychosocial history to assess the initial response. Initial responses to recurrence typically include insomnia, restlessness, anxiety, and poor concentration; however, depression and anxiety are the predominant responses.

Because these patients already have been through some type of cancer treatment, preparing for treatment again may be more difficult because they know what to expect. If patients had severe side effects with the initial treatment, they may need more encouragement or more aggressive symptom management. Patients with recurrence experience higher levels of symptom distress, particularly fatigue and pain (Mahon & Casperson, 1995). These patients also may face decisions regarding more aggressive treatment, such as stem cell transplants, immunotherapy, and/or clinical trials. These treatments may not have been considered the first time around, thus creating more unknowns (Pasacreta et al., 2001). In other cases, these therapies may have been offered at the time of initial treatment, and the patient may have decided on a more conservative approach. This can result in feelings of guilt or regret. Mahon et al. (1990) found that 80% of the patients facing recurrence in their sample believed they should have "fought the cancer more" following the initial diagnosis, and 50% believed they should have sought more opinions or more treatment with the initial diagnosis. This self-blame, anger, and guilt will contribute to patients' negative emotional responses.

The realization that treatment has failed can contribute to depression and a feeling of hopelessness. The patients' sense of hope may have provided the encouragement needed the first time around when a cure was anticipated. The loss of hope may contribute to the realization that one must consider the possibility of death. Holland (1998) described the existential crisis of recurrence as the individual having to consider for the first time that death could be the outcome and that one's goals may not be realized. Loss of confidence, increased fearfulness, and hopelessness are other reactions (Shell & Kirsch, 2001).

Loss of faith in the medical establishment may be a reaction as the individual realizes the initial treatment did not provide a cure. This can contribute to anger and consideration of alternative therapies or even to refusal of further therapy. Some individuals may experience a sense of personal failure in thinking that they have disappointed their physicians by not being cured. A sense of injustice, noted by a comment such as "it is not fair because I did everything they asked of me," can create more anxiety, anger, and helplessness.

Recurrence may present financial demands if the patient is considering aggressive or experimental treatment. An inability to work, problems with insurance coverage, and a need to relocate may contribute to this challenge and present additional stresses for patients and families. Another fear may be that of facing a more physically disabling illness as the disease progresses and treatment becomes more aggressive.

The Family's Response to Recurrence

As with the patient, family members must struggle with depression, anger, guilt, and the fear of death. Family members' responses also may be similar to their response at the time of initial diagnosis. However, the emotional climate of the family may be much different at the time of recurrence, especially if many disease-free years have passed. Changes in relationships caused by divorce or loss of family members may affect the family's emotional climate and the emotional support available for the patient.

Recurrence may create so much distress that family members and friends will react with detachment because they fear reinvesting in the patient's treatment when the outcome may be less positive. This particularly may be common when the patient experiences multiple remissions and exacerbations. The patient may wish to have less contact with family members and friends because of depression or fatigue (Mahon & Casperson, 1995). Maintaining a positive attitude may be more difficult for family members and friends, and providing emotional support to the patient could be more draining. On the other hand, family crises faced at the time of initial diagnosis may have strengthened the family members to better face this new challenge. Whereas in the past spouses or siblings may have thought that they never could have coped with a loved one having cancer, getting through the initial treatment may have given these individuals confidence in their ability to face whatever happens.

Weisman and Worden (1986) found that marriages that survived the challenges of the initial diagnosis mobilized well for the stressors of recurrence. However, Lewis and Deal (1995) found in their study that in 40% of couples facing recurrent breast cancer, one or more of the partners experienced depression. Northouse et al. (2002) reported that a family-based cancer care program resulted in more satisfaction and optimism and less uncertainty.

The response of parents to recurrence in a child may be very difficult as they realize that a cure may not be possible. Facing the realization that the situation is out of their control is particularly trying. Parents facing the news of recurrence have been found to curb their immediate response to the bad news to maintain hopefulness and to attempt to remain focused on curative therapy (Hinds et al., 1996).

Nursing's Response to Recurrence

Identifying how a patient coped at the time of initial diagnosis is an important early part of the treatment plan that may predict the patient's response to the news of recurrence. Knowing what physicians told patients also can provide important information to gauge the response. Reinforcement of hope may help to maintain emotional balance. Patients may fear abandonment by the healthcare team after "failing" the first-line treatment. Regardless of the treatment goal, physicians and nurses must present a treatment plan that communicates a continued commitment to patients.

Patients experiencing a recurrence will face many choices about treatment and need information to help them to make decisions. Mahon et al. (1990) found that 90% of their sample reported that healthcare professionals assumed patients had more knowledge about their disease and treatment than the patients felt they actually had. Also, 75% of their sample reported that professionals assumed that the patients were coping better than they actually were. This provides nurses with important information regarding the need to take the time to talk with patients about their coping as well as to reinforce teaching about the disease, treatment, and side effects. Making important treatment decisions during a time of emotional upheaval requires patients to have access to a variety of information at different times. Written material may be helpful for patients to review after receiving oral instructions. Access to alternative resources such as the Internet and cancer information hot lines may be useful as patients seek more opinions about their options.

Patients and family members need an opportunity to share fears in a safe environment. They may be reluctant to express their deepest fears to one another in order to provide a measure of "protection." The oncology nurse is in a key role to provide this important outlet.

Terminal Illness

Patients must face terminal illness when aggressive, curative treatment is no longer an option and the focus moves to palliative care. For some, this may come as a gradual awareness that the disease is progressing despite aggressive treatment. For others, this realization may be sudden. Some may continue to pursue aggressive treatment until the end, and others may reject treatment at the time of diagnosis. Still others may face life-threatening complications during active treatment. However the realization comes, it remains a difficult and emotional journey. At this time, patients and families experience many fears. Death is a threat with many common themes.

The Patient's Fears

Fear of the unknown: Death is one of the strongest fears of all human beings (Rando, 1984), and it presents the greatest "unknown" for many people. Questions such as what will happen to my family, my life plans, my life's work, and my body are difficult to face, and they are difficult questions for others, such as family members, to hear. Some of these thoughts can be acknowledged by talking about the concerns and making preparations to care for loved ones or to achieve a hoped-for goal. Other questions can be acknowledged only in a supportive environment. Spiritual support may provide some comfort.

Fear of pain and suffering: Pain is one of the most common and greatest fears for those at the end of life (Ng & von Gunten, 1998). Many individuals believe dying must mean terrible pain, loss of dignity, and uncontrollable suffering. Patients may have images of relatives screaming in torment while dying of cancer. The majority of people with terminal illness can obtain relief (Paice & Fine, 2001). However, the patient may need to be more sedated to obtain this relief in some cases (Panke, 2003). Unfortunately, this fear becomes a reality for some patients when healthcare professionals provide inadequate analgesia. Patients and their caregivers need to be educated about the options for pain control. Pain can produce feelings of guilt for patients who view pain as a cause of suffering for their family. Other common symptoms that cause suffering include dry mouth, shortness of breath, and lack of energy (McMillan & Small, 2002).

Fear of abandonment: As patients weaken and begin to lose some control, the fear that others involved in the care may abandon them can be intense. Patients may particularly fear abandonment by their physicians when the focus of care moves away from aggressive treatment. Physicians may have said, "There is nothing more I can do," which reinforces this fear. In most cases, physicians' continued involvement during the terminal stage is an important part of supportive care. Even when patients are under hospice care, attending physicians usually remain actively involved. Individuals who feel helpless and anxious around a dying patient may need encouragement to maintain their involvement with the patient to alleviate the patient's fears of being left alone.

Loss of control: When advancing cancer causes progressive weakness, fatigue, and confusion, patients have less opportunity to maintain control of the environment and what is happening to them (American Medical Association Council on Scientific Affairs, 1996). Because American society values self-reliance and independence, this loss can be humiliating and provoke anxiety. Loss of control can induce feelings of guilt because patients may feel uncomfortable relying on others and can maintain a belief of needing to be strong. Others inadvertently can add to this fear by taking over decision making and other responsibilities for patients out of a desire to help. Advancing disease that treatment can no longer control represents a loss of patients' power over the cancer. The act of stopping aggressive treatment may represent a major loss of control as patients feel they are "giving in" to the cancer.

Encouraging the completion of advanced directives and estate planning to ensure that personal wishes are known by others and will be followed can help patients to maintain a sense of control. Caregivers can be sensitive to the urge to take over for patients when they are still able to complete tasks. Helping patients to conserve energy and establish priorities in order to focus on things that are the most important can enhance a sense of control.

Loss of identity: As the individual becomes weaker, more aspects of self can be lost as the patient can no longer maintain skills, interests, and relationships. Individuals' abilities often define and affirm who they are, and when this is lost, they can feel more distressed and confused. Loss of dignity as patients become more dependent may increase this fear. Those patients with enough energy can leave a legacy by making video or audio recordings, which helps them to achieve a desired goal and enhances a sense of purpose and identity. For others, maintaining their self-respect and dignity by acknowledging their value as a person can address this fear.

Loss of body image/self: Valued physical traits may be lost as weakness and emaciation occur. Patients may be less able to complete normally important personal care routines (e.g., shaving, applying makeup). An individual may no longer be recognized as the same person by others. This can cause patients to feel shame or that they are not lovable. Maintaining patients' dignity, respecting modesty, and assisting with personal care are all important supportive care measures.

Loss of loved ones: Perhaps one of the most poignant fears that patients encounter is facing the loss of relationships with loved ones. Just as family members anticipate losing the patient, the patient, too, is anticipating separation and loneliness (Worden, 2000). For some people, the opportunity to acknowledge the grief, complete unfinished business with important people in their lives, and spend time with loved ones reminiscing about past joys and sorrows all can be therapeutic to patients and family members. Recognizing the limited time one has to right wrongs with a loved one or achieve forgiveness is a struggle for some. Borneman and Brown-Saltzman (2001) defined forgiveness as letting go of expectations that one will be vindicated for pain and loss. It can provide an opportunity for healing and possible reconciliation.

Loss of hope: Hope is a natural part of human existence. When hope for a cure is no longer possible, individuals often are able to alter wishes for the future. Hope can thrive in the presence of terminal illness even with the realization that cure is no longer possible (Ersek, 2001). Patients may begin to hope for an easy death, to resolve a conflict with an estranged relative, or to believe one's spouse will be prepared to face life alone. To help patients to reframe hope by focusing on the present and specifics, rather than vague uncertainties in the future, can be helpful.

The Family's Fears

Loss of the relationship: Anticipating the loss of the patient is the beginning of the grieving process, which includes facing sadness, struggling with anger, and anticipating life without this loved one. If the dying person is part of a family member's everyday life, as with a spouse or parent who lives with the family, the loss is more intense. During the dying process, family members begin to realize what life will be like as the patient weakens, is sleeping more, and is less a part of the daily routine. The patient may turn more inward, and there can be less emotional contact for the family (Davies, 2001). The approach of death may generate an awareness of losing a special relationship (e.g., a daughter losing her father who has always been her protector), loss of a part of oneself (e.g., losing one's wife means giving up a role as husband), or empathy and concern for others (e.g., the adult child who sees his or her parent anticipating facing life alone).

As family members realize that they are losing the relationship, they may fear that if the patient is too sedated to interact, they will be faced with the loss more quickly. Although family members may want the patient to be comfortable, they may try to keep him or her awake out of fear of having to face the painful realization of the loss of the relationship. Helping family members to acknowledge this fear and to reinforce the need to grieve this loss can be helpful along with reassuring them of the patient's need to be comfortable.

Loss of control: As with the patient, family members must face the loss of control when they can do nothing to stop the disease. This can generate many feelings, with anger often being the most pronounced. As a way to maintain some control, this anger may be expressed to physicians for not doing enough for the patient or to nurses whose actions are viewed as unhelpful (e.g., not being able to restart an IV on the first try, not bringing a medication immediately). For individuals who have never faced the death of a loved one before, this can be a particularly difficult experience because the sense of loss of control can be overwhelming. Helping family members to face the losses, acknowledging their efforts to advocate for the patient, and helping them to identify ways to maintain some control can be useful interventions. Family members may be facing loss of control in other areas of their lives as schedules are disrupted, sleep is interrupted, and conflicts arise with relatives and friends—all perhaps occurring at the same time. Some family members may need to maintain a job or child care while simultaneously helping to care for a dying loved one. Loved ones may need to take on a more proactive role as decision makers as the patient deteriorates (Zhang & Siminoff, 2003).

Fear of sorrow: The growing realization of the impending loss may generate intense emotions that are frightening to some individuals. Family members may have used avoidance as a means of protection from feeling pain. Once it is experienced, depression, anger, preoccupation, irritability, and difficulty making decisions can occur. This is part of the grieving process. As the patient grows more ill and eventually begins to withdraw from day-to-day life, the reality of the impending loss intensifies. This may be felt more strongly if the family member had protected himself or herself by using denial or avoidance. Helping the family member to be open to the grieving process and providing support and acceptance regardless of the reaction are very important. Family members also must recognize and help children in the family through their grief regardless of age (Hames, 2003).

Fear of pain and suffering: Family members may anticipate that the patient will have to endure much suffering during the dying process. This may cause them to seek assistance related to dying, such as physician-assisted suicide or euthanasia. The thought of seeing their loved one suffer can be so overwhelming that some individuals may act rashly to avoid even the remotest possibility of this happening. Education of the family about the dying process must begin early. This should include encouraging family members to express their fears about what they think will happen and then providing information to alleviate those fears. Koop and Strang (2003) found that family caregivers had improved bereavement outcomes when they felt they had accomplished something valuable by providing comfort and caring for their loved one.

The Role of the Oncology Nurse in End-of-Life Care

Cancer is now the leading cause of death in the United States for people younger than 85 years of age (Jemal et al., 2005). Therefore, it is vital for oncology nurses in all settings to be skillful in addressing the fears of patients and families when cancer is progressing. As part of the interdisciplinary team, the oncology nurse often is a leader in identifying palliative interventions and support needs for these patients.

Survivorship

Survivorship has become an important area of study for oncology professionals (Dow, 2003; Holland, 2002). The National Coalition for Cancer Survivorship (2004) defined a cancer survivor as "any individual that has been diagnosed with cancer, from the time of discovery and for the balance of life." Survivors comprise a significant segment of society, but survivorship is a relatively new concept to oncology. With the advances in treatment, people with a cancer diagnosis are now living longer, and because of the aggressiveness of the treatment approaches, physical and psychological aftereffects are common. These changes have contributed to the development of the concept of survivorship to encompass the phases and changes the individual experiences after a cancer diagnosis (see Chapter 2).

Until the 1990s, relatively little research examined this period for patients with cancer, particularly in regard to the psychosocial sequelae (Quigley, 1989). This may be because of the assumption that quality of life returns to normal after treatment (Ferrans, 1994). Leigh (1997) postulated that in the past it was thought that recovery from a once-fatal illness was reward enough, so no need existed to study the quality of survivors' lives. However, growing evidence has suggested that the effects of treatment, both physically and emotionally, remain long after therapy is completed (Dow, 2003). Dow noted that the National Cancer Institute has identified cancer survivorship as a major area of research.

Survivorship is a dynamic, lifelong process (Pelusi, 1997) that is viewed as a continuum or ongoing role rather than an event that occurs at some designated point in time (e.g., five years). The perception of the quality of one's life as a survivor may change over time as new symptoms or treatment effects recede or increase or as one's coping abilities change. This definition not only includes people with no evidence of disease but also those living with cancers not associated with cure or cancers controlled by treatment but that periodically progress. Leigh (1997) noted that survivors also are called victors, graduates, and veterans. These all are terms that connote power rather than implying dependency (e.g., patient, victim).

Personal Growth for Cancer Survivors

Survivors often report positive outcomes, including a heightened sense of appreciation of family members and friends, feelings of being a better person for having gone through this difficult experience, and the changing of priorities in life for the better. Some studies of survivors have revealed an increased desire to be of service to others, and many survivors volunteer to help other patients with cancer (Ferrans,

1994; Pelusi, 1997; Wyatt, Kurtz, & Liken, 1993). Living through a life-threatening cancer experience can increase one's desire to move quickly to accomplish one's goals because of a heightened sense of the preciousness of life and how quickly it can be altered. Others may make difficult decisions more easily (e.g., leaving a destructive relationship, completing work toward a degree) because of a sense of urgency created by having a potentially fatal illness.

Quality of Life for Cancer Survivors

The World Health Organization (1993) defined quality of life as individuals' perceptions of their position in life in the context of the culture and value system in which they live and in relation to their goals, standards, and concerns. Grant and Dean (2003) identified the domains of quality of life to include physical health, emotional state, level of independence, social relationships, environment, and spiritual state. Initially included as part of clinical trials, the measurement of quality of life in oncology now is being used to compare types of treatment, side effects, and the consequences of cancer treatment. How each individual cancer survivor perceives the effects of the cancer and its treatment on day-to-day life is a very personal experience. A person's subjective perception and expectations create the actual quality of life experienced. Coping with limitations such as lymphedema, chronic pain, sexual dysfunction, and fears about the disease can greatly affect one's perception of health and satisfaction with his or her life. Individuals may make decisions about whether to seek more aggressive treatment based not just on prolonging life but on the risk of creating more of a burden related to their quality of life. Although grateful to be alive, survivors may have difficulty adjusting to the trade-offs of survival, including the long-term and potentially unknown late effects of the disease and treatment. Ferrell et al. (1998) noted that breast cancer survivors continue to experience fatigue, pain, fear of breast cancer recurrence, fear of breast cancer in female relatives, and the stress of living with uncertainty and maintaining hope. Psychological well-being is influenced by the ability to maintain a sense of control in the face of a potentially life-threatening illness and can contribute to problems such as anxiety, mood swings, and depression. Ferrell, Smith, Cullinane, and Melancon (2003) found that women who survived ovarian cancer demonstrated resourcefulness and perseverance by sharing coping mechanisms and survival strategies. Social well-being involves family issues, including sexual and marital problems, adjustment of children, work-related problems, and financial concerns. Factors affecting spiritual well-being include the ability to maintain hope and derive meaning from the cancer experience, which is characterized by uncertainty. Any change in one domain will affect other domains. For example, problems with fertility will affect the emotional, spiritual, and social domains.

Cancer as a Chronic Illness

For survivors who experience advancing cancer or the ongoing effects of or disabilities from cancer and its treatment, survivorship may include the challenge of living with a chronic illness. Nail (1997) noted that the public generally does not view cancer as a chronic illness, so when cancer treatment is over, survivors are expected to move on with their lives. Yet, because of long-term, late effects of the disease and treatment, survivors may have to continue dealing with the illness. Rather than being encouraged to move on with their lives, survivors may need support in managing the chronic aspects of the condition. Often, the support that patients received at the time of diagnosis and treatment becomes less available once they enter extended survivorship.

The Oncology Nurse's Role in Survivorship

In whatever setting a nurse works, cancer survivors will be part of the patient population. Educating survivors and potential survivors about what to expect is a key role for oncology nurses. "The individual's experience with cancer and quality of life is profoundly influenced by nursing care" (Ferrell, 1996, p. 915). In addition to being educators about survivorship issues, oncology nurses need to consider sharing knowledge about the impact of survivorship with nononcology nurse colleagues, who will be the nurses more likely to see survivors after treatment.

Cancer survivors need information about the psychological changes that will occur, the long-term physical effects of treatment, reentering the work world, the financial impact of the disease, and the effect of the disease on the family. Preparing the survivor for the anxiety that is associated with follow-up medical appointments, self-monitoring of symptoms, the end of treatment, reactions when returning to work, and anniversary-related emotions can provide important support and reassurance for patients experiencing these feelings. Providing encouragement to continue medical follow-up and support group involvement is another role for nurses. See Appendix for resource information.

Family members and friends also need preparation and education about the process of survivorship. Members of the patient's support system may assume that life will return to normal. Nurses need to encourage them to recognize that the individual's ongoing need to share his or her memories or feelings can be important to recovery.

Recognizing the uniqueness of the cancer experience for each individual is an important element to remember when assessing survivors. Each individual will respond differently to this process. Some may easily talk about it; others may avoid bringing up the topic of cancer for fear of "jinxing" themselves, whereas others may become anxious and depressed. Each individual interprets the disease and circumstances around it to fit his or her perception of the world.

Cancer survivorship has emerged as an important area for oncology professionals. Professional organizations, including the Oncology Nursing Society and the American Society of Clinical Oncology, have recognized and supported the needs of survivors. The National Cancer Institute has established the Office of Cancer Survivorship to create more recognition of the issues faced after cancer treatment. The quality of life of cancer survivors needs to be the focus of future research, and the oncology nurse has a key role in this area.

Conclusion

A cancer diagnosis clearly has significant physical effects on an individual—effects that result from the disease itself and its treatment. Few other diseases, however, wreak the additional psychosocial havoc that cancer does. The psychosocial ramifications are serious, long-lasting, and broad, and they affect not only individuals with cancer but also their extended network of family, friends, and acquaintances. At every stage along the cancer continuum, the care delivered must address physical aspects of the illness in addition to the mental health and coping strengths of the patient and family. Nurses are very much partners in this endeavor, taking their place beside physicians and other allied healthcare providers. The oncology nursing specialist, as well as any nurse caring for patients with cancer, cannot be effective without a respect for and a command of a broad range of psychosocial nursing skills. In no other specialty is nursing quite so instrumental in facilitating emotional care.

References

American Medical Association Council on Scientific Affairs. (1996). Good care of the dying patient. *JAMA, 275,* 474–478.

Beauchamp, T.L., & Childress, J.F. (2001). *Principles of biomedical ethics* (5th ed.). New York: Oxford University Press.

Bedell, C.H. (2003). A changing paradigm for cancer treatment: The advent of new oral chemotherapy agents. *Clinical Journal of Oncology Nursing, 7*(Suppl. 6), 5–9.

Borneman, T., & Brown-Saltzman, K. (2001). Meaning in illness. In B.R. Ferrell & N. Coyle (Eds.), *Textbook of palliative nursing* (pp. 415–424). New York: Oxford University Press.

Borneman, T., Chu, D.Z.J., Wagman, L., Ferrell, B., Juarez, G., McCahill, L.E., et al. (2003). Concerns of family caregivers of patients with cancer facing palliative surgery for advanced malignancy. *Oncology Nursing Forum, 30,* 997–1005.

Buckman, R. (1992). *Breaking bad news: A guide for healthcare professionals.* Baltimore: Johns Hopkins University Press.

Dankert, A., Duran, G., Engst-Hastreiter, U., Keller, M., Waadt, S., Henrich, G., et al. (2003). Fear of progression in patients with cancer, diabetes mellitus, and chronic arthritis. *Rehabilitation, 42,* 155–163.

Davies, B. (2001). Supporting families in palliative care. In B.R. Ferrell & N. Coyle (Eds.), *Textbook of palliative nursing* (pp. 363–373). New York: Oxford University Press.

Dias, L., Chabner, B.A., Lynch, T.J., & Penson, R.T. (2003). Breaking bad news: A patient's perspective. *Oncologist, 8,* 587–596.

Dow, K.H. (2003). Challenges and opportunities in cancer survivorship research. *Oncology Nursing Forum, 30,* 455–469.

Dunn, S.M., Patterson, P.U., & Butow, P.N. (1993). Cancer by any other name: A randomized trial of the effects of euphemism and uncertainty in communicating with cancer patients. *Journal of Clinical Oncology, 11,* 989–996.

Ersek, M. (2001). The meaning of hope in the dying. In B.R. Ferrell & N. Coyle (Eds.), *Textbook of palliative nursing* (pp. 339–351). New York: Oxford University Press.

Ferrans, C.E. (1994). Quality of life through the eyes of survivors of breast cancer. *Oncology Nursing Forum, 21,* 1645–1651.

Ferrell, B.R. (1996). The quality of lives: 1,525 voices of cancer. *Oncology Nursing Forum, 23,* 909–916.

Ferrell, B.R., Grant, M.M., Funk, B.M., Otis-Green, S.A., & Garcia, N.J. (1998). Quality of life in breast cancer survivors: Implications for developing support systems. *Oncology Nursing Forum, 25,* 887–895.

Ferrell, B.R., Smith, S.L., Cullinane, C.A., & Melancon, C. (2003). Psychological well being and quality of life in ovarian cancer survivors. *Cancer, 98,* 1061–1071.

Freedman, T.G. (1994). Social and cultural dimensions of hair loss in women treated for breast cancer. *Cancer Nursing, 14,* 334–341.

Fried, T.R., Bradley, E.H., & O'Leary, J. (2003). Prognosis communication in serious illness: Perceptions of older patients, caregivers, and clinicians. *Journal of the American Geriatrics Society, 51,* 1398–1403.

Frost, M.H., Suman, V.J., Rummans, T.A., Dose, A.M., Taylor, M., Novotny, P., et al. (2000). Physical, psychological, and social well-being of women with breast cancer. *Psycho-Oncology, 9,* 221–231.

Gill, K.M., Mishel, M., Belyea, M., Germino, B., Germino, L.S., Porter, L., et al. (2004). Triggers of uncertainty about recurrence and long-term treatment side effects in older African American and Caucasian breast cancer survivors. *Oncology Nursing Forum, 31,* 633–639.

Girgis, A., & Sanson-Fisher, R.W. (1995). Breaking bad news: Consensus guidelines for medical practitioners. *Journal of Clinical Oncology, 13,* 2449–2456.

Given, B., Wyatt, G., Given, C., Sherwood, P., Gift, A., DeVoss, D., et al. (2004). Burden and depression among caregivers of patients with cancer at the end of life. *Oncology Nursing Forum, 31,* 1105–1117.

Glajchen, M. (1999). Psychosocial issues in cancer care. In C. Miaskowski & P. Buchsel (Eds.), *Oncology nursing: Assessment and clinical care* (pp. 305–317). St. Louis, MO: Mosby.

Glajchen, M. (2004). The emerging role and needs of family caregivers in cancer care. *Journal of Supportive Oncology, 2,* 145–155.

Grant, M.M., & Dean, G.E. (2003). Evolution of quality of life in oncology and oncology nursing. In C.R. King & P.S. Hinds (Eds.), *Quality of life from nursing and patient perspectives* (2nd ed., pp. 3–27). Sudbury, MA: Jones and Bartlett.

Greenberg, D.B. (1998). Radiotherapy. In J.C. Holland (Ed.), *Psycho-oncology* (pp. 269–276). New York: Oxford University Press.

Hames, C.C. (2003). Helping infants and toddlers when a family member dies. *Journal of Hospice and Palliative Nursing, 5,* 103–110.

Hilton, B.A. (1996). Getting back to normal: The family experience during early stage breast cancer. *Oncology Nursing Forum, 23,* 605–614.

Hinds, P.S., Birenbaum, L.K., Clarke-Steffen, L., Quargnenti, A., Kreissman, S., Kozik, A., et al. (1996). Coming to terms: Parental response to a first cancer recurrence in their child. *Nursing Research, 45,* 148–153.

Holland, J.C. (1998). Clinical course of cancer. In J.C. Holland (Ed.), *Psycho-oncology* (pp. 3–15). New York: Oxford University Press.

Holland, J.C. (2002). History of psychosocial oncology: Overcoming attitudinal and conceptual barriers. *Psychosomatic Medicine, 64,* 206–221.

Holland, J.C. (2003). American Cancer Society Award lecture. Psychological care of patients: Psycho-oncology contribution. *Journal of Clinical Oncology, 21*(Suppl. 23), 253s–265s.

Jacobsen, P.B., Roth, A.J., & Holland, J.C. (1998). Surgery. In J.C. Holland (Ed.), *Psycho-oncology* (pp. 257–268). New York: Oxford University Press.

Jemal, A., Murray, T., Ward, E., Samuels, A., Tiwari, R., Ghafoor, A., et al. (2005). Cancer statistics, 2005. *CA: A Cancer Journal for Clinicians, 55,* 10–30.

Katz, J. (1984). *The silent world of doctors and patients.* New York: Free Press.

King, P. (2003). Listen to the children and honor their pain. *Oncology Nursing Forum, 30,* 797–800.

Knobf, M.T. (1998). Chemotherapy. In J.C. Holland (Ed.), *Psycho-oncology* (pp. 277–288). New York: Oxford University Press.

Koop, P.M., & Strang, V.R. (2003). The bereavement experience following home-based family care-giving for persons with advanced cancer. *Clinical Nursing Research, 12,* 127–144.

Kristjanson, L.J., & Ashcroft, T. (1994). The family's cancer journey: A literature review. *Cancer Nursing, 17,* 1–17.

Lampic, C., Thurfjell, E., Bergh, J., Carlsson, M., & Sjoden, P.O. (2003). Attainment and importance of life values among patients with primary breast cancer. *Cancer Nursing, 26,* 295–304.

Lederberg, M.S. (1998). The family of the cancer patient. In J.C. Holland (Ed.), *Psycho-oncology* (pp. 982–993). New York: Oxford University Press.

Leigh, S.A. (1997). Quality of life for life: Survivors influencing research. *Quality of Life, 5*(1), 58–65.

Lewis, F.M., & Deal, L.W. (1995). Balancing our lives: A study of the married couple's experience with breast cancer recurrence. *Oncology Nursing Forum, 22,* 943–953.

Mahon, S.M. (1991). Management of psychosocial consequences of cancer recurrences: Implications for nurses. *Oncology Nursing Forum, 18,* 577–583.

Mahon, S.M., & Casperson, D.S. (1995). Psychosocial concerns associated with recurrent cancer. *Cancer Practice, 3,* 372–380.

Mahon, S.M., Cella, D.F., & Donovan, M.I. (1990). Psychosocial adjustment to recurrent cancer. *Oncology Nursing Forum, 17*(Suppl. 3), 47–60.

McMillan, S.C., & Small, B.J. (2002). Symptom distress and quality of life in patients with cancer newly admitted to hospice home care. *Oncology Nursing Forum, 29,* 1421–1428.

Mood, D.W. (1996). The diagnosis of cancer: A life transition. In R. McCorkle, M. Grant, M. Frank-Stromborg, & S. Baird (Eds.), *Cancer nursing: A comprehensive textbook* (2nd ed., pp. 298–314). Philadelphia: Saunders.

Munkres, A., Oberst, M.T., & Hughes, S.H. (1992). Appraisal of illness, symptom distress, self-care burden, and mood states in patients receiving chemotherapy for initial and recurrent cancer. *Oncology Nursing Forum, 19,* 1201–1209.

Nail, L.M. (1997). Interviews with oncology nurse cancer survivors. *Oncology Nursing Society 1997 Annual Congress Symposia Highlights,* p. 31.

Nail, L.M. (2001). I'm coping as fast as I can: Psychosocial adjustment to cancer and cancer treatment. *Oncology Nursing Forum, 28,* 967–970.

National Coalition for Cancer Survivorship. (2004). *Glossary.* Retrieved February 15, 2005, from http://canceradvocacy.org/resources/glossary.aspx

Ng, K., & von Gunten, C.F. (1998). Symptoms and attitudes of 100 consecutive patients admitted to an acute hospice and palliative care unit. *Journal of Pain and Symptom Management, 16,* 307–316.

Northouse, L.L. (2005). Helping families of patients with cancer. *Oncology Nursing Forum, 32,* 743–750.

Northouse, L.L., Cracchiolo-Caraway, A., & Appel, C.P. (1991). Psychological consequences of breast cancer on the partner and family. *Seminars in Oncology Nursing, 7,* 216–223.

Northouse, L.L., Mood, D., Kershaw, T., Schafenacher, A., Mellon, S., Walker, J., et al. (2002). Quality of life of women with recurrent breast cancer and their family members. *Journal of Clinical Oncology, 20,* 4050–4064.

Northouse, L.L., & Northouse, P.G. (1996). Interpersonal communication systems. In R. McCorkle, M. Grant, M. Frank-Stromborg, & S.B. Baird (Eds.), *Cancer nursing: A comprehensive textbook* (2nd ed., pp. 1211–1222). Philadelphia: Saunders.

Novack, D.H., Plumer, R., & Smith, R.L. (1978). Changes in physicians' attitudes toward telling the cancer patient. *JAMA, 241,* 897–900.

Oken, D. (1961). What to tell cancer patients: A study of medical attitudes. *JAMA, 175,* 1120–1128.

Paice, J.A., & Fine, P.G. (2001). Pain at the end of life. In B.R. Ferrell & N. Coyle (Eds.), *Textbook of palliative nursing* (pp. 76–90). New York: Oxford University Press.

Panke, J.T. (2003). Difficulty in managing pain at the end of life. *Journal of Hospice and Palliative Nursing, 5,* 83–90.

Pasacreta, J.V., Minarik, P.A., & Nield-Anderson, L. (2001). Anxiety and depression. In B.R. Ferrell & N. Coyle (Eds.), *Textbook of palliative nursing* (pp. 269–289). New York: Oxford University Press.

Pelusi, J. (1997). The lived experience of surviving breast cancer. *Oncology Nursing Forum, 24,* 1343–1353.

Quigley, K.M. (1989). The adult cancer survivor: Psychosocial consequences of cure. *Seminars in Oncology Nursing, 5,* 63–69.

Rabow, M.W., & McPhee, S.J. (1999). Beyond breaking bad news: How to help patients who suffer. *Western Journal of Medicine, 171,* 260–263.

Rando, T.A. (1984). *Grief, dying, and death.* Champaign, IL: Research Press Company.

Rawl, S.M., Given, B.A., Given, C.W., Champion, V.L., Kozachik, S.L., Barton, D., et al. (2002). Intervention to improve psychological functioning for newly diagnosed patients with cancer. *Oncology Nursing Forum, 29,* 967–975.

Sarna, L., Brown, J.K., Cooley, M.E., Williams, R.D., Chernecky, C., Padilla, G., et al. (2005). Quality of life and meaning of illness of women with lung cancer [Online exclusive]. *Oncology Nursing Forum, 32,* E9–E19.

Schofield, P.E., Butow, P.N., Thompson, J.F., Tattersall, M.H., Beeney, L.J., & Dunn, S.M. (2003). Psychological responses of patients receiving the diagnosis of cancer. *Annals of Oncology, 14,* 48–56.

Schulz, R., Williamson, G.M., Knapp, J.E., Bookwala, J., Lave, J., & Fello, M. (1995). The psychologic, social, and economic impact of illness among patients with recurrent cancer. *Journal of Psychosocial Oncology, 13*(3), 21–45.

Shell, J.A., & Kirsch, S. (2001). Psychosocial issues, outcomes, and quality of life. In S.E. Otto (Ed.), *Oncology nursing* (4th ed., pp. 948–972). St. Louis, MO: Mosby.

Tulsky, J.A. (1998). Teaching physicians to deliver bad news: Some practical advice. *Journal of Palliative Medicine, 1,* 423–426.

Vickberg, S.M. (2001). Fears about breast cancer recurrence. *Cancer Practice, 9,* 237–243.

Walker, B.L., Nail, L.M., Larsen, L., Magill, J., & Schwartz, A. (1996). Concerns, affect, and cognitive disruption following completion of radiation therapy for localized breast or prostate cancer. *Oncology Nursing Forum, 23,* 1181–1187.

Weisman, A.D., & Worden, J.W. (1976–1977). The existential plight in cancer: Significance of the first 100 days. *International Journal of Psychiatry in Medicine, 7,* 1–15.

Weisman, A.D., & Worden, J.W. (1986). The emotional impact of recurrent cancer. *Journal of Psychosocial Oncology, 3*(4), 5–16.

Worden, J.W. (2000). Towards an appropriate death. In T.A. Rando (Ed.), *Clinical dimensions of anticipatory mourning* (pp. 267–277). Champaign, IL: Research Press.

World Health Organization. (1993). *Study protocol for the World Health Organization project to develop a quality of life assessment instrument.* Geneva, Switzerland: Author.

Wyatt, G., Kurtz, M.E., & Liken, M. (1993). Breast cancer survivors: An exploration of quality of life issues. *Cancer Nursing, 16,* 440–448.

Zhang, A.Y., & Siminoff, L.A. (2003). The role of the family in treatment decision making by patients with cancer. *Oncology Nursing Forum, 30,* 1022–1028.

CHAPTER 2

Survivorship

DEBORAH A. BOYLE, RN, MSN, AOCN®, FAAN

Cancer therapists talk in terms of a "five-year survival rate," by which they mean the number of patients with a given tumor who will live five years beyond the time of diagnosis. It is an arbitrary way of measuring human existence but useful for scoring the likelihood of escape from cancer. In mid-March 1980, I tiptoed past the invisible line and into the future.

—Fitzhugh Mullan, 1983

As an evolving focus in clinical practice, education, and research, cancer survivorship has emerged as a prominent yet enigmatic milestone within the cancer trajectory. Not afforded the intensity of study nor the rigor of public attention as cancer treatment and, more recently, end-of-life care, living beyond a diagnosis of cancer often is deemed a privilege not deserving of query despite its numerous quandaries.

More than two decades have passed since the phenomenon of cancer survivorship began to gain prominence in the lay public and within professional venues. Progress has been made in the arenas of advocacy and lobbying for research funding to advance the fledgling evidence base addressing life after cancer (Clark & Stovall, 1996; Ganz, 2001). It is timely to review the state of the science of cancer survivorship with particular emphasis on its psychosocial challenges. Controversies and possibilities for the future will be proposed as oncology nurses play a major role in this expanding paradigm of cancer care (Ferrell, Virani, Smith, & Juarez, 2003).

Definitional Dilemmas

The historical construct of survivorship was associated with living through extraordinary life situations such as fires, floods, earthquakes, volcanic eruptions, wars, and concentration camps (Dow, 1990). In the mid-1900s, when cancer uniformly was deemed an incurable disease, family members were considered survivors following the death of a loved one (Leigh, 1994). Since the more recent inception of the cancer survivorship movement, semantics have been debated. Prompting this deliberation was an evolving consensus that the historic medical model used to identify cancer survivors was unsuitable. Izsak and Medalie (1971) were first credited with bringing this contention to notoriety.

> Survival rates, while justifiably important in themselves, cover only a portion of the total problem. These rates do not relate to how the patient survives, at what cost to his physical functioning, how he adapted to his condition from a psychological point of view, and how he is fulfilling his roles in his family, at work, among friends, and in the wider society. (pp. 179–180)

More than a decade later, Mullan (1985), a physician and cancer survivor, wrote a poignant editorial to colleagues in the *New England Journal of Medicine* addressing the inadequacies of the definitional paradigm at that time. He suggested that there was no "moment of cure" or "invisible line" that a patient traversed to become a survivor.

> During these years I frequently wondered when I could safely declare victory. When could I say simply that I was cured? Actuarial and population-based figures give us survival estimates for various cancers, but those figures do not speak to the individual patient whose experience is unique and not determined or described by aggregate data. Many patients are 'cured' long before they pass the five-year mark and others go well beyond the five-year point with overt or covert disease that removes them from the ranks of the 'cured' no matter how well they feel. Survival is a much more useful concept because it is a generic idea that applies to everyone diagnosed as having cancer, regardless of the course of illness. (pp. 270–271)

Mullan (1985) formulated a new theory about cancer survival. He proposed that patients transition through phases of acute, extended, and permanent survival, each characterized by distinct coping agendas. Figure 2-1 compares Mullan's conceptualization with the medical model, correlating permanent survival with the classic distinction of "being cured." The National Coalition of Cancer Survivorship (NCCS) adopted this construct and delineated components of survivorship as

- The act of living on, no matter what happens
- Beginning the moment the patient is told he or she has cancer and continuing for the rest of the patient's life
- Extending far beyond the restrictions of time and treatment
- A dynamic concept with no artificial boundaries
- A process of "going through," suggesting movement through phases
- A continued or ongoing process rather than a stage of survival
- A healing process
- Not dependent on biology or medical outcomes, but reflecting quality of life
- The experience of living with, through, or beyond cancer (Leigh, 2001).

A cancer survivor then is any person who has been diagnosed with cancer, from the time of discovery and for the balance of life (NCCS, 2004). For the purposes of this chapter, however, extended and permanent survival are the foci of analysis.

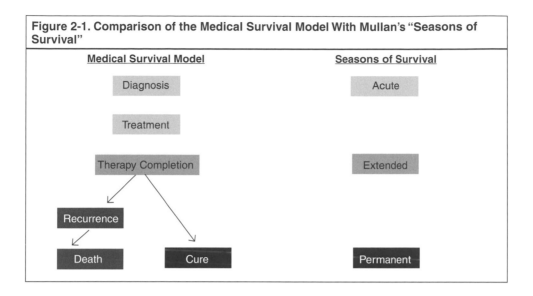

Figure 2-1. Comparison of the Medical Survival Model With Mullan's "Seasons of Survival"

Scope of Survivorship

The burgeoning attention to cancer survivorship can be linked with two significant corollaries. First, advances in cancer treatment have facilitated long-term survival in a greater number of patients with a variety of tumor types. These success stories have challenged the long-standing notion that a cancer diagnosis equates with inescapable death (Loescher, Clark, Atwood, Leigh, & Lamb, 1990). This growing number of people living with a history of cancer has prompted recognition of a new subset of patients we know little about. Consider the following (Boyle, 2002; Dow, 2003; Jemal et al., 2005; Leigh, 1992; Rowland, Aziz, Tesauro, & Feuer, 2001; Stat Bite, 2004).

- Over the past three decades, the number of cancer survivors has increased from three million in 1971 to 9.8 million in 2001.
- Sixty percent of adults and 77% of children diagnosed with cancer will survive more than five years.
- Fourteen percent of survivors were diagnosed more than two decades ago.
- Sixty percent of cancer survivors are age 65 or older.
- Approximately 71% of female cancer survivors have histories of breast, gynecologic, or colorectal primaries.
- Nearly two-thirds (63%) of male cancer survivors have had malignancies of the prostate, other genitourinary sites (e.g., testicular, renal), or the lower bowel (e.g., colon, rectum).
- Estimation of the numbers of secondary cancer survivors (i.e., family members) is unattainable.

Second, increasing concern over long-term effects of aggressive therapies instituted in the 1970s and early 1980s has warranted regard for the development of organ compromise and treatment-related second cancers (Matesich & Shapiro, 2003; Theodoulou & Seidman, 2003).

Little doubt exists that the number of Americans with and at risk for cancer will grow exponentially because of the increasing number of older adults who are most vulnerable to cancer (Boyle, 2003a). This projection, along with continued progress in treating cancer, will engender a larger cohort of survivors who are living longer with a history of cancer (Yabroff, Lawrence, Clauser, Davis, & Brown, 2004). These survivors also will face an increased risk for the development of second and third malignancies (Kattlove & Winn, 2003). The prominence of coexisting chronic illness with advanced age may complicate early symptom recognition. Additionally, the ethnicity profile of survivors will change as American society grows into a more heterogeneous cultural mix. Attention to ethnicity profile is imperative as culturally prescribed norms may affect health-seeking behavior, symptom verbalization, self-care practices, and the provision of family support (Ashing-Giwa, Padilla, Tejero, & Kim, 2004; Dirksen & Erickson, 2002; Farmer & Smith, 2002; Gil-Fernandez et al., 2003). A paucity of studies have addressed cultural diversity within the construct of cancer survivorship (Aziz & Rowland, 2002; Gotay, Holup, & Pagano, 2002). Yet significant research is needed to plan post-therapy and long-term interventions, especially in the field of ethnogeriatrics (Baider et al., 2004; Schultz, Stava, Beck, & Vassilopoulou-Sellin, 2004).

The most comprehensive body of evidence concerning the physical and emotional ramifications of living with a history of cancer has focused on survivors who historically were the first to benefit from aggressive chemotherapy that evolved in the 1970s. These patient cohorts include childhood survivors of acute leukemia and young adult survivors of Hodgkin lymphoma and testicular cancer (Clift & Thomas, 2004; Fizazi, Chen, & Logothetis, 2002; Fleer, Hoekstra, Sleijfer, & Hoekstra-Weebers, 2004; Ganz, 2003; Hale et al., 1999; Jenkinson et al., 2004; Levin, Brown, Pawletko, Gold, & Whitt, 2000; Metayer et al., 2000; Mykletun et al., 2005; Nyandoto, Muhonen, & Joensuu, 1998; Shusterman & Meadows, 2000; Stevens, Mahler, & Parkes, 1998; Zebrack et al., 2002). More recently, survivorship following breast cancer has received considerable attention largely because of this malignancy's growing incidence and its prominence within public venues (Beaver & Luker, 2005; Ganz et al., 2002, 2004; Lindsey, Waltman, Gross, Ott, & Twiss, 2004; Mandelblatt, Armetta, Yabroff, Liang, & Lawrence, 2004; Schover, 2004). General implications of surviving cancer can be imposed upon subsets of cancer survivors. However, more in-depth investigations are necessary to fully understand the scope and intensity of issues germane to tumor type, treatment, patient age, and a host of other variables (Kattlove & Winn, 2003).

Psychosocial Correlates of Surviving Cancer

In the late 1970s, Veronesi and Martino (1978) published their revelation of an unrecognized problem in the continuing management of cancer. They called attention to cancer's long-term social consequences and stressed the pervasiveness of patient anxiety and feelings of isolation during the latter phase of the cancer continuum. The prevalence and intensity of these issues frequently were underestimated by oncology professionals. These Italian cancer specialists made recommendations to reconfigure the long-term care of patients and address gaps in service. Of particular note was the following statement.

> One of the most important tasks of medicine and society is to do all that is possible to make the patient's life after treatment the most normal possible and similar to that led before the dramatic event. However, to obtain satisfactory results in this direction, a complete change of all the approaches to the problem of cancer would be necessary. (p. 349)

That same year, Woods and Earp (1978) published their findings of breast cancer survivors. They documented the relationship between persistent physical disability (e.g., lymphedema, restricted hand motion, reduced strength in the affected arm) and incidence of depression in women who were considered cured following mastectomy. The study also described an association between women's need to communicate their concerns and the families' desire to avoid such dialogue. Termed "conversational isolationism," this phenomenon exemplified how the women triggered emotional distress in their families by disclosing their fears about cancer recurrence and the possibility of dying prematurely. The families responded by deterring or avoiding these conversations, which ultimately left the women feeling isolated and without significant support during critical times of need. In a similar context, today's cancer survivors may be reticent to voice concerns that arise during long-term survival for fear of appearing less than grateful for their newfound positive bill of health (Turner et al., 2005).

At each phase of the cancer journey, coping challenges can be considered analogous to "parachuting into a jungle with no survival skills" (Ferrell & Dow, 1996, p. 76). With little or misleading information to guide adaptation, patients and families often face this life-threatening experience feeling ill-equipped to master this new challenge. The literature on emotional ramifications of coping during long-term survival following cancer can be clustered into seven themes. These include reactions of loss and grief, recurrence anxiety, feelings of isolation and abandonment, coping with transitional crisis, dilemmas associated with reentry and work, reevaluation of life priorities, and family coping. A number of mediating or enhancing factors influence these responses, such as patient age, family unit stability, degree of social support and spiritual orientation, evidence of concurrent family stressors, premorbid history of mental illness, nature and degree of role responsibilities, communication style, information requirements, and access to resources to aid coping (Ferrell, Smith, Juarez, & Melancon, 2003; Halstead & Fernsler, 1994; Matthews, 2003; Mellon, 2002; Mellon & Northouse, 2001; Sammarco, 2001; Sapp et al., 2003; Vachon, 2001; Varni, Katz, Colegrove, & Dolgin, 1994). Because quality of survival is in the eye of the beholder, it is imperative that survivors' needs are carefully and individually assessed (Leigh, 1992). This includes determination of interventions to enhance the quality of long-term survivorship and the identification of potential or real pathologies that may compromise continued coping (Hewitt & Rowland, 2002; Kornblith & Ligibel, 2003; Ross et al., 2003; Saleeba, Weitzner, & Meyers, 1996; Spijker, Trijsburg, & Duivenvoorden, 1997). "Flashing back," a survivor-specific emotional response similar to a post-traumatic stress disorder, also must be considered (Amir & Ramati, 2002; Carter, 1993; Kwekkeboom & Seng, 2002; Yehuda, 2002). Figure 2-2 lists coping agendas associated with long-term survivorship in relation to other phases of the cancer continuum.

Although nonpsychological implications of cancer survivorship are not the focus of this chapter, it must be emphasized that coping is appended to the incidence and

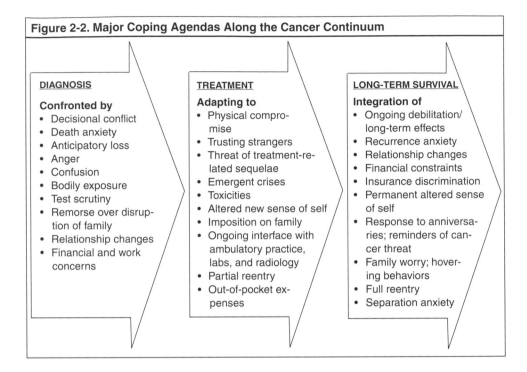

Figure 2-2. Major Coping Agendas Along the Cancer Continuum

DIAGNOSIS

Confronted by
- Decisional conflict
- Death anxiety
- Anticipatory loss
- Anger
- Confusion
- Bodily exposure
- Test scrutiny
- Remorse over disruption of family
- Relationship changes
- Financial and work concerns

TREATMENT

Adapting to
- Physical compromise
- Trusting strangers
- Threat of treatment-related sequelae
- Emergent crises
- Toxicities
- Altered new sense of self
- Imposition on family
- Ongoing interface with ambulatory practice, labs, and radiology
- Partial reentry
- Out-of-pocket expenses

LONG-TERM SURVIVAL

Integration of
- Ongoing debilitation/long-term effects
- Recurrence anxiety
- Relationship changes
- Financial constraints
- Insurance discrimination
- Permanent altered sense of self
- Response to anniversaries; reminders of cancer threat
- Family worry; hovering behaviors
- Full reentry
- Separation anxiety

intensity of physiologic long-term sequelae. The enduring demands of physiologic compromise can affect survivors' emotional status (Dorval, Maunsell, Deschenes, Brisson, & Masse, 1998; Redaelli, Stephens, Brandt, Botteman, & Pashos, 2004; Schimmer et al., 2001; Yabroff et al., 2004). Physiologic compromise includes both the effects of cancer therapy and the development of secondary cancers resulting from curative modalities (Bhatia & Sklar, 2002; Deniz, O'Mahoney, Ross, & Purushotham, 2003; Matesich & Shapiro, 2003; Syrjala et al., 2004; Theodoulou & Seidman, 2003). For example, the growing body of evidence concerning the prominence of fatigue following cancer therapy may influence the stamina required to cope during protracted survivorship (Bower et al., 2000; Cella, Davis, Breitbart, & Curt, 2001; Gelinas & Fillion, 2004; Gross, Ott, Lindsey, Twiss, & Waltman, 2002; Knobel et al., 2001; Mast, 1998a; Ruffer et al., 2003). Cognitive impairment, which may interfere with memory and interpersonal communication, has become a focus of study in the evaluation of adult long-term effects (Ahles & Saykin, 2001; Harder et al., 2002; Schagen, Hamburger, Muller, Boogerd, & van Dam, 2001; Tannock, Ahles, Ganz, & van Dam, 2004; Wefel, Lenzi, Theriault, Buzdar, et al., 2004). Knowledge resulting from neuro-oncology and other pediatric trials where cranial radiation was delivered has been applied to adult populations (Anderson et al., 2001; Brown et al., 2003; Challinor, Miaskowski, Moore, Slaughter, & Franck, 2000; Jansen, Miaskowski, Dodd, & Dowling, 2005; Lilja, Portin, Hamalainen, & Salminen, 2001; Meyers, Geara, Wong, & Morrison, 2000; Salminen et al., 2003). Most recently, cognitive impairment has been correlated with the receipt of adjuvant chemotherapy in women with breast cancer and also has been associated with long-term effects following bone marrow transplantation and immunotherapy (Ahles et al., 2002; Harder et al.; Kirkwood et al., 2002; O'Shaughnessy, 2003; Rugo & Ahles, 2003; Wefel, Lenzi, Theriault, Davis, & Meyers, 2004). Subsequent information derived from ongoing clinical trials will further delineate how altered cognition affects long-term quality of life.

The course of patients' survival continuum influences coping. Consider the following trajectories as possibilities (Welch-McCaffrey, Hoffman, Leigh, Loescher, & Meyskens, 1989).

- Live cancer-free for many years
- Live many years cancer-free but die rapidly of a late recurrence
- Live cancer-free following the first cancer but then develop a second primary cancer
- Live with intermittent periods of active disease
- Live with persistent disease
- Live on after expected death

The psychosocial demands related to each of these trajectories impose unique burdens of anxiety, emotional lability, and fear in both survivors and their families. Uncertainty is a nebulous stress that frequently prompts these responses and predominates over time (Mishel, 1997; Nelson, 1996). Waiting, a major theme evident throughout cancer, prompts uncertainty and its resultant psychosocial sequelae (Gaudine, Sturge-Jacobs, & Kennedy, 2003; Wallace, 2003).

Loss and Grief

Givens are no longer certainties; life is no longer infinite; health is no longer assumed. Death is not for someone else but for everyone. (A patient quoted in Lewis, 1993)

Loss is germane to the entire populace of cancer survivors. Although loss frequently is related to a concrete entity, such as a material possession, loved one, or body part or function, the conception of loss is much broader than this. It may relate to a diminished sense of oneself as healthy, fit, young, attractive, strong, adaptable, sexual, a compatible partner and provider, resourceful, dependable, or employable (Rudberg, Nilsson, & Wikblad, 2000; Wilmoth, 2001). Grief also may be voiced over the loss of how life used to be before the intrusion of cancer (Ferrell & Dow, 1996). Responses of grief and loss earlier in the cancer trajectory may transcend extended or permanent survival, especially if they were not addressed or resolved around their time of presentation. The acute treatment phase of cancer survivorship requires that targeted attention be focused on mastering the therapies employed to treat one's cancer and to adapt to the aftereffects of these therapies. Hence, some issues of loss and grief may have been discounted during this time frame. The reality of loss may only surface when treatment is completed and the permanence of cancer-imposed modifications become realized. Some patients describe this phenomenon as surreal, almost dreamlike, as the acuity and intensity of earlier phases of cancer treatment preclude one's true grasp of what transpired.

Because children and young adults were the focus of early research about survivorship, reproductive compromise has generated considerable interest over time. Loss of fertility in the prime of life has been deemed a significant consequence of successful treatment for cancer (Averette, Mirhashemi, & Moffat, 1999; Huyghe et al., 2004). Despite decades of study, conflicting reports prevail about the potential of conception following aggressive cancer therapy, particularly with alkylating antineoplastics and pelvic fields of radiation (Aisner, Wiernik, & Pearl, 1993; Moore & Foster, 2000; Puscheck, Philip, & Jeyendran, 2004). Additionally, the long-term emotional ramifications of infertility have not been fully explored (Braun, Hasson-Ohayon, Perry, Kaufman, & Uziely, 2005; Weigers, Chesler, Zebrack, & Goldman, 1998; Zebrack, Casillas, Nohr, Adams, & Zeltzer, 2004). Safety concerns of pregnancy following successful treatment of a hormone-related tumor continue to be debated (Blakely et al., 2004; Surbone & Petrek, 1997). Ethical dilemmas also may arise as the mother's longevity and health of the fetus are deliberated (Kenney et al., 1996; Petrek, 1994).

Recurrence Anxiety

I still don't renew subscriptions for three years, just annually. (A patient quoted in Wyatt, Kurtz, & Liken, 1993)

Recurrence anxiety is worry focused on the possibility that the cancer will return. It is a pervasive and, at times, overwhelming dread experienced by families as well as patients (Dow, 1992; Welch-McCaffrey et al., 1989). It is the coping response that all survivors can expect to experience. Recurrence anxiety can be described as, "Walking through life with a dark cloud hanging over your head, never knowing if or when the cancer will recur," or "Sitting on a powder keg waiting for it to go off" (Schmale et al., 1983, p. 166). Early work by Shanfield (1980) described the cancer experience.

> The experience of having had cancer is a permanent one, character-
> ized by an easy access to the initial affect associated with the illness
> and the recovery period, a continuing concern about one's mortality,
> and an enduring sense of vulnerability. (p. 133)

The usual pattern of recurrence anxiety is erratic with the exception of the immediate period following treatment completion. The first year following therapy cessation generally is associated with the most intense concerns about recurrence (Cella & Tross, 1986; Fobair & Mages, 1981; Hayden et al., 2004; Kornblith & Ligibel, 2003). Recurrence anxiety resurfaces when unusual symptoms are noted and at times of health surveillance and follow-up (Boyle, 1999; Vickberg, 2001; Wenzel et al., 2002). It can produce two distinct behaviors. Hypochondriasis may evolve, as the survivor suspects that any somatic change or new symptom portends the cancer's return. Recurrence anxiety also can elicit avoidance behaviors whereby physician contact is circumvented for fear that physical follow-up could diagnose the malignancy's reappearance. Episodic worry incited by symptom suspicion, return doctor visits, or exposure to fellow survivors with progressive cancer can evoke chronic anxiety in cancer survivors (Powel & McFadden, 1995). Recurrence anxiety also may prevail in families, prompting "hovering behaviors" and persistent scrutiny of the survivor's physical status. This may solicit conflict within the couple or family unit as the survivor attempts to minimize or dismiss cancer's presence in his or her life while the family maintains focus on its possible return. However, over time, recurrence anxiety usually diminishes, with periodic episodes resurfacing around physician visits and the presence of unusual somatic complaints (Gil et al., 2004; Langeveld, Grootenhuis, Voute, de Haan, & van den Bos, 2004).

Isolation and Abandonment

> *I also cried because I would not be coming back to that familiar table where I had been comforted and encouraged. Instead of joyous, I felt lonely, abandoned and terrified. This was the rocky beginning of cancer survivorship for me.* (A patient quoted in McKinley, 2000)

The aloneness associated with survivorship can be a horrific part of the cancer journey (Bushkin, 1993). The sense of detachment may emanate from feeling different, uniquely vulnerable, or stigmatized. It also may originate from survivors' fears that their social support network will withdraw or ultimately detach completely (Pedro, 2001). Ambulatory, healthy-appearing survivors may be refused the intensity of indulgence given initially around diagnosis and active therapy. Yet ongoing emotional concerns may persist long term.

As therapy ends, survivors may experience separation anxiety (Lethborg, Kissane, Burns, & Snyder, 2000; Ward, Viergutz, Tormey, DeMuth, & Paulen, 1992). This distancing from the treatment team can be quite traumatic. Although patients generally are happy about completing therapy, the lack of contact with and exposure to the treatment team frequently prompts concern. With close contact gone, worry may emanate about whom to go to with questions or concerns, especially if the fear of recurrence predominates. Recurrence anxiety is especially intense in the absence of active therapy to manage the malignancy.

Relationship changes may ensue in both social and intimate contexts. Family caregivers may not anticipate being stigmatized in their own social circles (Boyle et al., 2000). Friends and coworkers may treat family members differently based on their proximity to the person facing life-threatening cancer. One wife reported, "When I returned to work after my husband's treatment was over, my coworkers acted like I was the one who had cancer. They avoided me like the plague" (H. Katz, personal communication, 1994). Identification with the family member may prompt an existential crisis heralded by the predominance of death anxiety, highly correlated with a diagnosis of cancer (Amir & Kalemkerian, 2003; Rawnsley, 1994).

> Our fear of death makes it essential to maintain a distance between ourselves and anyone who is threatened by death. Denying our connection to the precariousness of others' lives is a way of pretending that we are immortal. Yet, cancer connects us to one another because having cancer is an embodiment of the existential paradox that we all experience: We feel that we are immortal, yet we know that we will all die. (Trillin, 1981, p. 699)

Alterations in intimacy and sexuality also enhance feelings of isolation (Dorval, Maunsell, Taylor-Brown, & Kilpatrick, 1999; Dow, 1995; Ganz, 2001; Ganz et al., 2002; Zebrack, Casillas, et al., 2004). Unable to decipher the root cause of change as being fatigue, worry, or newfound unattractiveness, both survivors and family members despair that the security associated with prior close relationships may be permanently jeopardized. Hence, at a time when both the survivor and primary caregiver need support and emotional connectivity, detachment rather than closeness may become the norm.

Transitional Crisis

He just doesn't seem as though he can forget about it and just lead a normal life. It's curtailing our life. It's something I wish that he would get over but I don't think that he is going to. (Family member quoted in Little, Paul, Jordens, & Sayers, 2002)

A transition implies moving from one relatively stable state, with an experience of disorganization and upheaval during the process, toward another stable state (Clarke-Steffen, 1993). Transitions generally are considered stressful because they impose adaptational challenges, evoke anxiety, and require a period of readjustment (MacLean, Foley, Ruccione, & Sklar, 1996). It has been widely acknowledged that chronically ill children require help with major life transitions (Hobbie & Ogle, 2001; Konsler & Jones, 1993). Developmentally tailored clinics, educational workshops, and outreach community-based support provide interventions to master new transitions within the context of pediatric oncology. However, comparable needs of adults transitioning through various phases of illness are infrequently acknowledged.

Major adjustments within the cancer experience include changes in one's sense of self from well person to sick patient (upon cancer diagnosis), ill patient to well person (upon successful completion of therapy), and episodic well person to ill patient (when follow-up testing is performed, reinforcing the sick role during intermittent hospitalizations, or when recurrence becomes a suspicion or is diagnosed). Additionally, age-specific implications of survivorship must be considered as supportive care interventions are planned (President's Cancer Panel, 2004; Utley, 1999; Weekes & Kagan, 1994). Table 2-1 outlines some examples of developmental challenges during various periods of transition in survivorship.

Table 2-1. Developmental Challenges During Transitional Crises in Survivorship

Age Group	Parental Separation	Survivor Guilt	Reentry	Role Change	Discrimination/ Isolation
Pediatrics	X		X		X
Adolescence	X	X	X	X	X
Young Adult	X	X	X	X	X
Middle Age		X	X	X	X
Older Adult		X		X	X

Another major transition for all survivors and their loved ones has received attention primarily in pediatric oncology settings. The family unit's attempts to "get back to normal" following treatment are, in fact, impossible. The intrusion of cancer causes permanent change in how survivors and families respond and cope. A new norm must be constructed for the family unit to move forward (see Figure 2-3). Families facing cancer must reconstruct reality and change its future orientation, manage information, assign meaning to illness, reorganize roles, manage therapeutic regimens, and evaluate and shift priorities (Clarke-Steffen, 1993). Although originally designed to depict family coping requirements during childhood cancer, this model has equivalent meaning within the adult cancer experience.

Figure 2-3. Elements of Rehabilitative Interventions to Enhance Long-Term Cancer Survival

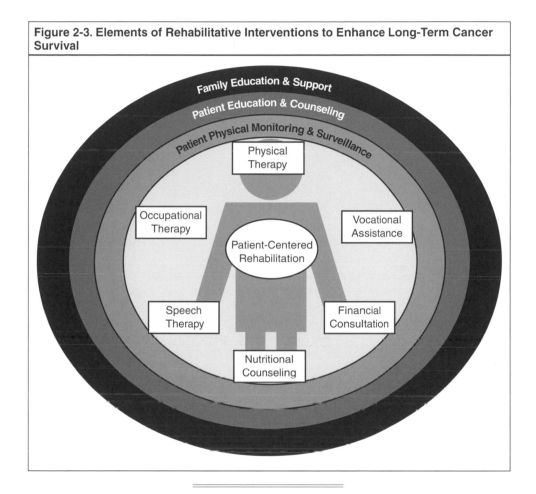

Reentry and Work

I lost my breast, not my brain. (Anonymous)

Regardless of age, some degree of cancer-related stigma should be expected and frequently makes reentry problematic. Going back to school is considered a stressful time for children with a history of cancer that is well served by professional support and advocacy, whereas adults are expected to return to work and family life without comparable aid.

Reestablishing oneself back into precancer lifestyle norms may occur gradually during the course of active cancer therapy or abruptly following completion of treatment depending upon individual requirements for hospitalization and recovery. Coworkers and colleagues usually expect compromise in physical functioning during active therapy but may be unaware of comparable needs long term. Survivors themselves may have misconceptions about their ability to resume pretreatment work patterns following treatment. Even young adult, childhood, and adolescent cancer survivors have noted work- and school-related functional impairment upon reentry. Needing to work fewer hours, taking on lighter job responsibilities, or requiring more frequent breaks are a few examples of adaptations required (Bloom et al., 1993; Helder et al., 2004; Joly et al., 1996).

Concern over employment discrimination is significant (Boyle, 1996). Discrimination in the workplace may include "shunning," a concerted effort to avoid contact with the survivor (Berry, 1993). Feeling "job lock" (the inability to pursue other employment options as a result of cancer-related bias) and problems with obtaining health insurance or experiencing a loss of benefits are real concerns for cancer survivors (Christ, Lane, & Marcove, 1995; Langeveld et al., 2004). Survivors may be bypassed for promotions or job transfers because they may be considered incapable or have questionable longevity. Additionally, job termination remains a fear in today's workplace (Schultz, Beck, Stava, & Sellin, 2002). Regardless of positive trends in dispelling myths about survivors' work performance, many supervisory personnel continue to believe that upon return to work, survivors may no longer be able to perform their job adequately or may not take their job seriously (Stat Bite, 1993). More than one-half of patients with cancer ultimately will survive long term, yet it appears that many employers remain entrenched in the old paradigm that equates cancer with a death sentence. The Americans with Disabilities Act (ADA) can protect survivors from discriminatory practices by employers and can lobby for accommodation of disability in the workplace (Bradley & Bednarek, 2002; Hoffman, 1997). Yet, the ADA's power to eliminate discrimination rarely has been tested (Arnold, 1999). As perceptions change about the uniform lethal nature of cancer, so may work-related stigma. Recent reports of the absence of discrimination at work are indeed promising (Maunsell et al., 2004).

Reevaluating Life Priorities

Face it. You've got to be like me to really appreciate how silly it is to read a letter from Dear Abby's column about a woman upset because her neighbor hasn't returned her salad bowls. It's like, "Oooooh lady, how can you stand it?" (Bombeck, 1989, p. xxi)

Empirical evidence exists about the positive nature of living through and beyond cancer. The threat of death followed by recovery often prompts cancer survivors to reexamine life's meaning. Deemed a secondary benefit of having cancer, life review frequently reconfigures personal measures of quality of life (Gotay, Isaacs, & Pagano, 2004). Life review often results in minimization of minor anxieties that, following diagnosis, appear inconsequential when compared to the threat of cancer (Maher, 1982; Tomich & Helgeson, 2002). A philosophic reflection on the meaning of life may result in the reexamination of the role of spirituality in everyday life, past coping styles, and precipitants of emotional crisis (Vickberg et al., 2001). Younger survivors may find this introspection most beneficial (Schroevers, Ranchor, & Sanderman, 2004).

Family Coping

We do a lot of waiting, a lot of resting, a lot of waiting and a lot of resting. When you love someone, you just kind of hang in there and let whatever the course is take hold. (Family member quoted in Boyle et al., 2000)

Cancer is a family disease (Boyle, 2003b; Moulton, 2000; Rowland et al., 2001). Considered "secondary survivors," families have unique issues and provocations as they cope with life after cancer (Boyle et al., 2000; Mellon, 2002). Families must integrate and synthesize information often of a secondhand nature, monitor and supervise ongoing care requirements, and worry in isolation about what the future holds. Guilt may prevail. (Could I have recognized the symptoms earlier? Should I have forced him to go to the doctor even though he resisted? How could I have been so consumed with the kids that I did not see his weight loss?) These enduring feelings can plague families long term. Families experience frustration and feel isolated, confused, and tired in response to the competing demands of providing usual family care in conjunction with accommodating survivor needs. More in-depth investigation of family issues during survivorship is required because the future portends the addition, rather than the detraction, of caregiving expectations that are imposed on families.

Intervention Considerations

To address the perception of being "caught in a black hole of system unresponsiveness," more comprehensive care is required for adult survivors in both the extended and permanent phases of survival (Belec, 1992; Gray, 1992). Such care should model programs that are offered for cardiac and stroke rehabilitation because these illnesses are considered chronic conditions rather than fatal ones. Follow-up care should be more than the routine testing that currently is provided to detect recurrence, second primaries or other complications (Beaver & Luker, 2005; Bhatia & Sklar, 2002; Deniz et al., 2003; Matesich & Shapiro, 2003).

Just as cancer treatment is tailored to patients' needs within acute survival, follow-up care also should be customized and individualized. In many cases, interventions during permanent survival will be comparable to what is provided during extended survival. Hence, interventions appropriate to both of these phases require contemplation.

Follow-up care should be rendered as an extension of services provided by the cancer care team. This team, unlike community-based generalists, knows the survivor over time and the natural history of the malignancy (Adewuyi-Dalton, Ziebland, Grunfeld, & Hall, 1998; Oeffinger et al., 2004). This continued relationship with the core team fosters trust and enhances communication as a result of the longevity of this affiliation. Some new healthcare providers with complementary skills and knowledge will need to be added to the team during extended and permanent survival (e.g., physical therapist). Of benefit is the review of pediatric follow-up programs that have been operational for decades and thus may serve as a template for adult-focused program development. The specific domains within extended and permanent survival that require intervention include (Kattlove & Winn, 2003)

- Surveillance to detect recurrent cancer
- Assessment of genetic susceptibility to cancer (both survivors and family members)
- Detection of a second primary malignancy
- Monitoring of treatment complications
- Dealing with physiologic alterations related to cancer or its treatment
- Support for psychosocial problems.

Again, separation of physiologic and psychosocial issues is formidable. Thus, comprehensive follow-up programs that offer myriad interventions during protracted survival are required (Boyle, 2003b). Any attempt to provide novel follow-up services for adult survivors must be accompanied by companion assistance for families. Additionally, data that demonstrate value-added benefit, cost effectiveness, and improved quality-of-life outcomes will substantiate program viability.

Physiologic Surveillance

Planning for monitoring physiologic problems during survivorship should be tumor-, treatment-, and age-specific. Tumor-related issues pertain to the natural history of the malignancy with specific concern about metabolic compromise, usual patterns of metastases, and recurrence trajectories (Emens & Davidson, 2003; Mahon, Williams, & Spies, 2000; Nuver, Smit, Postma, Sleijfer, & Gietema, 2002; Svobodnik et al., 2004). Consideration of tumor type and cancer stage is important because it influences both the type and frequency of surveillance. Treatment type dictates surveillance of specific organs or physiologic processes (Theodoulou & Seidman, 2003). Age-related factors may heighten awareness of comorbidity in symptom presentation. Both empirical and evidence-based findings have driven recommendations for follow-up care (Christianson & Anderson, 2003; Evans, 2002; Kattlove & Winn, 2003; Kondagunta, Sheinfeld, & Motzer, 2003; Meyerhardt & Mayer, 2003; Patel, Zagars, & Pisters, 2003; Pfister, Benson, & Somerfield, 2004; Smith, 2003; Vaughn, Gignac, & Meadows, 2002; Vaidya & Curtin, 2003; Wooldridge & Link, 2003; Yao & DiPaola, 2003). As a result of the growing volume of breast cancer survivors, most research has focused on their long-term symptom distress and requirements for continued follow-up care (Bottomley et al., 2005; Burstein & Winer, 2000; Carpenter et al., 2004; Chlebowski, Kim, & Col, 2003; Collins, Bekker, & Dodwell, 2004; Emens & Davidson; Eversley et al., 2005; Mast, 1998b; Partridge, Winer, & Burstein, 2003; Schover, 2004; Utley, 1999). Testing of these recommendations is necessary to formulate evidence-based guidelines that provide cancer care providers with an organized strategy for surveillance (Ganz, 2001; Loprinzi, 1995). Such guidelines would dictate the timing of physiologic examination, the type and scope of diagnostic testing and screening evaluations, and the nature of needed psychosocial support.

Psychosocial Support

Emotional, family, and work-related concerns must be addressed with comparable rigor as physiologic compromise. A broader range and frequency of interventions will be required during the "first year out" as the stresses of reentry and recurrence anxiety predominate during this time frame (Boyle, 1999). The provision of psychosocial support generally depends more upon survivor preference and acceptance than on physiologically based surveillance interventions (see Appendix for examples). Possible support options within the psychosocial realm include the following.

1. Educational forums to minimize uncertainty, dispel misconceptions, and enhance coping skills during long-term survival should be offered with equal intensity as those provided prior to the initiation of new cancer therapy (Mullan, 1984). These offerings may include individual sessions, workshops, and small group teaching for both survivors and families. Additionally, written and Internet-based materials from reputable sources that address expectations during survivorship are needed to augment formal teaching sessions (Boyle, 1999; Sharp, 1999; Tesauro, Rowland, & Lustig, 2002).

2. Counseling to enhance mastery of common emotional sequelae is germane to long-term survivorship. Individual sessions, groups, marital counseling, and peer support for both survivors and families are required. Anticipation of survivor-specific coping themes (e.g., recurrence anxiety, reentry problems, workplace discrimination, infertility, relationship changes) is important. By emphasizing personal strengths and the benefits of positive reappraisal, quality of life can be improved (Dorval et al., 1999; Dow, 1995; Fiore, 1979; Kessler, 2002; O'Connor & Wicker, 1995; Rauch, Miny, Conroy, Neyton, & Guillemin, 2004; Welch-McCaffrey et al., 1989).

Issues related to planning physiologic follow-up and psychosocial care present uncertainty, such as when to educate the patient and family about post-therapy expectations. In cases where education regarding survivor issues was provided prior to the end of treatment, the majority of patients frequently did not remember the content of these discussions (Boyle et al., 2000). Around the end of active therapy, patients and families may be consumed with getting through treatment; hence, reception of new information about life after treatment may be limited. Patients thus require significant reinforcement of teaching and should not be expected to easily retain information about follow-up care.

Finally, long-term screening of adults with a history of childhood cancer remains in question. The questions of how much, how long, and by whom require answers along with factors that promote adherence with surveillance guidelines (Kadan-Lottick et al., 2002; Yeazel et al., 2003; Zebrack, Eshelman, et al., 2004).

Rehabilitation Programs

Within the auspices of health promotion and wellness resides an important but neglected opportunity to foster living well with a history of cancer—rehabilitation. In considering the acceptance of rehabilitation as a component of follow-up care for patients with cardiac disease, the absence of such in cancer care suggests pervasive negativism and bias about the utility and efficacy of rehabilitation.

Rehabilitation is the bridge that leads a person from a condition of diversity to a condition of normality (Veronesi & Martino, 1978). It is a practical attempt to maximize independence and dignity in individuals who have had cancer (Watson, 1992). A rehabilitation program for cancer survivors should be individually planned with attention to minimizing deficits and reinforcing strengths (Mellette, 1993). Its correlation with improved long-term outcomes requires intensive study (Holmes, Chen, Feskanich, Kroenke, & Colditz, 2005). Some rehabilitation interventions include (see Figure 2-3)

- Physical, occupational, and speech therapy
- Psychosocial, vocational, financial, and nutritional counseling.

Additional rehabilitation team members augment the expertise of the cancer team with the use of their specialty knowledge (Wells, 1990). For example, physical therapists can address deconditioning and reduced endurance while increasing strength and compensating for functional decline. Nutritional counselors can foster a sense of control to navigate survivors toward long-term wellness (Chlebowski, 2003; Demark-Wahnefried & Rock, 2003). Occupational therapists can recommend energy-conserving techniques in the home to decrease debilitating fatigue. Attention to issues involved with returning to work is an important component of societal reintegration of cancer survivors (Spelten, Sprangers, & Verbeek, 2002). Programs that focus on recovery give survivors and caregivers a strong message of hope. These programs acknowledge that living on following a cancer diagnosis is a realistic option. Education, emotional support, and exercise with intensive follow-up can foster patients' quality of life while contributing to physiologic and psychosocial wellness (Courneya & Friedenreich, 1999; Courneya et al., 2003; Cox & Wilson, 2003; Gambosi & Ulreich, 1990; Jacobs & Hobbie, 2002; Pinto, Eakin, & Maruyama, 2000; Pinto & Maruyama, 1999; Pinto & Trunzo, 2004). This becomes increasingly important as cancer survivorship becomes recognized as a distinct clinical entity within cancer care (Kattlove & Winn, 2003).

Research

Evidence is required to drive innovation within the survivorship paradigm. Acknowledging the critical role of family survivors in the research agenda is imperative (Moulton, 2000). The trend of heightened acuity and greater intensity of cancer therapies will require continued investigation of the long-term burden of cancer and its treatment (Schimmer et al., 2001; Yabroff et al., 2004). Positive outcomes of survivor research can enhance lobbying for programmatic insurance coverage when reduced debilitation and quicker return to work can be quantified. Figure 2-4 lists some examples of research questions that require attention. Investigation of these issues is best served by interdisciplinary inquiry and research designs, and consensus with primary and secondary survivors on the meaning of findings. Concern about special, at-risk survivor populations also mandates investigation of oncology nurses and physicians who themselves survive cancer or survive the cancer experience as family members (Welch-McCaffrey, 1984). How this personal experience impacts professional retention and interaction with patients and families requires extensive study.

Figure 2-4. Themes for Cancer Survivor Research Focusing on Psychosocial Challenges

- Quality of life related to
  - Impact of various therapies long term
  - Baseline performance status and prognostic indicators
  - Surviving second cancers
  - Ethnicity
  - Socioeconomic status
  - Marital status
  - Presence of concurrent comorbid illness
- Long-term effects on families
- Education and support preferences based on age, "time out" post-therapy completion, and type of treatment
- Scope and nature of employment and workplace barriers to successful reentry
- Impact of nurse-led education, support, and surveillance during patient transition into the phase of extended survival
- Impact of intensive psychosocial follow-up with patients having precancer histories of emotional illness
- Recurrence anxiety
  - Prompts and reinforcers for health-seeking behaviors and health surveillance
  - Characteristics over time
  - Patient variables associated with hypochondriasis and physician avoidance

Note. Based on information from Dow, 2003; Gibson, 2004; Gotay & Muraoka, 1998; Helder et al., 2004; Lindsey et al., 2004; Moore et al., 2002; Svobodnik et al., 2004.

Conclusion

Survivorship is the challenge faced daily by millions who are engaged in defiance of cancer and in the affirmation of life (Mullan, 1996). In a variety of instances, however, advances in cancer therapies have added years to life but not necessarily life to years. The dilemmas and challenges of survivorship are multiple and require significant practice innovations based on the science of research findings. In today's cancer care paradigm, survivorship is a life lived in a context of evolving knowledge (Little et al., 2002).

Survivorship is a nurse-intensive phenomenon (Ferrell, Virani, et al., 2003). Oncology nurses are a critical influence on patients' ability to transition through the cancer continuum. Wilmoth (2001) described one element of this as helping survivors to move to a new level of equilibrium following a cancer-related crisis. Both patients and families who evolve through the cancer trajectory could benefit from the long-term support, education, and advocacy that the same oncology nurses they trusted in earlier phases of their cancer experience could provide during long-term survivorship. This, however, requires oncology nurses to expand their body of knowledge to encompass the recognition and management of unique issues pertinent to living with a history of cancer. In the future, its significance will grow as education, support, advice, symptom scrutiny, and a holistic orientation to care for survivors and their families will be expected. Poletti (1985) poignantly described that the role of the oncology nurse is to help the patient to be a fully functioning person first and a patient with cancer second. This is the essence of nursing expertise and scholarship following life after cancer.

References

Adewuyi-Dalton, R., Ziebland, S., Grunfeld, E., & Hall, A. (1998). Patients' views of routine hospital follow-up: A qualitative study of women with breast cancer in remission. *Psycho-Oncology, 7,* 436–439.

Ahles, T.A., & Saykin, A. (2001). Cognitive effects of standard-dose chemotherapy in patients with cancer. *Cancer Investigation, 19,* 812–820.

Ahles, T.A., Saykin, A.J., Furstenberg, C.T., Cole, B., Mott, L.A., Skalla, K., et al. (2002). Neuropsychological impact of standard-dose systemic chemotherapy in long-term survivors of breast cancer and lymphoma. *Journal of Clinical Oncology, 20,* 485–493.

Aisner, J., Wiernik, P.H., & Pearl, P. (1993). Pregnancy outcomes in patients treated for Hodgkin's disease. *Journal of Clinical Oncology, 11,* 503–512.

Amir, M., & Kalemkerian, G.P. (2003). Run for your life: The reactions of some professionals to a person with cancer. *Journal of Clinical Oncology, 21,* 3696–3699.

Amir, M., & Ramati, A. (2002). Post-traumatic symptoms, emotional distress and quality of life in long-term survivors of breast cancer: A preliminary research. *Journal of Anxiety Disorders, 16,* 195–206.

Anderson, D.M., Rennie, K.M., Ziegler, R.S., Neglia, J.P., Robison, L.R., & Gurney, J.G. (2001). Medical and neurocognitive late effects among survivors of childhood central nervous system tumors. *Cancer, 92,* 2709–2719.

Arnold, K. (1999). The American with Disabilities Act: Do cancer patients qualify as disabled? *Journal of the National Cancer Institute, 91,* 822–825.

Ashing-Giwa, K.T., Padilla, G.V., Tejero, J.S., & Kim, J. (2004). Breast cancer survivorship in a multiethnic sample. *Cancer, 101,* 450–465.

Averette, H.E., Mirhashemi, R., & Moffat, F.L. (1999). Pregnancy after breast carcinoma: The ultimate medical challenge. *Cancer, 85,* 2301–2304.

Aziz, N., & Rowland, J. (2002). Cancer survivor research among ethnic minorities and medically underserved groups. *Oncology Nursing Forum, 29,* 788–801.

Baider, L., Andritsch, E., Goldzweig, G., Uziely, B., Ever-Hadani, P., Hofman, G., et al. (2004). Changes in psychological distress of women with breast cancer in long-term remission and their husbands. *Psychosomatics, 45,* 58–68.

Beaver, K., & Luker, K.A. (2005). Follow-up in breast cancer clinics: Reassuring for patients rather than detecting recurrence. *Psycho-Oncology, 14,* 94–101.

Belec, R.H. (1992). Quality of life: Perceptions of long-term survivors of bone marrow transplantation. *Oncology Nursing Forum, 19,* 31–37.

Berry, D.L. (1993). Return-to-work experiences of people with cancer. *Oncology Nursing Forum, 20,* 905–911.

Bhatia, S., & Sklar, C. (2002). Second cancers in survivors of childhood cancer. *Nature Reviews Cancer, 2,* 124–132.

Blakely, L.J., Buzdar, A.U., Lozada, J.A., Shullaih, S.A., Hoy, E., Smith, T.L., et al. (2004). Effects of pregnancy after treatment for breast carcinoma on survival and risk of recurrence. *Cancer, 100,* 465–469.

Bloom, J.R., Fobair, P., Gritz, E., Wellisch, D., Spiegel, D., Varghese, A., et al. (1993). Psychosocial outcomes of cancer: A comparative analysis of Hodgkin's disease and testicular cancer. *Journal of Clinical Oncology, 11,* 979–988.

Bombeck, E. (1989). *I want to grow hair, I want to grow up, I want to go to Boise.* New York: Harper & Row.

Bottomley, A., Therasse, P., Piccart, M., Efficace, F., Coens, C., Gotay, C., et al. (2005). Health-related quality of life in survivors of locally advanced breast cancer: An international randomized controlled phase III trial. *Lancet Oncology, 6,* 287–294.

Bower, J.E., Ganz, P.A., Desmond, K.A., Rowland, J.H., Meyerowitz, B.E., & Belin, T.R. (2000). Fatigue in breast cancer survivors: Occurrence, correlates and impact on quality of life. *Journal of Clinical Oncology, 18,* 743–753.

Boyle, D.A. (1999). Fear of recurrence: It's a normal side effect of cancer. *COPING, 13*(3), 19.

Boyle, D.A. (2002). Families facing cancer: The forgotten priority [Editorial]. *Clinical Journal of Oncology Nursing, 6,* 1–2.

Boyle, D.A. (2003a). Establishing a nursing research agenda in geriatric oncology. *Critical Reviews in Hematology/Oncology, 48,* 103–111.

Boyle, D.A. (2003b). Psychological adjustment to the melanoma experience. *Seminars in Oncology Nursing, 19,* 70–77.

Boyle, D.A., Blodgett, L., Gnesdiloff, S., White, J., Bamford, A.M., Sheridan, M., et al. (2000). Caregiver quality of life after autologous bone marrow transplantation. *Cancer Nursing, 23,* 193–205.

Boyle, G.C. (1996). Legal barriers against employment discrimination for the breast cancer patient. *Innovations in Breast Cancer Care, 2,* 13–16.

Bradley, C.J., & Bednarek, H.L. (2002). Employment patterns of long-term survivors. *Psycho-Oncology, 11,* 188–198.

Braun, M., Hasson-Ohayon, I., Perry, S., Kaufman, B., & Uziely, B. (2005). Motivation for giving birth after breast cancer. *Psycho-Oncology, 14,* 282–296.

Brown, P.D., Buckner, J.C., O'Fallon, J.R., Iturria, N.L., Brown, C.A., O'Neill, B.P., et al. (2003). Effects of radiotherapy on cognitive function in patients with low-grade glioma measured by the Folstein Mini-Mental State examination. *Journal of Clinical Oncology, 21,* 2519–2524.

Burstein, H.J., & Winer, E.P. (2000). Primary care for survivors of breast cancer. *New England Journal of Medicine, 343,* 1086–1094.

Bushkin, E. (1993). Signposts of survivorship. *Oncology Nursing Forum, 20,* 869–874.

Carpenter, J.S., Elam, J.L., Ridner, S.H., Carney, P.H., Cherry, G.J., & Cucullu, H.L. (2004). Sleep, fatigue, and depressive symptoms in breast cancer survivors and matched healthy women experiencing hot flashes. *Oncology Nursing Forum, 31,* 591–598.

Carter, B. (1993). Long-term survivors of breast cancer: A qualitative descriptive study. *Cancer Nursing, 16,* 354–361.

Cella, D., Davis, K., Breitbart, W., & Curt, G. (2001). Cancer-related fatigue: Prevalence of proposed diagnostic criteria in a United States sample of cancer survivors. *Journal of Clinical Oncology, 19,* 3385–3391.

Cella, D.F., & Tross, S. (1986). Psychological adjustment to survival from Hodgkin's disease. *Journal of Consulting and Clinical Psychology, 54,* 616–622.

Challinor, J., Miaskowski, C., Moore, I., Slaughter, R., & Franck, L. (2000). Review of research studies that evaluated the impact of treatment for childhood cancers on neurocognition and behavioral social competence: Nursing implications. *Journal of the Society of Pediatric Nursing, 5,* 57–74.

Chlebowski, R.T. (2003). The American Cancer Society guide for nutrition and physical activity for cancer survivors: A call to action for clinical investigators. *CA: A Cancer Journal for Clinicians, 53,* 266–267.

Chlebowski, R.T., Kim, J.A., & Col, N.F. (2003). Estrogen deficiency symptom management in breast cancer survivors in the changing context of menopausal hormone therapy. *Seminars in Oncology, 30,* 776–788.

Christ, G.H., Lane, J.M., & Marcove, R. (1995). Psychosocial adaptation of long-term survivors of bone carcinoma. *Journal of Psychosocial Oncology, 13*(4), 1–22.

Christianson, D.F., & Anderson, C.M. (2003). Close monitoring and lifetime follow-up is optimal for patients with a history of melanoma. *Seminars in Oncology, 30,* 369–374.

Clark, E.J., & Stovall, E.L. (1996). Advocacy: The cornerstone of cancer survivorship. *Cancer Practice, 4,* 239–244.

Clarke-Steffen, L. (1993). A model of family transition to living with childhood cancer. *Cancer Practice, 1,* 285–292.

Clift, R.A., & Thomas, E.D. (2004). Follow-up 26 years after treatment for acute myelogenous leukemia. *New England Journal of Medicine, 351,* 2456–2457.

Collins, R.F., Bekker, H.L., & Dodwell, D.J. (2004). Follow-up care of patients treated for breast cancer: A structured review. *Cancer Treatment Reviews, 30,* 19–35.

Courneya, K.S., & Friedenreich, C.M. (1999). Physical exercise and quality of life following cancer diagnosis: A literature review. *Annals of Behavioral Medicine, 21,* 171–179.

Courneya, K.S., Friedenreich, C.M., Quinney, H.A., Fields, A.L., Jones, L.W., & Fairey, A.S. (2003). A randomized trial of exercise and quality of life in colorectal cancer survivors. *European Journal of Cancer Care, 12,* 347–357.

Cox, K., & Wilson, E. (2003). Follow-up for people with cancer: Nurse-led services and telephone interventions. *Journal of Advanced Nursing, 43,* 51–61.

Demark-Wahnefried, W., & Rock, C.L. (2003). Nutrition-related issues for the breast cancer survivor. *Seminars in Oncology, 30,* 789–798.

Deniz, K., O'Mahoney, S., Ross, G., & Purushotham, A. (2003). Breast cancer in women after treatment for Hodgkin. *Lancet Oncology, 4,* 207–214.

Dirksen, S.R., & Erickson, J.R. (2002). Well-being in Hispanic and non-Hispanic white survivors of breast cancer. *Oncology Nursing Forum, 29,* 820–826.

Dorval, M., Maunsell, E., Deschenes, L., Brisson, J., & Masse, B. (1998). Long-term quality of life after breast cancer: Comparison of 8-year survivors with population controls. *Journal of Clinical Oncology, 16,* 487–494.

Dorval, M., Maunsell, E., Taylor-Brown, J., & Kilpatrick, M. (1999). Marital stability after breast cancer. *Journal of the National Cancer Institute, 91,* 54–59.

Dow, K.H. (1990). The enduring seasons of survival. *Oncology Nursing Forum, 17,* 511–516.

Dow, K.H. (1992). On the nature and meaning of locally recurrent breast cancer. *Quality of Life—A Nursing Challenge, 1,* 27–34.

Dow, K.H. (1995). A review of late effects of cancer in women. *Seminars in Oncology Nursing, 11,* 128–136.

Dow, K.H. (2003). Challenges and opportunities in cancer survivorship research. *Oncology Nursing Forum, 30,* 455–469.

Emens, L.A., & Davidson, N.E. (2003). The follow-up of breast cancer. *Seminars in Oncology, 30,* 338–348.

Evans, C.P. (2002). Follow-up surveillance strategies for genitourinary malignancies. *Cancer, 94,* 2892–2905.

Eversley, R., Estrin, D., Dibble, S., Wardlaw, L., Pedrosa, M., & Favita-Penney, W. (2005). Post-treatment symptoms among ethnic minority breast cancer survivors. *Oncology Nursing Forum, 32,* 250–260.

Farmer, B.J., & Smith, E.D. (2002). Breast cancer survivorship: Are African American women considered? A concept analysis. *Oncology Nursing Forum, 29,* 779–788.

Ferrell, B.R., & Dow, K.H. (1996). Portraits of cancer survivorship: A glimpse through the lens of survivors' eyes. *Cancer Practice, 4,* 76–80.

Ferrell, B.R., Smith, S.L., Juarez, G., & Melancon, C. (2003). Meaning of illness and spirituality in ovarian cancer survivors. *Oncology Nursing Forum, 30,* 249–258.

Ferrell, B.R., Virani, R., Smith, S., & Juarez, G. (2003). The role of oncology nursing to ensure quality care for cancer survivors: A report commissioned by the National Cancer Policy Board and Institute of Medicine [Online exclusive]. *Oncology Nursing Forum, 30,* E1–E11.

Fiore, N. (1979). Fighting cancer—One patient's perspective. *New England Journal of Medicine, 300,* 284–289.

Fizazi, K., Chen, I., & Logothetis, C.J. (2002). Germ-cell tumor survivors: The price for cure. *Annals of Oncology, 13,* 187–189.

Fleer, J., Hoekstra, H.J., Sleijfer, D.T., & Hoekstra-Weebers, J.E. (2004). Quality of life of survivors of testicular germ cell cancer: A review of the literature. *Supportive Care in Cancer, 12,* 476–486.

Fobair, P., & Mages, N.L. (1981). Psychological morbidity among cancer patient survivors. In P. Ahmed (Ed.), *Living and dying with cancer* (pp. 285–308). New York: Elsevier.

Gambosi, J.R., & Ulreich, S. (1990). Recovering from cancer: A nursing intervention program recognizing survivorship. *Oncology Nursing Forum, 17,* 215–219.

Ganz, P.A. (2001). Late effects of cancer and its treatment. *Seminars in Oncology Nursing, 17,* 241–248.

Ganz, P.A. (2003). Why and how to study the fate of cancer survivors: Observations from the clinic and research laboratory. *European Journal of Cancer, 39,* 2136–2141.

Ganz, P.A., Desmond, K.A., Leedham, B., Rowland, J.H., Meyerowitz, B.E., & Belin, T.R. (2002). Quality of life in long-term, disease-free survivors of breast cancer: A follow-up study. *Journal of the National Cancer Institute, 94,* 39–49.

Ganz, P.A., Kwan, L., Stanton, A.L., Krupnick, J.L., Rowland, J.H., Meyerowitz, B.E., et al. (2004). Quality of life at the end of primary treatment of breast cancer: First results from the moving beyond cancer randomized trial. *Journal of the National Cancer Institute, 96,* 376–387.

Gaudine, A., Sturge-Jacobs, M., & Kennedy, M. (2003). The experience of waiting and life during breast cancer follow-up. *Research and Theory for Nursing Practice, 17,* 153–168.

Gelinas, C., & Fillion, L. (2004). Factors related to persistent fatigue following completion of breast cancer therapy. *Oncology Nursing Forum, 31,* 269–278.

Gibson, F. (2004). Surveillance and follow-up in cancer care: Meaning and purpose [Editorial]. *European Journal of Oncology Nursing, 8,* 105–106.

Gil, K.M., Mishel, M.H., Belyea, M., Germino, B., Porter, L.S., LaNey, I.C., et al. (2004). Triggers of uncertainty about recurrence and long-term treatment side effects in older African American and Caucasian breast cancer survivors. *Oncology Nursing Forum, 31,* 633–639.

Gil-Fernandez, J., Ramos, C., Tamayo, T., Tomas, T., Figuera, A., Arranz, R., et al. (2003). Quality of life and psychological well-being in Spanish long-term survivors of Hodgkin's disease: Results of a controlled pilot study. *Annals of Hematology, 82,* 14–18.

Gotay, C.C., Holup, J., & Pagano, I.S. (2002). Ethnic differences in quality of life among early breast and prostate cancer survivors. *Psycho-Oncology, 11,* 103–113.

Gotay, C.C., Isaacs, P., & Pagano, I. (2004). Quality of life in patients who survive a dire prognosis compared to control cancer survivors. *Psycho-Oncology, 13,* 882–892.

Gotay, C.C., & Muraoka, M.Y. (1998). Quality of life in long-term survivors of adult onset cancer. *Journal of the National Cancer Institute, 90,* 656–667.

Gray, R.E. (1992). Persons with cancer speak out: Reflections on an important trend in Canadian health care. *Journal of Palliative Care, 8*(4), 30–37.

Gross, G.J., Ott, C.D., Lindsey, A.M., Twiss, J.J., & Waltman, N. (2002). Postmenopausal breast cancer survivors at risk for osteoporosis: Physical activity, vigor, and vitality. *Oncology Nursing Forum, 29,* 1295–1300.

Hale, G.A., Marina, N.M., Jones-Wallace, D., Greenwald, C.A., Jenkins, J.J., Rao, B.N., et al. (1999). Late effects of treatment for germ cell tumors during childhood and adolescence. *Journal of Pediatric Hematology/Oncology, 21,* 115–122.

Halstead, M.T., & Fernsler, J.I. (1994). Coping strategies of long-term cancer survivors. *Cancer Nursing, 17,* 94–100.

Harder, H., Cornelissen, J.J., Van Gool, A.R., Duivenvoorden, H.J., Eijkenboom, W.M., & van den Bent, M.J. (2002). Cognitive functioning and quality of life in long-term adult survivors of bone marrow transplantation. *Cancer, 95,* 183–192.

Hayden, P.J., Keogh, F., Conghalle, M.N., Carroll, M., Crowley, M., Fitzsimon, N., et al. (2004). A single-centre assessment of long-term quality of life status after sibling allogeneic stem cell transplantation for chronic myeloid leukemia in first chronic phase. *Bone Marrow Transplantation, 34,* 545–556.

Helder, D.I., Bakker, B., de Heer, P., van der Veen, F., Vossen, J.M., Wit, J.M., et al. (2004). Quality of life in adults following bone marrow transplantation during childhood. *Bone Marrow Transplantation, 33,* 329–336.

Hewitt, M., & Rowland, J.R. (2002). Mental health service use among cancer survivors: Analyses of the National Health Interview Survey. *Journal of Clinical Oncology, 20,* 4581–4590.

Hobbie, W.L., & Ogle, S. (2001). Transitional care for young adult survivors of childhood cancer. *Seminars in Oncology Nursing, 17,* 268–273.

Hoffman, B. (1997). Is the Americans with Disabilities Act protecting cancer survivors from discrimination? *Cancer Practice, 5,* 119–121.

Holmes, M.D., Chen, W.Y., Feskanich, D., Kroenke, C.H., & Colditz, G.A. (2005). Physical activity and survival after breast cancer diagnosis. *JAMA, 293,* 2479–2486.

Huyghe, E., Matsuda, T., Daudin, M., Chevreau, C., Bachaud, J.M., Plante, P., et al. (2004). Fertility after testicular cancer treatments: Results of a large multicenter study. *Cancer, 100,* 732–737.

Izsak, F.C., & Medalie, J.H. (1971). Comprehensive follow-up of carcinoma patients. *Journal of Chronic Diseases, 24,* 179–191.

Jacobs, L.A., & Hobbie, W.L. (2002). The living well after cancer program: An advanced practice model of care. *Oncology Nursing Forum, 29,* 637–638.

Jansen, C.E., Miaskowski, C., Dodd, M., & Dowling, G. (2005). Chemotherapy-induced cognitive impairment in women with breast cancer: A critique of the literature. *Oncology Nursing Forum, 32,* 329–342.

Jemal, A., Murray, T., Ward, E., Samuels, A., Tiwari, R.C., Ghafoor, A., et al. (2005). Cancer statistics, 2005. *CA: A Cancer Journal for Clinicians, 55,* 10–30.

Jenkinson, H.C., Hawkins, M.M., Stiller, C.A., Winter, D.L., Marsden, H.B., & Stevens, M.C. (2004). Long-term population-based risks of second malignant neoplasms after childhood cancer in Britain. *British Journal of Cancer, 91,* 1905–1910.

Joly, F., Henry-Amar, M., Arveux, P., Reman, O., Tanguy, A., Peny, A., et al. (1996). Late psychosocial sequelae in Hodgkin's disease survivors: A French population-based case-control study. *Journal of Clinical Oncology, 14,* 2444–2453.

Kadan-Lottick, N.S., Robison, L.L., Gurney, J.G., Neglia, J.P., Yasui, Y., Hayashi, R., et al. (2002). Childhood cancer survivors' knowledge about their past diagnosis and treatment: Childhood Cancer Survivor Study. *JAMA, 287,* 1832–1839.

Kattlove, H., & Winn, R.J. (2003). Ongoing care of patients after primary treatment for their cancer. *CA: A Cancer Journal for Clinicians, 53,* 172–196.

Kenney, L.B., Nicholson, H.S., Brasseux, C., Mills, J.L., Robison, L.L., Zeltzer, L.M., et al. (1996). Birth defects in offspring of adult survivors of childhood acute lymphoblastic leukemia: A Children's Cancer Group/National Institutes of Health Report. *Cancer, 78,* 169–176.

Kessler, T.A. (2002). Contextual variables, emotional state, and current and expected quality of life in breast cancer survivors. *Oncology Nursing Forum, 29,* 1109–1116.

Kirkwood, J.M., Bender, C., Agarwala, S., Tarhini, A., Shipe-Spotloe, J., Smelko, B., et al. (2002). Mechanisms and management of toxicities associated with high-dose interferon alfa-2b therapy. *Journal of Clinical Oncology, 20,* 3703–3718.

Knobel, H., Loge, J.H., Lund, M.B., Forfang, K., Nome, O., & Kaasa, S. (2001). Late medical complications and fatigue in Hodgkin's disease survivors. *Journal of Clinical Oncology, 19,* 3226–3233.

Kondagunta, G.V., Sheinfeld, J., & Motzer, R.J. (2003). Recommendations of follow-up after treatment of germ cell tumors. *Seminars in Oncology, 30,* 382–389.

Konsler, G.K., & Jones, G.R. (1993). Transition issues for survivors of childhood cancer and their healthcare providers. *Cancer Practice, 1,* 319–324.

Kornblith, A.B., & Ligibel, J. (2003). Psychosocial and sexual functioning of survivors of breast cancer. *Seminars in Oncology, 30,* 799–813.

Kwekkeboom, K.L., & Seng, J.S. (2002). Recognizing and responding to post-traumatic stress disorder in people with cancer. *Oncology Nursing Forum, 29,* 643–650.

Langeveld, N.E., Grootenhuis, M.A., Voute, P.A., de Haan, R.J., & van den Bos, C. (2004). Quality of life, self-esteem and worries in young adult survivors of childhood cancer. *Psycho-Oncology, 13,* 867–881.

Leigh, S. (1992). Myths, monsters and magic: Personal perspectives and professional challenges of survival. *Oncology Nursing Forum, 19,* 1475–1480.

Leigh, S. (1994). Cancer survivorship: A consumer movement. *Seminars in Oncology, 21,* 783–786.

Leigh, S. (2001). The culture of survivorship [Preface]. *Seminars in Oncology Nursing, 17,* 234–235.

Lethborg, C.E., Kissane, D., Burns, W.I., & Snyder, R. (2000). "Cast adrift": The experience of completing treatment among women with early stage breast cancer. *Journal of Psychosocial Oncology, 18*(4), 73–90.

Levin, W., Brown, R.T., Pawletko, T.M., Gold, S.H., & Whitt, J.K. (2000). Social skills and psychological adjustment of child and adolescent cancer survivors. *Psycho-Oncology, 9,* 113–126.

Lewis, F.M. (1993). Psychosocial transitions and the family work in adjusting to cancer. *Seminars in Oncology Nursing, 9,* 127–129.

Lilja, A.M., Portin, R.I., Hamalainen, P.I., & Salminen, E.K. (2001). Short-term effects of radiotherapy on attention and memory performances in patients with brain tumors. *Cancer, 91,* 2361–2368.

Lindsey, A.M., Waltman, N., Gross, G., Ott, C.D., & Twiss, J. (2004). Cancer risk-reduction behaviors of breast cancer survivors. *Western Journal of Nursing Research, 26,* 872–890.

Little, M., Paul, K., Jordens, C.F., & Sayers, E.J. (2002). Survivorship and discourses of identity. *Psycho-Oncology, 11,* 170–178.

Loescher, L.J., Clark, L., Atwood, J.R., Leigh, S., & Lamb, G. (1990). The impact of the cancer experience on long-term survivors. *Oncology Nursing Forum, 17,* 223–229.

Loprinzi, C.L. (1995). Follow-up testing for curatively treated cancer survivors: What to do? *JAMA, 273,* 1877–1878.

MacLean, W.E., Foley, G.V., Ruccione, K., & Sklar, C. (1996). Transitions in the care of adolescent and young adult survivors of childhood cancer. *Cancer, 78,* 1340–1344.

Maher, E.L. (1982). Anomic aspects of recovery from cancer. *Social Science and Medicine, 16,* 907–912.

Mahon, S.M., Williams, M.T., & Spies, M.A. (2000). Screening for second cancers and osteoporosis in long-term survivors. *Cancer Practice, 8,* 282–290.

Mandelblatt, J., Armetta, C., Yabroff, K.R., Liang, W., & Lawrence, W. (2004). Descriptive review of the literature on breast cancer outcomes: 1990 through 2000. *Journal of the National Cancer Institute Monographs, 33,* 8–44.

Mast, M.E. (1998a). Correlates of fatigue in survivors of breast cancer. *Cancer Nursing, 21,* 136–142.

Mast, M.E. (1998b). Survivors of breast cancer: Illness uncertainty, positive reappraisal, and emotional distress. *Oncology Nursing Forum, 25,* 555–562.

Matesich, M.A., & Shapiro, C.L. (2003). Second cancers after breast cancer treatment. *Seminars in Oncology, 30,* 740–748.

Matthews, B.A. (2003). Role and gender differences in cancer-related distress: A comparison of survivor and caregiver self-reports. *Oncology Nursing Forum, 30,* 493–499.

Maunsell, E., Drolet, M., Brisson, J., Brisson, C., Masse, B., & Deschenes, L. (2004). Work situation after breast cancer: Results from a population-based study. *Journal of the National Cancer Institute, 96,* 1813–1822.

McKinley, E.D. (2000). Under toad days: Surviving the uncertainty of cancer recurrence. *Annals of Internal Medicine, 133,* 479–480.

Mellette, S.J. (1993). Cancer rehabilitation. *Journal of the National Cancer Institute, 85,* 781–784.

Mellon, S. (2002). Comparisons between cancer survivors and family members on meaning of the illness and family quality of life. *Oncology Nursing Forum, 29,* 1117–1125.

Mellon, S., & Northouse, L.L. (2001). Family survivorship and quality of life following a cancer diagnosis. *Research in Nursing and Health, 24,* 446–459.

Metayer, C., Lynch, C.F., Clarke, E.A., Glimelius, B., Storm, H., Pukkala, E., et al. (2000). Second cancers among long-term survivors of Hodgkin's disease diagnosed in childhood and adolescence. *Journal of Clinical Oncology, 18,* 2435–2443.

Meyerhardt, J.A., & Mayer, R.J. (2003). Follow-up strategies after curative resection of colorectal cancer. *Seminars in Oncology, 30,* 349–360.

Meyers, C.A., Geara, F., Wong, P.F., & Morrison, W.H. (2000). Neurocognitive effects of therapeutic irradiation for base of skull tumors. *International Journal of Radiation Oncology, Biology, Physics, 46,* 51–55.

Mishel, M.H. (1997). Uncertainty in illness. *Annual Review of Nursing Research, 15,* 57–80.

Moore, H.C., & Foster, R.S. (2000). Breast cancer and pregnancy. *Seminars in Oncology, 27,* 646–653.

Moore, S., Corner, J., Haviland, J., Wells, M., Salmon, E., Normand, C., et al. (2002). Nurse-led follow up and conventional medical follow up in the management of patients with lung cancer: A randomized trial. *BMJ, 325,* 1145–1151.

Moulton, G. (2000). Cancer survivor issues are all in the family. *Journal of the National Cancer Institute, 92,* 101–103.

Mullan, F. (1983). *Vital signs: A young doctor's struggle with cancer.* New York: Laurel Books.

Mullan, F. (1984). Re-entry: The educational needs of the cancer survivor. *Health Education Quarterly, 10*(Suppl.), 88–94.

Mullan, F. (1985). Seasons of survival: Reflections of a physician with cancer. *New England Journal of Medicine, 313,* 270–273.

Mullan, F. (1996). Survivorship: A powerful place. In B. Hoffman (Ed.), *A cancer survivor's almanac: Charting your journey* (pp. XV–XIX). Minneapolis, MN: Chronimed.

Mykletun, A., Dahl, A.A., Haaland, C.F., Bremnes, R., Dahl, O., Klepp, O., et al. (2005). Side effects and cancer-related stress determine quality of life in long-term survivors of testicular cancer. *Journal of Clinical Oncology, 23,* 3061–3068.

National Coalition for Cancer Survivorship. (2004). *Glossary.* Retrieved February 16, 2005, from http://www.canceradvocacy.org/resources/glossary.aspx

Nelson, J.P. (1996). Struggling to gain meaning: Living with the uncertainty of breast cancer. *Advances in Nursing Science, 18*(3), 59–76.

Nuver, J., Smit, A.J., Postma, A., Sleijfer, D.T., & Gietema, J.A. (2002). The metabolic syndrome in long-term survivors, an important target for secondary preventive measures. *Cancer Treatment Reviews, 28,* 195–214.

Nyandoto, P., Muhonen, T., & Joensuu, H. (1998). Second cancer among long-term survivors from Hodgkin's disease. *International Journal of Radiation Oncology, Biology, Physics, 42,* 373–378.

O'Connor, A.P., & Wicker, C.A. (1995). Clinical commentary: Promoting meaning in the lives of cancer survivors. *Seminars in Oncology Nursing, 11,* 68–72.

Oeffinger, K.C., Mertens, A.C., Hudson, M.M., Gurney, J.G., Casillas, J., Chen, H., et al. (2004). Health care of young adult survivors of childhood cancer: A report from the Childhood Cancer Survivor Study. *Annals of Family Medicine, 2,* 61–70.

O'Shaughnessy, J. (2003). Chemotherapy-related cognitive dysfunction in breast cancer. *Seminars in Oncology Nursing, 19*(4 Suppl. 2), 17–24.

Partridge, A.H., Winer, E.P., & Burstein, H.J. (2003). Follow-up care of breast cancer survivors. *Seminars in Oncology, 30,* 817–825.

Patel, S.R., Zagars, G.K., & Pisters, P.W. (2003). The follow-up of adult soft-tissue sarcomas. *Seminars in Oncology, 30,* 413–416.

Pedro, L.W. (2001). Quality of life for long-term survivors of cancer: Influencing variables. *Cancer Nursing, 24,* 1–11.

Petrek, J.A. (1994). Pregnancy safety after breast cancer. *Cancer, 74,* 528–531.

Pfister, D.G., Benson, A.B., & Somerfield, M.R. (2004). Surveillance strategies after curative treatment of colorectal cancer. *New England Journal of Medicine, 350,* 2375–2382.

Pinto, B.M., Eakin, E., & Maruyama, N.C. (2000). Health behavior changes after a cancer diagnosis: What do we know and where do we go from here? *Annals of Behavioral Medicine, 22,* 38–52.

Pinto, B.M., & Maruyama, N.C. (1999). Exercise in the rehabilitation of breast cancer survivors. *Psycho-Oncology, 8,* 191–206.

Pinto, B.M., & Trunzo, J.J. (2004). Body esteem and mood among sedentary and active breast cancer survivors. *Mayo Clinic Proceedings, 79,* 181–186.

Poletti, R. (1985). Living a full life with cancer. In F.J. Cleton, A.T. van Oosterom, & H.M. Pinedo (Eds.), *Clinical oncology and cancer nursing: Proceedings of the second European Conference on Clinical Oncology and Cancer Nursing, held in Amsterdam, 2–5 November 1983.* New York: Pergamon Press.

Powel, L., & McFadden, M.E. (1995). Repercussions of cancer treatment: Long-term physiological and psychological sequelae. *Quality of Life—A Nursing Challenge, 4*(2), 33–39.

President's Cancer Panel. (2004). *Living beyond cancer: Finding a new balance.* Bethesda, MD: U.S. Department of Health and Human Services, National Institutes of Health, National Cancer Institute.

Puscheck, E., Philip, P.A., & Jeyendran, R.S. (2004). Male fertility preservation and cancer treatment. *Cancer Treatment Reviews, 30,* 173–180.

Rauch, P., Miny, J., Conroy, T., Neyton, L., & Guillemin, F. (2004). Quality of life among disease-free survivors of rectal cancer. *Journal of Clinical Oncology, 22,* 354–360.

Rawnsley, M.M. (1994). Recurrence of cancer: A crisis of courage. *Cancer Nursing, 17,* 342–347.

Redaelli, A., Stephens, J.M., Brandt, S., Botteman, M.F., & Pashos, C.L. (2004). Short- and long-term effects of acute myeloid leukemia on patient health-related quality of life. *Cancer Treatment Reviews, 30,* 103–117.

Ross, L., Johansen, C., Dalton, S.O., Mellemkjaer, L., Thomassen, L.H., Mortensen, P.B., et al. (2003). Psychiatric hospitalizations among survivors of cancer in childhood or adolescence. *New England Journal of Medicine, 349,* 650–657.

Rowland, J.H., Aziz, N., Tesauro, G., & Feuer, E.J. (2001). The changing face of survivorship. *Seminars in Oncology Nursing, 17,* 236–240.

Rudberg, L., Nilsson, S., & Wikblad, K. (2000). Health-related quality of life in survivors of testicular cancer 3 to 13 years after treatment. *Journal of Psychosocial Oncology, 18*(3), 19–31.

Ruffer, J.U., Flechtner, H., Tralls, P., Josting, A., Sieber, M., Lathan, B., et al. (2003). Fatigue in long-term survivors of Hodgkin's lymphoma: A report from the German Hodgkin Lymphoma Study Group (GHSG). *European Journal of Cancer, 39,* 2179–2186.

Rugo, H., & Ahles, T. (2003). The impact of adjuvant therapy for breast cancer on cognitive function: Current evidence and directions for research. *Seminars in Oncology, 30,* 749–762.

Saleeba, A.K., Weitzner, M.A., & Meyers, C.A. (1996). Subclinical psychological distress in long-term survivors of breast cancer: A preliminary communication. *Journal of Psychosocial Oncology, 14*(1), 83–93.

Salminen, E., Portin, R., Korpela, J., Backman, H., Parvinen, L.M., Helenius, H., et al. (2003). Androgen deprivation and cognition in prostate cancer. *British Journal of Cancer, 89,* 971–976.

Sammarco, A. (2001). Psychological stages and quality of life of women with breast cancer. *Cancer Nursing, 24,* 272–277.

Sapp, A.L., Trentham-Dietz, A., Newcomb, P.A., Hampton, J.M., Moinpour, C.M., & Remington, P.L. (2003). Social networks and quality of life among female long-term colorectal survivors. *Cancer, 98,* 1749–1758.

Schagen, S.B., Hamburger, H.L., Muller, M.J., Boogerd, W., & van Dam, F.S. (2001). Neuropsychological evaluation of late effects of adjuvant high-dose chemotherapy on cognitive function. *Journal of Neuro-Oncology, 51,* 159–165.

Schimmer, A.D., Elliott, M.E., Abbey, S.E., Raiz, L., Keating, A., Bearlands, H.J., et al. (2001). Illness intrusiveness among survivors of autologous blood and marrow transplantation. *Cancer, 92,* 3147–3154.

Schmale, A.H., Morrow, G.R., Schmitt, M.H., Adler, L.M., Enelow, A., Murawski, B.J., et al. (1983). Well-being of cancer survivors. *Psychosomatic Medicine, 45,* 163–169.

Schover, L.R. (2004). Myth-busters: Telling the true story of breast cancer survivorship [Editorial]. *Journal of the National Cancer Institute, 96,* 1800–1801.

Schroevers, M.J., Ranchor, A.V., & Sanderman, R. (2004). The role of age at the onset of cancer in relation to survivors' long-term adjustment: A controlled comparison over an eight-year period. *Psycho-Oncology, 13,* 740–752.

Schultz, P.N., Beck, M.L., Stava, C., & Sellin, R.V. (2002). Cancer survivors: Work-related issues. *Journal of the American Association of Occupational Health Nurses, 50,* 220–226.

Schultz, P.N., Stava, C., Beck, M.L., & Vassilopoulou-Sellin, R. (2004). Ethnic/racial influences on the physical health of cancer survivors. *Cancer, 100,* 156–164.

Shanfield, S.B. (1980). On surviving cancer: Psychological considerations. *Comprehensive Psychiatry, 21,* 128–134.

Sharp, J.W. (1999). The Internet: Changing the way cancer survivors obtain information. *Cancer Practice, 7,* 266–269.

Shusterman, S., & Meadows, A.T. (2000). Long term survivors of childhood leukemia. *Current Opinion in Hematology, 7,* 217–222.

Smith, T.J. (2003). Evidence-based follow-up of lung cancer patients. *Seminars in Oncology, 30,* 361–368.

Spelten, E.R., Sprangers, M.A., & Verbeek, J.H. (2002). Factors reported to influence the return to work of cancer survivors: A literature review. *Psycho-Oncology, 11,* 124–131.

Spijker, A., Trijsburg, R.W., & Duivenvoorden, H.J. (1997). Psychological sequelae of cancer diagnosis: A meta-analysis review of 58 studies after 1980. *Psychosomatic Medicine, 59,* 280–293.

Stat Bite. (1993). Workplace attitudes toward cancer patients. *Journal of the National Cancer Institute, 85,* 771.

Stat Bite. (2004). Number of cancer survivors by sex and years since diagnosis. *Journal of the National Cancer Institute, 96,* 1414.

Stevens, M.C., Mahler, H., & Parkes, S. (1998). The health status of adult survivors of cancer in childhood. *European Journal of Cancer, 34,* 694–698.

Surbone, A., & Petrek, J.A. (1997). Childbearing issues in breast cancer survivors. *Cancer, 79,* 1271–1278.

Svobodnik, A., Yang, P., Novotny, P.J., Bass, E., Garces, Y.I., Jett, J.R., et al. (2004). Quality of life in 650 lung cancer survivors 6 months to 4 years after diagnosis. *Mayo Clinic Proceedings, 79,* 1024–1030.

Syrjala, K.L., Langer, S.L., Abrams, J.R., Storer, B., Sanders, J.E., Flowers, M.E., et al. (2004). Recovery and long-term function after hematopoietic cell transplantation for leukemia or lymphoma. *JAMA, 291,* 2335–2343.

Tannock, I.F., Ahles, T.A., Ganz, P.A., & van Dam, F.S. (2004). Cognitive impairment associated with chemotherapy for cancer: Report of a workshop. *Journal of Clinical Oncology, 22,* 2233–2239.

Tesauro, G.M., Rowland, J.H., & Lustig, C. (2002). Survivorship resources for post-treatment cancer survivors. *Cancer Practice, 10,* 277–283.

Theodoulou, M., & Seidman, A.D. (2003). Cardiac effects of adjuvant therapy for early breast cancer. *Seminars in Oncology, 30,* 730–739.

Tomich, P.L., & Helgeson, V.S. (2002). Five years later: A cross-sectional comparison of breast cancer survivors with healthy women. *Psycho-Oncology, 11,* 154–169.

Trillin, A.S. (1981). Of dragons and garden peas: A cancer patient talks to doctors. *New England Journal of Medicine, 304,* 699–701.

Turner, J., Zapart, S., Pedersen, K., Rankin, N., Luxford, K., & Fletcher, J. (2005). Clinical practice guidelines for the psychosocial care of adults with cancer. *Psycho-Oncology, 14,* 159–173.

Utley, R. (1999). The evolving meaning of cancer for long-term survivors of breast cancer. *Oncology Nursing Forum, 26,* 1519–1523.

Vachon, M.L. (2001). The meaning of illness to a long-term survivor. *Seminars in Oncology Nursing, 17,* 279–283.

Vaidya, A.P., & Curtin, J.P. (2003). The follow-up of ovarian cancer. *Seminars in Oncology, 30,* 401–412.

Varni, J.W., Katz, E.R., Colegrove, R., & Dolgin, M. (1994). Perceived stress and adjustment of long-term survivors of childhood cancer. *Journal of Psychosocial Oncology, 12*(3), 1–16.

Vaughn, D.J., Gignac, G.A., & Meadows, A.T. (2002). Long-term medical care of testicular cancer survivors. *Annals of Internal Medicine, 136,* 463–470.

Veronesi, U., & Martino, G. (1978). Can life be the same after cancer treatment? *Tumori, 64,* 345–351.

Vickberg, S.M. (2001). Fears about breast cancer recurrence. *Cancer Practice, 9,* 237–243.

Vickberg, S.M., Duhamel, K.N., Smith, M.Y., Manne, S.L., Winkel, G., Papadopoulos, E.B., et al. (2001). Global meaning and psychological adjustment among survivors of bone marrow transplant. *Psycho-Oncology, 10,* 29–39.

Wallace, M. (2003). Uncertainty and quality of life of older men who undergo watchful waiting for prostate cancer. *Oncology Nursing Forum, 30,* 303–309.

Ward, S.E., Viergutz, G., Tormey, D., DeMuth, J., & Paulen, A. (1992). Patients' reactions to completion of adjuvant breast cancer therapy. *Nursing Research, 41,* 362–366.

Watson, P.G. (1992). Cancer rehabilitation: An overview. *Seminars in Oncology Nursing, 8,* 167–173.

Weekes, D.P., & Kagan, S.H. (1994). Adolescents completing cancer therapy: Meaning, perception, and coping. *Oncology Nursing Forum, 21,* 663–670.

Wefel, J.S., Lenzi, R., Theriault, R., Buzdar, A.U., Cruickshank, S., & Meyers, C.A. (2004). 'Chemobrain' in breast carcinoma?: A prologue. *Cancer, 101,* 466–475.

Wefel, J.S., Lenzi, R., Theriault, R.L., Davis, R.N., & Meyers, C.A. (2004). The cognitive sequelae of standard-dose adjuvant chemotherapy in women with breast carcinoma. *Cancer, 100,* 2292–2299.

Weigers, M.E., Chesler, M.A., Zebrack, B.J., & Goldman, S. (1998). Self-reported worries among long-term survivors of childhood cancers and their peers. *Journal of Psychosocial Oncology, 16*(2), 1–23.

Welch-McCaffrey, D. (1984). Oncology nurses as cancer patients: An investigative questionnaire. *Oncology Nursing Forum, 11*(2), 48–50.

Welch-McCaffrey, D., Hoffman, B., Leigh, S.A., Loescher, L.J., & Meyskens, F.L. (1989). Surviving adult cancers. Part 2: Psychosocial implications. *Annals of Internal Medicine, 111,* 517–524.

Wells, R.J. (1990). Rehabilitation: Making the most of time. *Oncology Nursing Forum, 17,* 503–507.

Wenzel, L.B., Donnelly, J.P., Fowler, J.M., Habbal, R., Taylor, T.H., Aziz, N., et al. (2002). Resilience, reflection and residual stress in ovarian cancer survivorship: A Gynecologic Oncology Study Group study. *Psycho-Oncology, 11,* 142–153.

Wilmoth, M.C. (2001). The aftermath of breast cancer: An altered sexual self. *Cancer Nursing, 24,* 278–286.

Woods, N.F., & Earp, J.L. (1978). Women with cured breast cancer: A study of mastectomy patients in North Carolina. *Nursing Research, 27,* 279–285.

Wooldridge, J.E., & Link, B.K. (2003). Post-treatment surveillance of patients with lymphoma treated with curative intent. *Seminars in Oncology, 30,* 375–381.

Wyatt, G., Kurtz, M.E., & Liken, M. (1993). Breast cancer survivors: An exploration of quality of life issues. *Cancer Nursing, 16,* 440–448.

Yabroff, K.R., Lawrence, W.F., Clauser, S., Davis, W.W., & Brown, M.L. (2004). Burden of illness in cancer survivors: Findings from a population-based national sample. *Journal of the National Cancer Institute, 96,* 1322–1330.

Yao, S., & DiPaola, R.S. (2003). An evidence-based approach to prostate cancer follow-up. *Seminars in Oncology, 30,* 390–400.

Yeazel, M.W., Oeffinger, K.C., Gurney, J.G., Mertens, A.C., Hudson, M.M., Emmons, K.M., et al. (2003). The cancer screening practices of adult survivors of childhood cancer. *Cancer, 100,* 631–640.

Yehuda, R. (2002). Post-traumatic stress disorder. *New England Journal of Medicine, 346*, 108–114.

Zebrack, B.J., Casillas, J., Nohr, L., Adams, H., & Zeltzer, L.K. (2004). Fertility issues for young adult survivors of childhood cancer. *Psycho-Oncology, 13*, 689–699.

Zebrack, B.J., Eshelman, D.A., Hudson, M.M., Mertens, A.C., Cotter, K.L., Foster, B.M., et al. (2004). Health care for childhood cancer survivors. *Cancer, 100*, 843–850.

Zebrack, B.J., Zeltzer, L.K., Whitton, J., Mertens, A.C., Odom, L., Berkow, R., et al. (2002). Psychological outcomes in long-term survivors of childhood leukemia, Hodgkin's disease and non-Hodgkin's lymphoma: A report from the Childhood Cancer Survivor Study. *Pediatrics, 110*, 42–52.

SECTION II

Influences on the Psychosocial Experience

CHAPTER 3

Life's Meaning and Cancer

ROSE MARY CARROLL-JOHNSON, RN, MN

> *In spite of the illness, in spite of the archenemy sorrow, one can remain alive long past the usual date of disintegration if one is unafraid of change, insatiable in intellectual curiosity, interested in big things, and happy in small ways.*
>
> —Edith Wharton

Meaning evolves from the reality of one's life as perceived by one's mind and experienced by one's heart (Fife & Taylor, 1995). Hearing the news that one has cancer initially jolts a person's reality and stirs up thoughts of "What is happening to me? Why me?" Unexpected and negative life changes such as a cancer diagnosis precipitate a process of trying to make sense of the event and of attempting to integrate it into one's life. The process has been described as a search for meaning. The search for meaning is one's attempt to respond to questions such as "What is the significance of the event?" and "What does my life mean now?" (Taylor, 1983). As the treatment phase of an illness comes to a close, many patients find themselves dealing with thoughts such as "How do I get on with my life?"

The Concept of Meaning

"Meaning" as a concept is not easily explained; it frequently is embedded in one's private thoughts and, consequently, is difficult to discuss. It is a multidimensional concept with a variety of interpretations derived from fields of thought and inquiry, including psychology, philosophy, and spirituality. The search for meaning involves integrating an individual experience into the more cosmic view of human life as it fits into each idiosyncratic pattern. Frankl (1986) called it "the will to meaning" and saw it as a primary motivational force in humans. From these descriptions, one can ascertain that meaning is a multidimensional concept.

The Meaning of Illness

A classic article about suffering by Cassell (1982) demonstrated how meaning relates to illness. He described meaning as a fundamental dimension of person-hood and said that assigning meaning to illness is a way to ameliorate the suffering associated with it. The personal meaning of illness includes dimensions of intellect, emotion, body, and spirit. Others have conceived that the meaning one gives to an event such as a cancer diagnosis is an important part of the process of adaptation. Experiencing meaning is a positive occurrence that offers fulfillment in life and, when illness occurs, an opportunity to cope with the illness more effectively (Richer & Ezer, 2000).

Searching for Meaning in Illness

Many of the major tasks confronting a person with cancer are similar to those that concern patients with any serious chronic illness. After the initial shock of diagnosis, one attempts to understand the personal significance of the cancer diagnosis. One then needs some way to acknowledge the reality of the illness and find a framework that integrates personal events related to the illness into one's life in a purposeful way. This integration may involve the reworking and redefining of past meaning while looking for meaning in the current situation (O'Connor, Wicker, & Germino, 1990). Richer and Ezer's (2000) concept analysis of belief and meaning embedded in the cancer experience identified two types of meaning emerging from the literature: existential meaning (related to the individual's place in the world) and situation meaning (involving the way in which a person evaluates specific negative events).

Existential meaning probably is best exemplified by the groundbreaking work of Frankl (1963, 1986), who viewed the search for meaning as a primary force initiated by suffering. Armen and Rehnsfeldt (2003) addressed the role of suffering in their work with women with breast cancer. They identified a process by which the suffering evolves as individuals come to terms with the changes in their lives and their goals.

The search for meaning—a search that is unique and specific to each person—can result in self-transcendence, a component of the search for meaning. Self-transcendence is the ability to extend oneself beyond one's personal circumstance and take on broader life perspectives, activities, and purposes (Coward, 1990). It is an experience of meaning on a different plane that brings a person in touch with something greater than the here and now.

Degner, Hack, O'Neil, and Kristjanson (2003) have explored specific meanings of a cancer diagnosis based on the early work of Lipowski (1970). Lipowski identified eight categories of meaning of illness: challenge, enemy, punishment, weakness, relief, strategy, irreparable loss, and value. Degner et al. found that women with breast cancer who ascribed more positive meanings (e.g., challenge, value) had better psychological adjustment than those who had more negative meanings (e.g., enemy, loss, punishment). Those in the latter category experienced higher levels of depression and anxiety and poorer quality of life.

The Meaning of Illness as It Relates to Coping

The meaning that a person ascribes to an illness can have a profound impact on how that person copes. Meaning becomes truly significant in dealing with the disruption that illness imposes on everyday life and in finding the means to endure the stresses one encounters. As noted previously, Degner et al. (2003) found that women who ascribed positive meaning to breast cancer had less trait anxiety and depression and reported better emotional functioning and quality of life than women who gave their illness a negative meaning. Constructing meaning involves encouraging individuals to reorganize central aspects of their personal world, their identity, and their social world. According to Fife (1994), a person copes with illness using options to reformulate one's identity and one's hope for the future. For Vachon (2001), this is a process of survivorship, a component of becoming a survivor.

A person's self-identity is altered continually during a cancer experience. From the moment of hearing the word "cancer" at the time of diagnosis, through treatments that may change how one looks and feels, and on into recovery, a person continues to strive to feel normal again. Frank (1991), a sociologist who was diagnosed with and treated for a seminoma, noted that one "wears" cancer while enduring the physical changes of hair loss and an IV line during treatment. He was referring not only to a change in his appearance but also to a defect in his identity that he related to the stigma of cancer.

Vachon (2001), herself a cancer survivor and a nurse psychotherapist, noted that a diagnosis of cancer elicits the need to understand the meaning of the cancer to one's life followed by a process of finding a place for it in one's life. Utley (1999) found that the women in her study felt changed by the cancer experience and more appreciative of life and those in their lives. They went from an outsider perspective of cancer as sickness and death to a first-person sense of the reality of the experience. These women came away feeling that the cancer had transformed their lives for the better in many ways.

The Meaning of Illness as It Relates to Spirituality

Spirituality has been linked to the quest for meaning and purpose in life. The association between spirituality and searching for the meaning of an illness is evident when one considers the highly personal nature of the experience. When facing a life-threatening condition, people turn to inner resources such as faith, religion, and God for support.

A study of newly diagnosed patients with cancer showed that faith assisted individuals in their search for the meaning of their illness (O'Connor et al., 1990). The link between a spiritual experience and meaning is apparent in the words of a hospice patient and family members who described "experiences of the whole person that brought them in touch with something that they consider greater than or outside of themselves" (Steeves & Kahn, 1987, p. 115). Ferrell, Smith, Juarez, and Melancon (2003) also uncovered this connection between spirituality and meaning in women with ovarian cancer.

Albaugh (2003) explored this subject in a phenomenologic study of spirituality in patients with a variety of cancers. His subjects described the role of their spiritual beliefs in dealing with the diagnosis of cancer as being intrinsic. Their spirituality imparted a sense of meaning and comforted and strengthened them. They came to see the diagnosis as a "wake-up call" to clarify what was really important in life. Similar to the women patients in Utley's (1999) study, the diagnosis brought these patients to an appreciation of time with loved ones and time spent "living." Spiritual beliefs can provide the context for making some sense of a life-altering event such as a cancer diagnosis. See Chapter 7 for an expanded discussion of these concepts.

Cultural Influences on Meaning

Finding meaning in an illness is influenced by one's cultural heritage because different cultures view illness differently. The beliefs, values, customs, and patterns of behavior within a group provide direction for how a person responds to events in his or her life. Because cancer is viewed as life-threatening and is associated with prolonged and intense treatments, caregivers must take into account how these aspects of illness are perceived in the patient's culture. The force of cultural influences bears strongly on an individual's and the family's responses to a cancer diagnosis. The interpretations and attributions of the group to a cancer illness provide caregivers with a basis for understanding patient and family responses to illness-associated experiences. Richer and Ezer's (2000) concept analysis of meaning in the experience of cancer identified personal beliefs and situation and existential meaning as separate and important contributors to the concept. Culture shapes personal beliefs and supports existential meaning. The importance of a sense of spirituality to this process of determining meaning is not only real but may be more influential depending on race or culture. Healthcare providers must be open to and assess this influence.

Family Influences on Meaning

Family members are affected profoundly by and have a significant impact on the meaning of illness. In a study of newly diagnosed patients with cancer, O'Connor and Wicker (1989) found that social support from family members assisted individuals in their search for meaning. Subjects described the value of family closeness and of the love and care of family members. Family members themselves must integrate the changes brought on by the illness and, in doing so, discover what the illness means to them. A study examining the meaning of cancer for partners of newly diagnosed patients noted that their responses included feelings of uncertainty and change in relationships, a future without the partner, and a future of uncertainty (Germino, Fife, & Funk, 1995). Nursing efforts to address these family concerns can have a direct effect on patients' reactions.

Nursing Implications

Although nurses often may not address topics such as spirituality and meaning, it is important nonetheless to assess these aspects of patient coping and adjustment, to assist the patient to determine some of these elements, and then to support, if possible, the patient's search for understanding.

Assessment can begin with a few simple, straightforward questions. Determining answers to these questions may be the first steps in the patient's efforts to understanding (Richer & Ezer, 2000). Questions can be as simple as

- What does the word "cancer" bring to your mind?
- What do you think caused your cancer?
- What effect do these ideas have on your ability to deal with your diagnosis?
- How will these ideas influence your everyday life?

Asking these questions legitimizes their importance and lets patients know it is permissible to talk about these concerns.

Interventions can consist of usual techniques, such as patient education about general topics, or specific symptom concerns and advice regarding day-to-day functioning (Richer & Ezer, 2000). In addition, nurses should make a specific effort to create trusting relationships with patients to facilitate more in-depth discussions regarding meaning and coping (Richer & Ezer). Patients who express negative meanings (e.g., punishment) may need additional psychosocial intervention, particularly at crisis points in the course of the disease (Degner et al., 2003; Utley, 1999).

Creative work is another avenue to self-transcendence through which one may discover meaning in life (Frankl, 1986). Creative work includes reaching out to others who are in a similar situation. It can be one of the most meaningful aspects of life. A way of relating to others is through storytelling. At a time when storytelling continues to be emphasized and the lay literature abounds with personal accounts of people's experiences with illness, this represents a way of reaching out to a person who may be in a similar situation (Frank, 1995). Storytelling also helps a person to make sense of an illness experience. People tell their stories not just to work out their changing lives but also to guide others who will follow them. Stories are a way of finding new destinations. They are an opportunity to validate the experience of reconstructing one's life schemes. In addition, reciprocity exists in the use of storytelling—the storyteller offers himself or herself as a guide to the other's self-formation while the receiver of the guidance recognizes and values the storyteller.

Conclusion

The concept of meaning of illness is multidimensional, spanning the physical, social, psychological, cultural, and spiritual aspects of life experience. It is a continuing process of interweaving the present with the past and the future, with the hope of adding value and understanding to one's present life circumstance of illness. This search for meaning in the context of illness can lead to a transformation that allows the patient to transcend the suffering and ultimately cope better with the diagnosis and course of the illness. Healthcare professionals can be instrumental in facilitating exploration of these issues or in helping the patient to seek ways to find answers to the existential and situational dilemmas that a diagnosis of cancer inevitably creates. Albaugh (2003) added that by helping patients on this journey, nurses learn valuable life lessons in return.

Special thanks to Anne P. O'Connor, RN, MSN, AOCN®, who served as the author of this chapter in the first edition.

References

Albaugh, J. (2003). Spirituality and life-threatening illness: A phenomenologic study. *Oncology Nursing Forum, 30,* 593–598.

Armen, M., & Rehnsfeldt, A. (2003). The hidden suffering among breast cancer patients: A qualitative metasynthesis. *Qualitative Health Research, 13,* 510–527.

Cassell, E.J. (1982). The nature of suffering and the goals of medicine. *New England Journal of Medicine, 306,* 639–645.

Coward, D.D. (1990). The lived experience of self-transcendence in women with advanced breast cancer. *Nursing Science Quarterly, 3,* 162–169.

Degner, L., Hack, T., O'Neil, J., & Kristjanson, L. (2003). A new approach to eliciting meaning in the context of breast cancer. *Cancer Nursing, 26,* 169–178.

Ferrell, B.R., Smith, S.L., Juarez, G., & Melancon, C. (2003). Meaning of illness and spirituality in ovarian cancer survivors. *Oncology Nursing Forum, 30,* 249–257.

Fife, B.L. (1994). The conceptualization of meaning in illness. *Social Science and Medicine, 38,* 309–314.

Fife, B.L., & Taylor, E.J. (1995). The experience of cancer and its meaning. *Seminars in Oncology Nursing, 11,* 1–2.

Frank, A.W. (1991). *At the will of the body: Reflections on illness.* Boston: Houghton Mifflin.

Frank, A.W. (1995). *The wounded storyteller.* Chicago: University of Chicago Press.

Frankl, V.E. (1963). *Man's search for meaning.* New York: Pocket Books.

Frankl, V.E. (1986). *The doctor and the soul: From psychotherapy to logotherapy* (3rd ed.). New York: Vintage.

Germino, B.B., Fife, B.L., & Funk, S.G. (1995). Cancer and the partner relationship: What is its meaning? *Seminars in Oncology Nursing, 11,* 43–50.

Lipowski, Z.J. (1970). Physical illness, the individual, and the coping processes. *Psychiatry in Medicine, 1,* 91–102.

O'Connor, A.P., & Wicker, C.A. (1989). *A framework for understanding the cancer patient's search for meaning.* Unpublished master's thesis, University of North Carolina, Chapel Hill.

O'Connor, A.P., Wicker, C.A., & Germino, B.B. (1990). Understanding the cancer patient's search for meaning. *Cancer Nursing, 13,* 167–175.

Richer, M.C., & Ezer, H. (2000). Understanding beliefs and meanings in the experience of cancer: A concept analysis. *Journal of Advanced Nursing, 32,* 1108–1115.

Steeves, R.H., & Kahn, D.L. (1987). Experience of meaning and suffering. *Image: The Journal of Nursing Scholarship, 19,* 114–116.

Taylor, S. (1983). Adjustment to threatening events: A theory of cognitive adaptation. *American Psychologist, 38,* 1161–1173.

Utley, R. (1999). The evolving meaning of cancer for long-term survivors of breast cancer. *Oncology Nursing Forum, 26,* 1519–1523.

Vachon, M. (2001). The meaning of illness to a long-term survivor. *Seminars in Oncology Nursing, 17,* 279–283.

CHAPTER 4

Coping and Adaptation

NANCY JO BUSH, RN, MN, MA, AOCN®

Every tear I ever cried,
turned to pearl before it died.
Every pain that in me burned,
turned to wisdom I had earned.

—Joan Walsh Anglund

Coping is an integral part of everyday life. As people deal with daily hassles in their environment, they cope on many different levels. Hassles are those mundane, everyday challenges that can be considered minor annoyances or serious pressures. Coping is the response that people employ in an attempt to adapt to these stressors (Kohn, 1996). Daily stressors may consist of work dissatisfaction, family dysfunction, time pressures, and various other demands. These mundane stressors can adversely affect health, and, if cumulative, they may have a negative impact on physical and psychological well-being exceeding that of major life-changing stressors (Kohn). Therefore, the continuum of coping can range from confronting the stresses of everyday life to facing a chronic, life-threatening illness such as cancer. The patient experiencing cancer is attempting to cope not only with the daily stressors of living but, at the same time, is trying to integrate and adapt to a life-threatening illness (Nail, 2001). Normal demands of everyday life, such as child care, family and job responsibilities, and financial pressures, will be exaggerated in a time of crisis. For example, if marital discontent already exists, a cancer diagnosis may put additional pressure on the relationship, exceeding the personal coping resources the couple has available (Lewis, 2004). Individuals and families confronting cancer experience many changes in their day-to-day lives, incorporating illness and treatment-related demands into daily routines that may already be overwhelmed with hassles and everyday stressors (Nail).

Coping responses are complex phenomena. Many variables affect the way in which people respond to stress. The situation or context of the stressor is one important variable, in addition to personality traits. When conceptualizing coping, *contextual approaches* look at coping as a dynamic process, changing over time as the individual confronts different stressful demands (Holahan, Moos, & Schaefer, 1996; Nail, 2001). The intensity of stress incurred when juggling career and home is different than when these daily demands are combined with chemotherapy treatments for cancer. The challenges a person faces at the diagnostic stage of cancer will be different from those faced during treatment or at end of life. Therefore, the context of the stress will influence the individual's and family's coping responses. In addition, the coping responses that people habitually apply are influenced by their personality characteristics and past experiences. Coping also has been conceptualized from a *dispositional approach,* taking into account the consistent manner by which individuals adapt when confronted with stress (Holahan et al.; Kohn, 1996; Nail). For example, if one is prone to anxiety, confronting a stressful situation will heighten this emotional response.

Characteristics of personality and coping develop over a lifetime as a person moves toward emotional maturity. Cancer can strike, often without warning, anywhere along the continuum of psychosocial development. Although the individual confronts cancer with a preset repertoire of coping skills, these skills may not be adequate for the specific situation, or the cancer experience may tax the individual's emotional resources. In addition, the cancer diagnosis may be the first life-threatening stressor that the individual and family have had to face, calling upon the need for reinforcement of past coping styles and the need to form new coping strategies that fit the demands of the situation. Coping is, therefore, a complex, changing process influenced by the situation (context), individual differences (personality traits), and previous experiences. There is no "right" or "wrong" way to cope (Nail, 2001).

> Every person brings unique characteristics to dealing with illness; a particular personality, a way of coping, a set of beliefs and values, and a way of looking at the world. The goal is to take these qualities into consideration and make sure that they work in favor of the person at each point along the cancer journey. (Holland & Lewis, 2000, p. 3)

Definitions of Coping

Historically, coping had been viewed as an unconscious defense in response to intrapsychic conflict. Recently, coping has been conceptualized as an active, conscious response to stress (Lazarus, 2000). Several specific definitions exist to describe the function of coping mechanisms. Coping has been defined as a stabilizing factor that promotes adaptive functioning during stressful periods (Holahan et al., 1996) and as "any effort to manage external or internal demands that are appraised as negative or challenging" (Maes, Leventhal, & de Ridder, 1996, p. 226). The construct of coping has been interchanged with concepts such as adaptation, mastery, resiliency, and adjustment (Henderson, Gore, Davis, & Condon, 2003). Coping is an adaptive response to stress; a person attempts to restore equilibrium in response to stressful life events such as cancer (Henderson et al.). Within the framework of a self-regulation model of coping, Spencer, Carver, and Price (1998) defined coping as those behaviors and cognitive activities aimed at responding to and overcoming adversity. Adaptation is the result of effective coping and is a state of equilibrium, reflecting the individual's return to life activities, goals, and social functioning. Ineffective coping is disengagement from, or the inability to return to, the normal activities of life (Spencer et al.).

Situational Coping

Coping efforts aim to reduce or eliminate the stressful conditions one is facing in an attempt to minimize the inherent emotional distress that one is experiencing. Thus, "coping strategies" are defined as those behavioral and cognitive efforts that are shaped by the context in which they are generated (Lazarus, 1993). Therefore, coping effectiveness is best evaluated within the context of the challenges faced by the individual and family. These context-driven or contextual definitions of coping are based on the stressors (e.g., cancer) and the situational factors (e.g., chemotherapy, radiation) that shape an individual's coping mechanisms. When coping is assessed in relation to a specific context, the assessments become problem-specific, and outcomes are measured in regard to specific stressors (e.g., confronting the cancer, dealing with treatment) (Somerfield & Curbow, 1992). Within this framework, evaluation of coping effectiveness can be based upon outcomes rather than coping strategies per se, and interventions to enhance coping can focus on a modifiable stressor (Nail, 2001).

Dispositional Coping

Coping also has been defined within the framework of an individual's personality or habitual way of responding to stress, in other words, his or her coping style. Dispositional approaches to defining coping behaviors are based on evaluating the individual's inherently stable person-based traits or resources that influence the coping mechanisms chosen when facing stress (Holahan et al., 1996). Personality variables, such as optimism and pessimism, attitude or "fighting spirit," and locus of control, have been identified as influencing the coping strategies one chooses when confronting stress (Somerfield & Curbow, 1992; Spencer et al., 1998; Wilkes, O'Baugh, Luke, & George, 2003). Families also have personalities or traits that influence coping. The family stress theory contends that the family is a social system; stress in one family member has a reverberating effect on each family member in the system (Friedman, Bowden, & Jones, 2003). Families develop basic and unique strengths to protect their members from adverse events. Family communication, problem solving, and interpersonal relationships influence how families cope and adapt to stressful life experiences (Friedman et al.; McCubbin & McCubbin, 1996).

Summary

Two distinct ways of conceptualizing coping emerge: either as a disposition or trait that becomes a mode or pattern of coping for the person and family or as a process that the person and family carry out in response to a specific stressful experience (Cohen & Lazarus, 1979; Holahan et al., 1996). Inherently, one influences the other. Coping outcomes are based upon individual experiences and coping traits, and coping is a process that changes over time (Nail, 2001), dependent upon the challenges being faced. Coping can be conceptualized within a framework of adaptation—a positive, adaptive resource of all human beings (Rowland, 1989a). When faced with stressful experiences, an individual and family evaluate the stressors as challenges to be mastered to bring about adaptation and equilibrium.

Coping and Adaptation

Defining coping within an adaptational framework challenges healthcare professionals to identify and promote effective coping strategies that strengthen physical and psychosocial adaptation (Rowland, 1989a). Mastery, the successful conclusion of adaptive efforts (White, 1974), becomes a major goal when coping is conceptualized as a positive, conscious attempt toward resolution and adaptation (Pearlin & Schooler, 1978; White). Adapting to a cancer diagnosis has been known to present greater challenges than other life-threatening and debilitating diseases because of the negative connotations that society has placed on the illness. Cancer is thought of as a synonym for death—the catastrophic "big C" (Nail, 2001; Neilson-Clayton & Brownlee, 2002). Therefore, applying stress and coping theories to the experience of cancer often is limited and daunting. Nail warned that clinical application based upon coping research is challenging because of the following limitations: the diversity and complexity of conceptual coping models, assumptions underlying coping research, and a lack of clear implications for evidence-based interventions. Lewis (2004) concurred in a review of family-focused oncology nursing research. As an example, coping behaviors that underlie stress and adaptation theory have not always proved to be predictive of how the family actually responds and adjusts to the experience of breast cancer (Lewis). Conceptual theories provide a framework for the assessment of coping with cancer, yet one must proceed with caution.

For oncology nurses, it is imperative to understand how coping has been defined within the broader realm of human experience, to recognize the limitations of research and application, and then to evaluate the patient's and family's coping efficacy based on outcomes rather than adherence to a specific set of coping theories or strategies (Nail, 2001). For many patients, the experience of cancer is a crisis with such demands that their past coping repertoire is not sufficient to support them. It is no longer sufficient to assess patients' past coping mechanisms or coping habits and expect this pattern to fit the new and often threatening challenges they face. Personality-based traits must be evaluated yet reinforced with social and psychological resources that fit the situation or crisis the individual confronts. This demands not only an assessment of the contextual component of coping but also application of a developmental approach to evaluate effective responses.

Many authors (Holland, 1989; Mages & Mendelsohn, 1979; Sales, 1991; Sales, Schulz, & Biegel, 1992) have conceptualized coping as a developmental process in which individuals and families respond to the different demands and tasks inherent in the various stages of cancer. Yet, the experience of living with and surviving cancer may not fit into clearly defined transition points such as diagnosis, treatment, recurrence, and palliation (Lethborg, Kissane, Burns, & Snyder, 2000). Cessation of active cancer treatment brings forth its own set of stressors

(Lethborg et al.), and coping responses in the prediagnosis phase is an area that has not been investigated (Nail, 2001). The important issue concerns the "pattern of distress" over the course of the cancer trajectory (Spencer et al., 1998). Disease-related variables, such as the type of cancer, treatment requirements, and prognosis, also are important determinants to how individuals and families cope. If coping is a process that changes over time, then coping effectiveness will vary depending on the different clinical stages of cancer and the different illness-related demands. For example, denial and avoidant coping may be effective during the early stages of cancer to temper the threat and prevent the individual from becoming overwhelmed with anxiety. Yet, this coping strategy is less effective or maladaptive if prolonged into later stages of the disease continuum (Somerfield & Curbow, 1992; Spencer et al.).

For many, the experience of cancer may be a crisis added to another life-changing event (e.g., a comorbid illness, the recent death of a family member). These additional circumstances may overwhelm the patient and family as a result of an accumulation of stressors combined with a depleted level of psychosocial coping resources. In contrast, success in coping effectively with previous life stressors likely may influence adaptation and subsequent coping with the next stressful life event (Spencer et al., 1998). The chronicity of cancer leaves patients and families at risk for long-term depletion of emotional, social, and financial resources. Family-focused research has indicated that family relationships may worsen with long-term survival, and without appropriate interventions, the family may wear out over time (Kornblith, 1998; Lewis, 2004). Yet, some individuals have described the experience of cancer as one that has added meaning and perspective to their lives (Taylor, 1995). Some may view the journey as a challenging but positive life-changing event (Schnoll, Knowles, & Harlow, 2002).

Being aware of the dispositional, contextual, and developmental mechanisms underlying coping strategies prevents professionals from defining effective or adaptive coping for patients. Instead, a knowledge base about coping variables assists professionals in helping patients to identify their own coping strengths and weaknesses and to identify and provide appropriate resources (Nail, 2001). Oncology nurses are in a pivotal position to assess, intervene, and help strengthen coping mechanisms and, if necessary, refer patients for psychological counseling. A major goal when intervening is to promote adaptation by ensuring that patients and families move along the cancer continuum with the education, compassion, and support needed to secure or reinforce their own coping abilities. Thus, by helping patients to gain mastery over the challenges of the cancer experience, nurses can be instrumental in guiding patients to create strategies that can promote effective coping and bring about adaptation to chronic illness.

Conceptual Framework for Coping Assessment

Coping Strategies

A classic and commonly cited model for coping is the stress-coping framework (Lazarus, 2000; Lazarus & Folkman, 1984). This model presents coping as a dynamic process of appraisal and response that changes over time as individuals interact and confront stressors in their environment (Somerfield & Curbow, 1992). The underlying principle of the Lazarus-Folkman model is that an individual's emotional or behavioral responses to stress are determined by how the person evaluates or appraises the stressor (Maes et al., 1996). Lazarus (1982) asserted that people apply cognitive activities (e.g., evaluative perceptions, inferences) to interpret stressful experiences and that these evaluations guide their adaptational interchange with the environment. Within this framework, three major functions of coping have been identified: appraisal-focused coping, problem-focused or instrumental coping, and emotion-focused or palliative coping (Maes et al.; Rowland, 1989a). Researchers additionally have recognized avoidance-focused coping as a function of withdrawing from a threat (Spencer et al., 1998). Positive emotions result if the person appraises the stressor as a challenge; negative emotions occur if the stressor is appraised as threatening (Maes et al.). Most often, the person confronting cancer experiences a roller coaster of positive and negative emotions depending on the circumstances (Wilkes et al., 2003). People with cancer often appraise situations as both threatening (potential for harm) and challenging (potential for mastery) at the same time (Nail, 2001). Therefore, a combination of coping strategies that are individualized and driven by the patient's appraisal of the stressors often is the most effective.

Appraisal-focused coping: The appraisal or evaluation of the stressful event is a major determinant of coping responses. Lazarus and Folkman (1984) identified two types of appraisal processes: primary appraisal and secondary appraisal. *Primary appraisal* addresses the personal meaning of the stressful event and whether the threat is interpreted as negative or challenging. Most often, illnesses such as cancer are appraised as stressful and threatening; the threats of harm and loss, such as loss in self-esteem, role function, and independence, are anticipatory fears of most patients confronting cancer (Barry, 2002a). The ultimate threat is the fear of dying or the fear of dying in pain (Nail, 2001). *Secondary appraisal* incorporates the person's evaluation of his or her capability to reduce the threat or damage caused by the stressor. A common question is, "What can I do about it?" (Barry, 2002a). For the patient with cancer the question is often, "How can I take control of the situation?" (Wilkes et al., 2003). The individual's past experiences (e.g., with cancer) and personality (e.g., coping style) will influence how he or she will appraise the stressor. Other personality variables, such as self-efficacy, influence the appraisal process. The role of self-efficacy, an individual's confidence in his or her ability to carry out appropriate behaviors and skills, has been shown not only to influence the appraisal of a stressor but also to improve coping skills (Devins & Binik, 1996).

Problem-focused coping: Once the stressful situation is appraised, the patient directs problem-focused coping at the external event (e.g., cancer, chemotherapy). To problem solve, the person attempts to change the stressful situation by changing either his or her actions or the environment (Maes et al., 1996). Problem-focused coping is action oriented, and the goal is to solve the problem at hand. Two methods of problem-focused coping are information seeking and direct action. *Information seeking* serves as a basis for action (e.g., problem solving) by providing the knowledge necessary for a coping decision or for reappraisal of the threat. A cancer diagnosis is extremely threatening, but if the individual gains knowledge regarding the actual stage, treatment, and prognosis of the cancer, this information can be applied to the person's emotional reactions (e.g., dispelling the myths and fears with concrete information). Patients and families differ in the timing, type, and amount of information needed to support their coping efforts. Research has found that different *informational coping styles* exist (Nikoletti, Kristjanson, Tataryn, McPhee, & Burt, 2003). For example, much of the information imparted to patients at diagnosis is standard, disease-related content, is impersonal, and is given at a time when patients and families feel overwhelmed with anxiety and fear (Delbar & Benor, 2001). Information supports effective problem solving when it is tailored to the individual patient and family based upon their past history, life experiences, emotional needs, and education (Delbar & Benor; Nail, 2001; Nikoletti et al.). Disparity between the amount of information given and the individual's coping style can lead to increased distress (Nikoletti et al.).

Direct action includes any actions the person carries out, excluding cognitive means, to minimize the threat or danger of the stressor. The patient experiencing a breast lump may take direct action by obtaining a mammogram and following through with a breast biopsy. Taking direct action to confront the stressor gives patients confidence in their ability to control the situation, based upon knowing "what to expect" and "what to do if" (Delbar & Benor, 2001). Inherent in problem-solving coping is patients' and families' need to feel empowered and in control of the challenge at hand. Patients' taking control has been linked to having a positive attitude when fighting cancer (Wilkes et al., 2003). Understanding the concept of control is essential to support coping, but the individual's feeling of control will be personal and situational (Nail, 2001). For example, a patient who has a trusting relationship with his or her physician may seek his or her advice and allow the physician to make the treatment decision while the patient still maintains a sense of control (Nail). Overall, patients and families have reported that learning to control symptoms, reduce pain and discomfort, and improve quality of life creates a sense of control that enables them to believe in their ability to cope (Delbar & Benor; Redinbaugh, Baum, Tarbell, & Arnold, 2003). Supporting problem-focused strategies can help patients and families to feel in control and prevent them from feeling helpless or powerless, but resources must be made available to supplement their coping abilities.

Emotion-focused coping: Maintaining emotional equilibrium is another function of coping. Emotion-focused coping relies on *intrapsychic processes*, the varied cognitive processes that influence emotional responses (e.g., feelings, concerns, worries regarding the cancer) (Maes et al., 1996). To regulate emotional distress, the person attempts to manage the subjective and somatic components of stress-related emotions. In contrast to problem-focused and active coping, emotion-focused coping is viewed as passive or palliative coping. This does not imply that emotion-focused coping is negative or maladaptive. Emotional expression, such as crying, is a palliative coping measure that appropriately can serve the goal of regaining emotional balance. Expressing feelings such as anger and fear is important for healing, and studies have found diversions such as humor to be positive coping tactics (Johnson, 2002; Lethborg et al., 2000; Spencer et al., 1998). Emotion-focused coping encompasses defense mechanisms, such as denial, that a person may apply to seek emotional insulation from the threat. A newly diagnosed patient with cancer can become overwhelmed with fear and anxiety. Denial early in the cancer experience is a common protective mechanism that allows the patient time to integrate emotionally what is happening to him or her. This defense can be adaptive in the short run, but avoidance coping must be evaluated based upon the situation being confronted. For example, if a patient with cancer states that he or she is avoiding thinking about the disease in order to move forward, the nurse must determine whether this is denial or avoidant coping (Spencer et al.).

Avoidance-focused coping: Researchers have identified this method of coping as the person's attempt to disengage mentally or even physically from the threatening situation (Kohn, 1996; Spencer et al., 1998). Avoidance coping is the *inhibition of action* that may hamper coping effectiveness. The fear of cancer or fearing "the worst" may cause an individual to delay seeking medical advice. For patients with cancer, prolonging a diagnosis or refusing necessary treatment out of fear are inherently risky behaviors. Conceptually, avoidance-focused coping and denial are difficult to apply across gender, age, and cultural populations; the function these behaviors serve must be evaluated on an individual basis and within the context of the particular situation.

Summary

Research has shown that problem-focused coping strategies, such as changing one's lifestyle (e.g., smoking cessation) in response to diagnosis, facilitate adaptation among patients with cancer and survivors alike (Schnoll et al., 2002). Patients most often employ problem-focused coping in response to stressful experiences that are perceived as changeable (Kohn, 1996; Rowland, 1989a). The other two methods of coping, appraisal and emotion focused, commonly are implemented in situations appraised as uncontrollable, as often is the case when confronted with cancer (Rowland, 1989a). Although the diagnosis of cancer is not changeable, the inherent challenges can be modified, controlled, and met with courage and perseverance. Cancer demands the reordering of one's priorities and the revision of one's goals, often contributing to reappraisal of the event as an opportunity for growth rather than only as a loss (Nolen-Hoeksema, 2000).

Coping as a Process

Coping is not a static event; it is an ever-changing and expanding process that develops over time. When dealing with a stressful, life-threatening illness such as cancer, flexibility in coping will promote adaptation at different transition points during the illness (Cohen & Lazarus, 1979; Nail, 2001). Coping may be best conceptualized as a process of "two steps forward, one step back" (Murphy, 1974), one that is influenced by constantly changing variables. "Coping is not a single act but rather a constellation of many acts and thoughts, triggered by a complex set of demands that change with time" (Cohen & Lazarus, p. 225). Coping must be assessed within the reality of the illness and, most importantly, by accepting the reality of the person undergoing the experience (Mages & Mendelsohn, 1979; Nail). Furthermore, assessment must recognize the interpersonal relationships supporting the patient (e.g., family, social support). Understanding the many variables that follow and how they influence coping responses is vital for accurate assessment and to plan interventions based upon the individual coping needs of the patient and the family.

Nature of the Illness

Included in the contextual and personality-based dimensions that influence coping, researchers have identified specific variables that are important determinants of how one may cope with a stressful situation (see Figure 4-1). When discussing coping with cancer, Rowland (1989a) stated that the primary influence on coping is the nature of the stress. When evaluating how the individual is coping with a cancer diagnosis, determining the site, stage, and type of cancer; the course of treatment; and the prognosis is of the utmost importance. A woman who is diagnosed with stage I breast

Figure 4-1. Variables That Influence Coping
• Nature of the Illness • Phases of Illness • Personality Dimensions • Coping Styles • Cultural, Socioeconomic, and Gender Dimensions • Developmental Life Stage • Social Networks and Support • Family Coping • Personal Meaning, Spirituality, and Hope • Specific Coping Challenges

cancer will have a different coping response than a woman diagnosed with stage III disease that requires chemotherapy and radiation. The general stressor—confronting cancer—is the same, but the realities and the threat of each specific case will be entirely different. Disease and treatment variables, such as chemotherapy side effects, have been shown to change an individual's perception and experience of the illness (Lethborg et al., 2000; Maes et al., 1996). The stressful array of physical symptoms (e.g., alopecia, total body hair loss) have been reported to cause psychological trauma (Lethborg et al.). Table 4-1 outlines the side effects of cancer and treatment that influence coping.

Studies in the literature have reported numerous objective stressors that affect patients and families when attempting to cope with cancer. These include disease prognosis (Howell, Fitch, & Deanc, 2003), caregiving demands, the duration of the illness, and the patient's distress (Borneman et al., 2003; Given, Given, & Kozachik, 2001; Haley, 2003; Redinbaugh et al., 2003; Sales et al., 1992). Research indicates that caregiver strain correlates with helping patients with self-care and physical needs and with managing their treatments and symptoms. Also, the longer the duration of the illness, the more evidence of distress. When the continuum of cancer extends over long periods of time, personal and social resources needed to cope effectively may be depleted (Lewis, 2004; Rowland, 1989a).

Phases of Illness

Different stages or phases of the cancer continuum will present specific coping challenges. These phases most often are categorized as diagnostic, treatment, remission, recurrence, and terminal phases. Anxiety and worry are common emotional responses during the diagnostic phase of cancer. Weisman and Worden (1976–1977) termed the

Table 4-1. Treatment-Related Variables Influencing Coping

Treatment	Stressor	Coping Challenge
Surgery	Preoperative anxiety and fear Loss of body part Loss of body function	Integrate the functional and cosmetic deficits of surgery into body image, self-esteem, and sexuality.
Chemotherapy	Systemic side effects: nausea and vomiting, diarrhea, stomatitis, alopecia, and fatigue Length of treatment	Continue with role function and family/job responsibilities while undergoing treatment. Integrate changes in body image.
Radiation	Skin markings (tattooing) Site-specific side effects: nausea and vomiting, diarrhea, stomatitis, alopecia, and fatigue Length of treatment	Cope with visual signs of cancer. Continue with role function and family/job responsibilities while undergoing treatment.
Biotherapy	Side effects: fever, fatigue, malaise, and muscle/joint tenderness Neurologic effects: mood disturbances and changes in cognition	Incorporate rest periods into daily routine. Continue with role function and family/job responsibilities while undergoing treatment. Cope with mood changes, fatigue, and cognitive effects.

first 100 days after diagnosis as the "existential plight in cancer." Fear may give way to shock, numbness, and denial when a confirmation of cancer is made (Cloutier & Ferrall, 1996). A multitude of emotions may follow—sadness, anger, depression, and personal grief—but gradually reality must be incorporated into the person's psyche (Fawzy, Fawzy, Hyun, & Wheeler, 1997). The treatment phase will bring about a variety of emotional reactions, and the management of treatment side effects becomes a major coping challenge. Surgery can generate fear related to changes in body image or loss of bodily functions. Chemotherapy and radiation may cause anticipatory fear resulting from a lack of knowledge about the treatment (e.g., it is common for patients to fear that external radiation may cause them to be radioactive). Common side effects of treatment (e.g., relentless fatigue, nausea and vomiting, alopecia, the disruption of normal lifestyle) leave the patient vulnerable to feelings of anxiety and depression.

When treatment ends, patients may enter the remission phase with uncertainty. Feelings of fear and ambivalence regarding the future may surface at this time. The patient may feel a loss of control over the cancer when active treatment has ended and may feel that nothing is being done to keep the cancer at bay. The literature has described this transition point as being "cast adrift" (Lethborg et al., 2000). Fears of recurrence threaten cancer survivors, especially patients who have been treated for more advanced disease (Kornblith, 1998). If the fear becomes reality, the recurrence phase of cancer is especially difficult for patients and families. At this stage, the initial hope for cure is gone. Many of the feelings—shock, disbelief, anxiety, anger, and depression—are similar to those experienced in the diagnostic phase, but they usually are more intense (Borneman et al., 2003; Fawzy et al., 1997). Women experiencing recurrent ovarian cancer have reported a sense of desperation and difficulties coping with the side effects of progressive disease (Howell et al., 2003).

Even if the recurrence is limited and asymptomatic, the patient's hope, confidence, and future plans are shaken (Weisman & Worden, 1986). The coping challenge in the advanced or terminal phase is the evident progression of disease and the inevitable awareness of mortality (Borneman et al., 2003). As the cancer progresses, issues surrounding intimacy and dependency may cause patients to feel helpless (Cloutier & Ferrall, 1996). Hope shifts from hope for cure to hope for relief from suffering (Borneman et al.). Fears of abandonment, pain, and loss of dignity are common in the terminal phase of cancer (Fawzy et al., 1997).

Personality Dimensions

The personal meaning of illness and of cancer, specifically, will be incorporated into the person's appraisal of the diagnosis. Past experiences with cancer or a prior psychiatric history, in addition to other individual variables such as values, beliefs, and religious preference, will affect coping responses (Rowland, 1989a; Spencer et al., 1998). The individual may perceive the cancer diagnosis as punishment for wrongdoing or as a sign of weakness and failure. Some people confront cancer with a fighting spirit, interpreting the disease as the "enemy" and the treatment as the "battlefield" (Rowland, 1989a). Fighting spirit has been a variable reported to positively influence adaptation of patients with cancer (Spencer et al.). Intrinsic to these perceptual differences are the person's basic personality structure and life experiences.

One's personality includes the emotional or internal resources and cognitive characteristics that influence the appraisal and coping processes. Examples of such traits that may influence psychological adjustment to cancer include the individual's proneness to anxiety and depression, locus of control, optimism, hardiness, and ego strength. It has been reported that individuals who have a prior history of significant anxiety or depression are at the highest risk for emotional instability when confronting cancer (Pasacreta, Minarik, & Nield-Anderson, 2001). If a person has trait anxiety, he or she is predisposed to more frequent and intense reactions to stressful events (Gorman, Raines, & Sultan, 2002), and the normal anxieties experienced with cancer (e.g., apprehension, tension, nervousness, worry) may become exacerbated. Studies have demonstrated that heightened levels of arousal and anxiety proneness, as measured by the State-Trait Anxiety Inventory, have been associated with the diagnosis of cancer (Clark, 1993) (see Chapter 13).

Along with anxiety, depression has been described as one of the most common psychosocial responses to the cancer experience. Depression is a normal response to perceived loss. When assessing the losses incurred by cancer, an adjustment disorder with depressed mood is not an uncommon finding. This diagnosis must be differentiated from a predisposition to depression or a past history of depressive episodes that may be intensified by the illness. Depressed individuals are more likely to use emotional and avoidance-style coping strategies (Zeidner & Saklofske, 1996). Therefore, individuals with a history of anxiety and depression may be at a greater risk for appraising the stressor of cancer as more threatening and overwhelming than individuals without such a history (see Chapter 15).

Locus of control is a personality construct that has been applied to evaluating health outcomes. Internal locus of control has been defined as the belief that people have internal control or responsibility for their perception of life events and their reactions to them (Fernsler & Miller, 2000). When confronted with ambiguous or overwhelming situations, the individual with an internal locus of control is more likely to appraise the situation as challenging and controllable (Barsevick, Much, & Sweeney, 2000).

Patients experiencing cancer who have an internal locus of control may be more likely to be active participants in their care plan and use problem-focused coping. External locus of control is the individual's belief that life events and consequences are beyond personal control or are external to the individual (Fernsler & Miller). This trait in patients with cancer may cause them to displace blame for the onset of illness and displace responsibility for the success of treatment. The characteristic of internal/external locus of control can be compared to the construct of control versus helplessness/hopelessness, and hopelessness is a major determinant for ineffective coping (Barry, 2002b). Researchers have identified a relationship between helplessness and pessimism and poor mental and physical health in patients with cancer (Parle & Maguire, 1995).

Another innate trait that is reported to influence coping is optimism (Aspinwall & Brunhart, 2000; Nail, 2001; Schnoll et al., 2002; Spencer et al., 1998). "Optimism" refers to a person's generalized confidence and positive expectations of the future. Optimistic patients are more likely to cope in active, problem-focused ways, whereas pessimistic patients are more likely to apply passive or avoidant forms of coping (Aspinwall & Brunhart; Maes et al., 1996). Research has pointed to a relationship between optimism and a fighting spirit and positive outcomes of coping (Parle & Maguire, 1995; Spencer et al.). Research has found higher levels of optimism to be associated not only with lower levels of avoidant coping but also with overall improvement in mental and physical health (Schnoll et al.). Another variable closely related to optimism and pessimism is that of neuroticism. This broad personality trait of worry, distress, and pessimism about one's future also has been reported to negatively influence emotional adjustment (Spencer et al.).

Another personality characteristic, described as good ego strength (Rowland, 1989a), may buffer the effects of stressful life events and contribute positively to an individual's psychological hardiness or resilience to stress. Resiliency is a relatively new concept that addresses the ability to withstand and rebound from crises and adversity (Nolen-Hoeksema, 2000; Walsh, 1996). Resilience encompasses the use of effective coping styles (e.g., problem-focused, emotion-focused) and how one is able to adapt coping styles to specific situations (Hawley & DeHaan, 1996). In the area of developmental psychology, resilient children have been observed to be flexible in adapting their coping styles to specific situations in addition to evaluating the effectiveness of their coping efforts (Hawley & DeHaan). These same characteristics of resiliency can apply to adults. Ego strength is a resiliency trait that has been defined as an intrapsychic and unconscious response. It involves the use of defense mechanisms that the ego engages to master the stress being confronted (Barry, 2002b). If coping fails, self-control and ego strength give way to defenses such as displacement, heightened alertness, anxiety, panic attacks, and loss of control (Barry, 2002b). Rowland (1989a) pointed out that characteristics used to describe emotionally healthy individuals, or people with strong egos, are most likely the same personality traits that accompany the use of effective coping strategies and a more positive adaptation to illness. Researchers have described resiliency in families as consisting of action-oriented behaviors aimed to reduce stress, obtain resources, and manage tension within the family system when confronting stress and crises (Friedman et al., 2003; McCubbin & McCubbin, 1996).

Coping Styles

Certain personality characteristics, such as optimism and anxiety, have been found to contribute to habitual ways or styles of coping (see Figure 4-2). Research supports that avoidant and passive styles of coping, such as helplessness/hopelessness, correlate with poor disease outcomes (Aspinwall & Brunhart, 2000; Watson & Greer, 1998). Problem-solving coping, which includes characteristics such as having a fighting spirit, has been correlated with positive disease outcomes (Watson & Greer). Studies have demonstrated that an optimistic personality is associated with good health related to the optimists' more active coping efforts and lower levels of avoidant coping (Aspinwall & Brunhart).

Figure 4-2. Coping Styles

Fighting spirit—an active problem-solving coping style. Patient accepts the disease, is determined to fight, and actively takes part in treatment decisions. This style is associated with optimism.

Avoidance (denial)—an avoidance-style of coping in which the patient refuses to accept the diagnosis, denies the seriousness of the illness, or avoids thinking about it.

Fatalism (stoic acceptance)—a passive style of coping in which the patient accepts the diagnosis and becomes resigned and fatalistic in attitude.

Anxious preoccupation—an emotion-focused style of coping in which the patient anxiously worries about the cancer and is preoccupied with fears that any physical ailment is the return of the disease. The patient requires constant reassurance. This style may be associated with preexisting anxiety.

Hopelessness/helplessness—an emotion-focused coping style in which the patient feels overwhelmed and is engulfed by the illness and feels like giving up. This style is associated with pessimism.

Note. Based on information from Watson & Greer, 1998.

Cultural, Socioeconomic, and Gender Dimensions

A person's culture has been described as the lens through which he or she perceives the world (Barsevick et al., 2000). Cultural beliefs play a complex role in the stress-coping response (Helman, 2001). Different cultural groups exposed to similar stressors will appraise the situation through their "world view" (Helman), although cancer is one of the most feared diseases in every culture (Die-Trill, 1998). Culturally ascribed norms will influence the behaviors associated with coping (e.g., health-seeking behaviors) and the resources used for social support (e.g., family, community) (Barsevick et al.). Research is limited regarding the similarities and differences in coping strategies between ethnic groups (Spencer et al., 1998). For example, research supports that both African American and Caucasian women seek social support as a coping strategy, yet the sources of support differ between the two groups (Bourjolly & Hirschman, 2001; Henderson et al., 2003). African American women reported that God, prayer, and spirituality are their main sources of emotional support; Caucasian women reported relying more on their spouses, children, and friends (Bourjolly &

Hirschman; Henderson et al.). Understanding the factors that influence African American women's needs for coping support will provide nurses with research-based evidence for interventions (e.g., planning a faith-based support group for African American women fighting breast cancer) (Henderson et al.).

To provide culturally competent care, nurses must recognize the differences that exist when the experience of coping with cancer is framed within the cultural belief system of the individual. As with patients, family attitudes also are shaped by the cultural beliefs about the specific illness. Beliefs about cancer causation, communication and language barriers, truth-telling practices, and family roles in cancer care will differ across culturally diverse populations (Die-Trill, 1998). The Oncology Nursing Society (Brant et al., 2000) has provided guidelines that address cultural competence for nursing practice, education, and research (Cohen & Palos, 2001).

Socioeconomic status is linked closely to the cultural dimensions of coping. Minority populations have fewer financial and educational resources, and these factors will influence the appraisal and coping strategies employed by patients with fewer socioeconomic means (Barsevick et al., 2000). Factors that will negatively influence coping responses include limited access to care, lack of education, unemployment, and limited insurance. For example, fear of rising medical costs among blue-collar cancer survivors has forced them to stay in jobs that they are no longer able to perform (Spencer et al., 1998). Socioeconomic status and level of education may be predictors of the type of support available to minority populations (Bourjolly & Hirschman, 2001). Demographic and clinical variables shown to support coping have included higher income and level of education and a positive perception of one's health (Schnoll et al., 2002). Low socioeconomic status is predictive of avoidance-style coping, which may result in higher levels of emotional distress (Spencer et al.). Therefore, healthcare providers must aim interventions to support coping at the socioeconomic limitations faced by many minority groups, such as providing bus tokens or cab vouchers for transportation to treatment and free, culturally sensitive educational programs and support groups (Bourjolly & Hirschman).

Limitations in research and practice present additional barriers to appreciating the coping process across different disease sites and different genders. The majority of research has focused on women's adaptation to breast cancer, leaving a dearth of information necessary to understand coping strategies for other malignancies, and even less is known about adaptation for male patients (McGovern, Heyman, & Resnick, 2002; Spencer et al., 1998). Men may be at higher risk for poor adjustment to cancer. For example, research on coping has revealed that men tend to use more withdrawal behaviors, such as avoiding feelings, not reaching out for social support, and attempting to hide the level of stress they are facing from others (Friedman et al., 2003). Men may be more unwilling to attend support groups (McGovern et al.), and in a study regarding coping with incontinence after prostate surgery, only a minority of the men studied were able to describe explicitly the emotional effects of incontinence (e.g., depression) in comparison to the participants' ability to address the physical and practical problems they encountered (Palmer, Fogarty, Somerfield, & Powel, 2003). Further research is needed to elucidate not only gender differences in adjustment, but also gender differences related to specific malignancies and treatments (Kornblith, 1998).

Developmental Life Stage

Cancer can strike at any point in an individual's life cycle. Erikson (1963) described psychosocial development and the inherent tasks or challenges that the person must resolve at each stage of emotional growth. Disruption of these tasks will affect the ability to cope (Rowland, 1989a). Although the prescribed ages within Erikson's theoretical framework must be adapted to current societal norms, the identified stages and tasks are still pertinent (Barry, 2002b). For example, the task for puberty and adolescence is defined as "ego identity versus role confusion." Ego identity answers the question "Who am I?" A basic conflict of this psychosocial stage is the adolescent's identity formation contrasted with identity confusion. The late adolescent is asserting independence and confronting social demands, and these tasks will be challenged with a diagnosis of cancer. Dependency on parents, interruptions of social and role functions because of treatment, and the effects of body-image changes on sexuality are just a few examples of the identity confusion that can result when the adolescent faces cancer. For each psychosocial stage of development, from infancy to late adulthood, cancer can disrupt emotional development and the resolution of life goals. If cancer strikes in child-bearing years, the potential of treatment-induced infertility can create emotional distress and marital problems (Kornblith, 1998). Research has identified that in this aspect and in others (e.g., physical health, finances, employment), young people experiencing cancer reported greater adjustment problems and poorer quality of life than older people with cancer (Barsevick et al., 2000).

Social Networks and Support

Social support is another significant variable believed to be positively associated with coping and adapting to the stress of cancer (Blanchard, Albrecht, Ruckdeschel, Grant, & Hemmick, 1995; Schnoll et al., 2002). Social support encompasses family, personal relationships, community, church, and larger social systems (e.g., culture) (Guidry, Aday, Zhang, & Winn, 1997). Studies have shown that social support can buffer the negative impact of cancer as well as influence the manner in which individuals cope (Pierce, Sarason, & Sarason, 1996; Thoits, 1986). Social support can assist with coping by helping patients to reappraise the situation as less threatening, by helping patients to problem solve and make decisions, and by providing direct intervention through physical and emotional support (Rowland, 1989b; Schnoll et al.). Table 4-2 outlines the principal domains of social support. When evaluating social support for patients, it is important to remember that what and how strongly patients *perceive* their social support to be are critical factors (Hudek-Knezevic, Kardum, & Pahljina, 2002). For example, a patient may attend a cancer support group and yet not feel that it meets his or her personal needs, not an uncommon finding for minority populations (Henderson et al., 2003).

Overall, seeking out social support as a coping strategy is vital to coping with cancer. Schnoll et al. (2002) found that in the four domains of social support (informational, companionship, instrumental, and esteem) assessed by the Interpersonal Support Evaluation List tool, all four types of social support correlated strongly with positive adaptation to cancer survivorship—sexual, extended family, social, and psychological adjustment. Lastly, therapeutic support in the form of psychoeducational support has been shown to positively enhance psychological and physical well-being (Edelman,

Table 4-2. Functions and Components of Social Support

Functions of Support	Components of Support
Informational/educational	Provides necessary information, knowledge, and skills for decision making and coping
Emotional/affectional	Interpersonal relationships that provide love, nurturance, acceptance, intimacy, and caring support
Tangible/instrumental	Provides financial assistance, physical goods, or services
Affirmational	Provides the sense that one's feelings are accepted and understood
Affiliational	Provides a sense of belonging or social identity
Appraisal	Provides supportive feedback and validation to the patient

Note. Based on information from Hudek-Knezevic et al., 2002; Rowland, 1989b.

Craig, & Kidman, 2000; Neilson-Clayton & Brownlee, 2002), along with strengthening the immune system (Fawzy, Fawzy, Arndt, & Pasnau, 1995).

When evaluating the effectiveness of social support, consider intervening variables. First, the dynamics of family functioning and social support will vary across cultural groups. Oncology nurses need to understand and respect the diversity among ethnic populations and be aware that social support will be defined within their cultural perspective. For example, in Native American culture, the entire "family" is actively involved with the patient's treatment and recovery. In the Native American community, family is not restricted to blood relatives; therefore, from the Native Americans' perspective, family support comes from interpersonal ties and the "adoption" of extended fathers, mothers, sisters, and cousins (Burhansstipanov & Hollow, 2001). Minority populations may be unaware of support resources available to them. When investigating preferences for psychosocial interventions in a multiethnic population, Gotay and Lau (2003) found that only 10% of patients studied had received information about psychosocial counseling; mental health professionals were not routinely incorporated in the cancer care system for these patients (see Chapter 6).

Lastly, oncology nurses must recognize that different forms of social support are helpful for some patients and not for others, especially when taking into account different family functioning and gender differences in coping. Lewis (2004) pointed out that spouses coping with breast cancer have differing views of what constitutes supportive behavior (e.g., the husband may feel that trying to reassure his wife or cheer her up is the most helpful, whereas the wife may find that these behaviors avoid dealing with her emotions). Diminished social support from family and friends over time has been found to be a distressing hardship of long-term survivors (Kornblith, 1998). After the crises of diagnosis and treatment, many family and friends do not understand the residual physical and psychological effects of cancer and may unknowingly desire for the patient to "return to normal." But as one patient with cancer poignantly expressed, returning to normalcy does not mean returning to the same place or identity (Lethborg et al., 2000). Finally, the family's adjustment can positively or negatively support the patient's coping, depending upon the level of family functioning.

Family Coping

Adapting to the strain and ever-changing demands of cancer is as much a task for families as for patients. The emotional distress experienced by family members is not just caused by the patient's illness-related stressors but also results from redefined relationships and roles and the increased stress placed upon the family system (Given et al., 2001; Lewis, 2004; Neilson-Clayton & Brownlee, 2002). In a review of family-focused oncology nursing research, Lewis outlined pertinent findings that may be contrary to what professionals would expect in regard to family adaptation to breast cancer. A major finding is that long-term adjustment to breast cancer negatively affects marital quality, family members' ability to cope, the child's self-esteem, and the quality of the child-parent relationship. Lewis found that the coping behaviors of the family remained stable over time irrelevant of illness demands, and evidence of family burnout existed when confronted with long-term stressors. Research of other cancer sites (e.g., head and neck) has supported this worsening of family relationships resulting from the chronic nature of illness demands (Kornblith, 1998).

Using a family systems approach to cancer care will enhance both patient and family coping. Similar to the patient's experience, the family's emotions range from shock to despair, anxiety to anguish (Duhamel & Dupuis, 2004). Family members most often feel isolated and alone in their feelings and, in addition, rank their own emotional needs and physical health as a low priority (Nikoletti et al., 2003). Studies have found that perceived health is lower and depression is greater in family caregivers than in the general population, and the social impact of cancer on the family includes interpersonal losses of outside relationships, activities, and paid employment (Haley, 2003).

Family dynamics have been found to influence problem solving and treatment decision making (Zhang & Siminoff, 2003). Family caregivers who are emotionally involved with patients have been found to show empathy and support for patient decisions, whereas noncohesive families display more discordance about treatment decisions (Zhang & Siminoff). To support family coping, nurses must be aware of disparity between the patient's and family's emotions and needs and validate each person's feelings. Duhamel and Dupuis (2004) have identified four elements as essential for effective family coping: acknowledging the family's existence, experience, expertise, and their need to maintain hope amid the losses they are experiencing. The patient's coping responses are interdependent with the family's coping responses —one cannot be separated from the other.

Personal Meaning, Spirituality, and Hope

An important variable influencing coping and adaptation to cancer is that patients can find some positive meaning for their cancer when answering the question, "Why me?" (Taylor, 1995). The search for meaning is a significant part of the cancer experience, and, most often, the majority of patients with cancer ascribe positive meanings to their experience. These include reprioritization of life goals, changed lifestyles and personal values, increased appreciation for life, and spiritual development (Taylor). Gaining insight into the meaning of life and resilience and strength in the face of adversity also support coping in family members (Nolen-Hoeksema, 2000) (see Chapter 3).

Confronting the existential issues brought about by cancer can be a profound emotional experience contributing to these changed perspectives. Research has indicated that spirituality (defined as the metaphysical or transcendent aspects of life related to supernatural forces) may have a positive impact on the emotional adjustment of patients with cancer (Jenkins & Pargament, 1995). Spirituality encompasses organized religion in addition to the belief in a "higher power" or other philosophies. Religious practice and strong spirituality may promote effective coping by decreasing the intensity of symptoms (e.g., pain, anxiety) and social isolation (Jenkins & Pargament) (see Chapter 7). Hope or hopefulness is another variable thought to positively influence the cancer experience. Studies have associated a sense of hope with spiritual healing, improved quality of life, and more effective coping (Felder, 2004; Post-White et al., 1996) (see Chapter 8). Although defining the dimensions of personal meaning, spirituality, and hope is difficult, healthcare professionals should evaluate the influence of these variables on emotional responses for each patient and family experiencing cancer.

Specific Coping Challenges With Cancer

Different physiologic and psychological demands along the cancer continuum will present specific coping challenges. These demands may be illness- or treatment-related: fatigue, pain, cognitive changes, medication side effects, and grief and loss. Unrelenting fatigue has been the most frequently reported symptom of cancer and treatment, and patients have identified fatigue as having a negative effect on quality of life (Mock, 2001). Fatigue can increase feelings of distress while undergoing cancer treatment, can have a negative impact on cognitive function, and can contribute to anxiety and depression (see Chapter 11).

Pain is another subjective phenomenon that influences coping. Psychiatric diagnoses (e.g., adjustment disorder with depressed or anxious mood, major depression) increase in patients with cancer with uncontrolled pain (Breitbart & Payne, 1998), and severe pain increases anxiety, which, in turn, increases the perception of pain (Pasacreta et al., 2001). Severe, uncontrolled pain is also a major risk factor for cancer-related suicide (Breitbart & Payne) (see Chapters 9 and 15).

Cognitive changes in patients with cancer are a distressing challenge and may be the direct (e.g., primary brain tumors or metastatic disease) or indirect (e.g., metabolic or electrolyte imbalances, drug or radiation side effects, infection) effects of disease or treatment on the central nervous system (Walch, Ahles, & Saykin, 1998). Certain chemotherapeutic agents (e.g., vinca alkaloids) may contribute to depression and mood changes in addition to affecting cognition. Alcohol and drug abuse also may compromise the patient's cognitive abilities. Cognitive changes can impair general appearance and behavior, mood, affect, and thought content and can lead to more serious psychiatric diagnoses, such as dementia or delirium. Cognitive disabilities that range from the inability to concentrate to loss of memory and symptoms of dementia can contribute to feelings of powerlessness and loss of control and dignity.

Finally, grief and loss throughout the cancer continuum are major coping challenges. Beginning with diagnosis, patients constantly confront physical and psychological losses that must be successfully grieved to enable individuals to cope effectively. Physical changes, such as loss of a body part or function, will affect body image and self-esteem. Successful mourning must take place to enable the individual to incorporate a new sense of self. Psychological losses involve changes in role function, job security, financial security, and, if cancer recurs, constant readjustment of lifestyle and future goals. A necessary challenge for patients and families is to reorganize and readjust as they face the continued demands of chronic illness (Lewis, 2004). If resolution of loss does not happen, patients are vulnerable to psychiatric complications, such as major depression. The ultimate challenge is the anticipatory grieving experienced by patients and families when death is imminent. Healthcare professionals are in a unique position to help patients and families through anticipatory grieving, resolution of conflicts, and preparation for bereavement (Chockinov & Holland, 1989; Nolen-Hoeksema, 2000; Redinbaugh et al., 2003) (see Chapters 18 and 27).

Interventions to Support Coping

Psychosocial support should be an inseparable entity of the cancer treatment plan (Guidry et al., 1997). If not addressed, the acute and chronic stress associated with cancer can cause emotional distress for patients, interfere with life goals, and contribute to a lower quality of life (Anderson, 2003). When planning interventions, nurses must recognize that (a) no single coping response is more effective than another; (b) interventions must be individualized for the specific needs of the patient and family; and (c) it may be necessary to provide a variety of resources to meet different challenges as they emerge (Nail, 2001; Pearlin & Schooler, 1978; Walsh, 1996). Nurses should base interventions upon a thorough psychosocial assessment of the many variables that influence coping behaviors (see Figure 4-1). Interventions should target patients at high risk for coping difficulties (e.g., trait anxiety) and should target points of time when they are most needed (e.g., recurrence) (Nail). Healthcare professionals must assess patients' emotional reactions to cancer at the outset of the cancer experience. Research has shown that early reactions often are predictive of individuals at risk for later adaptation and psychiatric problems (e.g., anxiety, depression) (Pasacreta et al., 2001).

A major goal of supporting patient and family coping is to promote adaptation. The adaptive tasks of chronic illness include reducing environmental threats, tolerating negative events, maintaining a positive self-image, maintaining emotional equilibrium, and positively staying involved in interpersonal relationships (Cohen & Lazarus, 1979). Figure 4-3 outlines assessment criteria and interventions that support effective coping and adaptation for patients and families. The hallmark of successful adaptation has been described as "engagement": a full and enthusiastic return to the normal activities of life" (Spencer et al., 1998, p. 212). Interventions directed toward adaptation focus on assisting patients and families with choosing effective coping strategies, helping them to regain preillness equilibrium, and, if possible, helping them to integrate and find meaning in the experience. Overcoming the challenges of cancer can lead to emotional growth and can contribute to a positive change in self-perception and one's life (Nolen-Hoeksema, 2000). Nurses can support this healing process by identifying how each patient and family define what coping means to them, moving toward what Lewis (2004) poignantly termed "relational-focused care."

Figure 4-3. Assessment Criteria and Interventions to Support Effective Coping and Adaptation for the Patient and Family

Assessment Criteria for Patient and Family Coping
- Understand the patient's and family's appraisal of the situation; identify what is appraised as threatening and what is appraised as challenging.
- Identify the stressors confronting the individual and family as perceived by them, within their reality, and within the context of their situation/lives.
- Assess coping efficacy based upon their individual and family experiences, strengths, and coping traits.
- Acknowledge the patient's and family's experience of the illness. Allow them to tell their story and discover their feelings and the meaning that each person ascribes to the experience.

Interventions to Promote Effective Coping and Adaptation
- Incorporate a family systems approach. Acknowledge the family's existence, the family's experience, the family's expertise, and their need to maintain hope.
- Communicate basic but necessary information to support coping: your name, your credentials, your role in their care, and how and when they can contact you.
- Use simple gestures that acknowledge their presence: Address the patient and family by name, shake their hands, and include them in conversations.
- Recognize and respect cultural and religious belief systems in the delivery of care.
- Provide clear, concise information regarding the care plan, what patient-active approach is expected of the individual, and what the patient can expect of you.
- Enhance confidence and hope. Note the patient's and family's strengths and abilities, and support and reinforce their unique coping styles.
- Use evidence-based interventions that are appropriate to the goal of care and the individual situation.
- Do not overload the patient and family with information. Assess readiness to learn, and recognize that information seeking is different for each patient and family.
- Be aware of your professional presence and role and its effect on the patient.
- Communicate positivism. Encourage the patient and family to be positive, do not tell them. Respect the patient's and family's attitudes and perceptions.
- Validate your assessment of the situation with the patient and family. Do not assume that your evaluation is correct and in line with the patient's and family's perspectives.
- Evaluate outcomes based upon the individual's and family's coping efficacy and values, not based upon preconceived notions of what constitutes effective coping.

Note. Based on information from Duhamel & Dupuis, 2004; Nail, 2001; Wilkes et al., 2003.

To meet and adjust to the physical and emotional demands of cancer, patients and families must constantly reappraise the meaning of the experience in relation to their beliefs, values, and life goals. Nurses can support this appraisal-focused coping by encouraging patients and families to examine their internal feelings—thoughts and impulses that are influencing their emotional responses. A wide variety of interventions can help to reduce the anxiety and fears that patients with cancer most often experience, thus allowing more emotional energy to be directed toward cognitive restructuring and problem solving. Interventions used to manage emotional stress include relaxation training, guided imagery, hypnosis, exercise, and music and art therapy. Encouraging a positive and optimistic attitude also will promote adaptive coping. Encouraging patients and family members to focus on short-term, attainable goals will help them to positively reframe what they find threatening and uncontrollable. Role modeling a positive and optimistic attitude will not only promote more effective coping (Wilkes et al., 2003) but also will allow patients and families to define what these concepts mean to them. For example, is optimism seen as hope for cure, hope for pain relief, or hope for quality time with those they love? The meaning of a hopeful, fighting spirit—like coping—will be dynamic and will change over the continuum of the disease. Hopefulness can be present no matter what the stage of disease or the goals for cure (Nail, 2001). Inherent risks are involved if supportive resources are not provided for emotion-focused coping. Coping behaviors can remain unchanged over time, not meeting the emotional needs of those involved (Lewis, 2004).

In addition, coping interventions should be evidence based. Research has demonstrated that strategies promoting active problem-solving behaviors, in contrast to passive or avoidant styles, have consistently proved to be more effective (Schnoll et al., 2002). For example, encouraging the patient to become an active and informed part of the treatment plan will promote effective coping behaviors and increase the patient's sense of control. Information seeking is an identified coping strategy that provides patients and families with the knowledge needed for decision making. Independent of where patients are on the cancer continuum, health education regarding the disease and treatment is vital. Coping failure most often begins with a lack of the knowledge, skills, or experience needed to make competent decisions (Lazarus & Folkman, 1984). If the educational component of cancer care is missing, patients will feel overwhelmed and confused, leading to feelings of powerlessness (see Chapter 22). In a review of stress research and quality-of-life interventions, Anderson (2003) found that education stood out as a significant intervention for improvement in both physical and mental health for patients studied. Another coping strategy, direct action (e.g., deciding to enter a clinical trial), cannot take place without adequate knowledge and without understanding the personal risks and benefits involved. When providing information to patients and families, nurses must take into account information-coping styles and readiness to learn. Education also must be balanced with emotional support to help patients and families to deal effectively with the information and its implications (Nikoletti et al., 2003).

Helping patients to develop new strategies as they move along the cancer continuum is another necessity. Research has shown that individuals who have exhibited more flexibility in their coping efforts have been more resilient and better able to cope (Aspinwall & Brunhart, 2000). Provide patients and families with choices and alternatives, recognizing that just because one intervention is frequently used does not mean it is effective across the board (Nail, 2001). An understanding of what feeling in control means for patients and families is critical to support their coping (Nail). For example, employing simple but challenging interventions in a busy healthcare setting (e.g., allowing the patient to choose appointment times, structuring chemotherapy sessions for family members to be present) can be the difference between patients and family members feeling in control and supported or frustrated and unheard. Interventions should target the most pressing stressor, focusing on what can and cannot be changed. If the stressor cannot be changed or identified, then direct interventions toward modifying the response to the stressor (Nail). A cancer diagnosis cannot be changed, but symptom management during treatment can modify the impact on patients' quality of life. Lastly, nursing interventions using a self-care approach have been found to improve patients' coping abilities (Delbar & Benor, 2001). Teaching patients how to predict and manage their own symptoms promotes independence and an internal locus of control (Delbar & Benor).

To be successful, coping interventions should be constructed within a systems framework—incorporating family, community, and social support—while maintaining sensitivity to cultural and spiritual beliefs. Caring for the family supports the greatest resource the patient has in striving to cope with and adapt to cancer. In the construct of appraisal-focused coping, it has been found that family caregivers who are hopeful are better equipped to find meaning in their lives amid the challenges of cancer (Borneman et al., 2003). To support problem solving in families, nurses can facilitate communication between the patient and family members. Long-standing family roles and communication patterns influence the different perceptions of care needs and the different emotional responses of the patient and family during the cancer trajectory (Given et al., 2001). If these family roles and communication patterns go unrecognized, research has found that they can contribute to the caregiver's sense of burden, adding to family conflict and caregiver distress (Given et al.). Lewis (2004) has proposed a "healing paradigm" for evidence-based understanding and intervention to promote family coping (see Figure 4-4). Caregivers who are able to "reframe" coping by accepting their loved one's illness and who can redefine the illness demands in a more manageable way feel more capable to meet these challenges and thus experience less caregiver stress (Redinbaugh et al., 2003) (see Chapter 36).

Figure 4-4. Healing Paradigm for Family Coping

- Help the family to stabilize and maintain its core functions during stressful times.
- Sustain or enhance relationships among family members—as a family "unit," not as a family with cancer.
- Nurture the needs of individual members within the family, despite the cancer.
- Add to the family members' competencies; promote confidence to manage illness-related challenges based upon the family's definition of the stressor and their perception of the situation, not on the professional's assumptions.
- Help the family to reorganize routines around treatment, symptom management, long-term care, and survivorship while protecting "quality" family time apart from the cancer experience.
- Support family relationships by reconfiguring, stabilizing, protecting, and enhancing communication, especially for children and in the parent-child relationship.
- Provide safety for family members to express their feelings and thoughts about the cancer experience over time, and validate and normalize their feelings.

Note. Based on information from Lewis, 2004.

Finally, reinforcing social support strongly influences patients' and families' capacity to cope. Fawzy et al. (1995) recommended implementation of structured psychosocial interventions for the patients early in the course of cancer diagnosis and treatment. Figure 4-5 outlines components of a structured psychiatric intervention program for newly diagnosed patients and those in late stages of treatment. Enhancing problem-solving capabilities should include training in the following coping skills: (a) how to identify the most pressing stressor/problem, (b) how to brainstorm possible solutions, (c) how to select and implement appropriate strategies, and (d) how to evaluate outcomes and reappraise the situation (Fawzy et al., 1997). Skills training should include characteristics of effective coping styles (e.g., optimism, practicality, flexibility, resourcefulness). Support groups and psychoeducational support programs are examples of structured interventions that can provide patients with tools to enhance problem-focused coping. With appropriate education, patients are less apt to use avoidance-focused styles of coping.

Psychological support for patients can be provided in the form of crisis intervention, counseling, and psychotherapy. Crisis intervention models frequently are applied in the area of oncology. This type of practice model is short-term and involves (a) defining the threatening events, (b) assessing the patient's interpretation of the stressors, (c) assessing the patient's coping efforts and the resources available, and (d) assessing the patient's level of functioning. Family

Figure 4-5. Components of Structured Psychiatric Interventions
Newly diagnosed or early treatment stage • Health education • Stress management and behavioral training • Coping strategies, including problem solving • Psychosocial group support **Advanced metastatic disease or late treatment stage** • Weekly group support programs • Focus on daily coping • Pain management, symptom management • Existential issues related to death and dying
Note. Based on information from Fawzy et al., 1995.

crisis interventions follow the same principles to mobilize family coping capabilities as a whole (Friedman et al., 2003). Most often, patients experiencing cancer must deal with specific crisis events (e.g., diagnosis, recurrence), and the most beneficial interventions aim to help patients and families to deal effectively with the challenges that are most pressing.

More in-depth interpersonal interventions, such as counseling and psychotherapy, may be warranted if particular dynamics of the individual are not solved by crisis intervention or structured psychoeducational support. If an individual has difficulty coping because of underlying conflicts or personal agenda, interventions aimed at general populations may be inadequate (Lazarus & Folkman, 1984; Pasacreta et al., 2001). Individual therapy provides a safe forum for patients to work out intrapsychic conflicts that may be interfering with effective coping behaviors. If the patient has overwhelming anxiety or depression or a past history of psychiatric disorders, referral for psychotherapy is necessary. The goals of psychotherapy with a patient who has cancer focus on the illness and its consequences, exploring only the past and present issues that are affecting coping and adaptation to cancer (Massie, Holland, & Straker, 1989). Psychopharmacologic management of emotional distress, psychiatric symptoms (e.g., anxiety, depression), and disease-related symptoms (e.g., insomnia, pain) play an important role in the treatment plan (Massie & Lesko, 1989; Pasacreta et al.).

Social support and psychological resources must be a consistent and ongoing component of cancer care (see Appendix). Patients and families continue to process cancer as a major life experience even after completion of treatment and recovery. Patients have expressed a perceived reduction in supportive networks at this time, when they ask themselves, "What shall I do with my life now?" (Lethborg et al., 2000). Other patients have expressed that at stressful transition points, such as recurrence, communication and support between themselves and healthcare providers become strained, causing them to feel helpless and abandoned (Howell et al., 2003). The need for social support for men also must be recognized. Gender differences exist, and men have different yet equally pressing needs for social support networks (Poole et al., 2001). Men in support groups have been found to use coping styles with less hopelessness and helplessness and with more fighting spirit (McGovern et al., 2002).

Cultural differences exist as well, and social support networks should be made available to meet the needs of racially and ethnically diverse populations (Bourjolly & Hirschman, 2001; Gotay & Lau, 2003).

Lastly, social support should use a family systems approach. Solution-focused brief therapy is a viable approach with families (Neilson-Clayton & Brownlee, 2002). This approach helps families to recognize their strengths, coping abilities, and hopefulness toward solving problems and moving into the future (Neilson-Clayton & Brownlee). Northouse et al. (2002) studied the effectiveness of a family-based intervention program that incorporated both the Lazarus and Folkman (1984) stress-coping model and the McCubbin and McCubbin (1996) family stress and resiliency model. This family-based program for women with recurrent breast cancer outlines nursing interventions tailored to address each component of the FOCUS program—**f**amily involvement, **o**ptimistic attitude, **c**oping effectiveness, **u**ncertainty reduction, and **s**ymptom management. The core content of the program was tailored to meet the particular needs and strengths of each family involved. The program incorporated an essential principle that should underlie all interventions to enhance coping, which is to identify and base interventions on how patients and families function and cope within their "reality," not on how theories predict they should (Lewis, 2004; Nail, 2001). Evaluate outcomes based upon the coping efficacy of patients and family members, not on the specific coping strategies they employ (Nail). Nurses also must recognize research limitations. It is difficult to make conclusions regarding the effectiveness of psychological interventions for stress and coping because the majority of studies have focused on breast cancer populations and limitations resulting from the heterogeneity of the interventions studied (Anderson, 2003). Research including identifying the role of gender and minority differences within a stress/coping framework and longitudinal studies across varied cancer populations are needed to understand adaptation from prediagnosis to survivorship.

Conclusion

Nursing plays an integral role in helping patients and families to cope and adapt to cancer. The crux of nursing is a humanistic approach and nurturance of the human potential (Friedman et al., 2003). Supporting patient coping is congruent with the goals of oncology nursing care. From nurses at the bedside to those in advanced practice, nursing interventions to enhance coping occur across the cancer continuum. Interventions include patient and family education, symptom management, supporting and reinforcing effective coping strategies, and referring patients and families to appropriate resources if ineffective coping is identified. Intrinsic to all coping interventions are the goals of empowering patients and families and providing hope. Empowerment occurs when the necessary information, skills, and problem-solving methods are provided to build the self-esteem and self-confidence of patients and family members to successfully meet the challenges they face (Friedman et al.). Hope is a far less tangible goal, but one that may be an essential ingredient for coping effectively with cancer (Reading, 2004). Even during the terminal stage of illness, patients can hope for life goals, such as having the resources to finish their life business, being free of pain, and dying with dignity. Martocchio (1985) succinctly summed up the relationship between hope and coping: "Hoping is coping" (p. 297).

References

Anderson, B.L. (2003). Psychological interventions for cancer patients. In C.W. Given, B. Given, V.L. Champion, S. Kozachik, & D.N. DeVoss (Eds.), *Evidence based cancer care and prevention: Behavioral interventions* (pp. 179–217). New York: Springer.

Aspinwall, L.G., & Brunhart, S.M. (2000). What I do know won't hurt me: Optimism, attention to negative information, coping, and health. In J.E. Gillham (Ed.), *The science of optimism and hope: Research essays in honor of Martin E.P. Seligman* (pp. 163–200). Philadelphia: Templeton Foundation Press.

Barry, P.D. (2002a). Stress: Effective coping and adaptation. In P.D. Barry (Ed.), *Mental health and mental illness* (7th ed., pp. 157–170). Philadelphia: Lippincott.

Barry, P.D. (2002b). Theories and stages of personality development. In P.D. Barry (Ed.), *Mental health and mental illness* (7th ed., pp. 85–105). Philadelphia: Lippincott.

Barsevick, A.M., Much, J., & Sweeney, C. (2000). Psychosocial responses to cancer. In C.H. Yarbro, M.H., Frogge, M. Goodman, & S.L. Groenwald (Eds.), *Cancer nursing: Principles and practice* (5th ed., pp. 1529–1549). Sudbury, MA: Jones and Bartlett.

Blanchard, C.G., Albrecht, T.L., Ruckdeschel, J.C., Grant, C.H., & Hemmick, R.M. (1995). The role of social support in adaptation to cancer and to survival. *Journal of Psychosocial Oncology, 13*(1/2), 75–95.

Borneman, T., Chu, D.Z.J., Wagman, L., Ferrell, B., Juarez, G., McCahill, L.E., et al. (2003). Concerns of family caregivers of patients with cancer facing palliative surgery for advanced malignancies. *Oncology Nursing Forum, 30,* 997–1005.

Bourjolly, J.N., & Hirschman, K.B. (2001). Similarities in coping strategies but differences in sources of support among African American women coping with breast cancer. *Journal of Psychosocial Oncology, 19*(2), 17–38.

Brant, J., Ishida, D., Itana, J., Kagawa-Singer, M., Palos, G., Phillips, J., et al. (2000). *Multicultural outcomes: Guidelines for cultural competence.* Pittsburgh, PA: Oncology Nursing Society.

Breitbart, W., & Payne, D.K. (1998). Pain. In J.C. Holland (Ed.), *Psycho-oncology* (pp. 451–467). New York: Oxford University Press.

Burhansstipanov, L., & Hollow, W. (2001). Native American cultural aspects of oncology nursing care. *Seminars in Oncology Nursing, 17,* 206–219.

Chockinov, H., & Holland, J.C. (1989). Bereavement: A special issue in oncology. In J.C. Holland & J.H. Rowland (Eds.), *Handbook of psychooncology: Psychological care of the patient with cancer* (pp. 612–627). New York: Oxford University Press.

Clark, J.C. (1993). Psychosocial responses of the patient. In S.L. Groenwald, M.H. Frogge, M. Goodman, & C.H. Yarbro (Eds.), *Cancer nursing: Principles and practice* (pp. 449–467). Sudbury, MA: Jones and Bartlett.

Cloutier, A., & Ferrall, S. (1996). Psychosocial aspects of complex responses to cancer. In P.D. Barry (Ed.), *Psychosocial nursing care of physically ill patients and their families* (pp. 412–433). Philadelphia: Lippincott.

Cohen, F., & Lazarus, R.S. (1979). Coping with the stresses of illness. In G.C. Stone, F. Cohen, & N.E. Adler (Eds.), *Health psychology: A handbook. Theories, applications, and challenges of a psychological approach to the health care system* (pp. 217–254). San Francisco: Jossey-Bass.

Cohen, M.L., & Palos, G. (2001). Culturally competent care. *Seminars in Oncology Nursing, 17,* 153–158.

Delbar, V., & Benor, D.E. (2001). Impact of a nursing intervention on cancer patients' ability to cope. *Journal of Psychosocial Oncology, 19*(2), 57–74.

Devins, G.M., & Binik, Y.M. (1996). Facilitating coping with chronic physical illness. In M. Zeidner & N.S. Endler (Eds.), *Handbook of coping: Theory, research, applications* (pp. 640–696). New York: John Wiley.

Die-Trill, M. (1998). The patient from a different culture. In J.C. Holland (Ed.), *Psycho-oncology* (pp. 857–866). New York: Oxford University Press.

Duhamel, F., & Dupuis, F. (2004). Guaranteed returns: Investing in conversations with families of patients with cancer. *Clinical Journal of Oncology Nursing, 8,* 68–71.

Edelman, S., Craig, A., & Kidman, A.D. (2000). Group interventions with cancer patients: Efficacy of psychoeducational versus supportive groups. *Journal of Psychosocial Oncology, 18*(3), 67–85.

Erikson, E. (1963). *Childhood and society* (2nd ed.). New York: Norton.

Fawzy, F.I., Fawzy, N.W., Arndt, L.A., & Pasnau, R.O. (1995). Critical review of psychosocial interventions in cancer care. *Archives of General Psychiatry, 52,* 100–113.

Fawzy, F.I., Fawzy, N.W., Hyun, C.S., & Wheeler, J.G. (1997). Brief, coping-oriented therapy for patients with malignant melanoma. In J.L. Spira (Ed.), *Group therapy for medically ill patients* (pp. 133–163). New York: Guilford Press.

Felder, B.E. (2004). Hope and coping in patients with cancer diagnoses. *Cancer Nursing, 27,* 320–324.

Fernsler, J.I., & Miller, M.A. (2000). Factors affecting health behavior. In C.H. Yarbro, M.H. Frogge, M. Goodman, & S.L. Groenwald (Eds.), *Cancer nursing: Principles and practice* (5th ed., pp. 85–99). Sudbury, MA: Jones and Bartlett.

Friedman, M.M., Bowden, V.R., & Jones, E.G. (2003). *Family nursing: Research, theory, and practice* (5th ed.). Upper Saddle River, NJ: Prentice Hall.

Given, B.A., Given, C.W., & Kozachik, S. (2001). Family support in advanced cancer. *CA: A Cancer Journal for Clinicians, 51,* 213–231.

Gorman, L.M., Raines, M.L., & Sultan, D.F. (2002). *Psychosocial nursing for general patient care* (2nd ed.). Philadelphia: F.A. Davis.

Gotay, C.C., & Lau, A.K. (2003). Preferences for psychosocial interventions among newly diagnosed cancer patients from a multiethnic population. *Journal of Psychosocial Oncology, 20*(4), 23–37.

Guidry, J.J., Aday, L.A., Zhang, D., & Winn, R.J. (1997). The role of informal and formal social support networks for patients with cancer. *Cancer Practice, 5,* 241–246.

Haley, W.E. (2003). Family caregivers of elderly patients with cancer: Understanding and minimizing the burden of care. *Journal of Supportive Oncology, 1*(4 Suppl. 2), 25–29.

Hawley, D.R., & DeHaan, L. (1996). Toward a definition of family resilience: Integrating life-span and family perspectives. *Family Process, 35,* 283–298.

Helman, C.G. (2001). *Culture, health, and illness* (4th ed.). London: Arnold.

Henderson, P.D., Gore, S.V., Davis, B.L., & Condon, E.H. (2003). African American women coping with breast cancer: A qualitative analysis. *Oncology Nursing Forum, 30,* 641–647.

Holahan, C.J., Moos, R.H., & Schaefer, J.A. (1996). Coping, stress resistance, and growth: Conceptualizing adaptive functioning. In M. Zeidner & N.S. Endler (Eds.), *Handbook of coping: Theory, research, applications* (pp. 24–43). New York: John Wiley.

Holland, J.C. (1989). Clinical course of cancer. In J.C. Holland & J.H. Rowland (Eds.), *Handbook of psychooncology: Psychological care of the patient with cancer* (pp. 75–100). New York: Oxford University Press.

Holland, J.C., & Lewis, S. (2000). *The human side of cancer: Living with hope, coping with uncertainty.* New York: HarperCollins.

Howell, D., Fitch, M.I., & Deane, K.A. (2003). Women's experiences with recurrent ovarian cancer. *Cancer Nursing, 26,* 10–17.

Hudek-Knezevic, J., Kardum, I., & Pahljina, R. (2002). Relations among social support, coping, and negative affect in hospitalized and nonhospitalized cancer patients. *Journal of Psychosocial Oncology, 20*(2), 45–63.

Jenkins, R.A., & Pargament, K.I. (1995). Religion and spirituality as resources for coping with cancer. *Journal of Psychosocial Oncology, 13*(1/2), 51–74.

Johnson, P. (2002). The use of humor and its influence on spirituality and coping in breast cancer survivors. *Oncology Nursing Forum, 29,* 691–695.

Kohn, P.M. (1996). On coping adaptively with daily hassles. In M. Zeidner & N.S. Endler (Eds.), *Handbook of coping: Theory, research, applications* (pp. 181–201). New York: John Wiley.

Kornblith, A.B. (1998). Psychosocial adaptation of cancer survivors. In J.C. Holland (Ed.), *Psychooncology* (pp. 223–254). New York: Oxford University Press.

Lazarus, R.S. (1982). Stress and coping as factors in health and illness. In J. Cohen, J. Cullen, & T.R. Martin (Eds.), *Psychosocial aspects of coping* (pp. 163–190). New York: Raven Press.

Lazarus, R.S. (1993). Coping theory and research: Past, present, and future. *Psychosomatic Medicine, 55,* 234–247.

Lazarus, R.S. (2000). Evolution of a model of stress, coping, and discrete emotions. In V.H. Rice (Ed.), *Handbook of stress, coping, and health: Implications for nursing research, theory, and practice* (pp. 195–222). Thousand Oaks, CA: Sage Publications.

Lazarus, R.S., & Folkman, S. (1984). *Stress, appraisal, and coping.* New York: Springer.

Lethborg, C.E., Kissane, D., Burns, W.I., & Snyder, R. (2000). "Cast adrift": The experience of completing treatment among women with early stage breast cancer. *Journal of Psychosocial Oncology, 18*(4), 73–90.

Lewis, F.M. (2004). Family-focused oncology nursing research. *Oncology Nursing Forum, 31,* 288–292.

Maes, S., Leventhal, H., & de Ridder, D. (1996). Coping with chronic diseases. In M. Zeidner & N.S. Endler (Eds.), *Handbook of coping: Theory, research, applications* (pp. 221–251). New York: John Wiley.

Mages, N.L., & Mendelsohn, G.A. (1979). Effects of cancer on patients' lives: A personological approach. In G.C. Stone, F. Cohen, & N.E. Adler (Eds.), *Health psychology: A handbook. Theories, applications, and challenges of a psychological approach to the health care system* (pp. 255–284). San Francisco: Jossey-Bass.

Martocchio, B.C. (1985). Family coping: Helping families help themselves. *Seminars in Oncology Nursing, 1,* 292–297.

Massie, M.J., Holland, J.C., & Straker, N. (1989). Psychotherapeutic interventions. In J.C. Holland & J.H. Rowland (Eds.), *Handbook of psychooncology: Psychological care of the patient with cancer* (pp. 455–469). New York: Oxford University Press.

Massie, M.J., & Lesko, L.M. (1989). Psychopharmacological management. In J.C. Holland & J.H. Rowland (Eds.), *Handbook of psychooncology: Psychological care of the patient with cancer* (pp. 470–491). New York: Oxford University Press.

McCubbin, M.A., & McCubbin, H.I. (1996). Resiliency in families: A conceptual model of family adjustment and adaptation in response to stress and crises. In H.I. McCubbin, A.I. Thompson, & M.A. McCubbin (Eds.), *Family assessment: Resiliency, coping, and adaptation: Inventories for research and practice* (pp. 1–64). Madison, WI: University of Wisconsin.

McGovern, R.J., Heyman, E.N., & Resnick, M.I. (2002). An examination of coping style and quality of life of cancer patients who attend a prostate cancer support group. *Journal of Psychosocial Oncology, 20*(3), 57–68.

Mock, V. (2001). Fatigue management. *Cancer, 92*(Suppl. 6), 1699–1707.

Murphy, L.B. (1974). Coping, vulnerability, and resilience in childhood. In G.V. Coelho, D.A. Hamburg, & J.E. Adams (Eds.), *Coping and adaptation* (pp. 69–100). New York: Basic Books.

Nail, L.M. (2001). I'm coping as fast as I can: Psychosocial adjustment to cancer and cancer treatment. *Oncology Nursing Forum, 6,* 967–970.

Neilson-Clayton, H., & Brownlee, K. (2002). Solution-focused brief therapy with cancer patients and their families. *Journal of Psychosocial Oncology, 20*(1), 1–13.

Nikoletti, S., Kristjanson, L.J., Tataryn, D., McPhee, R., & Burt, L. (2003). Information needs and coping styles of primary family caregivers of women following breast cancer surgery. *Oncology Nursing Forum, 30,* 987–996.

Nolen-Hoeksema, S. (2000). Growth and resilience among bereaved people. In J.E. Gillham (Ed.), *The science of optimism and hope: Research essays in honor of Martin E.P. Seligman* (pp. 107–127). Philadelphia: Templeton Foundation Press.

Northouse, L.L., Walker, J., Schafenacker, A., Mood, D., Mellon, S., Galvin, E., et al. (2002). A family-based program of care for women with recurrent breast cancer and their family members. *Oncology Nursing Forum, 29,* 1411–1419.

Palmer, M.H., Fogarty, L.A., Somerfield, M.R., & Powel, L.L. (2003). Incontinence after prostatectomy: Coping with incontinence after prostate cancer surgery. *Oncology Nursing Forum, 30,* 229–238.

Parle, M., & Maguire, P. (1995). Exploring relationships between cancer, coping, and mental health. *Journal of Psychosocial Oncology, 13*(1/2), 27–50.

Pasacreta, J.V., Minarik, P.A., & Nield-Anderson, L. (2001). Anxiety and depression. In B.R. Ferrell & N. Coyle (Eds.), *Textbook of palliative nursing* (pp. 269–289). New York: Oxford University Press.

Pearlin, L.I., & Schooler, C. (1978). The structure of coping. *Journal of Health and Social Behavior, 19,* 2–21.

Pierce, G.R., Sarason, I.G., & Sarason, B.R. (1996). Coping and social support. In M. Zeidner & N.S. Endler (Eds.), *Handbook of coping: Theory, research, applications* (pp. 434–451). New York: John Wiley.

Poole, G., Poon, C., Achille, M., White, K., Franz, N., Jittler, S., et al. (2001). Social support for patients with prostate cancer: The effect of support groups. *Journal of Psychosocial Oncology, 19*(2), 1–16.

Post-White, J., Ceronsky, C., Kreitzer, M.J., Drew, D., Mackey, K.W., Koopmeiners, L., et al. (1996). Hope, spirituality, sense of coherence, and quality of life in patients with cancer. *Oncology Nursing Forum, 23,* 1571–1579.

Reading, A. (2004). *Hope and despair: How perceptions of the future shape human behavior.* Baltimore: Johns Hopkins University Press.

Redinbaugh, E.M., Baum, A., Tarbell, S., & Arnold, R. (2003). End-of-life caregiving: What helps family caregivers cope? *Journal of Palliative Medicine, 6,* 901–909.

Rowland, J.H. (1989a). Intrapersonal resources: Coping. In J.C. Holland & J.H. Rowland (Eds.), *Handbook of psychooncology: Psychological care of the patient with cancer* (pp. 44–57). New York: Oxford University Press.

Rowland, J.H. (1989b). Intrapersonal resources: Social support. In J.C. Holland & J.H. Rowland (Eds.), *Handbook of psychooncology: Psychological care of the patient with cancer* (pp. 58–71). New York: Oxford University Press.

Sales, E. (1991). Psychosocial impact of the phase of cancer on the family: An updated review. *Journal of Psychosocial Oncology, 9*(4), 1–17.

Sales, E., Schulz, R., & Biegel, D. (1992). Predictors of strain in families of cancer patients: A review of the literature. *Journal of Psychosocial Oncology, 10*(2), 1–26.

Schnoll, R.A., Knowles, J.C., & Harlow, L. (2002). Correlates of adjustment among cancer survivors. *Journal of Psychosocial Oncology, 20*(1), 37–59.

Somerfield, M., & Curbow, B. (1992). Methodological issues and research strategies in the study of coping with cancer. *Social Science and Medicine, 34,* 1203–1216.

Spencer, S.M., Carver, C.S., & Price, A.A. (1998). Psychological and social factors in adaptation. In J.C. Holland (Ed.), *Psycho-oncology* (pp. 211–219). New York: Oxford University Press.

Taylor, E.J. (1995). Whys and wherefores: Adult patient perspectives of the meaning of cancer. *Seminars in Oncology Nursing, 11,* 32–40.

Thoits, P.A. (1986). Social support as coping assistance. *Journal of Consulting and Clinical Psychology, 54,* 416–423.

Walch, S.E., Ahles, T.A., & Saykin, A.J. (1998). Neuropsychological impact of cancer and cancer treatments. In J.C. Holland (Ed.), *Psycho-oncology* (pp. 500–505). New York: Oxford University Press.

Walsh, F. (1996). The concept of family resilience: Crisis and challenge. *Family Process, 35,* 261–281.

Watson, M., & Greer, S. (1998). Personality and coping. In J.C. Holland (Ed.), *Psycho-oncology* (pp. 91–98). New York: Oxford University Press.

Weisman, A.D., & Worden, J.W. (1976–1977). The existential plight in cancer: Significance of the first 100 days. *International Journal of Psychiatry in Medicine, 7,* 1–15.

Weisman, A.D., & Worden, J.W. (1986). The emotional impact of recurrent cancer. *Journal of Psychosocial Oncology, 3*(4), 5–16.

White, R.W. (1974). Strategies of adaptation: An attempt at systematic description. In G.V. Coelho, D.A. Hamburg, & J.E. Adams (Eds.), *Coping and adaptation* (pp. 47–68). New York: Basic Books.

Wilkes, L.M., O'Baugh, J., Luke, S., & George, A. (2003). Positive attitude in cancer: Patients' perspectives. *Oncology Nursing Forum, 30,* 412–416.

Zeidner, M., & Saklofske, D. (1996). Adaptive and maladaptive coping. In M. Zeidner & N.S. Endler (Eds.), *Handbook of coping: Theory, research, applications* (pp. 505–531). New York: John Wiley.

Zhang, A.Y., & Siminoff, L.A. (2003). The role of the family in treatment decision making by patients with cancer. *Oncology Nursing Forum, 30,* 1022–1028.

CHAPTER 5

Gender and Age Differences in the Psychological Response to Cancer

Paula J. Anastasia, RN, MN, AOCN®, OCN®

We do not grow absolutely, chronologically. We grow sometimes in one dimension, and not in another, unevenly. We grow partially. We are relative. We are mature in one realm, childish in another. The past, present, and future mingle and pull us backward, forward, or fix us in the present. We are made up of layers, cells, constellations.

—Anais Nin

Nearly half of the people in the United States will be diagnosed with cancer during their lifetime (Jemal et al., 2005). Unfortunately, cancer not only affects the individual but also the family and support systems of the diagnosed individual. An estimated one in two men and one in three women will develop cancer (Jemal et al.). The most common malignancies in men are prostate, lung, and colorectal cancers. For women, breast cancer remains the most common cancer, followed by lung and colorectal cancers (Jemal et al.). In addition, cancer does not discriminate based on age. Although it remains true that the incidence of invasive cancer increases with age (see Table 5-1), cancer can occur at any time. Although relatively rare in children, cancer is the second leading cause of death, behind accidents, in children between the ages of 1 and 14 in the United States. The most common malignancies in children are leukemias and tumors of the central and sympathetic nervous system (Jemal et al.).

Table 5-1. Development Rates of Invasive Cancer by Gender and Age

Gender	Birth–39 Years	40–59 Years	60–79 Years	Birth to Death (%)
Male	1 in 71	1 in 12	1 in 3	1 in 2
Female	1 in 51	1 in 11	1 in 4	1 in 3

Note. Based on information from American Cancer Society, 2005.

Unquestionably, the impact of a cancer diagnosis will add stress to the affected patient. The majority of the literature addressing the psychological effects experienced by patients identifies the potential for altered coping mechanisms and role adjustments. Factors such as the patient's gender and age, support systems, and religious and cultural norms influence the complexity of understanding coping styles. This chapter focuses on gender and age and how they influence coping behaviors.

Stereotypes

Traditionally, mass media have portrayed men as strong, silent types who financially support their spouse and family. Men generally are viewed as more emotionally reserved and less communicative about feelings than women. Women are portrayed as more emotional and vulnerable to changing events. Women are perceived as the caretakers and nurturers, without having much responsibility for financial matters. Even though women comprise one-half of the workforce, these stereotypes still predominate (Courts, Newton, & McNeal, 2005; Stellman & Stellman, 1995). Men and women engage in social roles differently; therefore, psychological factors, such as stress and anxiety as a result of a cancer diagnosis, are likely to influence health behaviors differently.

A review of the literature concerning the stereotypes of gender revealed that men are described as dominant, rational, independent, and decisive, and women are described as submissive, emotional, dependent, sensitive, caring, and nurturing (Geis, 1993). In addition, women are more concerned about responding to the needs of others, a trait Gerber (1989) defined as "communion," whereas men are concerned with promoting themselves and asserting their power over others, a trait Gerber defined as "agency." However, when men and women were surveyed, both sexes responded that they had an equal balance of traits of agency and communion. Perhaps, men's and women's personalities are not so different, and societal stereotypes are what define a difference. The different roles that men and women play may lead people to believe that they have different personalities. Because of perceived stereotypes, when a man is told of a cancer diagnosis, people presume that he will act without emotion and remain in control. Conversely, when a woman is informed about a cancer diagnosis, a display of emotion is expected, and healthcare providers stand ready to offer comfort (Kronenwetter et al., 2005; Weidner & Collins, 1993).

Reactions to a cancer diagnosis vary greatly in regard to age. A child's reaction is hard to predict and, therefore, is less likely to be affected by stereotypes. It has been found that as the infant becomes able to differentiate between caregivers, the infant's expectations and reactions for the father's behavior are different from those for the mother. At six weeks, infants lifted their shoulders and eyebrows when their fathers appeared, whereas the same infants, appearing to expect routine, became more settled and less animated when they saw their mothers (Pruett, 2002). Studies have found that fathers interact differently, providing less rhythmic but more exciting physical and auditory stimulation (Lamb, 2004; Sahler & Wood, 2001). Regardless of age, reactions to a diagnosis will be influenced by developmental age, ability to understand the content of the message, parental or family reactions, the way in which the diagnosis is explained, and the individual's previous experience with and interpretation of the content.

Effects of Gender and Age on Coping

An individual's response to child-rearing modeling, values, and beliefs determine coping styles. Effective coping is achieved when short-term and long-term reductions of the stress and the coping task are complete. However, the effectiveness of the coping style is based on social and cultural norms, and what is adaptive for one person may be maladaptive for another (Levenson, 2003). Lazarus and Folkman (1984) identified two types of coping behavior—problem focused and emotion focused (see Figure 5-1). Problem-focused coping is directed at problem-solving strategies, whereas emotion-focused coping concerns maintaining emotional equilibrium during the stressful situation. Problem-focused strategies include identifying the problem and cognitively determining solutions to the problem. Problem-focused or cognitive appraisal strategies include assessing the problem, identifying the resources, evaluating the outcome, and eventually adapting to the stressor. This type of coping mechanism frequently is used by individuals who need to maintain control in their lives (Davison, Goldenberg, Gleave, & Degner, 2003). Emotion-focused coping uses mechanisms such as avoidance to reduce emotional distress (Barsevick, Much, & Sweeney, 2000). Mismatches between the individual's ability to process information and coping style may increase psychosocial distress.

Figure 5-1. Comparison of Stereotypical Problem- and Emotion-Focused Coping	
Problem-Focused	**Emotion-Focused**
• Identifies solutions through information seeking, education, and obtaining new skills • Active coping • External focus • Used often by men	• Maintains emotional equilibrium • Uses coping mechanisms such as avoidance, denial, and emotional expression (e.g., crying, laughing) • Passive coping • Internal focus • Used often by women
Note. Based on information from Barsevick et al., 2000; Lazarus & Folkman, 1984; Zeidner & Saklofske, 1996.	

Gender-Based Psychosocial Concerns

Simon (1995) examined male-female differences in work and family roles and found that married working mothers had more anxiety, distress, and somatic complaints than their spouses. Brown and Barbarin (1996) noted similar responses in parents who cared for a child with cancer. Women experienced more personal strain than men as a result of trying to maintain the household and job responsibilities while caring for a sick child. Women caregivers scored higher than male caregivers on cancer-related anxiety, fear of cancer recurrence, and uncertainty about the future (Matthews, 2003). Men saw themselves as less involved with the medical aspects of the illness but responsible for financial needs. Men employed more problem-solving skills and were less emotionally expressive than women. This may be interpreted in several ways. For many men, the threat of relinquishing control and independence may interfere with coping abilities

(Carmel & Bernstein, 2003; Courts et al., 2005; Simpson & Stroh, 2004). Men whose self-esteem is determined by their ability to provide financial support may be at risk for having a more difficult time adjusting to their new role as a patient with cancer.

Additional maladaptive behaviors may be observed if men are feeling insecure or vulnerable because of role changes or financial issues. The workplace serves many functions for people other than just being a source of income, such as helping to form one's identity in society and in social roles. A disability resulting from cancer may prevent patients from participating in social activities. Cancer may alter relationships with spouses or significant others. Spouses or friends may become caregivers, causing guilt or role conflict for patients (Germino et al., 1998; Matthews, 2003; Northouse, Mood, Templin, Mellon, & George, 2000). Similarly, women who feel too weak or fatigued from their disease and treatment to maintain their household role may be at risk for additional role conflict and feelings of guilt if someone else is managing the household responsibilities (Bower et al., 2000; Simpson & Stroh, 2004).

The ability to adjust to a cancer diagnosis varies greatly among individuals, and several factors are predictors of psychological adjustment, including an availability of social support, performance status, meaning of the diagnosis, and site of malignancy (Matthews, 2003). Relationships with family, coworkers, and friends make up the social sphere of a patient. Lack of adequate social support is a predictor of psychological morbidity following a life crisis. In a study of 520 patients with cancer interviewed eight weeks after diagnosis, men were just as likely as women to confide their feelings; however, men used only one confidant, whereas women used a larger circle of friends and family (Harrison, Maguire, & Pitceathly, 1995). A man who relies on his wife for psychological support and confidence may be at risk for psychological distress if his confidant, his wife, has cancer. He may internalize his distress because he feels he cannot share his stress with his confidant (Courts et al., 2005). He may hide his feelings or use avoidance as a coping behavior. Avoidance behavior often prevents the individual from facing the situation because it will increase stress. Avoiders usually believe that they have little control over or responsibility for improving the situation. Men generally use denial or avoidance and, therefore, may choose not to communicate feelings about treatment. Women, by contrast, typically are more verbal and communicative about their feelings (Davison et al., 2003; Levenson, 2003). Women use coping strategies that give them more control over their emotions, especially when cancer makes them feel as if they have little control (Caldwell et al., 2003; Kim, Yeom, Seo, Kim, & Yoo, 2002). Many women, therefore, may benefit from the sharing relationship found in a support group.

These gender differences in coping can be found in children also (Sahler & Wood, 2001). In a comparison of adolescent gender differences, Boekaerts (1996) noted that girls addressed problems immediately and talked within their social network to solve problems. Boys, however, did not address problems with as much urgency as the girls did and waited until problems were imminent before addressing the stressor. This reinforced the idea that girls identify with social support, whereas boys tend to solve the problem themselves. Coping behaviors learned as children often are the same strategies used in adulthood.

Age-Based Influences

Age and developmental status will influence one's coping with a diagnosis of cancer. Children react based on their ability to comprehend, and they evaluate occurrences in very personal ways (e.g., their physical reaction, what is interfered with in their lives). Adolescents react based on their level of maturity (Woodgate & Degner, 2003). During their adjustment to a cancer diagnosis, adolescents may reenact developmental tasks that they have not successfully achieved or mastered. For example, age 6–12 is the psychosocial stage where the child develops a sense of self and accomplishment. The ages of 12–18 are influenced by personal identity, autonomy, and sexual and emotional maturity. If these critical stages are interrupted by a cancer diagnosis and treatment, major developmental tasks may not be achieved, or at least are delayed (Woodgate, 2005). Many adolescents reported difficulty maintaining friendships in school and were often absent because of treatment. Some adolescents reported overprotective parents, which made it harder for them to gain independence (Hokkanen, Eriksson, Ahonen, & Salantera, 2004). In an interview, a 16-year-old female described the feeling of "body imprisonment" of not being able to walk to the bathroom by herself. This increased her stress when her family was asleep and she was dependent on their assistance. This adversely affected her sense of self and body image (Woodgate).

Erikson's (1963) theory of personality development continues to form the basis of understanding the age-related tasks or problems that each person struggles to master as he or she matures emotionally and psychologically. The impact of a cancer diagnosis will be experienced differently, to some extent, depending upon those life tasks the individual is struggling with at any given age (see Table 5-2). Many behaviors

Table 5-2. Erikson's Developmental Stages

Age	Psychosocial Stage	Main Developmental Tasks	Personality Outcomes
Birth–1 year	Trust versus mistrust	Establish a basic trust	Hope, faith, and optimism
1–3 years	Autonomy versus shame	Learn to control bodies, behavior, and their environment.	Self-control and will-power
3–6 years	Initiative versus guilt	Explore, imagine, and develop conscience.	Direction, purpose, and imagination
6–12 years	Industry versus inferiority	Work and produce; develop self-assurance.	Competence
12–18 years	Identity versus role confusion	Incorporate changes to the body; integrate concepts and values with society.	Devotion and fidelity
Early adulthood	Intimacy versus isolation	Develop intimate love and interpersonal relationships.	Affiliations, love, and mutuality
Young/middle adulthood	Generativity versus stagnation	Create and care for the next generation; nourish and nurture.	Care
Old age	Ego integrity versus despair	Become satisfied with life, and accept what has been.	Wisdom

Note. Based on information from Erikson, 1963.

are transmitted through modeling and social learning. Learning can occur through observation and imitation of others and by modifying behavior in accord with the reinforcements others receive (Sahler & Wood, 2001). Because the average age of cancer diagnosis is in the sixth decade of life, the risk for comorbid disease, decreased mobility, loss of partner, or limited finances may influence coping strategies. If the patient has a support network, good performance status, and purpose in life, the individual may have effective coping patterns.

Cancer-Specific Effects of Gender and Age

Males

For men, cancer is the second leading cause of death in the 35–54 age group, just slightly behind heart disease (Jemal et al., 2005) (see Table 5-3). Traditionally, men work outside the home and are the primary financial supporters of the family. Inside the family network, men may demonstrate many roles, including husband, father, and handyman. Time off from work for physician and office visits may result in financial hardship. Concern about job security and downsizing may interfere with men's ability to confide in their coworkers about an illness. Problem-solving skills may be based on how much time away from work the treatment will warrant (Bradley, Given, Given, & Kozachik, 2000). Nurses need to be cognizant of the needs of patients at different stages of the life span. Referral to a social worker is an appropriate intervention for problems that are beyond the training of oncology nurses.

The developmental stage of the person is an important factor when considering the emotional needs of the patient. For instance, testicular cancer generally is diagnosed in men between the ages of 20–40 (Bosl, Bajorin, Sheinfeld, Motzer, & Chaganti,

Table 5-3. Developmental Age and Deaths From Cancer in the United States, 2001

< 20 Years	20–39 Years	40–59 Years	60–79 Years	80+ Years
Males				
1. Leukemia	1. Leukemia	1. Lung	1. Lung	1. Lung
2. Brain	2. Brain	2. Colorectal	2. Colorectal	2. Prostate
3. Endocrine	3. Colon	3. Pancreas	3. Prostate	3. Colorectal
4. Bones and joints	4. NHL	4. Liver	4. Pancreas	4. Leukemia
5. Soft tissue	5. Lung	5. Esophagus	5. Leukemia	5. Bladder
Females				
1. Leukemia	1. Breast	1. Breast	1. Lung	1. Lung
2. Brain	2. Cervix	2. Lung	2. Breast	2. Colorectal
3. Endocrine	3. Leukemia	3. Colorectal	3. Colorectal	3. Breast
4. Bones and joints	4. Lung	4. Ovary	4. Pancreas	4. Pancreas
5. Soft tissue	5. Brain	5. Pancreas	5. Ovary	5. NHL

NHL—non-Hodgkin lymphoma

Note. Based on information from Centers for Disease Control and Prevention, 2002, 2004; Jemal et al., 2005.

2001). According to Erikson (1963), this is the stage of young adulthood when a man is beginning intimacy and career choices. His relationship with his partner will affect how he perceives his diagnosis. If he feels threatened in terms of his masculinity, he may develop maladaptive coping styles. If he is unmarried, worries about future acceptability as a mate may cause distress and poor judgment regarding treatment choices (Dahl et al., 2005; Reiker, 1996).

Prostate cancer generally is diagnosed after the age of 50, a time in most men's lives when their children are grown and career goals have been achieved. Men undergoing surgery for genitourinary cancers may experience altered self-esteem and body-image concerns related to incontinence and sexual dysfunction (Volk et al., 2004). Men with prostate cancer may elect not to have surgery because of undesirable side effects (O'Rourke, 2001). In a study by Volk et al., most husbands indicated they would be willing to trade some longevity to avoid complications of impotence and incontinence. These findings are consistent with those of Singer et al. (1991), who first reported that men view sexual dysfunction as a significant complication and would consider treatment options with a shorter survival benefit if their sexual functioning was maintained. Davison, Degner, and Morgan (1995) surveyed a group of men with prostate cancer and found that men tended to require more information about diagnostic tests, physical distress, and the effect of disease on their spouse, whereas women whose partner has prostate cancer needed more information about psychological well-being and the effect of the disease on the family.

Females

The multifaceted roles of a woman may include wife, mother, and financial contributor for many who work outside the home. Poor insurance coverage and loss of financial compensation are additional burdens that are magnified with a cancer diagnosis. Loss of a body part or reproductive function can be devastating for women. Although these issues appear to be similar for both men and women, women are more likely to communicate their distress. Women verbalize more concerns about body image and fertility, especially women of childbearing years (Maughan, 2003; Rowland et al., 2000).

Most research concerning the female response to cancer has involved women with breast cancer. Women being treated for this disease generally experience anxiety and distress, especially related to altered body image, regardless of the type of breast surgery. Younger women are more likely to report sexual problems and a sense of isolation, anxiety, and depression (Ganz et al., 2002). A focus group of 34 Asian women breast cancer survivors reported many concerns such as lack of knowledge and gender role and family obligations. They were concerned about their children and burdening the family (Ashing, Padilla, Tejero, & Kagawa-Singer, 2003). Younger women with ovarian cancer experienced more psychological distress and anxiety after treatment, whereas women with a strong marriage before treatment had less distress post-treatment (Caldwell et al., 2003). A literature review of the psychosocial impact of a woman's breast cancer diagnosis on her family reported that husbands generally experienced feelings of anxiety and distress (Northouse, 1995). Husbands who lacked social support reported more emotional distress. Younger spouses, regardless of gender, reacted more emotionally to a partner's illness than did older spouses (Walker, 1997).

In addition to the stress of the cancer diagnosis on women, cancer can transform family roles. Marriage is recognized as having a positive influence on emotional support and reduction of depression (Davies, Avison, & McAlpine, 1997; Desai & Jann, 2000). The degree of satisfaction in the marriage prior to the diagnosis influences the positive outcome of support (Walker, 1997; Whisman, 2001). Fear of cancer recurrence, anxiety and helplessness, and lack of information can cause distress for the partner or caregiver, although women tend to worry more about the impact on the family. The caregiver role can affect the family unit, resulting in emotional distress that is more severe for the caregiver than for the individual with cancer (Boehmer & Clark, 2001; Northouse et al., 2000; Walker). Research has shown that coping strategies that provide problem-solving plans reduce stress and empower the patient and/or caregiver (Bucher et al., 2001). This seems to be particularly true for men (Davison et al., 2003). Research has found that providing structured information supports more active decision making for patients and lower levels of distress for patients and spouses (Davison et al., 2003).

Culture and Gender

Gender is just one of the many considerations when trying to understand the patient with cancer. More than race and ethnicity, cultural practices provide individuals with beliefs and values. Individuals use ritualistic and familiar behaviors in times of stress that give security and meaning to uncontrolled and unforeseen events (Kagawa-Singer, 1995). Interpersonal relationships differ among cultures, and obtaining a professional interpreter (instead of using a family member) in cases involving a language barrier may be necessary so that information is not withheld or misunderstood. More specifically, when caring for Asian American and Latino families, nurses need to recognize the geographic varieties of these ethnic groups and differences involving geographic immigration. For example, in the traditional Latino family, status is typically from oldest to youngest, and from men to women. In times of grief, Latino women may respond by crying openly. Latino men are expected to be strong and often do not grieve openly; however, hugging and human touch are appropriate strategies for the healthcare team to use to show support to Latino individuals (Clements et al., 2003). In the Asian family, the husband maintains a role of leadership and dominance. The son sometimes performs this role as well. The wife is the homemaker and child caretaker. For Asians who are born in the United States or who immigrated years ago, cultural conflict or adaptation to less traditional roles may occur (Bjorck, Cuthbertson, Thurman, & Lee, 2001; Kim, Laroche, & Tomiuk, 2004).

Conclusion

The ability of the oncology team to recognize and identify individual psychosocial differences will assist in the understanding of patients' coping styles. Patients present to the clinician not just with a cancer diagnosis but also with a history of life lessons and influences that shape the individual's personality and coping style. Further research needs to examine differences among gender, developmental phases, and culture. The future of health care has moved from the hospital to the home. The role of the caregiver and family unit will be important assessments, as both the patient and the caregiver will be at risk for experiencing emotional and physical factors in response to the cancer diagnosis. Further research examining differences in gender-specific coping patterns, in addition to the developmental transitions for the aging process, will assist in the identification of at-risk maladaptive coping patterns. This will allow for appropriate and supportive nursing interventions and therapeutic outcomes for patients and families.

References

American Cancer Society. (2005). *Cancer facts and figures, 2005*. Atlanta, GA: Author.

Ashing, K.T., Padilla, G., Tejero, J., & Kagawa-Singer, M. (2003). Understanding the breast cancer experience of Asian American women. *Psycho-Oncology, 12*, 38–58.

Barsevick, A.M., Much, J., & Sweeney, C. (2000). Psychosocial response to cancer. In C.H. Yarbro, M.H. Frogge, M. Goodman, & S.L. Groenwald (Eds.), *Cancer nursing: Principles and practice* (5th ed., pp. 1529–1549). Sudbury, MA: Jones and Bartlett.

Bjorck, J.P., Cuthbertson, W., Thurman, J.W., & Lee, Y.S. (2001). Ethnicity, coping and distress among Korean Americans, Filipino Americans, and Caucasian Americans. *Journal of Social Psychology, 141*, 421–441.

Boehmer, U., & Clark, J.A. (2001). Communication about prostate cancer between men and their wives. *Journal of Family Practice, 50*, 226–231.

Boekaerts, M. (1996). Coping with stress in childhood and adolescence. In M. Zeidner & N.S. Endler (Eds.), *Handbook of coping* (pp. 452–484). New York: John Wiley.

Bosl, G.J., Bajorin, D.F., Sheinfeld, J., Motzer, R.J., & Chaganti, R.S.K. (2001). Cancer of the testis. In V.T. DeVita, Jr., S. Hellman, & S.A. Rosenberg (Eds.), *Cancer principles and practice of oncology* (6th ed., pp. 1491–1518). Philadelphia: Lippincott Williams and Wilkins.

Bower, J.E., Ganz, P.A., Desmond, K.A., Rowland, J.H., Meyerowitz, B.E., & Belin, T.R. (2000). Fatigue in breast cancer survivors: Occurrence, correlates, and impact on quality of life. *Journal of Clinical Oncology, 18*, 743–753.

Bradley, C.J., Given, B.A., Given, C.W., & Kozachik, S. (2000). Physical, economic, and social issues confronting patients and families. In C.H. Yarbro, M.H. Frogge, M. Goodman, & S.L. Groenwald (Eds.), *Cancer nursing: Principles and practice* (5th ed., pp. 1550–1564). Sudbury, MA. Jones and Bartlett.

Brown, K.A.E., & Barbarin, O.A. (1996). Gender differences in parenting a child with cancer. *Social Work in Health Care, 22*(4), 53–71.

Bucher, J.A., Loscalzo, M., Zabora, J., Houts, P.S., Hooker, C., & BrintzenhofeSzoc, K. (2001). Problem-solving cancer care education for patients and caregivers. *Cancer Practice, 9*, 66–70.

Caldwell, R., Classen, C., Lagana, L., McGarvey, E., Baum, L., Duenke, S., et al. (2003). Changes in sexual functioning and mood among women treated for gynecological cancer who receive group therapy: A pilot study. *Journal of Clinical Psychology in Medical Settings, 10*, 149–156.

Carmel, S., & Bernstein, J.H. (2003). Gender differences in physical health and psychosocial well being among four age groups of elderly people in Israel. *International Journal of Aging and Human Development, 56*, 113–131.

Centers for Disease Control and Prevention. (2002). *Mortality data from the National Vital Statistics System*. Retrieved June 14, 2005, from http://www.cdc.gov/nchs/about/major/dvs/mortdata.htm

Centers for Disease Control and Prevention. (2004). *Behavioral risk factor survey*. Atlanta, GA: National Center for Chronic Disease Prevention and Health Promotion, Centers for Disease Control and Prevention and Health Promotion.

Clements, P.T., Vigil, G.J., Manno, M.S., Henry, G.C., Wilks, J., Das, S., et al. (2003). Cultural response to death. *Psychosocial Nursing, 41*(7), 18–26.

Courts, N., Newton, A., & McNeal, L. (2005). Husbands and wives living with multiple sclerosis. *Journal of Neuroscience Nursing, 37*, 20–27.

Dahl, A.A., Haaland, C.F., Mykletun, A., Bremnes, R., Dahl, A., Klepp, O., et al. (2005). Study of anxiety disorder and depression in long-term survivors of testicular cancer. *Journal of Clinical Oncology, 23*, 2389–2395.

Davies, L., Avison, W.R., & McAlpine, D.D. (1997). Significant life experiences and depression among single and married mothers. *Journal of Marriage and Family, 59*, 294–308.

Davison, J.B., Degner, L.F., & Morgan, T.R. (1995). Information and decision-making preferences of men with prostate cancer. *Oncology Nursing Forum, 22*, 1401–1408.

Davison, J.B., Goldenberg, L., Gleave, M.E., & Degner, L.F. (2003). Provision of individualized information to men and their partners to facilitate treatment decision making in prostate cancer. *Oncology Nursing Forum, 30*, 107–114.

Desai, H., & Jann, M. (2000). Major depression in women: A review of the literature. *Journal of the American Pharmaceutical Association, 40*, 525–537.

Erikson, E.H. (1963). *Childhood and society* (2nd ed.). New York: Norton.

Ganz, P.A., Desmond, K.A., Leedham, B., Rowland, J.H., Meyerowitz, B.E., & Belin, T.R. (2002). Quality of life in long-term, disease-free survivors of breast cancer: A follow-up study. *Journal of the National Cancer Institute, 94*, 39–49.

Geis, F.L. (1993). Self-fulfilling prophecies: A social psychological view of gender. In A.E. Beall & R.J. Sternberg (Eds.), *The psychology of gender* (pp. 9–54). New York: Guilford Press.

Gerber, G.L. (1989). Gender stereotypes. In J. Offerman-Zuckerberg (Ed.), *Gender in transition: A new frontier* (pp. 47–66). New York: Plenum.

Germino, B.B., Mishel, M.H., Belyea, M., Harris, L., Ware, A., & Mohler, J. (1998). Uncertainty in prostate cancer. *Cancer Practice, 6*, 107–113.

Harrison, J., Maguire, P., & Pitceathly, C. (1995). Confiding in crisis: Gender differences in pattern of confiding among cancer patients. *Social Science and Medicine, 41*, 1255–1260.

Hokkanen, H., Eriksson, E., Ahonen, O., & Salantera, S. (2004). Adolescents with cancer: Experience of life and how it could be made easier. *Cancer Nursing, 27*, 325–335.

Jemal, A., Murray, T., Ward, E., Samuels, A., Tiwari, R., Ghafoor, A., et al. (2005). Cancer statistics, 2005. *CA: A Cancer Journal for Clinicians, 55*, 10–30.

Kagawa-Singer, M. (1995). Socioeconomic and cultural influences on cancer care of women. *Seminars in Oncology Nursing, 11*, 109–119.

Kim, C., Laroche, M., & Tomiuk, M.A. (2004). The Chinese in Canada: A study in ethnic change with emphasis on gender roles. *Journal of Social Psychology, 144*, 5–29.

Kim, H.S., Yeom, H.A., Seo, Y.S., Kim, N.C., & Yoo, Y.S. (2002). Stress and coping strategies of patients with cancer. A Korean study. *Cancer Nursing, 25*, 425–431.

Kronenwetter, C., Weidner, G., Pettengill, E., Marlin, R., Crutchfield, L., McCormac, M., et al. (2005). A qualitative analysis of interviews of men with early stage prostate cancer. *Cancer Nursing, 28*, 99–107.

Lamb, M.E. (2004). The role of the father: An overview. In M.E. Lamb (Ed.), *The role of the father in child development* (4th ed., pp. 283–297). New York: John Wiley.

Lazarus, R.S., & Folkman, S. (1984). *Stress, appraisal, and coping.* New York: Springer.

Levenson, J.L. (2003). Psychological factors affecting medical conditions. In R.E. Hales & S.C. Yudofsky (Eds.), *American Psychiatric Press textbook of clinical psychiatry* (4th ed., pp. 631–657). Washington, DC: American Psychiatric Publishing.

Matthews, B.A. (2003). Role and gender differences in cancer-related distress: A comparison of survivor and caregiver self-reports. *Oncology Nursing Forum, 30*, 493–499.

Maughan, K. (2003). Specific keynote: In the shadow of illness—Supporting women with ovarian cancer. *Gynecologic Oncology, 88*(1 Pt. 2), S129–S133.

Northouse, L.L. (1995). The impact of cancer in women on the family. *Cancer Practice, 3*, 134–142.

Northouse, L.L., Mood, D., Templin, T., Mellon, S., & George, T. (2000). Couples' patterns of adjustment to colon cancer. *Social Science and Medicine, 50*, 271–284.

O'Rourke, M.E. (2001). Decision making and prostate cancer treatment selection: A review. *Seminars in Oncology Nursing, 17*, 108–117.

Pruett, K.D. (2002). Family development and the roles of mothers and fathers in child rearing. In M. Lewis (Ed.), *Child adolescent psychiatry: A comprehensive textbook* (3rd ed., pp. 287–292). Philadelphia: Lippincott Williams & Wilkins.

Reiker, P. (1996). How should a man with testicular cancer be counseled and what information is available to him? *Seminars in Urologic Oncology, 14,* 17–22.

Rowland, J.H., Desmond, K.A., Meyerowitz, B.E., Belin, T.R., Wyatt, G.E., & Ganz, P. (2000). Role of breast reconstructive surgery in physical and emotional outcomes among breast cancer survivors. *Journal of the National Cancer Institute, 92,* 1422–1429.

Sahler, O.J., & Wood, B.L. (2001). Theories and concepts of development as they relate to pediatric practice. In R.A. Hoekelman, H.M. Adams, N.M. Nelson, M.L. Nicholas, M.L. Weitzman, & M.H. Wilson (Eds.), *Primary pediatric care* (4th ed., pp. 637–654). St. Louis, MO: Mosby.

Simon, R. (1995). Gender, multiple roles, role meaning, and mental health. *Journal of Health and Social Behavior, 36,* 182–194.

Simpson, P.A., & Stroh, L.K. (2004). Gender differences: Emotional expression and feelings of personal inauthenticity. *Journal of Applied Psychology, 89,* 715–721.

Singer, P., Tasch, E., Stocking, C., Rubin, S., Siefler, M., & Weichselbaum, R. (1991). Sex or survival: Trade-offs between quality and quantity of life. *Journal of Clinical Oncology, 9,* 328–334.

Stellman, J.M., & Stellman, S.D. (1995). Social factors: Women and cancer. *Seminars in Oncology Nursing, 11,* 103–108.

Volk, R., Cantor, S., Cass, A., Spann, S., Weller, S., & Krahn, M. (2004). Preferences of husbands and wives for outcomes of prostate cancer screening and treatment. *Journal of General Internal Medicine, 19,* 339–348.

Walker, B.L. (1997). Adjustment of husbands and wives to breast cancer. *Cancer Practice, 5,* 92–98.

Weidner, G., & Collins, R.L. (1993). Gender, coping, and health. In H.W. Krohne (Ed.), *Attention avoidance: Strategies in coping with aversiveness* (pp. 241–266). Seattle, WA: Hogrefe & Huber.

Whisman, M.A. (2001). Marital adjustment and outcome following treatments for depression. *Journal of Consulting and Clinical Psychology, 69,* 125–129.

Woodgate, R. (2005). A different way of being: Adolescents' experience with cancer. *Cancer Nursing, 28,* 8–15.

Woodgate, R.L., & Degner, L.F. (2003). Expectations and beliefs about children's cancer symptoms: Perspectives of children with cancer and their families. *Oncology Nursing Forum, 30,* 479–491.

Zeidner, M., & Saklofske, D. (1996). Adaptive and maladaptive coping. In M. Zeidner & N.S. Endler (Eds.), *Handbook of coping* (pp. 505–531). New York: John Wiley.

CHAPTER 6

Cultural Influences on the Psychosocial Experience

DeLois P. Weekes, RN, BS, MS, DNSc

We cannot live for ourselves alone. Our lives are connected by a thousand invisible threads, and along these sympathetic fibers, our actions run as causes and return to us as results.

—Herman Melville

Of all those invisible threads and sympathetic fibers that connect one life to another, culture is, perhaps, the most ubiquitous. Culture affects every action and response to the exigencies of life. Cultural fibers are the invisible threads that influence how individuals respond to a cancer diagnosis, treatment, side effects of treatment, living with the disease, and facing death.

Nishimoto and Foley (2001) reminded healthcare professionals that it is the empathetic appreciation of the patient's background and way of life that supports and enables the provision of culturally competent care. That is, what the cancer experience means to patients and their family cannot be interpreted or understood in isolation; rather, it must be viewed from the cultural context that frames responses to the cancer experience. In many ways, culture functions as a tool for the creation of one's reality and the definition of one's purpose in life within that reality. Culture plays a pivotal role in defining the proper way to behave in a particular situation to maintain integrity and self-respect (Kagawa-Singer, 1998).

The cultural background of an ethnic or racial group influences the knowledge, attitudes, and practices of the group members that, in large part, determine the way members respond to disease prevention, treatment, and health care. When oncology nursing fails to attend to patients' culture and ethnicity, patients can interpret the care as insensitive and inappropriate (Guidry & Walker, 1999).

Each person forms beliefs about health and illness from his or her unique cultural/racial background and experience. Therefore, knowledge of the cultural identity of patients with cancer and concomitant skill in providing culturally competent care are key because without understanding how culture and race affect patients' behavioral responses, oncology nurses cannot provide appropriate, competent care.

Culture and Psychosocial Responses to Cancer

Growth of cultural competence in oncology nurses is in many ways associated with the degree to which they are able to bridge the cultural divide that exists between cultures and integrate culturally relevant content into the health history (Watts, 2003). Bridging the divide is facilitated by openness and sensitivity to the patients' world views, cultural beliefs, health and illness conceptualization, and integration of race consciousness into practice. Watts described race consciousness as awareness of the historical journey of the cultural group, knowledge of disparities in health care, and self-appraisal of the nurse's own attitudes and biases toward the group. As the divide is bridged, the oncology nurse's consideration of the influence of culture on individual and family responses to the cancer experience (e.g., diagnosis, treatment, side effects, living with cancer, facing death) becomes an inherent part of his or her practice. Bridging the cultural divide enables oncology nurses to become client-centered versus disease-centered practitioners. As a client-centered practitioner, oncology nurses listen to how patients define the illness, the language and terms used by patients to express their psychosocial response to the illness, and their beliefs about what is causing the illness (Castillo, 1997).

Psychosocial responses are triggered by the patient's awareness of changes in how his or her body feels. After awareness, decisions are made about whether the body is in a state of sickness or illness (Kleinman, Eisenberg, & Good, 1978). Next, the patient or family initiates actions to effect recovery, which may include seeking advice from extended family, healers, the community, and medical professionals. Kleinman et al. indicated that this process occurs across ethnic, cultural, and racial groups. The rate at which the process occurs, the type and nature of sickness/illness, the level of family and community involvement, and the point at which medical professionals are consulted are culturally determined. The nature of the illness is further shaped by patients' expectations and perceptions of symptoms, meanings learned from culture, and the extent to which the type of sickness/illness is viewed as socially acceptable within the culture.

Development of culturally appropriate programs includes assessment to elicit culturally valid and reliable information upon which to base intervention plans. Panos and Panos (2000) offered a culturally sensitive assessment process that focuses on several qualitative domains: (a) assess one's own cultural identity to identify biases from own cultural background, similarities, and dissimilarities of personal cultural values to those of patients and those of the dominant culture; (b) assess patients' level of acculturation and language preference to obtain information about their time in the United States and the degree to which they have adopted values and norms of the dominant culture; (c) assess the impact of acculturative stress—stress resulting from adjusting to life changes, such as a new language, different customs, and norms for social interaction occurring after immigration to a new host country (Berry, 1997), and determine the impact of adjustments and transitions on patients' emotional and physical health; (d) assess patients' family relationships and social support to determine the family structure (e.g., authority, decision making, gender roles) and kin network; and (e) assess patients' views and concepts of health and illness to determine their definition of illness and health, beliefs about causes of illness, description of symptoms, and where they go for healing.

Understanding of a particular patient's beliefs, values, and practices is facilitated further by conducting an interview aimed at obtaining information to help to explain the patient's view and definition of the sickness/illness, as well as what he or she thinks should be done about it and by whom. Kleinman et al. (1978) developed an explanatory model interview that, since its inception, many practitioners have found to be of benefit in determining patients' beliefs and practices related to sickness/illness. Guided by this model, a simple interview has been developed that can be completed in five minutes that enables the nurse to access essential information about patients' cultural beliefs. Although psychosocial responses differ across cultural groups, some similarities exist; therefore, nurses may use the interview with most cultural groups (see Figure 6-1).

Figure 6-1. Health and Illness Beliefs Interview

- What do you call your problem?
- What would you say brought the problem on?
- When did you first notice the problem?
- How long have you had the problem?
- How long do you think the problem will last?
- Do you believe this to be a serious problem?
- How do you feel now compared to how you felt before you had the problem?
- What have you done to help make the problem go away or to help you to feel better?
- How do you think the problem should be handled and by whom?

Note. Based on information from Kleinman et al., 1978.

Overview of Major Cultural Groups

The population of the United States is a fluid and dynamic mix of cultural and ethnic groups. Diversity within groups, variance in levels of acculturation and adaptation, socioeconomic status, and religious backgrounds also contribute to this rich mosaic. As a result, oncology nurses will inevitably work with patients and clients from diverse cultural and ethnic backgrounds. Although this is exciting, it also is challenging because the population is ever growing, both in number and diversity. Many cultural subgroups exist; however, this discussion will focus on three primary cultural groups: African Americans, Asian Americans, and Latinos/Hispanics. Table 6-1 presents a comparison of the cultural values of these major groups.

African Americans

In 1990, African Americans constituted 11.7% of the U.S. population. By 2000, the population had increased to 33.9 million or 12.1% of the total U.S. population (U.S. Census Bureau, 2005). Over the past 10 years, the number of African Americans increased faster than the non-Hispanic white population, and they are the predominant minority group in the South, where they constitute 19% of the population. The next largest concentrations are in the Northeast (12%), the Midwest (11%), and the West (6%) (U.S. Census Bureau).

Table 6-1. Major Cultural Groups: Comparison of Cultural Values

Cultural Values	African Americans	Asian/Pacific Islanders	Latinos/Hispanics
Communication			
• Restrained		X	
• Indirect		X	
• Nonverbal		X	
• Verbal	X		X
Family			
• Dutifulness/familial piety/*respecto*		X	X
• Extended networks	X	X	X
• Multigenerational/interdependent	X	X	X
Collective versus individual		X	X
Gender roles			
• Male identity linked to ability to provide for family	X		
• Female identity linked to mother, nurturer, caretaker	X	X	X
• Patriarchal/male		X	X
Saving face; respect	X	X	X
Harmony with body and environment		X	X

Note. Based on information from Flanagan, 2002.

Provision of culturally competent care to African Americans demands an understanding of the historical and sociopolitical contexts that influenced the culture. Arguably, the seminal historical event that stamped the culture of African Americans is slavery. The African American culture was forged in the crucible of slavery, which brought about the transformation of Africans from diverse cultural backgrounds into African Americans—a group defined by the color of their skin and inextricably bound together by the common experience of being forcibly transplanted and made subservient to European Americans. This transformation involved the adoption of aspects of European American cultural, social, and political practices without total abandonment of African cultural values that persist today (Carson, 1993). Not only did Africans adopt European cultural practices, but they also infused the European culture with their own cultural and social practices. Then, as now, the institutionalization of the African American culture occurred largely through the church (Carson).

Slavery, the meaning attached to it, and skin color continue to influence African Americans as a cultural group. Race, racism, and racial discrimination are rooted in the legacy of slavery and color all facets of life for African Americans. These factors make the African American experience in America distinctively different from that of other immigrants or refugees (Watts, 2003). Unlike other immigrants or refugees who relocated to this country by choice, African Americans were transported without choice, chained together as human cargo (Thomas, 1997).

Because of slavery and skin color, many African Americans have had and expect to have a negative healthcare experience (Smedley, Stith, & Nelson, 2002). Knowledge of the dehumanization and exploitation of African Americans in matters of health has been transmitted through folklore and historical documentation across generations (Smedley et al.). The Tuskegee story continues to reverberate through African American communities. Historian Reverby (1999) described the Tuskegee study in which African Americans thought they were being treated for their syphilis but were intentionally not treated as an exemplar of medical arrogance and unethical behavior born of racism in research.

Fear of exploitation based on race and skin color has engendered distrust of the healthcare system and reluctance of African Americans to participate in research, especially health care (i.e., access, screening, and utilization) (Lavizzo-Mourey & Mackenzie, 1996). A report by the Commonwealth Fund (Collins et al., 2002) of a telephone survey of 6,722 Whites, African Americans, Hispanics, and Asian Americans conducted by Princeton Survey Research Associates examined four major categories in health care: patient-physician communication, cultural competence in healthcare services, quality of clinical care, and access to care. Those from minority backgrounds reported less satisfaction with communication with physicians, less confidence in the physician, being treated with less respect, not being understood, not being offered alternative therapies, and less overall satisfaction with care. The results support the need to address cultural barriers to health care for racial and ethnic minorities.

African American culture is distinct and unique as a result, in large part, to the experience of slavery and ongoing discrimination. Bobo (2001) postulated that even at the end of the 20th century, a more modern type of "laissez-faire racism" continues to foster stereotypical treatment of African Americans, particularly in health care.

Asian/Pacific Islanders

The term "Asian/Pacific Islanders" refers to people whose familial roots originate from 43 ethnic groups and cultures consisting of 28 Asian groups and 15 Pacific Islander groups (Flanagan, 2002). Clearly, this is a heterogeneous group, whose numbers in the United States increased from 6.9 million in 1990 to 10.5 million in 2000. More than half (60%) are foreign-born, with many settling in the United States after 1980. Slightly more than one-third (36%) reside in California; however, Asian Americans are moving into the South, the Midwest, and the Northeast. In general, Asian Americans are well-educated, with 42% having a bachelor's degree or higher compared to 28% for non-Hispanic whites. Three general ethnicities exist within the Asian/Pacific Islanders cultural group: (a) Pacific Islanders, mostly Hawaiians, Samoans, and Guamanians; (b) Southeast Asians, largely Indochinese from Vietnam, Thailand, Cambodia, Laos, and Burmese and Filipinos; and (c) East Asians, including Chinese, Japanese, and Koreans (Trueba, Cheng, & Ima, 1993).

These three large groups differ in sociocultural traits, and there is wide-ranging diversity within each group, making cross-cultural communication a fundamental issue. Thus, it is important not to generalize one set of cultural understandings from one group to another. Although Indochinese (the Vietnamese and Hmong) differ in their basic cultural patterns, many Vietnamese have Chinese ancestry and are literate with strong abilities to adapt to the market society. In contrast, the Hmong have no written language and no skills that are easily applicable to the American marketplace (Huang, 1993).

In general, within the Asian culture, family is pivotal, may be patriarchal (i.e., focus on male authority) with roles defined around the primary authority of the father, and if the father dies, the eldest son assumes authority (Kitano, 1997). Improper behavior reflects not only on the individual, but the entire family. Behavior is viewed as a reflection of harmony or disharmony. Conformance to the rule of *filial piety* (respect for and provision of material, emotional, and psychological support to parents) is not only an expectation, but a duty in the Asian/Pacific Islanders' culture (Flanagan, 2002). Communication may be restrained, indirect, and include more nonverbal behavior. Failure to control emotions may be viewed as improper or shameful, resulting in loss of face for the family.

Embedded within the culture of many diverse groups are subtle cues that guide, influence, and regulate behavior (Flanagan, 2002). Provision of culturally competent care necessitates learning how to read the unspoken cues that enable one to walk, talk, and move appropriately within the culture without giving offense. For example, in some cultures even though the wife is the patient, conversations about her care occur with the husband or another male relative. The nurse may only learn this information through observation versus being explicitly told. This point is illustrated in the following example: An oncology nurse visited a Vietnamese patient in her hospital room during her recovery from breast cancer surgery. The nurse sat down, crossing her legs with her foot pointing toward the patient. The nurse noted that the patient seemed upset and embarrassed, but had no idea why, so she went on explaining the reason for her visit. Later the nurse learned that within the Vietnamese culture, the foot is considered profane. Thus, crossing the legs and letting the foot point at the patient is insulting to some Southeast Asians (Lindsay, Narayan, & Rea, 1998).

Time is another aspect of the covert culture. Many Southeast Asians/Pacific Islanders have a polychromic time (P-time) framework, in contrast to the Western monochromic time (M-time) concept (Huang, 1993). Within a P-time framework, different social interactions can happen simultaneously, whereas M-time demands a linear scheduling of events. Healthcare providers operating from an M-time perspective may view the P-time cultural norm as disruptive of scheduled hospital routines and tests. In contrast, when healthcare providers operate from a P-time perspective, the patient may view the nurse's expectations related to meals and baths, for example, as disrespectful. An understanding of cultural differences related to time may help healthcare providers to facilitate interactions with the patient and family and avoid misunderstandings.

Another covert cultural dimension is communication. Problems in communication between healthcare providers and Asian/Pacific Islanders, if not thoughtfully dealt with, may mitigate access to health care for this group. For example, nodding of the head means one thing to Westerners and another to many Asian and Pacific Islanders. Consider, for example, when some Asian patients say "ya" after having a procedure explained, often "ya" is interpreted as "yes" and viewed as affirmation. However, for many Asians, "ya" indicates respect and not necessarily agreement or understanding;

rather, it means, "I am listening, and I respect what you are saying." In conversations, Asians tend to favor verbal hesitancy and ambiguity, the intent of which is to avoid being offensive (Lindsay et al., 1998). Thus, to gain a fuller understanding about how Asian patients are responding to the situation, nonverbal cues become very important. This is sometimes problematic because Westerners often attend to what is explicitly said, ignoring nonverbal cues, such as verbal hesitancy.

The overt culture is embedded in values and norms, language, religion, philosophy, custom, and social organization forms, such as family. Some East Asians reflect both the Chinese tradition and Indian Buddhism. In comparison, Pacific Islanders historically have struggled to preserve their identity in the face of ongoing colonial oppression, giving them a unique and rich tribal cultural heritage (Trueba et al., 1993).

In summary, the Asian/Pacific Islander culture stems, in part, from the combined influence of Confucianism and Buddhism (Lee, 1996). As a result, the culture places emphasis on the collective or family unit, instead of the individual. Individual behavior is viewed as a reflection of the entire family system as well as the ancestral lineage (Flanagan, 2002). Maintenance of harmony is believed to be essential to health. Communication tends to be restrained, indirect, and nonverbal.

Latinos/Hispanics

The terms "Latino" and "Hispanic" are labels used to describe people from diverse settings and sociopolitical histories. They include Cubans, Chicanos, Mexicans, Argentineans, Colombians, Dominicans, Brazilians, Guatemalans, Costa Ricans, Nicaraguans, Salvadorians, and other nationalities from South America, Central America, and the Caribbean (Garcia-Preto, 1996). Because it affirms their native, pre-Hispanic identity, many Spanish-speaking immigrants from Latin America prefer the term "Latino" (Falicov, 1998). The term "Hispanic" is associated with political conservative groups who regard Spanish European ancestry as superior to the indigenous, native groups in the Americas (Falicov). Therefore, many Spanish-speaking groups view the term with disdain. Nevertheless, the U.S. Census Bureau employs the term "Hispanic" as a general rubric when referencing individuals living in the United States who have descendants from Spanish-speaking Latin American countries or from Spain.

According to the 2000 census, the Latino/Hispanic population has increased from 22 million in 1990 to 35 million in 2000, surpassing African Americans. Traditionally, the Latino/Hispanic groups were concentrated in the Southwest and West and a few areas such as New York, New Jersey, and Chicago. However, by 2000, the Census Bureau reported that Latinos/Hispanics were dispersing to smaller cities and rural areas in the Midwest, the South, and the Northeast (U.S. Census Bureau, 2005).

Distinctive models of family interaction have been developed and retained within the Latino/Hispanic culture. In the main, one of the most significant cultural values for Latinos/Hispanics is family unity, commitment, and obligation (Garcia-Preto, 1996). In some instances, the traditional model has been combined with values and norms acquired in the United States, resulting in a blended model. Nevertheless, family reflects strong family ties (blood and fictive kin [i.e., individuals viewed and treated as members of one's family]), living in proximity to one another, economic and social support to extended family, caring for ill or dependent family members, and emphasis on respect for elders (Garcia-Preto). This family interdependence and inclusiveness is referred to as *familismo* (Falicov, 1998). In some Latino/Hispanic family units, the *compadres* (godparents) may be quite prominent, providing economic and emotional assistance to the family (Garcia-Preto). The practice of *hijos de crianza*, transferring children from one nuclear family to extended family in times of crisis, is characteristic of some Latino/Hispanic families (Garcia-Preto). Gender roles may be organized around *machismo* (male authority in the family) and *marianismo* (female obedience to husband and nurturance of children) (Green, 1999). *Respecto* or dutifulness is owed to parents (Falicov).

Health and Illness Beliefs

Although patients experience myriad psychosocial responses to cancer screening, diagnosis, and treatment, most emanate from the health and illness beliefs embedded in the cultural, ethnic, and racial backgrounds of the particular group. Traditional explanatory models of health and illness often contain supernatural, magical, and moral injunctions and explanations that become the basis for treatment and intervention. When the culturally derived beliefs about health and illness are not considered and integrated into health care, patients may ignore, misuse, or complain about the nature and quality of the care and treatment they receive. For example, a 46-year-old Mexican-American woman who had lived in the United States for 15 years was diagnosed with intestinal cancer, treated with chemotherapy and surgery, and had no oral intake. Because she was no longer taking food by mouth, disrupting the hot/cold balance of nutrients that is the basis of the traditional health beliefs of the folk system in which she grew up, she believed that her doctors had given up on her. In response to this belief, she refused to cooperate with any aspect of treatment, did not communicate, and simply waited to die (Smiley, McMillan, Johnson, & Ojeda, 2000).

Kleinman et al. (1978) suggested that physicians typically operate from a disease-oriented explanatory model that focuses on the diagnosis and treatment of malfunctioning or maladaptive biologic and psychophysiologic processes. Patients experience illness as a subjective, intrapersonal event that emerges from their racial, ethnic, and cultural background and experience, which often has little to do with biologic or physiologic processes. When discord exists between the health and illness beliefs of the patient and provider, tension arises between the physician's prescribed treatment and the patient's perception of its relative efficacy. Patients frequently seek assistance from biomedical professionals to alleviate their symptoms and from folk healers to deal with the root cause of the illness. Therefore, oncology nurses must understand culturally influenced schemas of health and illness (Flanagan, 2002; Pachter, 1994).

As indicated earlier, considerable variance exists among and within the three major cultural groups, and concomitant variation is present in the health and illness beliefs held by each group. Yet, because of several common underlying themes, similarities also exist (Hufford, 1997). A common theme is that disease etiology usually is attributed to (a) some sort of imbalance or disharmony, including sin, personal relationships, and spiritual and environmental elements; (b) the patient's interrelationship with his or her body, community, or physical environment, and personal responsibility; and (c) energies that influence harmony and balance, exemplified in the Latino/Hispanic culture by the belief that if they eat too much hot food, illness will occur unless there is counterbalance with cold foods. A comparison of the health and illness beliefs of the three major cultures relative to the underlying themes appears in Table 6-2.

Table 6-2. Health and Illness Beliefs: Comparison of Major Cultural Groups

Health/Illness Belief	African Americans	Asian/Pacific Islanders	Latinos/Hispanics
Etiology of disease			
• Energies that influence harmony or balance			
- Hot and cold foods		X	X
- Energy fields: elements of the universe (e.g., fire, water, wind) and body	X	X	
• Imbalance or lack of harmony			
- Personal and social relationships	X	X	X
- Community interactions		X	
- Body and physical environment	X	X	
- Spiritual relationships (e.g., sin, evil spirits)	X	X	X
- Ancestral relationships		X	
- Body and mind (Yin-Yang with disruption of qi)		X	

Note. Based on information from Flanagan, 2002.

Cultural Influences on Responses to the Cancer Experience

Clinicians practicing in ethnically diverse settings generally agree that patients' ethnicity and culture affect the experience of illness and the response to treatment. Many sociologists describe culture as the learned, shared behavior of the members of a society. Culture also may be seen as beliefs, values, and morals passed on by significant others (e.g., teachers, parents, other family members). Culture is a very important factor that permeates and determines patients' and providers' responses to all life experiences (Prior, 1996).

Family and community are critically important in all three major cultural groups. Examples of the influence of family and community within the cultures on responses to cancer screening, diagnosis, and treatment are reflected in findings from selected studies. In a study of well-being in Hispanic and non-Hispanic survivors of breast cancer, Dirksen and Erickson (2002) found that social support from significant others (i.e., family) was a positive predictor of resourcefulness and well-being for Hispanic women. Social support was found to mitigate uncertainty for the Hispanic women. This finding is in concert with the value of family (blood relatives and fictive kin) in the Latino/Hispanic culture. These findings reinforce the importance of determining whom the cultural group views as supportive and of ensuring that patients have access to those individuals as needed. Social support also was a positive predictor of well-being for non-Hispanic white women. The researchers concluded that helpful support from others strongly affects well-being.

Katapodi, Facione, Miaskowski, Dodd, and Waters (2002) conducted a study of the influence of social support, defined as exchange of resources between at least two individuals (provider and recipient), to determine whether an improvement occurred in the well-being of the recipient. The researchers concluded that healthcare professionals often fail to acknowledge the importance of social support networks to the well-being of Hispanic patients.

In a study examining social support among Japanese women with breast cancer, Makabe and Hull (2000) found that Japanese women described three distinct experiences of social support. "Simply do it," occurring during the diagnostic phase of the cancer diagnosis, referred to advice from others that encouraged them to avoid delaying treatment. "Doing with/being with" occurred during hospitalization and was the physical presence of another person without verbal communication. "Doing for" occurred during treatment and recovery and referred to the supportive presence of another who took on responsibilities typically carried out by the woman. These findings are congruent with the Asian/Pacific Islanders' cultural value of nonverbal communication and support the importance of family and community to patients from diverse cultural groups. Jens, Chaney, and Brodie (2001) admonished oncology nurses to ask assessment questions about patients' home community. This kind of assessment reveals the degree of separation patients might experience as a result of the cancer diagnosis. Separation of patients from a community that provides cultural and contextual supports in the form of relatives, religious, and spiritual connections may adversely affect patients' acceptance of the diagnosis and treatment (Jens et al.).

Cultural predispositions that are deeply rooted and a lack of family support play pivotal roles in the degree to which people from multicultural populations participate in the early detection and prevention of cancer, as well as in cancer treatment programs. Indeed, when approached from a cultural perspective, people from these populations are difficult to reach and often are distrustful of the dominant group for cultural and linguistic reasons (Walters & Ankomah, 1996). Many programs aimed at fostering increased cancer screening participation by individuals from multicultural backgrounds continue to achieve limited success. As a result, during the past two decades, despite improved methods for early detection, little improvement has occurred in cancer mortality rates for many racial groups (e.g., African Americans, Latinos) (Webber, Fox, Zhang, & Pond, 1996). Factors accounting for the miniscule improvement include disruptions in communication between providers and patients, individual decision making and fatalism, differential treatment, growth in the racial and ethnic composition of the U.S. population, varying organizational follow-up methods, and lack of trust in medical tests (Phillips, Cohen, & Moses, 1999; Smith, Phillips, & Price, 2001).

In a study of access to care and stage at diagnosis of breast cancer in African American and Caucasian women, Bibb (2001) found that African American women from low socioeconomic backgrounds reported experiencing more access barriers and thus had more delays in diagnosis. The findings are congruent with those of Zaloznik (1997). Hunter et al. (1993) found a significant association between race and stage at diagnosis. As indicated earlier, primarily because of race, historical experience, and skin color, African Americans are a unique cultural group. The African American experience in America is distinctively different from that of other cultural groups (Watts, 2003).

Almost any discussion of cancer statistics observed for minority populations includes the term "barriers," which typically refers to poor accessibility and availability of healthcare services, the negative influences of poverty, limited knowledge, and deeply rooted distrust of the nation's healthcare systems. Many of the barriers are based on a person's perceptual world view, which, in part, is based on past experience. Past experience plays a significant role in influencing African Americans' present perceptions. Because of the unethical, inappropriate, and deadly experiments conducted in the 1930s, African Americans generally are wary of the healthcare system and believe that they have little chance of receiving honest information and treatment that will increase their chances of survival. So-called prevailing attitudes of pessimism and fatalism regarding cancer among minority populations also act as barriers. Although minority members may acknowledge and accept the severity of cancer, they are pessimistic about curing cancer, underestimate the incidence of the disease, and generally are hesitant to seek medical advice when symptoms suggestive of cancer appear (Guidry et al., 1996).

The Practice Imperative

A practice imperative exists for maintaining a multicultural perspective in practicing cancer care. Without this perspective, cultural and racial differences between nurses and patients may continue to engender poor communication and interpersonal tensions. These cultural differences may lead to inaccurate assessments of patients' needs and result in inappropriate intervention. Cultural "myopia" interferes with recognition of the realistic barriers that impede the use of healthcare services. Indeed, the failure of many prevention and early detection programs may be a result of ignorance about the depth of cultural difference, the perceived threats inherent in the system, the culturally generated symbolic meanings attached to these threats, and the degree to which they discourage participation. Robinson, Kimmel, and Yasko (1995) suggested that, to reduce the disparity in cancer incidence and mortality rates between whites and nonwhites, innovative, culturally appropriate prevention and early detection programs must be developed and implemented.

Religious Preferences

Religious affiliations often are part of patients' cultural responses to the cancer experience. In some religions, it is considered sacrilegious to disturb the body after death, which may determine views on postmortem examinations. Religious practices influence patients' receptivity to transplantation (e.g., bone marrow transplantation). Cultural heritage and religion help to form the meaning of the cancer diagnosis and beliefs about the causes of cancer. Based on meaning and perceived causes, patients may view cancer as a predestination to be accepted with fateful resignation. Other values and beliefs, such as disclosure of cancer diagnosis and the acceptability of the expression of anger, are part of patients' cultural responses to the cancer experience.

Braun, Mokuau, Hunt, Kaanoi, and Gotay (2002), in a study of supports and obstacles to cancer survival for Hawaii's native people, found that the majority of survivors perceived spirituality to play a critical role in their cancer experience. For example, some reported being inspired by the Holy Spirit to seek cancer screening, and many prayed before surgery and were prayed for by family members. Some nurses and physicians offered or were asked to pray with the patient before treatment. Some of the study participants expressed belief that they were expected to rise to "God's challenge" and seek treatment, rather than delaying treatment and presuming that it was their time to die. The researchers concluded that the spiritual beliefs held by the study participants obviated potential fatalist attitudes. However, participants felt that some Native Hawaiians might hold such views. Prayer also is frequently used by African Americans as a coping strategy (Henderson, Gore, Davis, & Condon, 2003). According to Barg and Gullatte (2001), faith-based support groups are effective in assisting African American patients with cancer with psychosocial and educational needs and concerns. Prayer and praying to the saints (*espiritismo* or spiritism, belief that saints or spirits have an influence on the living) is a common, traditional practice in the Latino/Hispanic culture (Pachter, Cloutier, & Berstein, 1995).

For many African Americans, religion is a key cultural influence on their response to a cancer diagnosis and cancer treatment. For example, beliefs may include that a direct connection exists between the human body and the forces of nature. Illness and other events often are attributed to either "natural" or "unnatural" causation (Diversity Resources, 2000). Natural events are those that operate in accordance with God's plan, and they help to maintain the balance and harmony of nature. Conversely, unnatural events are the work of the devil that upset the balance or harmony of nature (Diversity Resources). When balance and harmony in nature are disrupted, illness occurs and can only be cured when balance and harmony are restored.

In certain geographic regions of the United States, some African Americans ascribe illness to natural causes such as "cold" and improper conduct. Cold is thought to enter the body when it is most vulnerable (e.g., after childbirth, during menstruation). Improper conduct is strongly associated with the religious belief that sin, the root cause of illness, is reflective of divine punishments for one's misdeeds. Cure can only be achieved through repentance and contact with God either directly or through the intercessory activity of a faith healer (Diversity Resources, 2000).

The importance of religion as a cultural influence relates to the patient's belief in and use of icons. Other religious implications may include who within the family circle assumes the spiritual leadership during times of crisis and how spirituality is expressed within and outside of the family circle. Traditional health beliefs and essential activities that maintain health and prevent illness emerge, in part, from religious tenets and dictums.

Culturally Competent Care

It is impossible to overemphasize the importance of culture in determining patients' responses to the cancer experience; culture cannot be even minimally understood without careful, valid assessment. No care provider is exempt from responsibility and accountability to give culturally competent care. The need to increase diversity in the oncology nursing workforce is ever before us. That fact notwithstanding, oncology nurses from all cultural backgrounds must hone and develop cultural assessment skills to communicate in culturally appropriate ways.

Cultural assessment is not merely an assessment of patients but an assessment of self, family, and support people who may be involved in patients' care. Therefore, nurses must explore their own world views and determine which explanatory models of disease and illness they favor. They must examine their own personal cultural beliefs, values, biases, and prejudices before attempting to understand the patients' (Nagia, 1996).

To provide culturally competent care, nurses must possess certain basic understandings, such as the following.

- All people have value and are worthy of respect.
- All people, regardless of socioeconomic status, educational background, or race, have strengths that, if sought, may be found and built upon.
- Illness is a patient-defined subjective experience; thus, the patient is the only one able to tell the provider about it.
- Disease is a biomedical event that is diagnosed and defined by the providers within the context of the healthcare system.
- Patients' responses to the cancer experience are determined by illness and disease; therefore, both patients and healthcare providers participate in the process of assessment, problem identification, planning, and evaluation so as to formulate mutual goals and health outcomes.
- Culturally competent care can only be provided in the context of a multicultural model that builds upon the unique strengths of both patients and providers and includes ongoing, sensitive dialogue among all participants.
- Continuous cultural self-monitoring by oncology nurses is the most effective strategy to prevent erosion of cultural competence in the provision of oncology nursing care to people from multicultural populations.
- Regardless of the nurse's race or ethnicity, the combined concepts of culture, perceptual world view, and health illness beliefs are fundamental to the provision of culturally competent oncology nursing care.

Conclusion

Oncology nurses who adopt the principles of culturally competent care will be less vulnerable to the natural tendencies of ethnocentrism and stereotyping. They will be more likely to engage in ongoing, open communication that fosters valid assessment of culture and its relative influence on patients' responses to the cancer experience. As the diversity of the United States increases, the need for culturally competent care is even more critical, yet progress toward this goal is slow. Oncology nurses must resolve to do things differently and to make culturally competent care in oncology nursing practice a priority and a reality for all people with cancer.

References

Barg, F.K., & Gullatte, M.M. (2001). Cancer support groups: Meeting the needs of African Americans with cancer. *Seminars in Oncology Nursing, 17,* 171–178.

Berry, J.W. (1997). Immigration, acculturation and adaptation. *Applied Psychology: An International Review, 46,* 5–34.

Bibb, S. (2001). The relationship between access and stage at diagnosis of breast cancer in African American and Caucasian women. *Oncology Nursing Forum, 28,* 711–719.

Bobo, L.D. (2001). Racial attitudes and relations at the close of the twentieth century. In N.J. Smelser, W.J. Wilson, & F. Mitchell (Eds.), *America becoming: Racial trends and their consequences, Vol. 1* (pp. 264–301). Washington, DC: National Academies Press.

Braun, K.L., Mokuau, N., Hunt, G.H., Kaanoi, M., & Gotay, C.C. (2002). Supports and obstacles to cancer survival for Hawaii's native people. *Cancer Practice, 10,* 192–200.

Carson, C. (1993). African Americans. In J. Krieger (Ed.), *Oxford companion to politics of the world* (pp. 1–6). New York: Oxford University Press.

Castillo, R.J. (1997). *Culture and mental illness: A client-centered approach.* Pacific Grove, CA: Brooks/ Cole.

Collins, K., Hughes, D., Doty, M., Ives, B., Edwards, J., & Tenney, K. (2002). *Diverse communities, common concerns: Assessing health care quality for minority Americans.* New York: The Commonwealth Fund.

Dirksen, S.R., & Erickson, J.R. (2002). Well-being in Hispanic and non-Hispanic white survivors of breast cancer. *Oncology Nursing Forum, 29,* 820–826.

Diversity Resources, Inc. (2000). *What language does your patient hurt in? A practical guide to culturally competent care.* Amherst, MA: Author. Retrieved August 3, 2004, from http://www.diversityresources. com/rc21d/african.html

Falicov, C. (1998). *Latino families in therapy: A guide to multicultural practice.* New York: Guilford Press.

Flanagan, A.Y. (2002). *Cultural awareness and diversity: Health and illness.* Retrieved November 1, 2003, from http://www.nursingceu.com/RCEU/courses/diversity/

Garcia-Preto, N. (1996). Latino families: An overview. In M. McGoldrick, J. Giordano, & J.K. Pearce (Eds.), *Ethnicity and family therapy* (2nd ed., pp. 141–154). New York: Guilford Press.

Green, J.W. (1999). *Cultural awareness in the human services: A multi-ethnic approach* (3rd ed.). Boston: Allyn and Bacon.

Guidry, J.J., Greisinger, A., Aday, L.A., Winn, R.J., Vernon, A., & Throckmorton, T.A. (1996). Barriers to cancer treatment: A review of published research. *Oncology Nursing Forum, 23,* 1373–1398.

Guidry, J.J., & Walker, V.D. (1999). Assessing cultural sensitivity in printed materials. *Cancer Practice, 7,* 291–296.

Henderson, P.D., Gore, S.V., Davis, B.L., & Condon, E.H. (2003). African American women coping with breast cancer: A qualitative analysis. *Oncology Nursing Forum, 30,* 641–647.

Huang, G. (1993). *Beyond culture: Communicating with Asian American children and families.* New York: ERIC Clearinghouse on Urban Education. (ERIC Document Reproduction Service No. ED366673)

Hufford, D.J. (1997). Folk medicine and health culture in contemporary society. *Primary Care, 24,* 723–741.

Hunter, C.P., Redmond, C.K., Chen, V.W., Austin, D.F., Greenberg, R.S., Correa, P., et al. (1993). Breast cancer: Factors associated with stage at diagnosis in black and white women. *Journal of the National Cancer Institute, 85,* 1125–1137.

Jens, G.P., Chaney, H.S., & Brodie, K.E. (2001). Family coping styles and challenges. *Nursing Clinics of North America, 36,* 795–807.

Kagawa-Singer, M. (1998). A multicultural perspective on death and dying. *Oncology Nursing Forum, 25,* 1752–1756.

Katapodi, M.C., Facione, N.C., Miaskowski, C., Dodd, M.J., & Waters, C. (2002). The influence of social support on breast cancer screening in a multicultural community sample. *Oncology Nursing Forum, 29,* 845–852.

Kitano, H.H. (1997). *Race relations* (5th ed.). Upper Saddle River, NJ: Prentice Hall.

Kleinman, A., Eisenberg, L., & Good, B. (1978). Culture, illness, and care: Clinical lessons from anthropologic and cross-cultural research. *Annals of Internal Medicine, 88,* 251–258.

Lavizzo-Mourey, R.J., & Mackenzie, E.R. (1996). Cultural competence: Essential measurements of quality for managed care organizations. *Annals of Internal Medicine, 124,* 912–919.

Lee, E. (1996). Asian American families: An overview. In M. McGoldrick, J. Giordano, & J.K. Pearce (Eds.), *Ethnicity and family therapy* (2nd ed., pp. 227–248). New York: Guilford Press.

Lindsay, J., Narayan, M.C., & Rea, K. (1998). The Vietnamese client. *Home Healthcare Nurse, 16,* 693–700.

Makabe, R., & Hull, M.M. (2000). Components of social support among Japanese women with breast cancer. *Oncology Nursing Forum, 27,* 1381–1390.

Nagia, S.A. (1996). Providing culturally sensitive care to Egyptians with cancer. *Cancer Practice, 4,* 212–215.

Nishimoto, P.W., & Foley, J. (2001). Cultural beliefs of Asian Americans associated with terminal illness and death. *Seminars in Oncology Nursing, 17,* 179–189.

Pachter, L.M. (1994). Culture and clinical care: Folk illness beliefs and behaviors and their implications for health care delivery. *JAMA, 271,* 690–695.

Pachter, L.M., Cloutier, M.M., & Berstein, B.A. (1995). Ethnomedical (folk) remedies for childhood asthma in a mainland Puerto Rican community. *Archives of Pediatrics and Adolescent Medicine, 149,* 982–989.

Panos, P.T., & Panos, A.J. (2000). A model for a culture-sensitive assessment of patients in health care settings. *Social Work in Health Care, 31*(1), 49–62.

Phillips, J.M., Cohen, M.Z., & Moses, G. (1999). Breast cancer screening and African American women: Fear, fatalism, and silence. *Oncology Nursing Forum, 26,* 561–571.

Prior, L. (1996). Caring for patients from ethnic minority groups. *British Journal of Theatre Nursing, 6*(3), 28–30.

Reverby, S.M. (1999). Rethinking the Tuskegee Syphilis Study: Nurse Rivers, silence and the meaning of treatment. *Nursing History Review, 7,* 3–28.

Robinson, K.D., Kimmel, E.A., & Yasko, J.M. (1995). Reaching out to the African American community through innovative strategies. *Oncology Nursing Forum, 22,* 1989–1991.

Smedley, B.D., Stith, A.Y., & Nelson, A.R. (2002). *Unequal treatment: Confronting racial and ethnic disparities in healthcare.* Washington, DC: National Academies Press.

Smiley, M.R., McMillan, S.C., Johnson, S., & Ojeda, M. (2000). Comparison of Florida Hispanic and non-Hispanic Caucasian women in their health beliefs related to breast cancer and health locus of control. *Oncology Nursing Forum, 27,* 975–984.

Smith, E.D., Phillips, J.M., & Price, M.M. (2001). Screening and early detection among racial and ethnic minority women. *Seminars in Oncology Nursing, 17,* 159–170.

Thomas, H. (1997). *The slave trade.* New York: Touchstone.

Trueba, H.T., Cheng, L.L., & Ima, K. (1993). *Myth or reality: Adaptive strategies of Asian Americans in California.* Washington, DC: Falmer Press.

U.S. Census Bureau. (2005, January). *United States Census 2000.* Retrieved February 25, 2005, from http://www.census.gov/main/www/cen2000.html

Walters, J.F., & Ankomah, A. (1996). Community control of health services for Canadian Indians. *World Health Forum, 17,* 242–245.

Watts, R. (2003). Race consciousness and the health of African Americans. *Online Journal of Issues in Nursing, 8*(1). Retrieved February 25, 2005, from http://nursingworld.org/ojin/topic20/tpc20_3.htm

Webber, P.A., Fox, P., Zhang, X., & Pond, M. (1996). An examination of differential follow-up rates in breast cancer screening. *Journal of Community Health, 21,* 123–132.

Zaloznik, A.J. (1997). Breast cancer stage at diagnosis: Caucasians versus Hispanics. *Breast Cancer Research and Treatment, 42,* 121–124.

CHAPTER 7

Spirituality and Spiritual Nurture in Cancer Care

ELIZABETH JOHNSTON TAYLOR, PhD, RN

And almost every one when age,
Disease, or sorrows strike him,
Inclines to think there is a God,
Or something very like Him.

—Arthur Hugh Clough

Personal spirituality greatly influences one's response to the psychosocial and physical experiences of living with cancer; likewise, the psychosocial and physical sequelae of cancer greatly influence a person's spirituality. This chapter briefly describes spirituality and explains why it is essential to nursing care for patients with cancer. After presenting spiritual responses to living with cancer from the perspectives of the patient, the family caregiver, and the oncology nurse, the chapter will discuss evidence supporting selected approaches to nurturing the spirit.

What Is Spirituality?

Spirituality is "the life principle that pervades a person's entire being and that integrates and transcends one's biological and psychological nature," according to the North American Nursing Diagnosis Association (NANDA, 1999, p. 67). Another often-cited nurse scholar's definition of spirituality described it as the "the propensity to make meaning through a sense of relatedness to dimensions that transcend the self in such a way that empowers and does not devalue the individual" (Reed, 1992, p. 350). Reed posited that this relatedness involves intra-, inter-, and transpersonal connectedness. Spirituality, therefore, is an aspect of being that is deeply and uniquely human; it is universal and innate.

Martsolf and Mickley (1998) identified the salient attributes of spirituality: meaning (having purpose, making sense of life), value (having cherished beliefs and standards), and becoming (allowing life to unfold and knowing who one is). Goldberg's (1998) concept analysis of spirituality concluded that aspects of spirituality included meaning, presencing, empathy and compassion, giving hope, love, religion and transcendence, and touch and healing.

In addition to identifying components of spirituality, nurse authors have developed many terms for concepts related to spirituality, including spiritual well-being, spiritual need, spiritual distress, spiritual disequilibrium, spiriting, inspiriting, spiritual perspective, spiritual quality of life, and spiritual pain (Taylor, 2002). Spirituality and its related concepts clearly are broad in nature. Nursing literature, however, consistently differentiates religiousness from spirituality. "Religiousness" refers to an expression of spirituality. A religion offers an individual a specific world view—an explanation that seeks to provide answers to the questions of ultimate meaning. It recommends how one is to live harmoniously with oneself, others, nature, and God. Such explanations and recommendations are presented in a religion's belief system (e.g., myths/stories, doctrines, dogmas) and are remembered and appreciated through rituals and other religious practices or observances. An individual's religion may or may not be of an institutional nature (Taylor, 2002).

Why Is Spirituality Important in Oncology Nursing Care?

Several arguments support the importance of addressing spirituality in oncology nursing care.

Spirituality as Part of the Whole

Nursing prides itself on being a profession that cares for the whole person. Consequently, if a nurse accepts the philosophical presuppositions that a spiritual dimension exists in all people and that this dimension integrates and relates to the other dimensions of being human, then caring for the spirit is essential to ethical nursing care (Dossey, Keegan, & Guzzetta, 2000). Since 1978, NANDA International (2005) implicitly has supported this notion by including the diagnosis of "spiritual distress" in its formulary. Subsequently, NANDA International has added related diagnoses such as "impaired religiosity." The International Council of Nurses (2000) Code of Ethics for Nurses and nursing school accrediting bodies' mandates to prepare students to address the spiritual dimension further show nursing's commitment to caring for the whole person (Taylor, 2002).

Increased Spiritual Awareness as Life Is Threatened

The cancer experience increases one's sense of vulnerability and mortality, typically creating varying degrees of suffering and loss. By nature, such effects increase patients' spiritual awareness and sensitivity (Taylor, 2000a). Indeed, research has demonstrated that illness is accompanied by an increased spiritual awareness and frequent use of spiritual coping strategies (Halstead & Hull, 2001; Lengacher et al.,

2002; Tatsumura, Maskarinec, Shumay, & Kakai, 2003; Taylor & Outlaw, 2002; Thomas & Retsas, 1999). If nurses are to appreciate the varied responses and coping resources of patients with cancer, they must not neglect those that are spiritual.

Empirical Evidence

Several empirical studies have demonstrated significant relationships between spirituality and other health-related variables among people with cancer. For instance, spiritual well-being correlated with positive mood and hope and inversely with depression and negative mood in a sample of 100 older adults with cancer (Fehring, Miller, & Shaw, 1997). In a study of 1,610 patients with cancer, Brady, Peterman, Fitchett, Mo, and Cella (1999) observed that spiritual well-being correlated with and predicted overall quality of life. Likewise, Cotton, Levine, Fitzpatrick, Dold, and Targ (1999) reported on a study with 142 patients with breast cancer that demonstrated a negative correlation between spiritual well-being and anxiety and helplessness/hopelessness. This study also demonstrated a predictive relationship between spiritual well-being and quality of life. If nurses are interested in addressing factors that relate directly to health and quality of life, then they must address patients' spirituality.

The link between spirituality and physical health has received much more attention from researchers. Analyses of the multitude of empirical studies investigating how religiosity affects health have consistently suggested that there *may* be a health benefit from being religious—enough suggestion from the data to warrant further investigation (Powell, Shahabi, & Thoresen, 2003; Seeman, Dubin, & Seeman, 2003). When evaluating the strength of such evidence, however, Powell et al. found that the only hypothesis supported by persuasive evidence was that religious service attendance delays death. Other hypotheses, such as spirituality protecting against cancer mortality or spirituality slowing the progression of cancer, have inadequate or failed evidence.

Pragmatic Reasons

Pragmatic reasons exist for including spiritual care in nursing. The Joint Commission on Accreditation of Healthcare Organizations (JCAHO, 2004) has mandated since the early 2000s that spiritual beliefs and practices be assessed and that spiritual support is available in the institutions that it accredits. JCAHO particularly emphasizes the need for spiritual care for those facing imminent death. Nurturing the spirit also has marketing value. Today's consumers are interested in healthcare providers who care for the body, mind, and spirit. It is not unusual to find advertisements for healthcare institutions that proclaim they care for the body and soul. Although evidence is scanty and weak, spiritual care may save healthcare dollars. For example, Harris et al. (1999) conducted a randomized double-blind experiment to determine outcomes of intercessory prayer (i.e., petitioning God on behalf of others). They found that cardiac patients receiving intercessory prayer had an 11% reduction of overall adverse events during the course of hospitalization. Presumably, patients with fewer adverse outcomes reduce healthcare costs.

Although healthcare facilities typically have relegated spiritual care to chaplains, this compartmentalization of services is inadequate for several reasons.
- Spiritual needs can surface at any time and often are best cared for if addressed immediately.

- Spiritual needs do not occur in isolation or only during a pastoral visit.
- Many people are unable to benefit from spiritual care from a chaplain because of negative associations with organized religion.
- Much of spiritual caregiving requires rapport and a good relationship, which are difficult to achieve when patients are isolated or receive only brief chaplain visits.

However, the role of nursing lends itself well to at least an initial level of spiritual caregiving (e.g., nurses are in a position to develop rapport, nurses' constant presence allows them to witness spiritual needs). Indeed, many nursing theories implicitly or explicitly include spirituality as a dimension of nursing care (Martsolf & Mickley, 1998; Taylor, 2002).

Spiritual Responses to the Cancer Experience

The Patient's Perspective

Both quantitative and qualitative research reports offer insight into spiritual responses to the cancer experience from the patient's perspective. Some researchers have described specific aspects of spirituality among people with cancer, such as searching for meaning (Halstead & Hull, 2001; Taylor, 2000b), maintaining hope (Ebright & Lyon, 2002; Eliott & Olver, 2002), seeking forgiveness (Mickley & Cowles, 2001), and self-transcendence (Coward, 2003). Some researchers have categorized the observed "spiritual needs" of patients with cancer, which are summarized in Table 7-1. Most of these studies are qualitative, offering in-depth descriptions of these spiritual phenomena.

Other researchers have reported that people with cancer cope by using their existing spiritual or religious resources, such as faith and prayer (Gall & Cornblat, 2002; Lengacher et al., 2002; Schnoll, Harlow, & Brower, 2000; Tatsumura et al., 2003; Taylor & Outlaw, 2002). A myriad of descriptive, correlational studies about spiritual coping strategies among patients with cancer provide moderately strong evidence that they are prevalent, highly valued, and often associated with various forms of emotional well-being (Pargament, 1997). A patient's spiritual beliefs, however, do not necessarily ameliorate the distress of living with cancer. Little evidence shows that when patients have religious discontent (e.g., wonder if God has abandoned them or if God loves them) they have poorer life satisfaction and self-esteem (Gall, de Renart, & Boonstra, 2000) and are at increased risk for death (Pargament, Koenig, Tarakeshwar, & Hahn, 2001).

The literature describing the spirituality of patients with cancer indicates that positive as well as negative spiritual responses occur. These opposite responses can occur concurrently. For example, although the diagnosis of cancer may provoke spiritually painful questions and doubts, it also may bring the spiritual joy of learning how much the patient is loved.

Negative or distressing spiritual responses to cancer include having doubts about religious beliefs or the presence or nature of God, feeling isolated because of the inability to participate in religious practices, feeling guilt about being punished, and so forth. Few studies, however, explore this painful—and often unspeakable—aspect

Table 7-1. Spiritual Needs of Patients With Cancer

Author	Method	Spiritual Needs
Highfield & Cason (1983)	Condensed the categories of spiritual needs identified by pastoral counselor Howard Clinebell and provided illustrations from clinical observations	• Need to give love • Need to receive love • Need for hope and creativity • Need for meaning and purpose
Greisinger et al. (1997)	Interviews with 120 terminally ill patients with cancer	• Existential needs: to have hope, to know life has meaning and purpose, to know life has been productive • Spiritual needs: to find strength in beliefs, to find comfort in faith

Moadel et al. (1999)	Quantitative survey of 248 ethnically diverse patients; categories of spiritual need were identified a priori	• Prevalence of needs
		  - Would like help with overcoming fears (51%)
		  - Would like help with finding hope (42%)
		  - Finding meaning in life (40%)
		  - Finding spiritual resources (39%)
		  - Would like to talk about finding peace (43%)
		  - Would like to talk about meaning of life (28%)
		  - To talk about dying (25%)

Hermann (2001)	Qualitative research with 19 mostly white and Protestant hospice patients in the United States	• Need for involvement and control • Need for companionship • Need to finish business • Need for religion • Need to experience nature • Need for positive outlook

Taylor (2003b)	Qualitative interviews with 21 patients with cancer and 7 family caregivers	• Need to
		  - Relate to Ultimate Other (e.g., need to know God's will, feel that there is something out there looking after you/your loved one)
		  - Have positivity, gratitude, and hope (e.g., have hope that you/your loved one will be well, count your blessings)
		  - Give and receive love from other people (e.g., return others' kindnesses, protect your family from seeing you suffer)
		  - Review beliefs (e.g., wonder if your beliefs about God are correct, ask "why?")
		  - Create meaning, find purpose (e.g., get over or get past asking "why me?", try to make life count)
		  - Be religious (e.g., read scripture or spirit-nurturing material, have quiet time or space to reflect or meditate)
		  - Prepare for death (e.g., balance thoughts about dying with hoping for health)

of the cancer experience (Ferrell, Smith, Juarez, & Melancon, 2003; Taylor, Outlaw, Bernardo, & Roy, 1999).

Positive spiritual responses to living with cancer include strengthened faith, more motivation and time to pray or meditate, increased self-awareness and spiritual awareness, reprioritization of values, a heightened sense of pleasure for nature, and an intensified sense of joy about life (Taylor, 2000b; Taylor & Outlaw, 2002). The positive spiritual responses often appear to be preceded or accentuated by spiritual distress. A large number of descriptive studies of patients with cancer (the majority of which sampled women with breast cancer) have documented how many patients are plagued by the unanswerable question, "Why?" Some patients appear to get "stuck" searching for meaning, whereas many process this spiritual pain and are transformed by it (Carpenter, Brockopp, & Andrykowski, 1999; Taylor, 2000b). The challenge and struggle of living with cancer often functions as a catalyst for spiritual transformation.

The Family Caregiver's Perspective

Being the family caregiver for an individual with cancer can be emotionally and physically exhausting. Spirituality can be a resource for this stressful role (Petrie, Logan, & DeGrasse, 2001). Family caregivers' spiritual responses may include, "Why does my loved one have to suffer?"; "Where can I get my need for love filled when all I do is give care?"; and "What did I do to deserve this?" (Taylor, 2003b). Findings from two studies (Mellon, 2002; Taylor, 2003b) suggested there may be little difference between the spiritual needs of patients with cancer and their family caregivers. Harrington, Lackey, and Gates (1996) documented that 55 family caregivers surveyed ranked spiritual needs second only to informational needs in importance. However, family caregivers may receive spiritual nurture from their nurses less often than their loved ones, according to two descriptive Scandinavian studies (Kuuppelomaki, 2002; Strang, Strang, & Ternestedt, 2001).

Although several studies have documented increased mood disturbance, such as heightened anxiety, among family caregivers of patients with cancer, very few studies have investigated aspects of spirituality among this group. A few studies have suggested that family caregivers' sense of meaningfulness and spiritual well-being is associated with emotional health (Ferrell, Ervin, Smith, Marek, & Melancon, 2002; Strang & Strang, 2001). Much more research is needed not only to identify the specific spiritual needs of family caregivers but also to explore how spirituality affects mood, burden, and other aspects of family caregiving.

The Oncology Nurse's Perspective

Inherent in oncology nursing is sharing with patients the profound and humbling experiences of life, the sacred and the profane. This role can be burdensome and draining; it also can be a privilege. A survey of 813 hospice and oncology nurses revealed that most acknowledged that working with patients with cancer had influenced their own spirituality a great deal (65%) or somewhat (24%) (Highfield, Taylor, & Amenta, 2000). Although working with patients influences nurses, hospice and oncology nurses' personal spirituality and religiousness also influence if and how spiritual care is delivered to patients. Taylor, Highfield, and Amenta (1999) found that self-reported spirituality and attitudes about spiritual care were predictors of how frequently and how comfortably cancer nurses provided spiritual care.

Spiritual Caregiving

What Is Spiritual Care?

Spiritual care has been defined as "the health-promoting attendance to responses to stress that have an impact on an individual's or group's spiritual perspective" (Taylor, Amenta, & Highfield, 1995, p. 31). Wright's (2002) phenomenologic study of 16 palliative care providers concluded that spiritual care "seeks to affirm the value of each and every person based on nonjudgmental love" (p. 130). A number of descriptive nursing studies have explored nurses' perspectives about providing spiritual care; several of these investigated oncology, hospice, and palliative care nurses (Kristeller, Zumbrun, & Schilling, 1999; Kuuppelomaki, 2001; Sellers & Haag, 1998; Strang, Strang, & Ternestedt, 2002; Taylor, Highfield, et al., 1999; Wright). Although research about oncology nurses' spiritual caregiving typically predetermines specific activities or interventions that constitute spiritual care, many oncology nurses recognize that spiritual care often involves more than overt acts such as talking about spirituality or praying with a patient. In addition to these methods, spiritual care involves subtle ways of being that nurture the spirit.

Many specific approaches to spiritual caregiving have been described in the healthcare literature (Taylor, 2002). Approaches that transcend gender, cultural, or religious differences include activities and cognitive reframing that create meaningfulness; experiences that allow patients to identify or express themselves through art, literature, personal journal writing, or music; dream analysis; forgiveness therapy; religious or nonreligious rituals; meditation and prayer; being with nature; facilitation of religious practices; reading of spiritual material; storytelling; presencing (i.e., being there, being fully present); and referrals to experts (see Figure 7-1). A survey conducted by Sellers and Haag (1998) of 208 oncology, hospice, and parish nurses showed that these nurses could identify 95 different interventions. The most frequent included different types and methods of prayer, active listening, referral to spiritual care experts, facilitating and validating clients' (patients and caregivers) feelings and thoughts, conveying a nonjudgmental attitude, instilling hope, clarifying values and experiences, presence, touch, and referral to community or healthcare resources.

Oncology Nurses' Provision of Spiritual Care

Minimal and possibly contradictory evidence exists regarding how frequently oncology and hospice nurses provide spiritual care. Findings from an often-cited study (Taylor et al., 1995; Taylor, Highfield, & Amenta, 1994) revealed that oncology nurses agreed rather strongly that spiritual care was an important part of their role. However, when asked to indicate the frequency of their spiritual caregiving on a scale of 1 (never) to 5 (every day), these 181 nurses provided an average response of 2.8. In a subsequent analysis, Taylor, Highfield, et al. (1999) observed a difference between oncology and hospice nurses with regard to how frequently they offer spiritual care,

---

Figure 7-1. Approaches to Spiritual Caregiving

The nurse can nurture spiritual well-being by encouraging or facilitating the following.
- Activities and cognitive reframing that create meaningfulness
  - Altruistic activities (i.e., unselfish acts of kindness)
  - Dedication to a scientific, social, religious, or political cause
  - Hedonistic activities (i.e., highly pleasurable activities)
- Experiences that allow self-expression or enhance self-understanding
  - Visual art
  - Literature (e.g., writing poetry, bibliotherapy)
  - Journal writing
  - Music
  - Kinesthetic arts (e.g., dance)
  - Other "art" forms (e.g., cooking, flower arranging)
- Dream analysis (i.e., exploring the significance of dreams, learning about the spiritual life by being attentive to messages found in dreams)
- Forgiveness therapy
- Religious or nonreligious rituals
- Meditation and prayer
- Being with nature
- Religious practices
- Reading sacred writings or other spiritual material
- Storytelling (i.e., allowing a life review)
- Presencing (i.e., being there, being fully present)
- Referrals to spiritual care experts (e.g., clergy, pastoral counselors, chaplains)

Note. Based on information from Taylor, 2002.

---

with hospice nurses self-reporting providing spiritual care rather frequently (average of 3.4). Nearly half of the 267 nurses in a study by Kristeller et al. (1999) reported viewing themselves as the primary spiritual caregiver, with quite a few reporting that they would discuss a spiritual issue in depth (39%) or make a referral (37%). Only 8.5% indicated they would typically not address spiritual distress. Kuuppelomaki's (2001, 2002) surveys of Finnish nurses documented that half rarely offered spiritual care to patients with cancer, and 64% rarely or never offered it to family members. Sellers and Haag (1998) observed that 14% of their sample could not identify any nursing intervention for spiritual care. Apparently, some oncology nurses still fail to address their clients' spirituality.

Research has identified reasons for oncology nurses' neglect of patients' spiritual needs. These reasons or barriers to spiritual care include the nurses' lack of time; ambiguity and personal "baggage" about religion and spirituality; lack of knowledge about spirituality and spiritual caregiving; the belief that spiritual care is not within the domain of nursing; the implicit emphasis on providing physical care; and difficulty having an environment conducive to spiritual care (Kuuppelomaki, 2001; Wright, 2002).

A few of these studies about the spiritual care practices of oncology nurses explored selected factors that may be associated with the frequency of providing spiritual care. To summarize, scant but moderately strong evidence has indicated that nurses who are older, are diploma-prepared, work in hospice, attend religious services frequently, and perceive themselves as considerably spiritual are those most likely to provide spiritual care (Kuuppelomaki, 2002; Taylor et al., 1995; Taylor, Highfield, et al., 1999). American oncology nurses also may have more positive attitudes toward spiritual care and provide it more frequently than their counterparts in some other cultures, such as Israel and Finland (Kuuppelomaki, 2002; Musgrave & McFarlane, 2003). It is easy to assume that a society's mores about spirituality would influence the way its nurses practice spiritual care.

Another factor that may influence if and how a nurse provides spiritual care is the type of spiritual interventions being considered. Some fairly strong evidence from descriptive research has shown that nurses are more likely to offer interventions that are less intimate and less apt to cause embarrassment. The interventions that oncology nurses most frequently offer include praying privately for a patient, making a referral, informing the patient about resources, instilling hope, conveying acceptance, and listening and talking about a spiritual concern expressed by the client (Kristeller et al., 1999; Sellers & Haag, 1998; Taylor, Highfield, et al., 1999).

Given this empirical evidence about nurses and spiritual caregiving, the following recommendations are made for nurses in leadership positions.

- Nurture the spiritual well-being of nursing staff. This factor, more than any studied thus far, predicts the provision of spiritual care.
- Educate younger, less–spiritually sensitive or religious, and less-educated nurses about the benefits and methods of spiritual care; they are the staff least likely to deliver spiritual care.
- Recognize that nurses with high levels of spiritual well-being or who are considerably religious are more likely to provide spiritual care. Although this is natural, nurse leaders may need to educate staff regarding unethical proselytizing. That is, nurses should not share their own religious beliefs without a client's consent.
- Eliminate the barriers to spiritual caregiving: Teach how spirituality and religion are different, how to assess spiritual need, how to provide care in a time-efficient manner, and so forth. Also, allow nurses to reflect on their own spirituality and reasons for their perspectives about spiritual caregiving.

Cancer Care Recipients' Perspectives

Although a number of studies have explored oncology nurses' perspectives about providing spiritual care, very little research has explored patients' and their family members' perspectives about receiving spiritual care from nurses. A handful of qualitative studies have suggested that patients appreciate nurses' spiritual caregiving efforts. However, little evidence exists that challenges these findings (Taylor, 2003a). Two dated studies with very small samples indicated that these patients with cancer ranked nurses fourth, after family, friends, and clergy/chaplains, as the primary spiritual care provider (Taylor, 2003a). Another survey of 100 patients with cancer indicated which spiritual interventions from nurses were most accepted; the top-ranked interventions were less intimate, including making a referral for spiritual care and allowing them time for personal prayer (28% and 20%, respectively) (Reed, 1991).

Taylor's (2003a) qualitative study of 28 patients and family caregivers observed that some immediately recognized their spiritual needs and desired spiritual nurturing from a nurse, whereas others were unable to identify any need and/or disliked the notion of nurses providing spiritual care. The spiritual care these participants desired from a nurse included kindness and respect (foremost); talking and listening; prayer; connecting—with a sense of mutuality and equality in the relationship, with authenticity, and with physical presence; quality nursing care in general; and having nurses mobilize religious or spiritual resources. Unpublished quantitative data from the author's study of 224 patients with cancer and caregivers indicated that these clients' most preferred nurse-provided spiritual care interventions included using humor, helping them to have quiet time or space, and offering to pray privately for them. No significant differences were found between patient and caregiver preferences. A low correlation ($r = .29$) was observed between the frequency of attendance at religious services and the participants' increased preference for nursing spiritual care. These findings indicated that for both patients and caregivers, nurses must be sensitive to providing spiritual care in ways that are welcomed. These findings suggested that the interventions cancer nurses offer most frequently may be the sort of interventions preferred by care recipients (i.e., interventions that are less intimate, commonly used, and not overtly religious).

Spiritual Care Interventions

Although nursing literature often describes approaches to nurturing the spirit as "interventions," Mayer (1992) counseled that this term often is inappropriate in the context of spiritual care. "Interventions" suggests doing, rather than being, and implies that nurses are superior as they try to fix someone who is spiritually inferior. Such a stance is incongruent with spiritual care, which requires symmetry and respect in the nurse-client relationship.

A more in-depth discussion of a few of the most frequently nurse-provided or client-desired spiritual care interventions will be presented. These include prayer, empathic listening, presencing, and making a referral. Having established the fairly strong empirical basis supporting the provision of spiritual care, the evidence presented here will be about each specific intervention. For more detailed information about how to provide spiritual care, consult a text about spiritual caregiving (Burkhardt & Nagai-Jacobson, 2002; Taylor, 2002; Wilt, Smucker, Groer, & Wagner, 2001).

Prayer: Approximately 90% of Americans believe in prayer (Gallup, 1996), and 70% reported praying often for the health of a family member (Kalb, 2003). For some people with cancer, the intensity and frequency with which they pray increases after a diagnosis of cancer (Taylor & Outlaw, 2002). Much descriptive evidence supports the fact that individuals use prayer to cope with the cancer experience. The evidence supporting the efficacy of prayer in terms of physically healing patients, however, is inconclusive (Roberts, Ahmed, & Hall, 2000). The scientific testing of whether prayer "works" may be inappropriate, if given the belief that prayer is about encountering God (or a higher power), not controlling or manipulating God via prayer (Cohen, Wheeler, Scott, Edwards, & Lusk, 2000).

Although some evidence has supported the judicious use of prayer in clinical practice, little evidence is available to guide nurses in how to introduce this intervention. The author's unpublished data suggested that some patients prefer to be prayed for privately by the nurse. Another study of how patients with cancer use prayer to cope indicated that for some, beliefs about prayer can contribute to spiritual distress, such as questions about why God does not "answer" or about whether God exists (Taylor, Outlaw, et al., 1999). Poloma and Gallup's (1991) research indicated that various types of prayer experiences exist (see Table 7-2), and only certain types are associated with quality-of-life indicators. That is, meditational—and conversational, to a lesser

Table 7-2. Types of Prayer Experience

Type of Prayer	Description	Examples
Ritual	Habitual, recited, memorized prayer; useful during times of spiritual dryness or crisis (when one cannot concentrate or compose prayer)	"Hail Mary . . ." "Lord's Prayer" "Now I lay me down to sleep . . ."
Petitionary	Petitioning or asking the divine for something	"Dear Jesus, make me well!" "God, take the pain away."
Conversational/ colloquial	Speaking (verbally or with thought) to the divine as in conversation with a friend	"Lord, here I am . . . not feeling good . . . wondering what is going on . . . wishing I could feel your presence more . . . worrying about my family . . ."
Meditational	Encountering the divine without an agenda; being receptive, still, quiet; listening to that "still, small voice"	Centering prayer Meditating on word/phrase/sacred story Prayer of silence

Note. Based on information from Poloma & Gallup, 1991.

extent —approaches to prayer were associated with greater well-being than petitionary and ritual forms of prayer. This evidence suggested the following.

- Nurses may introduce prayer initially by offering to pray privately for a client.
- Nurses may need to explore the spiritual pain of clients who sense their prayers are unanswered or unheard or who encounter other spiritual doubts or conflicts while praying. This often requires a referral to a spiritual care specialist.
- Nurses can educate clients about the benefits and methods of meditational prayer and facilitate such experiences by allowing quiet time.

Empathic listening: The most empathic listener will listen not only intellectually to the words spoken but also for feelings, bodily expressions, and physical responses. The most astute listener will be aware of the spiritual dimension present (Taylor, 2002).

Myers' (2000) in-depth interviews with patients undergoing psychotherapy revealed several factors that make a client feel truly heard. Empathic therapists (a) allowed clients to hear themselves, (b) did not "flinch" when clients expressed various pains, (c) made clients feel accepted, even while aware of their undesirable characteristics, (d) helped clients to make sense of their own confusion, (e) made clients feel that their stories were valuable, and (f) provided feedback to clients (e.g., by asking questions and paraphrasing or summarizing their comments). Myers concluded that what makes a therapist ultimately effective is the quality of the connection built between the client and therapist.

Presencing: Fredriksson (1999) described "being present," "being there," and "being present" as a "gift of self" that is given by the nurse who maintains an attitude of attentiveness to the client. Pettigrew's (1990) landmark discussion of this intervention identified four components of presencing: a client's **vulnerability**, which demands a nurse's vulnerability as she or he comes alongside (i.e., is with the client physically); **silence** that allows listening; an **invitation** from the client to witness his or her suffering; and **privilege** that requires a client to be courageous enough to reveal vulnerabilities and losses.

Although research about nurses' presencing is scarce, some nurse scholars have delineated levels of presencing (Fredriksson, 1999; Snyder, Brandt, & Tseng, 2000). Osterman and Schwartz-Barcott (1996) proposed four ways of being present for clients (see Table 7-3).

Referral: A nurse is a spiritual care generalist (Taylor, 2002). At times (because of lack of time, energy, or expertise), the nurse must initiate a referral so that a client's spiritual concerns are addressed by an expert. In addition to chaplains and clergy (e.g., rabbi, priest, minister, lay spiritual leader), other spiritual counselors, folk healers, or mentors may be appropriate. Synagogues and churches increasingly are gaining the services of parish nurses who sometimes have training in theology as well as nursing. Other referral resources may include counselors at spiritual retreat centers.

Table 7-3. Levels of Presencing

Level	Characteristics	Example
Physical presence	Nurse is physically present, but not focused on the client.	Nurse watching television in a client's room with no interaction
Partial presence	Nurse is physically present, attends to some tasks, and relates to client only superficially.	Nurse silently changing an IV catheter while thinking about a dinner party
Full presence	Nurse is mentally, emotionally, and physically present and intentionally focuses on the client.	Nurse observing and listening fully to assist the client to problem solve
Transcendent presence	Nurse is physically, mentally, emotionally, and spiritually present; involves a transpersonal and transforming experience.	Nurse practicing therapeutic touch, co-meditation, or prayer, or nurse silently, purposefully, intentionally, and whole-heartedly staying with a client who is in severe pain

Note. Based on information from Osterman & Schwartz-Barcott, 1996.

Conclusion

Spirituality is an innate and global human dimension. Because of the intimate and continuous contact nurses have with patients with cancer and because of nurses' role in facilitating coping and improving quality of life, it is logical and important for nurses to include spiritual care as one of their responsibilities. This chapter's discussion of empirical evidence about spirituality and spiritual care from the perspectives of oncology nurses, patients with cancer, and family caregivers provides information and insight to guide effective and ethical spiritual caregiving.

References

Brady, M.J., Peterman, A.H., Fitchett, G., Mo, M., & Cella, D. (1999). A case for including spirituality in quality of life measurement in oncology. *Psycho-Oncology, 8,* 417–428.

Burkhardt, M.A., & Nagai-Jacobson, M.G. (2002). *Spirituality: Living our connectedness.* Albany, NY: Delmar/Thomson Learning.

Carpenter, J.S., Brockopp, D.Y., & Andrykowski, M.A. (1999). Self-transformation as a factor in the self-esteem and well-being of breast cancer survivors. *Journal of Advanced Nursing, 29,* 1402–1411.

Cohen, C.B., Wheeler, S.E., Scott, D.A., Edwards, B.S., & Lusk, P. (2000). Prayer as therapy: A challenge to both religious belief and professional ethics. *Hastings Center Report, 30*(3), 40–47.

Cotton, S.P., Levine, E.G., Fitzpatrick, C.M., Dold, K.H., & Targ, E. (1999). Exploring the relationships among spiritual well-being, quality of life, and psychological adjustment in women with breast cancer. *Psycho-Oncology, 8,* 429–438.

Coward, D.D. (2003). Facilitation of self-transcendence in a breast cancer support group: II. *Oncology Nursing Forum, 30,* 291–300.

Dossey, B.M., Keegan, L., & Guzzetta, C.E. (Eds.). (2000). *Holistic nursing: A handbook for practice* (3rd ed.). Gaithersburg, MD: Aspen.

Ebright, P.R., & Lyon, B. (2002). Understanding hope and factors that enhance hope in women with breast cancer. *Oncology Nursing Forum, 29,* 561–568.

Eliott, J., & Olver, I. (2002). The discursive properties of "hope": A qualitative analysis of cancer patients' speech. *Qualitative Health Research, 12,* 173–193.

Fehring, R., Miller, J., & Shaw, C. (1997). Spiritual well-being, religiosity, hope, depression, and other mood states in elderly people coping with cancer. *Oncology Nursing Forum, 24,* 663–671.

Ferrell, B.R., Ervin, K., Smith, S., Marek, T., & Melancon, C. (2002). Family perspectives of ovarian cancer. *Cancer Practice, 10,* 269–276.

Ferrell, B.R., Smith, S.L., Juarez, G., & Melancon, C. (2003). Meaning of illness and spirituality in ovarian cancer survivors. *Oncology Nursing Forum, 30,* 249–257.

Fredriksson, L. (1999). Modes of relating in a caring conversation: A research synthesis on presence, touch, and listening. *Journal of Advanced Nursing, 30,* 1167–1176.

Gall, T.L., & Cornblat, M.W. (2002). Breast cancer survivors give voice: A qualitative analysis of spiritual factors in long-term adjustment. *Psycho-Oncology, 11,* 524–535.

Gall, T.L., de Renart, R.M.M., & Boonstra, B. (2000). Religious resources in long-term adjustment to breast cancer. *Journal of Psychosocial Oncology, 18*(2), 21–37.

Gallup, G.H., Jr. (1996). *Religion in America.* Princeton, NJ: Princeton Religion Research Center.

Goldberg, B. (1998). Connection: An exploration of spirituality in nursing care. *Journal of Advanced Nursing, 27,* 836–842.

Greisinger, A.J., Lorimor, R.J., Aday, L., Winn, R.J., & Baile, W.F. (1997). Terminally ill cancer patients: Their most important concerns. *Cancer Practice, 5,* 147–154.

Halstead, M.T., & Hull, M. (2001). Struggling with paradoxes: The process of spiritual development in women with cancer. *Oncology Nursing Forum, 28,* 1534–1544.

Harrington, V., Lackey, N.R., & Gates, M.F. (1996). Needs of caregivers of clinic and hospice cancer patients. *Cancer Nursing, 19,* 118–125.

Harris, W.S., Gowda, M., Kolb, J.W., Strychacz, C.P., Vacek, J.L., Jones, P.G., et al. (1999). A randomized, controlled trial of the effects of remote, intercessory prayer on outcomes in patients admitted to the coronary care unit. *Archives of Internal Medicine, 159,* 2273–2278.

Hermann, C.P. (2001). Spiritual needs of dying patients: A qualitative study. *Oncology Nursing Forum, 28,* 67–72.

Highfield, M.E.F., Taylor, E.J., & Amenta, M.O. (2000). Preparation to care: The spiritual care education of oncology and hospice nurses. *Journal of Hospice and Palliative Nursing, 2,* 53–63.

Highfield, M.F., & Cason, C. (1983). Spiritual needs of patients: Are they recognized? *Cancer Nursing, 6,* 187–192.

International Council of Nurses. (2000). *The ICN code of ethics for nurses.* Geneva, Switzerland: Author. Retrieved March 1, 2001, from http://www.icn.ch/icncode.pdf

Joint Commission on Accreditation of Healthcare Organizations. (2004). *Comprehensive accreditation manual for hospitals: The official handbook.* Oakbrook Terrace, IL: Author.

Kalb, C. (2003, November 10). Faith and healing. *Newsweek,* 44–50, 53–54, 56.

Kristeller, J.L., Zumbrun, C.S., & Schilling, R.F. (1999). "I would if I could": How oncology nurses address spiritual distress in cancer patients. *Psycho-Oncology, 8,* 451–458.

Kuuppelomaki, M. (2001). Spiritual support for terminally ill patients: Nursing staff assessments. *Journal of Clinical Nursing, 10,* 660–670.

Kuuppelomaki, M. (2002). Spiritual support for families of patients with cancer: A pilot study of nursing staff assessments. *Cancer Nursing, 25,* 209–218.

Lengacher, C.A., Bennett, M., Kip, K.E., Keller, R., LaVance, M.S., Smith, L.S., et al. (2002). Frequency of use of complementary and alternative medicine in women with breast caner. *Oncology Nursing Forum, 29,* 1445–1452.

Martsolf, D.S., & Mickley, J.R. (1998). The concept of spirituality in nursing theories: Differing world-views and extent of focus. *Journal of Advanced Nursing, 27,* 294–303.

Mayer, J. (1992). Wholly responsible for a part, or partly responsible for a whole? The concept of spiritual care in nursing. *Second Opinion, 17*(3), 26–55.

Mellon, S. (2002). Comparisons between cancer survivors and family members on meaning of the illness and family quality of life. *Oncology Nursing Forum, 29,* 1117–1125.

Mickley, J.R., & Cowles, K. (2001). Ameliorating the tension: Use of forgiveness for healing. *Oncology Nursing Forum, 28,* 31–37.

Moadel, A., Morgan, C., Fatone, A., Grennan, J., Carter, J., Laruffa, G., et al. (1999). Seeking meaning and hope: Self-reported spiritual and existential needs among an ethnically-diverse cancer patient population. *Psycho-Oncology, 8,* 378–385.

Musgrave, C.F., & McFarlane, E.A. (2003). Oncology and nononcology nurses' spiritual well-being and attitudes toward spiritual care: A literature review. *Oncology Nursing Forum, 30,* 523–527.

Myers, S. (2000). Empathic listening: Reports on the experience of being heard. *Journal of Humanistic Psychology, 40,* 148–173.

NANDA International. (2005). *NANDA nursing diagnoses: Definitions and classification, 2005–2006.* Philadelphia: Author.

North American Nursing Diagnosis Association. (1999). *NANDA nursing diagnosis: Definitions and classification, 1999–2000.* Philadelphia: Author.

Osterman, P., & Schwartz-Barcott, D. (1996). Presence: Four ways of being there. *Nursing Forum, 31*(2), 23–30.

Pargament, K.I. (1997). *The psychology of religion and coping: Theory, research, practice.* New York: Guilford Press.

Pargament, K.I., Koenig, H.G., Tarakeshwar, N., & Hahn, J. (2001). Religious struggle as a predictor of mortality among medically ill patients: A 2-year longitudinal study. *Archives of Internal Medicine, 161,* 1881–1885.

Petrie, W., Logan, J., & DeGrasse, C. (2001). Research review of the supportive care needs of spouses of women with breast cancer. *Oncology Nursing Forum, 28,* 1601–1607.

Pettigrew, J. (1990). Intensive nursing care: The ministry of presence. *Critical Care Nursing Clinics of North America, 2,* 503–508.

Poloma, M.M., & Gallup, G.H., Jr. (1991). *Varieties of prayer: A survey report.* Philadelphia: Trinity Press International.

Powell, L.H., Shahabi, L., & Thoresen, C.E. (2003). Religion and spirituality: Linkages to physical health. *American Psychologist, 58*(1), 36–52.

Reed, P.G. (1991). Preferences for spiritually related nursing interventions among terminally ill and nonterminally ill hospitalized adults and well adults. *Applied Nursing Research, 4,* 122–128.

Reed, P.G. (1992). An emerging paradigm for the investigation of spirituality in nursing. *Research in Nursing and Health, 15,* 349–357.

Roberts, L., Ahmed, I., & Hall, S. (2000). Intercessory prayer for the alleviation of ill health. *Cochrane Database Systematic Review, 2,* CD000368.

Schnoll, R.A., Harlow, L.L., & Brower, L. (2000). Spirituality, demographic and disease factors, and adjustment to cancer. *Cancer Practice, 8,* 298–304.

Seeman, T.E., Dubin, L.F., & Seeman, M. (2003). Religiosity/spirituality and health: A critical review of the evidence for biological pathways. *American Psychologist, 58*(1), 53–63.

Sellers, S.C., & Haag, B.A. (1998). Spiritual nursing interventions. *Journal of Holistic Nursing, 16,* 338–354.

Snyder, M., Brandt, C.L., & Tseng, Y. (2000). Use of presence in the critical care unit. *AACN Clinical Issues: Advanced Practice in Acute and Critical Care, 11,* 27–33.

Strang, S., & Strang, P. (2001). Spiritual thoughts, coping and 'sense of coherence' in brain tumour patients and their spouses. *Palliative Medicine, 15,* 127–134.

Strang, S., Strang, P., & Ternestedt, B.M. (2001). Existential support in brain tumour patients and their spouses. *Supportive Care in Cancer, 9,* 625–633.

Tatsumura, Y., Maskarinec, G., Shumay, D.M., & Kakai, H. (2003). Religious and spiritual resources, CAM, and conventional treatment in the lives of cancer patients. *Alternative Therapies in Health and Medicine, 9*(3), 64–71.

Taylor, E.J. (2000a). Spiritual and ethical end-of-life concerns. In C.H. Yarbro, M.H. Frogge, M. Goodman, & S.L. Groenwald (Eds.), *Cancer nursing: Principles and practice* (5th ed., pp. 1565–1578). Sudbury, MA: Jones and Bartlett.

Taylor, E.J. (2000b). Transformation of tragedy among women surviving breast cancer. *Oncology Nursing Forum, 27,* 781–788.

Taylor, E.J. (2002). *Spiritual care: Nursing theory, research, and practice.* Upper Saddle River, NJ: Prentice Hall.

Taylor, E.J. (2003a). Nurses caring for the spirit: Patients with cancer and family caregiver expectations. *Oncology Nursing Forum, 30,* 585–590.

Taylor, E.J. (2003b). Spiritual needs of cancer patients and family caregivers. *Cancer Nursing, 26,* 260–266.

Taylor, E.J., Amenta, M.O., & Highfield, M.F. (1995). Spiritual care practices of oncology nurses. *Oncology Nursing Forum, 22,* 31–39.

Taylor, E.J., Highfield, M., & Amenta, M. (1994). Attitudes and beliefs regarding spiritual care: A survey of cancer nurses. *Cancer Nursing, 17,* 479–487.

Taylor, E.J., Highfield, M.F., & Amenta, M.O. (1999). Predictors of oncology and hospice nurses' spiritual care perspectives and practices. *Applied Nursing Research, 12,* 30–37.

Taylor, E.J., & Outlaw, F.H. (2002). Use of prayer among persons with cancer. *Holistic Nursing Practice, 16*(3), 46–60.

Taylor, E.J., Outlaw, F.H., Bernardo, T., & Roy, A. (1999). Spiritual conflicts associated with praying about cancer. *Psycho-Oncology, 8,* 386–394.

Thomas, J., & Retsas, A. (1999). Transacting self-preservation: A grounded theory of the spiritual dimensions of people with terminal cancer. *International Journal of Nursing Studies, 36,* 191–201.

Wilt, D.L., Smucker, C.L., Groer, M.W., & Wagner, J.W. (2001). *Nursing the spirit: The art and science of applying spiritual care.* Washington, DC: American Nurses Association.

Wright, M.C. (2002). The essence of spiritual care: A phenomenological enquiry. *Palliative Medicine, 16,* 125–132.

CHAPTER 8

The Influence of Hope on the Psychosocial Experience

PHYLLIS GORNEY COOPER, RN, MN

Hope is the thing with feathers
That perches on the soul
And sings the tune without the words
And never stops
At all.

—Emily Dickinson

Rachel Remen, MD (1996), author of *Kitchen Table Wisdom,* wrote the following about hope and cancer.

> In my experience, a diagnosis is an opinion and not a prediction. What would it be like if more people allowed for the presence of the unknown and accepted the words of their medical experts in this same way? The diagnosis is cancer. What that will mean remains to be seen. (p. 67)

Hope

Hope is a multifaceted, fundamental phenomenon of human life. Hope has been variably referred to as the drive to survive, the reason to be, and the difference between life and death (Dufault & Martocchio, 1985; Herth, 1989; Owen, 1989; Stephenson, 1991; Stotland, 1969). Fromm (1968) regarded hope as the activating force of the human spirit. Within the context of the cancer experience, hope has been recognized as an important factor in the well-being of individuals. MacDonald (1982) noted that hope is an important and viable "drug" in the treatment of cancer. Simonton, Matthews-Simonton, and Creighton (1978) illustrated the importance of hope in healing and illness recovery.

Hope is an important element in survival for the patient with cancer. Indeed, hopelessness and helplessness are frequent precursors of cancer. The hope we try to impart is essentially a stance towards life. It is not just a matter of philosophy, but of survival. For each patient, the process of getting well includes redefining his or her stance toward the experience of a life-threatening disease so that there is hope. (p. 73)

Dimensions of Hope

Although no overall description or model of hope exists, hope generally has been described as an emotion, a behavior, a disposition, and a cognition (Averhill, Catlin, & Chon, 1990). Positive emotions usually associated with hope include love, comfort, and inspiration. As an emotion, hope can function as a motivator to achieve goals (Stotland, 1969). Behaviors that manage negative situations or involve interpersonal relationships can result in a greater sense of hope (Ebright & Lyon, 2002; Marcel, 1967; Post-White et al., 1996). The disposition to hope can be viewed as a personal state (i.e., feelings attached to a specific situation) or a personal trait (i.e., a more permanent view or personality type) (McGee, 1984). Hope, as a cognitive process, functions to change perceptions about a specific circumstance, such as a positive outlook to redirect a sense of despair (Lynch, 1965).

Hope has been likened to experiences such as anticipation, belief, confidence, contemplation, desire, expectation, faith, optimism, and trust (Ebright & Lyon, 2002; Kipfer, 1992). Stephenson (1991) proposed that hope is an anticipation of a positive future desire or expectation. Stotland (1969) described hope as a motivational dimension that solves problems and fulfills goals. The deliverance from a negative situation through patience and confidence defines Marcel's (1967) view of hope. Similarly, Lynch (1965) described hope as a positive and necessary factor to manage despair. Morse and Doberneck (1995) outlined a definition of hope as a response to a threat that uses internal and external resources, as well as reevaluation, to endure to reach an outcome.

Central to the study of emotions, spirit, and health is work by Mate (2003) on stress and disease. Building on the classic work of Selye (1978), Mate noted that the literature consistently identifies three factors that lead to stress: uncertainty, the lack of information, and the loss of control. Therefore, the perception of threat greatly influences the perceiver. If the person feels mastery over the threat, a feeling of control exists and the impact of the stress on the body will be less than if the person feels unable to manage the threat. Physical problems and disease are the most challenging to this personal sense of control. Cancer, a disease caused by cellular lack of control, threatens this process of personal stress management at the core of the person's biopsychosocial/spiritual self. Cancer causes fear and an increase in emotional stress, but people with cancer often live long lives after initial and repeated episodes with the disease. The advances in prevention, management, and cure of cancer offer people concerned with or experiencing this disease hope for the present and future.

Nursing literature has presented various models of hope. Miller (1983) described hope in association with a general sense of faith. Faith is the basis of hope that promotes self-actualization and coping. The model of hope described by McGee (1984) contended that hope and hopelessness are opposites, noting that individual state-trait variables influence the level of hope or hopelessness at any given time. Dufault and

Martocchio (1985) identified two related but distinct components of hope: generalized hope, which relates to a broad, positive view of life, and particularized hope, which is concerned with specific outcomes.

Owen's (1989) conceptual model of hope included the unifying element of energy. In this model, the preservation or loss of hope was associated with energy exchange or transformation. The process of maintaining hope also was illustrated in Ersek's (1992) model, which outlined two components: "dealing with it" and "keeping it in its place." Patients used these process components to maintain hope through confronting and managing aspects of a cancer illness. Post-White et al.'s (1996) circular model proposed five themes of hope (see Figure 8-1). In this model, hope is sustained by

Figure 8-1. Themes of Hope

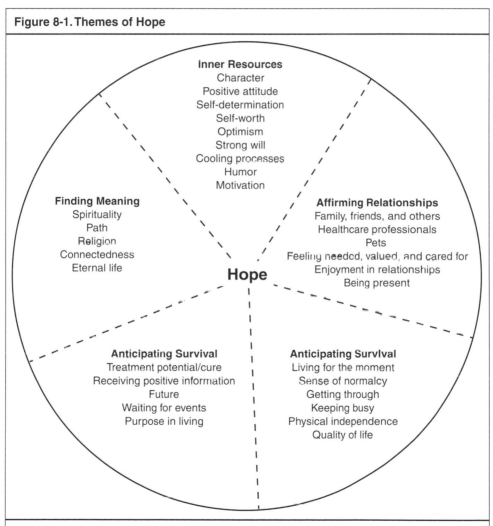

Note. From "Hope, Spirituality, Sense of Coherence, and Quality of Life in Patients With Cancer," by J. Post-White, C. Ceronsky, M.J. Kreitzer, K. Nickelson, D. Drew, K.W. Mackey, et al., 1996, *Oncology Nursing Forum, 23,* p. 1576. Copyright 1996 by the Oncology Nursing Society. Reprinted with permission.

common attributes, but patients with cancer use strategies in multiple ways to foster hope to meet their individual needs.

Hope Versus Hopelessness

To understand hope better, it is important to compare it to the concept of hopelessness. Generally, hopelessness is a negative view of the future with a sense of the impossible (Stephenson, 1991). Stotland (1969) noted that a person without hope is dull and listless and only oriented to the present. Hopelessness may manifest in an individual as frequent sighing, decreased activity level, lack of motivation, and feelings of helplessness that lead to a sense of a future with nothing (Poncar, 1994).

Hopelessness that is prolonged or is characterized by persistent symptoms may lead to depression or suicide. Nurses must attune themselves to an individual manifesting protracted hopelessness and intervene with referrals to appropriate services and treatment. Specifically, in patients with cancer and family caregivers of patients who are terminally ill, studies have found hopelessness to be related to physical or emotional isolation, fatigue, physical deterioration, and poor symptom control (Herth, 1990, 1993).

Hope and hopelessness can coexist, but these concepts represent opposite characteristics. Thus, hope and hopelessness conceptually can be visualized at a distance from each other with layers or phases of the two concepts filling in the center of a continuum. This view of hope and hopelessness lends credibility to why hope can still be found in "hopeless" situations.

Assessment

Nurses must be aware of methods to assess hope to implement appropriate nursing interventions to support hope. As noted previously, hope is a multidimensional concept with various definitions. Thus, an initial step in assessing hope is to select a description of hope that is appropriate to the clinical context and the purpose of the assessment. Nurses must consider patients' clinical conditions (e.g., energy levels, attention span, emotional ability) when assessing hope (Herth, 1993; Owen, 1989). To gain pertinent patient information regarding hope, nurses need to communicate carefully through written or oral means. Nurses need to be aware of patients' individual situations, such as cultural perspectives, clinical conditions, or education levels, that warrant adapting or revising interview methods concerning patient perceptions of hope (Farran, Herth, & Popovich, 1995). The selection of appropriate research instruments will facilitate collection of meaningful data about hope. For example, the Herth Hope Scale (Herth, 1991), the Herth Hope Index (Herth, 1992), and the Nowotny Hope Scale (Nowotny, 1989) have been developed and used in populations of individuals with cancer. Figure 8-2 lists questions for assessing hope in a clinical environment.

Farran, Wilken, and Popovich (1992) outlined a helpful framework for assessing hope. Using "hope" as an acronym, they devised the following list of elements to consider.

    H = Health
    O = Others
    P = Purpose
    E = Engaging process

Figure 8-2. Hope Assessment Tool

---

1. What gives you hope?
2. What inner resources (e.g., spirituality, meditation, visualization, prayer, daydreaming) do you use to sustain hope?
3. What external resources (e.g., family, friends, pets, living arrangement, community resources, income) do you use to sustain hope?
4. What is your current energy level/health level?
5. Currently, what are you hoping for?
6. What do you feel you can do to influence your level of hope?
7. What can others do to influence your level of hope?

Researchers have noted that health can be related to hope (Gaskins & Forte, 1995). With certain health problems, actual or perceived adversity may affect hope (Dufault & Martocchio, 1985; Herth, 1989, 1990; Hinds, 1988; Marcel, 1967). A suggested assessment question is "How has your health affected your feelings of hope?"

The maintenance or enhancement of hope has been strongly connected to relationships and social support (Herth, 1989, 1990, 1993; Miller, 1985; Poncar, 1994; Post-White et al., 1996; Raleigh, 1992). Asking "Do you have supportive others in your life?" will assess for the presence of significant relationships in the patient's life.

Purpose in life is interwoven with the concept of hope (Vaillot, 1970). Also, one's purpose in life may be founded on a spiritual or religious base. A useful assessment question is "What gives you hope?" If the reply indicates spiritual or religious contexts, a more formal spiritual assessment may be indicated.

The engaging process includes strategies of setting goals, taking action, maintaining control, and monitoring time (Farran et al., 1992). Within this context, suggested assessment questions might include "What do you hope will happen in the future?", "What action is needed to meet your future aims?", "Do you perceive control in your situation?", and "What gives you hope today?"

Influence of Culture

Nurses must be aware of various cultural interpretations of hope. Interview techniques and assessment tools in regard to hope must be applied carefully and appropriately in cultural contexts (Farran et al., 1995). Patients from certain cultures may find it difficult or taboo to discuss their hopes or sense of hope for fear of cultural or spiritual consequences. For example, American society places a high value on succeeding at all costs; thus, a sense of giving up or losing hope may leave the patient feeling physically and/or emotionally weak. Hispanic Americans have been reported to be more optimistic than Americans of other cultural-spiritual groups (Mickley & Soeken, 1993). Seeking resources and validating cultural contexts of hope are challenges facing nurses in various care arenas (see Chapter 6).

Hope-Inspiring Strategies

Because cancer is a chronic disease, nurses spend a significant amount of time with patients and their families. They are, therefore, in a unique position to foster hope

---

in patients. As with any nursing intervention, strategies to promote hopefulness and minimize hopelessness must be individualized. Hope-fostering strategies gleaned from various studies include the energy/stress management processes described. In addition, the presence of trusting relationships, adequate resources (e.g., financial, medical, living arrangements), illness management, realistic aims, and spiritual beliefs are significant adjuncts to how body energy is used (Cutcliffe, 1995; Ersek, 1992; Gaskins & Forte, 1995; Herth, 1990, 1993; Poncar, 1994; Post-White et al., 1996; Raleigh, 1992; Yates, 1993).

A critical component of hope is the presence of a caring, shared relationship (Cutcliffe, 1995; Herth, 1990; Post-White et al., 1996; Raleigh, 1992; Yates, 1993). Within a context of caring, nurses can influence a sense of connectedness through being present, using active listening, and using sensory stimulation practices. Respect and compassion for patients' personal dignity and worth communicate a sense of hope (Post-White et al.). Assisting patients to explore ways of maintaining and fostering relationships is helpful in renewing hope. Not only human relationships foster hope; pets also can fill this need. Teaching patients' family members and friends about strategies such as presencing, touch, privacy, conversation, and sensory stimulation may facilitate hope in both patients and significant others (Herth, 1990, 1993).

Patients may have a difficult time sustaining hope without adequate resources. Nurses may be pivotal in helping patients to identify and mobilize resources to positively influence patients' sense of hope (Gaskins & Forte, 1995; Herth, 1989, 1990, 1993; Poncar, 1994; Post-White et al., 1996; Raleigh, 1992). In addition, nurses must be aware of available external resources, such as support groups and volunteer programs. The availability and use of internal resources (e.g., emotions, psychological state, beliefs) and external resources help patients to maintain control and promote action.

A major role of oncology nurses is to minimize physical manifestations of disease with the overall goal of effective symptom management. As noted by Herth (1990, 1993), poorly controlled disease symptoms, such as severe pain and intractable vomiting, caused patients and caregivers to experience fear with ensuing fatigue and hopelessness. Additionally, a sense of abandonment and isolation because of minimal communication with nurses heightened patients' feelings of frustration and hopelessness. When symptoms of cancer cannot be eliminated with medical interventions, open, honest communication about medical treatments and alternative nursing interventions exhibits a caring, compassionate approach that renews hope (Herth, 1990, 1993; Poncar, 1994; Post-White et al., 1996).

Helping patients and significant others to develop attainable short-term, temporary goals that can be revised as the situation warrants supports a sense of control and hope (Herth, 1990, 1993). With this process, however, nurses must distinguish between realistic and false hopes (Herth, 1990). Careful communication used to highlight patients' assets, to build on specific progress and energy management skills, and to clarify information facilitates a sense of realistic hope. Further, the nurse's own sense of hope regarding patient goals is important (Farran et al., 1995).

Concepts of spirituality and personal meaning are common threads in many studies concerning hope (Dufault & Martocchio, 1985; Gaskins & Forte, 1995; Herth, 1989, 1990, 1993; Mickley & Soeken, 1993; Miller, 1989; Poncar, 1994; Post-White et al., 1996; Raleigh, 1992). Post-White et al. noted that spirituality, religion, faith, and belief in eternal life enhanced hope by assisting individuals with cancer to discover meaning in their lives. According to Vaillot (1970), the ability to hope is based on having meaning and purpose in one's life. With this in mind, hope becomes more than a conviction that something will turn out well; it is the certainty that something makes sense and has meaning regardless of how it turns out. Hickey (1986) noted that values clarification and self-reflection can facilitate one's sense of meaning in life. Strategies to support spiritual and personal meaning include coordinating resources to allow patients to express spirituality, encouraging journal writing, using energy balancing practices, suggesting the enjoyment of small everyday events (e.g., sunrises, tending plants, watching children play, favorite foods, birds singing, healing sounds), and helping patients to see the joys of favorite objects that instill hope (e.g., statues, photos, quilts).

Study and experimentation have revealed the importance of the mind and spirit relative to the body and its existence (Chopra, 1990, 2003; Mate, 2003). For some, this work will facilitate the fostering of hope and an increased sense of control over fears and stresses.

Much of the core work in stress management is based on the advances in science dealing with the fundamental essence of life—how our atoms, molecules, body systems, and hormones come together and create and maintain life. Chopra (1990) explained how all people are linked through a universal energy, the energy within our bodies and the energy we share with all others in the universe. This energy is constantly influenced by all internal and external stimuli. Cancer cells are internal stimuli initiated by some energy imbalance causing certain cells of the body to go out of control. Recent work in energy balancing by Chopra (2003) and Mate (2003) demonstrated that stimulation of the senses and body energies with healing energy can make changes in the body's immune system, its responses to cancer cells, and even the existence of the cancer cells.

These energy-influencing sensory stimuli added to other energy-balancing practices, such as prayer, meditation, guided imagery, and physical treatment, can increase the feelings of hopefulness in an individual. Researchers (Lengacher et al., 2002) and theorists (Dossey, Keegan, & Guzzetta, 2004) are using the energy-balancing practices and documenting the helpful outcomes in both case studies and experimental work. If one's hope is to be healed, the use of healing resources and practices can increase the healing energy in the body and promote the feeling of hope in the person.

The healing sensory stimuli are aromatherapy for smell; positive visual images and visualizations for sight; healthy foods and drinks; clean mouth for taste; human contact from loving, caring, healing individuals for touch; and mantras, energy sounds (Chopra, 2003), and music (Chopra, 2003; Guzzetta, 2005; Mate, 2003) for hearing. The outcome of the practices designed to stimulate all these senses is profound, particularly if started early and continued as a daily practice, not only when disease or health problems occur but more so as a daily health practice.

The most profound impact comes from the use of music/sound on the body energy and the healing process (Guzzetta, 2005; Healing Music Organization, 2003). Music can make us happy, sad, comfortable, agitated, or energized. Through healing sounds and music, the cells of the body at the atomic level are influenced just as our mind is (Healing Music Organization). Hope can be restored or maintained through energy work with all the senses. However, most people respond to sounds that are pleasing to them: using the basic healing sounds, music the person feels peaceful with can be a natural, noninvasive adjunct to other healing practices. According to the Healing Music Organization, sound and music can be the basis of healing and healthy living as well as generating healthy cells to attack the cells that are out of control.

Other available and relatively simple strategies have the potential to support the development of trusting patient-caregiver relationships and foster a sense of hopefulness. Remen (1996) related a story about a woman physician who bought some grow lights and started raising plants in her office, an otherwise sterile room without windows. The plants had done well, and her patients seemed to take great interest in the plants. She incorporated the plants into her therapy session, working with the patients to care for the plants prior to each session. After time, the patients wanted to take home cuttings to grow at home and would bring back to the physician stories of how well the plants were doing.

The plants came to represent hope. The physician's patients found her tending plants in an environment that was inhospitable to growth. As they watched the plants grow, they began to hope. Patients began to see there was a way to grow despite difficulties and limitations.

Conclusion

Hope is a vital component of the human experience. Hope is a feeling that manifests in a behavior, a disposition, or a cognition. Hope has achieved much status as healthcare professionals gain clarity related to the energy of a biopsychosocial/spiritual existence. Practices that enhance hope can be used to provide patients with some control and thus maintain a measure of health despite a serious illness.

Special thanks to Daniel L. Cooper, MS, for his assistance with the preparation of this chapter, and to Susan M. Schlesselman Buzhardt, RN, MSN, OCN®, who served as the author of this chapter in the first edition.

References

Averhill, J.R., Catlin, G., & Chon, K.K. (1990). *Rules of hope.* New York: Springer.

Chopra, D. (1990). *Quantum healing.* New York: Bantam Books.

Chopra, D. (2003, December 8). *The soul of healing* [Television broadcast]. Los Angeles: KOCE-TV.

Cutcliffe, J.R. (1995). How do nurses inspire and instill hope in terminally ill HIV patients? *Journal of Advanced Nursing, 22,* 888–895.

Dossey, B.M., Keegan, L., & Guzzetta, C. (Eds.). (2004). *Holistic nursing: A handbook for practice* (4th ed.). Sudbury, MA: Jones and Bartlett.

Dufault, K., & Martocchio, B. (1985). Symposium on compassionate care and the dying experience. Hope: Its spheres and dimensions. *Nursing Clinics of North America, 20,* 379–391.

Ebright, P.R., & Lyon, B. (2002). Understanding hope and factors that enhance hope in women with breast cancer. *Oncology Nursing Forum, 29,* 561–572.

Ersek, M. (1992). The process of maintaining hope in adults undergoing bone marrow transplantation. *Oncology Nursing Forum, 19,* 883–889.

Farran, C.J., Herth, K.A., & Popovich, J.M. (1995). *Hope and hopelessness: Critical clinical constructs.* Thousand Oaks, CA: Sage.

Farran, C.J., Wilken, C.S., & Popovich, J.M. (1992). Clinical assessment of hope. *Issues in Mental Health Nursing, 13,* 129–138.

Fromm, E. (1968). *The revolution of hope, toward a humanized technology.* New York: Harper and Row.

Gaskins, S., & Forte, L. (1995). The meaning of hope: Implications for nursing practice and research. *Journal of Gerontological Nursing, 21,* 1724.

Guzzetta, C. (2005). Music therapy: Hearing the melody of the soul. In B.M. Dossey, L. Keegan, & C. Guzzetta (Eds.), *Holistic nursing: A handbook for practice* (4th ed., pp. 617–640). Sudbury, MA: Jones and Bartlett.

Healing Music Organization. (2003). *Welcome to the Healing Music Organization.* Retrieved December 12, 2003, from http://www.healingmusic.org

Herth, K.A. (1989). The relationship between level of hope and level of coping response and other variables in patients with cancer. *Oncology Nursing Forum, 16,* 67–72.

Herth, K.A. (1990). Fostering hope in terminally ill people. *Journal of Advanced Nursing, 15,* 1250–1259.

Herth, K.A. (1991). Development and refinement of an instrument to measure hope. *Scholarly Inquiry for Nursing Practice, 5,* 39–51.

Herth, K.A. (1992). An abbreviated instrument to measure hope: Development and psychometric evaluation. *Journal of Advanced Nursing, 17,* 1251–1259.

Herth, K.A. (1993). Hope in the family caregiver of terminally ill people. *Journal of Advanced Nursing, 18,* 538–548.

Hickey, S.H. (1986). Enabling hope. *Cancer Nursing, 9,* 133–137.

Hinds, P.S. (1988). Adolescent hopefulness in illness and health. *Advances in Nursing Science, 10,* 79–88.

Kipfer, B.A. (1992). *Roget's 21st century thesaurus in dictionary form.* New York: Dell.

Lengacher, C.A., Bennett, M.P., Kip, K., Keller, R., LaVance, M., Smith, L.S., et al. (2002). Frequency of use of complementary and alternative medicine in women with breast cancer. *Oncology Nursing Forum, 29,* 1445–1452.

Lynch, W.F. (1965). *Images of hope: Imagination as healer of the hopeless.* Baltimore: Helicon.

MacDonald, J. (1982). *When cancer strikes: A book for patients, families, and friends.* Englewood Cliffs, NJ: Prentice-Hall.

Marcel, G. (1967). Desire and hope. In N. Lawrence & D. O'Connor (Eds.), *Readings in existential phenomenology* (pp. 277–285). Englewood Cliffs, NJ: Prentice-Hall.

Mate, G. (2003). *When the body says no.* Hoboken, NJ: John Wiley.

McGee, R. (1984). Hope: A factor influencing crisis resolution. *Advances in Nursing Science, 6,* 34–44.

Mickley, J., & Soeken, K. (1993). Religiousness and hope in Hispanic and Anglo-American women with breast cancer. *Oncology Nursing Forum, 20,* 1171–1177.

Miller, J.F. (1983). *Coping with chronic illness: Overcoming powerlessness.* Philadelphia: F.A. Davis.

Miller, J.F. (1985). Inspiring hope. *American Journal of Nursing, 85,* 22–25.

Miller, J.F. (1989). Hope-inspiring strategies of the critically ill. *Applied Nursing Research, 2,* 23–29.

Morse, J.M., & Doberneck, B. (1995). Delineating the concept of hope. *Image: The Journal of Nursing Scholarship, 27,* 277–285.

Nowotny, M. (1989). Assessment of hope in patients with cancer: Development of an instrument. *Oncology Nursing Forum, 16,* 57–61.

Owen, D. (1989). Nurses' perspectives on the meaning of hope in patients with cancer: A qualitative study. *Oncology Nursing Forum, 16,* 75–79.

Poncar, P.J. (1994). Inspiring hope in the oncology patient. *Journal of Psychosocial Nursing, 32*(1), 33–38.

Post-White, J., Ceronsky, C., Kreitzer, M.J., Nickelson, K., Drew, D., Mackey, K.W., et al. (1996). Hope, spirituality, sense of coherence, and quality of life in patients with cancer. *Oncology Nursing Forum, 23,* 1571–1579.

Raleigh, E. (1992). Sources of hope in chronic illness. *Oncology Nursing Forum, 19,* 443–448.

Remen, R. (1996). *Kitchen table wisdom: Stories that heal.* New York: Riverhead Books.

Selye, H. (1978). *The stress of life* (Rev. ed.). New York: McGraw-Hill.

Simonton, O.C., Matthews-Simonton, S., & Creighton, J.L. (1978). *Getting well again: A step-by-step, self-help guide to overcoming cancer for patients and families.* Toronto, Canada: Bantam Books.

Stephenson, C. (1991). The concept of hope revisited for nursing. *Journal of Advanced Nursing, 16,* 1456–1461.

Stotland, E. (1969). *The psychology of hope.* San Francisco: Jossey-Bass.

Vaillot, M.C. (1970). Living and dying. Hope: The restoration of being. *American Journal of Nursing, 70,* 268–273.

Yates, P. (1993). Towards a reconceptualization of hope for patients with a diagnosis of cancer. *Journal of Advanced Nursing, 18,* 701–706.

CHAPTER 9

The Psychosocial Impact of the Pain Experience

CAROL P. CURTISS, RN, MSN

> *Pain is the common companion of birth and growth, disease and death, and is a phenomenon deeply intertwined with the very question of human existence. It is among the most salient of human experiences, and it precipitates questioning the meaning of life itself.*
>
> —David Bakan

Pain is one of the most feared symptoms associated with cancer (American Cancer Society [ACS], 2001; Paice, 2004). Pain increases distress and suffering and is a significant threat to quality of life in adults and children (Chang, Hwang, Feuerman, & Kasimis, 2000; Chapman & Garvin, 1999; Loeser & Melzack, 1999; Paice). Epidemiologic evidence indicates that cancer pain adds substantially to the already considerable national disease burden of cancer (National Institutes of Health [NIH], 2002). Although pain is one of the most common symptoms reported by people with cancer (National Comprehensive Cancer Network [NCCN], 2002), published studies are virtually restricted to prevalence data; no reliable incidence studies exist (NIH). Estimates of prevalence range from 14%–100% (NIH).

Pain may occur anywhere in the illness trajectory from prediagnosis through end of life, as well as in survivors of cancer of all ages who may experience persistent pain as a long-term complication of otherwise curative therapy (ACS, 2001; Amichetti & Caffo, 2003; Jacox et al., 1994; Ryan et al., 2003). Cancer pain can be relieved or controlled for nearly everyone (American Pain Society [APS], 2003; Cherny, 2000), yet unrelieved cancer pain is a continuing significant public health problem and causes needless suffering for patients and their families. New mandates (Joint Commission on Accreditation of Healthcare Organizations, 2003) require all healthcare organizations to systematically screen for pain, assess pain when present, and develop a plan of care to manage pain as a core part of basic clinical care for everyone. Figure 9-1 presents a list of principles for managing pain effectively.

Figure 9-1. Principles for Managing Pain Effectively

- Ask about pain regularly; believe the person with pain.
- Complete a thorough history and physical examination.
- Assess pain, pain relief, the effects of pain on the person, and side effects of pain-relief measures.
- Reassess at each visit, with new pain, when pain changes, at transitions in health care, and with procedures that cause pain.
- Use medicines in a systematic, organized way.
- Anticipate and treat side effects aggressively.
- Increase doses of opiates to provide maximum relief and minimum side effects.
- Use the oral route unless contraindicated.
- Use nonpharmacologic interventions.
- Evaluate the effectiveness of the pain-relief plan routinely.
- Keep the plan simple.

Note. Based on information from Jacox et al., 1994; Pasero et al., 1999.

Pain is a subjective, complex, unique, individual experience. The International Association for the Study of Pain (1979) defined pain as "an unpleasant sensory and emotional experience associated with actual or potential tissue damage or defined in terms of such damage" (p. 249). McCaffery (1968) defined pain as whatever the person says it is, occurring whenever the person says it occurs. However pain is defined, the best indicator of pain and pain relief is self-report of the individual experiencing pain (ACS, 2001; APS, 2003; Jacox et al., 1994). Clinicians must accept verbal reports from the person in pain as the "gold standard" for understanding pain and pain relief (ACS; APS, 2003; Jacox et al.; NCCN, 2002). Pain and pain perception are different for each person, even when the source of the pain is similar. Interventions that work for one person may be ineffective for another person with similar pain. Therefore, all pain management plans must be developed based on a comprehensive assessment of each individual, using self-report as a guide whenever possible.

Pain and Quality of Life

Unrelieved pain is all-consuming and threatens every aspect of quality of life. Pain causes multiple losses for individuals and families and increases caregiver burden (Bostrom, Sandh, Lundberg, & Fridlund, 2003; Chang, Hwang, & Kasimis, 2002). Pain is multidimensional and has a physical, psychological, social, and spiritual or existential impact (Ferrell, 1995). Overall, people with cancer accompanied by pain report significantly worse quality of life than those without pain (Chang et al., 2002; Ferrell, Rhiner, Cohen, & Grant, 1991; Madison & Wilkie, 1995; Wells, Murphy, Wujcik, & Johnson, 2003). Quality of life is affected by pain throughout the illness trajectory and, for some, persistent pain lingers long after treatment is complete. Figure 9-2 presents a framework for examining the impact of pain on quality of life.

Physical Effects of Pain on Quality of Life

Unrelieved pain negatively affects every body system and results in multiple physical problems for people with cancer. Pain interrupts sleep, diminishes appetite, and decreases mobility, endurance, and energy. Pain-related symptoms such as fatigue, depression, constipation, anorexia, and decreased functional ability further strain individual resources. Pain also may impair immune response (American Academy of Pediatrics & Canadian Paediatric Society, 2000; Chong & Bajwa, 2003; Page, 1996). Overall, individuals with pain report significantly poorer levels of physical well-being, nutritional status, and quality of life than those who are pain free (Burrows, Dibble, & Miaskowski, 1998; Madison & Wilkie, 1995; Miaskowski & Lee, 1999). Unrelieved pain may cause permanent damage to the nervous system. When pain persists, pain impulses are permanently embedded in the central nervous system, causing hypersensitivity to additional painful stimuli and a decrease in antinociceptive mechanisms (APS, 2003; Baron, 2000; Regan & Peng, 2000). Pain impulses may continue even after healing occurs.

Psychological Effects of Unrelieved Pain

Dealing with persistent pain is an emotional challenge. Unrelieved cancer pain is associated with higher levels of depression, fatigue, anxiety, distress, and total mood disturbance (Glover, Dibble, & Miaskowski, 1995; Meuser et al., 2001; Poulos, Gertz,

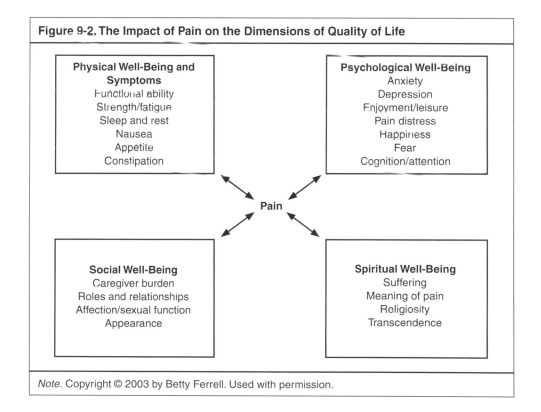

Figure 9-2. The Impact of Pain on the Dimensions of Quality of Life

Physical Well-Being and Symptoms
Functional ability
Strength/fatigue
Sleep and rest
Nausea
Appetite
Constipation

Psychological Well-Being
Anxiety
Depression
Enjoyment/leisure
Pain distress
Happiness
Fear
Cognition/attention

Pain

Social Well-Being
Caregiver burden
Roles and relationships
Affection/sexual function
Appearance

Spiritual Well-Being
Suffering
Meaning of pain
Religiosity
Transcendence

Note. Copyright © 2003 by Betty Ferrell. Used with permission.

Pankratz, & Post-White, 2001). Individuals with persistent pain describe diminished self-worth; loss of control; guilt; anger; helplessness; a negative impact on overall coping; and decreased ability to participate in leisure and work activities (Ferrell, 1995).

Unrelieved cancer pain is a primary risk factor for developing depressive disorders (Depression Guideline Panel, 1993; NIH, 2002). People with cancer are three times more likely than the general population and almost twice as likely than other medically hospitalized patients to develop depression (Arolt, Fein, Driessen, Dorlochter, & Maintz, 1998). Prevalence studies of depression in people with cancer range from 1%–42% (NIH). According to Bottomley (1998), approximately 20%–25% of all people with cancer will experience depression in the course of illness, and the prevalence increases in those with advanced disease. As pain worsens, depressive symptoms increase and quality of life decreases (Chang et al., 2000; Kelson et al., 1995). Although suicidal ideation does not occur frequently in people with cancer, some people hold suicide as an option when severe pain is unrelieved, but often reconsider when pain is treated effectively (Filiberti & Ripamonti, 2002). No data exist on the prevalence of pain and depression for long-term survivors of cancer, but depression is a major component of untreated, persistent pain in other disease states.

Poorly managed pain may distort mood and personality (Meuser et al., 2001; Miaskowski & Dibble, 1995). Family members may describe changes in patients' personality (e.g., "He is not the same person I knew because of the pain"). Unrelieved pain affects enjoyment, lifestyle, and relationships with others. In addition, if pain is poorly managed, personal control is undermined, taxing coping skills and emotional well-being. The sense of hopelessness, vulnerability, and fear that accompanies unrelieved pain may add to and exaggerate pain and contribute to the overall suffering (Ferrell, 1995).

Anxiety, like depression, may cause pain to feel worse (Keogh & Cochrane, 2002). The presence of pain may precipitate or intensify anxiety. Muscle tension caused by anxiety or fear further aggravates the problem. Treatment for anxiety disorders can help to relieve pain, and managing pain can reduce anxiety. Patient anxiety also influences family judgment about pain. Madison and Wilkie (1995) suggested that when the levels of anxiety increase in people with pain, family members underestimate pain intensity. Conversely, when anxiety is lower, family members overestimate pain intensity. This potential discrepancy in perceptions of pain can threaten relationships, trust, and family harmony and contribute to poor pain control.

Fear is a powerful emotion that increases pain perception. People with cancer and their families are frightened by pain and concerned that pain will be worse with time. They worry that treatments will be ineffective. Families sometimes see pain as a metaphor for death (Ferrell, 1995). Fear of addiction to opioid medications is one of the primary reasons people abandon therapy and do not obtain adequate pain control. Physicians, nurses, and other healthcare providers are reluctant to suggest adequate doses of opioids, and people with pain may be afraid to take medicines for comfort (American Geriatrics Society [AGS] Panel on Persistent Pain in Older Persons, 2002; APS, 2003; Jacox et al., 1994). Failure to understand that the physical symptoms of tolerance and dependence are different syndromes from psychological addiction continues to compromise adequate pain relief (American Academy of Pain Medicine, APS, & American Society of Addiction Medicine, 2001; APS, 2003, 2005). Jacox et al., the most recent APS guidelines, and the consensus statement just cited provide recommendations for differentiating, understanding, and managing each of these syndromes.

A person's understanding of pain, pain relief, and the meaning attributed to pain influences the experience of pain. For some, pain is a constant reminder of illness and death. For others, pain is seen as being a punishment, an enemy, a challenge, or as giving a sense of purpose. People who have had poor experiences with pain relief are more likely to be anxious and fearful with new pain. Comprehensive interdisciplinary assessment and a team approach to pain management help to address individual differences (APS, 2005).

Social Effects of Unrelieved Pain

Unrelieved pain causes many social losses, including changes in lifestyle, roles and relationships, and the ability to work, play, and socialize. Pain influences sexuality, intimacy, and the ability to give and receive affection (Ferrell, 1995; NIH, 2002). Chronic pain can cause changes in appearance and diminished self-esteem. Persistent pain forces some people to remain at home, being unable to resume work or education and becoming socially isolated. For long-term survivors of cancer, persistent pain from cancer or cancer treatment may last a lifetime after curative therapy for cancer.

Pain is a family experience, and patient comfort is a high priority for family members. Family caregivers feel helpless, frustrated, heartbroken, frightened, and overwhelmed when a loved one has pain (Ferrell et al., 1991). Family members often see pain as the indicator of overall health status and a sign of progression of disease. Loved ones share the suffering, loss of control, and impaired quality of life caused by pain and also experience psychological and social distress (Ferrell et al., 1991). Family caregivers have the additional burden of experiencing interrupted sleep, learning to make decisions about pain assessment and management, and dealing with medicines and technology at home. Other burdens include financial burdens from costs of therapy, loss of employment, and lost time from work for the patient or family members.

Effects of Unrelieved Pain on Spirituality

Unrelieved pain causes suffering for individuals and families and often results in a reevaluation of spiritual values and beliefs. Some people derive existential meaning from pain and suffering, describing positive life changes, opportunities for transcendence, increased control or power, and an enhanced sense of purpose (Cusick, 2003; Ferrell, 1995). Others experience pain as punishment, a test, or an existential crisis that adds to additional pain and suffering. Pain and suffering are not the same concepts, although they often are interrelated. Pain can be managed with relative ease for most people by using medications and simple nondrug interventions. Suffering, however, is far more complex and requires a more in-depth approach (see Chapters 7 and 10).

Developmental Issues Related to Pain Control

Infants and Children

Children are at risk for poorly managed pain throughout the cancer experience (American Academy of Pediatrics & APS, 2001; Anand & International Evidence-Based

Group for Neonatal Pain, 2001; APS, 2005; Cleeland et al., 1994; Jacox et al., 1994). Some studies indicated that children with cancer had substantial suffering in the last month of life (Foley & Gelbrand, 2001; Wolfe et al., 2000). Severe pain in children with cancer is an emergency and should be dealt with expeditiously (World Health Organization [WHO], 1998). Pain in children with cancer may arise from the disease, from diagnostic procedures, or from treatments. As with adults, non–cancer-related sources also can cause pain. Prevention of pain is key. Pain sensation, perception, and management are similar in children and adults, but children may experience increased physiologic and psychological trauma from cancer, diagnostic procedures, unfamiliar settings, and separation from family. Pain affects concentration, social development, and the ability to learn and play. Neonates are able to remember sensations, and infants can remember painful experiences by six months of age. Most four-year-olds can provide a self-report of pain using age-appropriate assessment tools. The child's developmental level, emotional and cognitive state, physical condition, family attitudes and beliefs, and previous pain experiences influence responses to pain. A child's pain has a profound impact on the entire family, with parents or caregivers experiencing an overwhelming sense of devastation and helplessness (Ferrell, Rhiner, Shapiro, & Dierkes, 1994).

Children's cancer pain can be relieved using strategies similar to those used with adults. Appropriate preparation for and adequate prevention of pain are critical. When healthcare providers anticipate and prevent pain from occurring, children are less fearful, tense, and anxious and feel more in control (Jacox et al., 1994). Information about the child's, parent's, and family's beliefs and expectations; the illness; and the child's environment are needed to prevent and control pain adequately. Self-report is the primary source of information for older children, whereas keen observational skills and developmentally appropriate assessment tools are required to assess children who are nonverbal or preverbal (APS, 2003; Jacox et al.; WHO, 1998). Initially, acute pain in nonverbal or preverbal children elicits crying with physical withdrawal from the stimuli, but children with long-term pain may appear depressed and withdrawn instead (Anand & International Evidence-Based Group for Neonatal Pain, 2001; Finley & McGrath, 1998). As pain continues, responses are further blunted.

Parents or caregivers can provide information and help children to feel comforted and more secure. A child-centered environment with familiar people, objects, and toys provides comfort during stressful periods. Family support throughout the experience is key. Accurate and ongoing assessment and a comprehensive plan that integrates nondrug interventions, emotional support, and appropriately selected medications titrated to each child's needs are vital.

Pain in Older Adults

Older adults also are vulnerable to undertreatment of pain (AGS, 2002). AGS identified the following consequences of untreated pain among older people: depression, anxiety, decreased socialization, sleep disturbances, impaired mobility, and increased healthcare utilization. Common myths leading to poor management in older adults are that pain is a normal process of aging, that tolerance to pain sensations increases with aging, and that opioids cannot be used safely with older adults. Clinical experience and limited research do not support these misconceptions (AGS; Jacox et al., 1994; Stein, 1996). Effective pain control improves mood, physical function, and quality of life for older people (AGS; Ferrell, Ferrell, & Rivera, 1995; Jakobsson, Klevsgard, Westergren, & Hallberg, 2003).

Principles for assessing and managing pain in older adults are the same as in other adults, except for several adaptations. A comprehensive assessment includes a medical evaluation and physical examination, thorough pain history, evaluation of the effects of pain on functional ability, evaluation of the effects of pain on the primary caregiver and family, psychosocial and financial issues, history of trauma or falls, and a complete evaluation of current medications, herbs, and dietary supplements. Accommodations should be made for visual and auditory deficits.

Many cognitively impaired people with cancer can complete assessment tools used to report current pain (Ferrell et al., 1995; Fuchs-Lacelle & Hadjistavropoulos, 2004; Hadjistavropoulos, von Baeyer, & Craig, 2001; Horgas, McLennon, & Floetke, 2003; Manz, Mosier, Nusser-Gerlach, Bergstrom, & Agrawal, 2000; Taylor & Herr, 2003), but even those who are able to use assessment tools require consistent, keen evaluation and observation. Pain behavior is more difficult to identify in the cognitively impaired and may include belligerence, withdrawal, restlessness, and other symptoms not commonly associated with pain. Some cognitive changes can be caused by unrelieved pain and may improve with adequate pain control. If pain is suspected, a systematic trial of pain relief interventions helps to differentiate between pain-induced cognitive impairment and other causes.

WHO's analgesic ladder for treating pain (WHO Expert Committee on Cancer Pain Relief and Supportive Care, 1990) needs only minor adaptation for use with older adults (AGS, 2002; Jacox et al., 1994). Older adults may be more sensitive to the peak effects and duration of analgesics because of changes in metabolism and slower excretion of medicines. "Start low and go slow" when titrating analgesics in the older adult (AGS). Begin dose escalation at the lower end of the spectrum, and raise doses slowly and carefully. Monitor and assess for pain relief, and aggressively anticipate and manage side effects frequently (AGS).

As the population ages, as more people live longer, and as society becomes more mobile, older adults often are the primary caregivers for other older adults. Fatigue, lack of energy, sleep deprivation, worry, hopelessness, and frustration are common problems of both the patients with unrelieved pain and the caregivers. Attentive pain management can ease the burden and promote physical and psychosocial well-being.

The Effects of Culture on Pain and Pain Relief

People from minority cultures often are treated inadequately for pain (Anderson et al., 2000; Bonham, 2001). Cleeland et al. (1994) identified minority status as a primary risk factor for poorly treated pain in outpatients with cancer. In addition, Anderson et al. found that pain was poorly controlled in minority patients with cancer, and the majority of minority patients wanted more information about their pain medications. Todd, Deaton, D'Adamo, and Goe (2000) found that African American and Hispanic patients in emergency departments were significantly less likely to receive analgesics than Caucasians for the same diagnosis, despite similar reports of pain in the medical record. Healthcare providers must examine personal values, beliefs, communication skills, and negotiating skills to provide competent, culturally sensitive care (Lipson, Dibble, & Minarik, 1996; Smedley, Stith, & Nelson, 2003) (see Chapter 6).

People universally perceive pain but react to it with individual emotions and behaviors. The experience of pain, methods to control pain, and reactions to pain each are learned experiences influenced by cultural expectations, values, and beliefs. These influences determine whether pain is reported, how it is reported, how it is expressed, and willingness to accept or reject a treatment plan. For example, some data indicate that culture, family beliefs, and religion contribute significantly to the management and expression of pain by Hispanic patients and caregivers (Bonham, 2001; Juarez, Ferrell, & Borneman, 1998). In this population, pain was viewed with stoicism, and the most common reason for noncompliance was an inability to understand instructions. The way in which a culture treats and regards cancer can influence the quality and tolerance of cancer-related pain. For example, when cancer is viewed as a punishment, pain may be seen as a necessary problem to endure. If cancer is a taboo subject in a culture, cancer pain may not be acknowledged at all. Understanding values, beliefs, and cultural influences helps caregivers to address individual needs fully and effectively. Some cultural variables that influence pain and pain control include the meaning of pain; religious beliefs, rituals, and values; methods of acceptable pain expression and pain tolerance; comfort with the use of medications (some cultures prefer externally applied medicines, such as salves and ointments, versus internally applied medicines, such as pills or injections); culturally acceptable coping styles and levels of anxiety in the presence of pain; significance of pain to the person; the body part involved; use of folk or non-Western medicine; concepts of illness and health; age; sex; and degree of acculturation (Clyde & Kwiatkowski, 2002).

Healthcare providers must learn about and consider personal preferences and diversity in the methods used to communicate information about pain (Last Acts Diversity Committee, 2001). For instance, the current focus on individual autonomy in health care is a Western value that does not transcend to cultures in which decisions are determined based on the needs and ideas of the group. In some cultures, the individual's wants and desires are secondary to group needs, making it inappropriate for an individual to make decisions about pain management without including other significant people in the process. Eye contact also is a Western value. Other cultures see direct eye contact as disrespectful or threatening. A pause or silence before responding to a question can be a cultural expectation. Healthcare providers lose valuable information and respect by failing to wait a sufficient amount of time for a response. Specific words used to describe pain differ from culture to culture, and some languages do not have a word for pain (Lasch, 2000).

Some cultures find it rude and disrespectful to question someone in authority, even when disagreement exists. In this case, the person may respond "yes," "no," or "all right" or simply nod, but he or she will not adhere to recommendations if they are inconsistent with his or her values and beliefs. The decision of whether to report pain also can be culturally based. The person's definition of pain may determine the amount of pain that is tolerated. If an individual believes pain should be endured, the patient may not express pain even when asked about it. Remembering that each person responds to pain as an individual, even in the presence of strong cultural ties, is important. Accurate and complete assessment and frequent reassessment of pain, including the person's beliefs, understanding, values, experiences with pain and pain relief, and the actual words they use to describe pain, will assist healthcare providers in delivering comprehensive pain management to individuals of many cultures (APS, 2005; Burrows et al., 1998).

Conclusion

Most pain can be relieved using the principles in current published standards and guidelines. But in spite of these and other resources, unrelieved pain continues to burden people with cancer and their families. The unnecessary burden of unrelieved pain in people with cancer adds needless discomfort and suffering to an already difficult situation and profoundly diminishes quality of life. In the United States, healthcare professionals have the knowledge, skills, medications, and, when needed, technology to manage most cancer pain. Nurses have a professional responsibility to aggressively identify pain and attentively control it. Spross (1985) said, "Pain is an emergency for the person experiencing it regardless of the underlying pathology. . . . We must apply the science and art of pain relief as though a life depended on it. Certainly, the quality of life does" (p. 31).

References

American Academy of Pain Medicine, American Pain Society, & American Society of Addiction Medicine. (2001). *Definitions related to the use of opioids for the treatment of pain: A consensus document.* Glenview, IL: American Pain Society.

American Academy of Pediatrics & American Pain Society. (2001). The assessment and management of acute pain in infants, children and adolescents. *Pediatrics, 108,* 793–797.

American Academy of Pediatrics & Canadian Paediatric Society. (2000). Prevention and management of pain and stress in the neonate. *Pediatrics, 105,* 454–461.

American Cancer Society. (2001). *American Cancer Society's guide to pain control.* Atlanta, GA: Author.

American Geriatrics Society Panel on Persistent Pain in Older Persons. (2002). The management of persistent pain in older persons: Clinical practice guideline. *Journal of the American Geriatrics Society, 50,* 1–20.

American Pain Society. (2003). *Principles of analgesic use in the treatment of acute pain and cancer pain* (5th ed.). Glenview, IL: Author.

American Pain Society. (2005). *Guidelines for the management of cancer pain in adults and children.* Glenview, IL: Author.

Amichetti, M., & Caffo, O. (2003). Pain after quadrantectomy and radiotherapy for early-stage breast cancer: Incidence, characteristics and influence on quality of life. Results from a retrospective study. *Oncology, 65,* 23–28.

Anand, K.J.S., & International Evidence-Based Group for Neonatal Pain. (2001). Consensus statement for the prevention and management of pain in the newborn. *Archives of Pediatrics and Adolescent Medicine, 155,* 173–180.

Anderson, K., Mendoza, T., Valero, V., Richman, S., Russell, C., Hurley, J., et al. (2000). Minority cancer patients and their providers: Pain management attitudes and practice. *Cancer, 88,* 1929–1938.

Arolt, V., Fein, A., Driessen, M., Dorlochter, L., & Maintz, C. (1998). Depression and social functioning in general hospital in-patients. *Journal of Psychosomatic Research, 45,* 117–126.

Baron, R. (2000). Peripheral neuropathic pain: From mechanism to symptoms. *Clinical Journal of Pain, 16*(Suppl. 2), S12–S20.

Bonham, V.L. (2001). Race, ethnicity, and pain treatment: Striving to understand the causes and solutions to the disparities in pain treatment. *Journal of Law, Medicine and Ethics, 29,* 52–68.

Bostrom, B., Sandh, M., Lundberg, D., & Fridlund, B. (2003). A comparison of pain and health-related quality of life between two groups of cancer patients with differing average levels of pain. *Journal of Clinical Nursing, 12,* 726–735.

Bottomley, A. (1998). Depression in cancer patients: A literature review. *European Journal of Cancer Care, 7,* 181–191.

Burrows, M., Dibble, S.L., & Miaskowski, C. (1998). Type of cancer pain influences patient outcomes. *Oncology Nursing Forum, 25,* 735–741.

Chang, V.T., Hwang, S.S., Feuerman, M., & Kasimis, B.S. (2000). Symptoms and quality of life of medical oncology patients at a Veterans Affairs medical center. *Cancer, 88,* 1175–1183.

Chang, V.T., Hwang, S.S., & Kasimis, B. (2002). Dynamic cancer pain management outcomes: The relationship between pain severity, pain relief, functional interference, satisfaction and global quality of life over time. *Journal of Pain and Symptom Management, 23,* 190–200.

Chapman, C.R., & Garvin, J. (1999). Suffering: The contributions of persistent pain. *Lancet, 353,* 2233–2237.

Cherny, N.I. (2000). The management of cancer pain. *CA: A Cancer Journal for Clinicians, 50,* 70–116.

Chong, M.S., & Bajwa, Z.H. (2003). Diagnosis and treatment of neuropathic pain. *Journal of Pain and Symptom Management, 25*(Suppl. 5), S4–S11.

Cleeland, C.S., Gonin, R., Hatfield, A.K., Edmonson, J.H., Blum, R.H., Stewart, J.A., et al. (1994). Pain and pain treatment in outpatients with metastatic cancer: The Eastern Cooperative Oncology Group's outpatient pain study. *New England Journal of Medicine, 330,* 592–596.

Clyde, C.L., & Kwiatkowski, K. (2002). Cultural perspective and pain. In B. St. Marie (Ed.), *Core curriculum for pain management nursing* (pp. 9–30). Philadelphia: Saunders.

Cusick, J. (2003). Spirituality and voluntary pain. *APS Bulletin, 13*(5). Retrieved October 24, 2003, from http://www.ampainsoc.org/pub/bulletin/sep03/path1.htm

Depression Guideline Panel. (1993). *Depression in primary care. Volume 1: Detection and diagnosis.* Rockville, MD: Agency for Health Care Policy and Research, U.S. Department of Health and Human Services, Public Health Service.

Ferrell, B.A., Ferrell, B.R., & Rivera, L. (1995). Pain in cognitively impaired nursing home patients. *Journal of Pain and Symptom Management, 10,* 591–595.

Ferrell, B.R. (1995). The impact of pain on quality of life: A decade of research. *Nursing Clinics of North America, 30,* 609–624.

Ferrell, B.R., Rhiner, M., Cohen, M.Z., & Grant, M. (1991). Pain as a metaphor for illness. Part 1: Impact of cancer pain on family caregivers. *Oncology Nursing Forum, 18,* 1303–1309.

Ferrell, B.R., Rhiner, M., Shapiro, B., & Dierkes, M. (1994). The experience of pediatric cancer pain. Part 1: Impact of pain on the family. *Journal of Pediatric Nursing, 9,* 368–379.

Filiberti, A., & Ripamonti, C. (2002). Suicide and suicidal thoughts in cancer patients. *Tumori, 88,* 193–199.

Finley, G.A., & McGrath, P.J. (1998). *Measurement of pain in infants and children* (Vol. 10). Seattle, WA: IASP Press.

Foley, K.M., & Gelbrand, H. (Eds.). (2001). *Improving palliative care for cancer: A summary report.* Washington, DC: National Academies Press.

Fuchs-Lacelle, S., & Hadjistavropoulos, T. (2004). Development and preliminary validation of the Pain Assessment Check List for Seniors with Limited Ability to Communicate (PACSLAC). *Pain Management Nursing, 5,* 37–49.

Glover, J., Dibble, S., & Miaskowski, C. (1995). Mood states of oncology outpatients. Does pain make a difference? *Journal of Pain and Symptom Management, 10,* 120–128.

Hadjistavropoulos, T., von Baeyer, C., & Craig, K.D. (2001). Pain assessment in persons with limited ability to communicate. In D.C. Turk & R. Melzack (Eds.), *Handbook of pain assessment* (2nd ed., pp. 134–149). New York: Guilford Press.

Horgas, A.L., McLennon, S.M., & Floetke, A.L. (2003). Pain management in persons with dementia. *Alzheimer's Care Quarterly, 4,* 297–311.

International Association for the Study of Pain. (1979). Pain terms: A list with definitions and notes on usage. *Pain, 6,* 249.

Jacox, A., Carr, D.B., Payne, R., Berded, C.B., Brietbart, W., Cain, J.A., et al. (1994). *Management of cancer pain: Clinical practice guideline no. 9.* Rockville, MD: Agency for Health Care Policy and Research, U.S. Department of Health and Human Services, Public Health Service.

Jakobsson, U., Klevsgard, R., Westergren, A., & Hallberg, I.R. (2003). Old people in pain: A comparative study. *Journal of Pain and Symptom Management, 26,* 625–636.

Joint Commission on Accreditation of Healthcare Organizations. (2003). *Approaches to pain management: An essential guide for clinical leaders.* Chicago: Joint Commission Resources.

Juarez, G., Ferrell, B., & Borneman, T. (1998). The influence of culture on cancer pain management in Hispanic patients. *Cancer Practice, 6,* 262–269.

Kelson, D.P., Portenoy, R.K., Thaler, H.T., Niedzwiecki, D., Passik, S.D., Tao, Y., et al. (1995). Pain and depression in patients with newly diagnosed pancreas cancer. *Journal of Clinical Oncology, 13,* 748–755.

Keogh, E., & Cochrane, M. (2002). Anxiety, sensitivity, cognitive biases, and the experience of pain. *Journal of Pain, 3,* 320–329.

Lasch, K.E. (2000). Culture, pain, and culturally sensitive pain care. *Pain Management Nursing, 1*(Suppl. 1), 16–22.

Last Acts Diversity Committee. (2001). *Last Acts statement on diversity and end of-life care.* Washington, DC: Last Acts National Program Office.

Lipson, J.G., Dibble, S.L., & Minarik, P.A. (1996). *Culture and nursing care: A pocket guide.* San Francisco: University of California, San Francisco Nursing Press.

Loeser, J., & Melzack, R. (1999). Pain: An overview. *Lancet, 353,* 1607–1609.

Madison, J.L., & Wilkie, D.J. (1995). Family members' perception of cancer pain. *Nursing Clinics of North America, 30,* 625–645.

Manz, B.D., Mosier, R., Nusser-Gerlach, M.A., Bergstrom, N., & Agrawal, S. (2000). Pain assessment in the cognitively impaired and unimpaired elderly. *Pain Management Nursing, 1,* 106–115.

McCaffery, M. (1968). *Nursing practice theories related to cognition, bodily pain, and man-environment interactions.* Los Angeles: University of California, Los Angeles Students' Store.

Meuser, T., Pietruck, C., Radbruch, L., Stute, P., Lehmann, K.A., & Grond, S. (2001). Symptoms during cancer pain treatment following WHO-guidelines: A longitudinal follow-up study of symptom prevalence, severity and etiology. *Pain, 93,* 247–257.

Miaskowski, C., & Dibble, S.L. (1995). The problem of pain in outpatients with breast cancer. *Oncology Nursing Forum, 22,* 791–797.

Miaskowski, C., & Lee, K.A. (1999). Pain, fatigue, and sleep disturbances in oncology patients receiving radiation therapy for bone metastases: A pilot study. *Journal of Pain and Symptom Management, 17,* 320–332.

National Comprehensive Cancer Network. (2002). *NCCN clinical practice guidelines in oncology v.1.2002.* Jenkintown, PA: Author.

National Institutes of Health. (2002). NIH State-of-the-Science Statement on symptom management in cancer: Pain, depression, and fatigue. *NIH Consensus and State-of-the-Science Statements, 19*(4), 1–29.

Page, G.G. (1996). The medical necessity of adequate pain management. *Pain Forum, 5,* 227–233.

Paice, J.A. (2004). Pain. In C.H. Yarbro, M.H. Frogge, & M. Goodman (Eds.), *Cancer symptom management* (3rd ed., pp. 77–93). Sudbury, MA: Jones and Bartlett.

Pasero, C., Portenoy, R.K., & McCaffery, M. (1999). Opioid analgesics. In M. McCaffery & C. Pasero (Eds.), *Pain: Clinical manual* (2nd ed., pp. 161–299). St. Louis, MO: Mosby.

Poulos, A.R., Gertz, M.A., Pankratz, V.S., & Post-White, J. (2001). Pain, mood disturbance, and quality of life in patients with multiple myeloma. *Oncology Nursing Forum, 28,* 1163–1171.

Regan, J.M., & Peng, P.P. (2000). Neurophysiology of cancer pain. *Cancer Control, 7,* 111–118.

Ryan, M., Stainton, M.C., Jaconelli, C., Watts, S., MacKenzie, P., & Mansberg, T. (2003). The experience of lower limb lymphedema for women after treatment for gynecologic cancer. *Oncology Nursing Forum, 30,* 417–423.

Smedley, B.D., Stith, A.Y., & Nelson, A.R. (Eds.). (2003). *Unequal treatment: Confronting racial and ethnic disparities in health care.* Washington, DC: National Academies Press.

Spross, J.A. (1985). Cancer pain and suffering: Clinical lessons from life, literature, and legend. *Oncology Nursing Forum, 12*(4), 23–31.

Stein, W.M. (1996). Cancer pain in the elderly. In B.R. Ferrell & B.A. Ferrell (Eds.), *Pain in the elderly: A report of the Task Force on Pain in the Elderly of the International Association for the Study of Pain* (pp. 69–80). Seattle, WA: IASP Press.

Taylor, L.J., & Herr, K. (2003). Pain intensity assessment: A comparison of selected pain intensity scales for use in cognitively intact and cognitively impaired African American older adults. *Pain Management Nursing, 4,* 87–95.

Todd, K.H., Deaton, C., D'Adamo, A.P., & Goe, L. (2000). Ethnicity and analgesic practice. *Annals of Emergency Medicine, 35,* 11–16.

Wells, N., Murphy, B., Wujcik, D., & Johnson, R. (2003). Pain-related distress and interference with daily life of ambulatory patients with cancer with pain. *Oncology Nursing Forum, 30,* 977–986.

Wolfe, J., Grier, H.E., Klar, N., Levin, S.B., Ellenbogen, B.A., Salem-Schatz, S., et al. (2000). Symptoms and suffering at the end of life in children with cancer. *New England Journal of Medicine, 342,* 326–333.

World Health Organization. (1998). *Cancer pain relief and palliative care in children with cancer.* Geneva, Switzerland: Author.

World Health Organization Expert Committee on Cancer Pain Relief and Supportive Care. (1990). *Cancer pain relief and palliative care: Technical report series 804.* Geneva, Switzerland: World Health Organization.

CHAPTER 10

Suffering

BETTY R. FERRELL, PhD, FAAN, AND VIRGINIA SUN, MSN, RN

Out of suffering have emerged the strongest souls.

—E.H. Chapin

In 1982, Cassell challenged the separation of illness into physical and psychological states in his classic paper "The Nature of Suffering and the Goals of Medicine." He asserted that "suffering is experienced by persons, not merely by bodies" (p. 639) and suggested that understanding the place of the person in human illness requires a rejection of the historical dualism of mind and body. According to Cassell (1999), suffering occurs when the intactness or integrity of an individual is threatened or disrupted. It involves some symptom or process (physical or otherwise) that poses a threat, the meaning of that threat, fear, and concerns about the future.

Cassell's classic work has served as a guiding force in challenging the medical profession to examine its goals and to recognize the moral mandate to attend not only to physical illness but also to the suffering that accompanies it. Nurses, perhaps, have been less inclined to consider a mind and body separation because they have recognized and embraced their professional domain to encompass the whole person. The vision and standards of oncology nursing are embedded in recognition of cancer as a life-threatening illness with dimensions of physical, psychological, social, and spiritual well-being (Ferrell, 1996). Oncology nurses consider the profession to be family-centered, acknowledging that cancer affects not one individual but the entire family.

Thus, for oncology nurses, recognition of suffering is not a novel notion but a reaffirmation of the importance of holistic care amid a rapidly changing healthcare environment. Nurses are faced with increasingly depersonalized cancer care characterized by high-tech treatments, invasive and aggressive care, and a frontier of scientific strides, including gene therapy, transplantation, and surgical approaches to eradicate disease. At the same time, nursing as a profession is rapidly moving toward a managed-care environment that has many potentially threatening components, including decreased staffing, reliance on assistive personnel, and transfer of even the most intensive care to family caregivers at home. The need to explore the basis of suffering is based on a reaffirmation of nursing's commitment to the wholeness of the patient and the existential crisis of a cancer diagnosis. This chapter explores what Cassell referred to as the nature of suffering, as well as the goals of oncology nursing.

The Nature of Suffering in Patients With Cancer

Suffering is discussed in oncology literature as a component of quality of life (QOL). A diagnosis of cancer and subsequent treatment profoundly influence QOL. Patients with cancer have described seeing their image in a mirror and reflecting on the physical devastation of disease and treatment, as well as the insult to the spirit. This recognition of decreased QOL leads the patient to become aware of the disease's devastation and an altered life that has diminished meaning. As many previous theorists (Copp, 1974; Frankl, 1963) have described, this decreased meaning leads to suffering. Relief of suffering thus is seen as a critical QOL intervention, particularly when the patient has advanced disease and the goals of care shift to comfort rather than cure. Suffering is included in the domain of spiritual well-being as an aspect of QOL, but it also is a component that transcends the other domains of physical, psychological, and social well-being (Ferrell, 1996). This model has been applied to patients with advanced cancer who are experiencing pain (Ferrell, Wisdom, Wenzl, & Schneider, 1989; Padilla, Ferrell, Grant, & Rhiner, 1990); survivors of bone marrow transplant (Ferrell et al., 1992; Grant et al., 1992), breast cancer (Dow, Ferrell, Leigh, Ly, & Gulasekaram, 1996), ovarian cancer (Ersek, Ferrell, Dow, & Melancon, 1997), and thyroid cancer (Dow, Ferrell, & Annelo, 1997); and other long-term survivors of cancer (Ferrell, Dow, Leigh, Ly, & Gulasekaram, 1995). These QOL studies have included varying populations across the cancer trajectory, and suffering is evident as a component in each. Suffering begins not at the transition from chronic illness to terminal illness but rather at the moment of diagnosis.

As an elusive and abstract concept, suffering often has been confused with other psychological constructs. Morse and Carter (1996) studied the essence of the concept of enduring and expressions of suffering and used narratives of illness experiences to analyze them. They defined three types of enduring: enduring to survive, enduring to live, and enduring to die. Suffering was defined as an emotional response to that which was endured, to the changed present, or to anticipating a changed future.

In another study, Morse, Bottorff, and Hutchinson (1995) examined the paradox of comfort. This conceptualization is applicable to cancer because cancer causes significant physical deterioration and symptoms. Eight themes of discomfort emerged in this study: the diseased body, the disobedient body, the deceiving body, the vulnerable body, the violated body, the resigned body, the enduring body, and the betraying body. The authors concluded that illness places patients' bodies in the foreground, dominating their lives.

Frankl (1963), another classic contributor to the field of suffering, developed a psychotherapy modality known as logotherapy. Logotherapy attempted to help individuals to find meaning in their experiences. Following his experiences as a concentration camp prisoner, Frankl applied his observations and experiences to individuals who survive life-threatening illnesses. Frankl observed that prisoners like himself, who had a will to live or a purpose to sustain themselves, were able to find meaning in their suffering and, thus, to survive. In applying these lessons to therapeutic relationships, Frankl contended that the clinician's role is to assist the person in finding meaning in suffering.

Just as nursing has a unique role in and contribution to cancer care, nursing also has a unique contribution to the relief of suffering. Copp (1974, 1990a, 1990b), a pioneer in applying the concept of suffering to the nursing profession, defined "suffering" as a state of anguish in one who bears pain, injury, or loss. Her classic work challenges nurses to assess and intervene in suffering.

Oncology nurses are intimately involved in the cancer journey, traversing the phases of cancer survivorship. Nurses are present during the shock and suffering associated with a new diagnosis, through the trials of aggressive treatment, the uncertainty and apprehension of remission, the devastation of recurrence, and the suffering associated with facing death from advanced disease. Nurses are instrumental in moving patients from the anguish of suffering to an experience of deriving meaning from suffering.

Recognizing the trajectory of cancer, Reich (1987, 1989) described the experience of suffering through the metaphor of language. He described the sufferers' struggle to discover a voice that would express the search for the meaning of suffering in three phases: mute suffering, expressive suffering, and new identity. In mute suffering, patients are so affected by their circumstances that they cannot verbally express their needs. This is not suffering in silence, however, because these individuals may be screaming in pain. The scream of pain may be the expression of mute suffering. In expressive suffering, the sufferer seeks a language to express the suffering. The language may be one of lament (complaint), story (in telling their story they gain voice, transform the suffering, or gain distance), or interpretation (often through metaphor). The third phase is new identity or having a voice of one's own. This occurs through experiencing solidarity with compassionate others and by taking on a language of suffering through reforming one's story, which then identifies the new self.

Sources of Suffering

A major source of suffering recognized in oncology has been that of uncontrolled symptoms. The side effects of cancer treatment often are reported to be more debilitating than the disease itself. The suffering from uncontrolled pain such as peripheral neuropathy has been described by patients with ovarian cancer as both severe and lingering (Ferrell, Smith, Cullinane, & Melancon, 2003b). Research in the area of fatigue has revealed that symptoms previously viewed as only physical problems also are associated with suffering. The experience of fatigue is a reminder of patients' many losses and results in the inability to participate in life activities. Patients often suffer from guilt and frustration because fatigue affects their need to take care of their families (Ferrell, Smith, Ervin, Itano, & Melancon, 2003).

Wolfe et al. (2000) examined the relationship of symptoms and suffering in children with cancer. Overall, 89% of the children experienced a great deal of suffering from at least one symptom, and 51% experienced three or more symptoms. Fatigue, pain, dyspnea, and poor appetite were the most commonly reported symptoms. Those children who died of a treatment-related complication suffered more symptoms than those who died of progressive disease.

Kuuppelomaki and Sirkka (1998) examined the nature, content, and meaning of suffering in patients with incurable cancer. Fifty percent of subjects experienced intense suffering, and 80% reported moderate suffering. Physical factors that led to intense suffering included pain, fatigue, and side effects of chemotherapy.

Benedict (1989) studied patients with lung cancer to explore the physical, psychological, and interactional aspects of lung cancer. Only 10% of the subjects reported experiencing no suffering, whereas 50% of the subjects reported experiencing the highest degree of suffering. The sources of greatest suffering in this study were disability, pain, anxiety, changed activities, and weakness/fatigue.

Throughout the literature, one commonly sees the terms "pain" and "suffering." It often is implied that these terms are synonymous or that they always are experienced together. These experiences are closely akin and, yet, also are quite separate. Many patients endure significant pain with little suffering, whereas others may experience extreme suffering even in the absence of pain.

Beyond physical symptoms lie the psychological aspects of the cancer diagnosis as sources of suffering. Suffering is intensified as patients recognize that their cancer will not be cured and, thus, serves no meaning. As Frankl (1963) stated, "Suffering ceases to be suffering . . . at the moment it finds meaning" (p. 113). Suffering creates one of the greatest challenges to uncovering meaning. This search for meaning is not a stagnant process but changes as each day unfolds and occurrences are interpreted (Borneman & Brown-Saltzman, 2001).

Specific events related to cancer are recognized as sources of suffering. One of the hallmarks of the cancer experience is that of loss. Patients with cancer experience phenomenal sacrifice, beginning with the physical losses associated with cancer treatment, such as loss of the breast or hair. Continued illness involves losses of relationships, responsibilities, and autonomy and the threat of loss of life itself. Many patients have described their experiences as a gradual unraveling in which one layer of their lives is removed at a time. Patients have described their loss of a sense of health once this devastating diagnosis was made. Many survivors of cancer experiencing long-term remission have discussed the loss of their future because they believe that the physical effects of the illness and treatment, despite a good prognosis, mean that they will not live a long life. Suffering is intensified when life priorities are altered and patients recognize what is truly important but then face the dilemma of limited time to enjoy those priorities and altered life goals.

Suffering Across the Cancer Trajectory

Suffering is evident in all phases of cancer, and the needs for nursing care vary across the phases. At the time of initial diagnosis, the psychological needs of patients are profound as they confront what often is the worst experience of their lives. Many patients equate their diagnosis with an inevitable death sentence, and this life-threatening disease instantly transformed them from healthy individuals to patients with cancer (Ferrell, Smith, Cullinane, & Melancon, 2003a). During cancer treatment, patients' physical needs become more intense as they experience the effects of surgery, chemotherapy, or radiation. The degree of physical symptoms experienced from cancer treatments tremendously affects suffering at this stage of the cancer trajectory. Patients describe the suffering associated with remission as they regain physical strength and health, yet they often have intense psychological distress as they adjust to living beyond the cancer diagnosis. The completion of active treatment frequently is accompanied by suffering related to uncertainty of the future and distress that nothing is being actively done to fight the disease (Ferrell et al., 2003a). The phase of recurrence has been described as one of the most intense times of suffering (Dow, Ferrell, Haberman, & Eaton, 1999; Ferrell et al., 2003a). For many, recurrence creates an awareness that, in fact, the treatment did not offer cure, and, thus, the patient now is living with a terminal illness rather than only a chronic one. For those who are still struggling with the effects of initial treatment, recurrence means having to cope with renewed physical and psychological distress. During the final phase of advanced disease or terminal illness, spiritual needs may become more intense as patients question the meaning of their lives and transcendence beyond death (Ferrell, 1993; Ferrell & Dean, 1995).

Suffering Across the Life Span

The experience of a cancer diagnosis is similar, but also profoundly different, across various age groups. A child with leukemia may struggle less with life's meaning but may be more overwhelmed by the unknown and uncertainty of illness and a disruption of all that has created security for the child (Shapiro, 1996). Research has shown that children might suffer more because they frequently are treated with highly aggressive regimens (Wolfe et al., 2000). The developmental tasks of adolescence and normal struggles to gain identity and autonomy become complicated by the diagnosis of an illness that often is perceived as reserved for the old. Young adults' experiences of cancer sharply contrast the developmental tasks of autonomy and pursuing life goals and cause suffering. Patients may perceive cancer at this period of life as an ultimate punishment as one is robbed of life goals and dreams before they can begin. Suffering associated with cancer for middle-aged adults may involve the struggle to maintain the roles and relationships of spouse, parent, and productive adult. Cancer in older adults and the associated suffering has widely diverse meanings. In many studies, older adults have been identified as a population for whom cancer caused less suffering because these patients perceived the disease as a normal occurrence and an end to life that was seen as inevitable in the near future.

Across the life span, suffering associated with cancer can be related to the losses that are associated with that phase of life. It also is closely associated with one's current roles and relationships. A young mother's anguish and suffering at the diagnosis of breast cancer may primarily focus on the reality that this will disrupt her role as a mother. The suffering associated with breast cancer in a middle-aged woman may center on the conflict of the unfairness of receiving the diagnosis just as she has completed the responsibilities of raising her children and now feels robbed of the much-anticipated time in her life when she could focus on her own needs.

Although the patient's chronologic age provides valuable information, one's psychological place in life also provides insight into suffering. Understanding what gives life meaning for an individual at any age is an important aspect of assessment. Ferrell (1996) interviewed an older woman with breast cancer whose entire life had centered around caring for her family and mentally disabled daughter. Providing physical care to her daughter had consumed this mother's life since age 40 to her current age of 75. The woman found a breast lump and, although she was aware that it was cancer, she chose not to seek any health care at all. To do so, she felt, would put her ability to continue her caregiving responsibilities in jeopardy. The physical pain and deterioration she endured from an untreated cancer was less important than the loss of meaning she would have experienced in "abandoning" her daughter and giving up her caregiver role. For this woman, continuing to do what was meaningful lessened the severe physical pain and fear of her own approaching death.

Similar to other aspects of oncology nursing, a need exists for heightened sensitivity and intervention when caring for those in vulnerable populations. Young children and frail older adults are less able to express their needs and are most vulnerable to suffering, just as they are most vulnerable to other untreated physical symptoms (Shapiro, 1996).

The cancer experience varies greatly among a mother observing her adult daughter with breast cancer, a preschool-aged child confused by the changes in his father who has been diagnosed with leukemia, the husband caring for his wife of 50 years, and a teenager accompanying her younger sibling to radiation therapy for treatment of a brain tumor. Reich's (1989) metaphor of "giving voice" applies to recognition of suffering across the age continuum because those who are most vulnerable to unrelieved suffering may be least able to articulate their needs.

Cultural Considerations

One's culture significantly influences one's reaction to a diagnosis of cancer or any illness. Culture provides the foundation for all life experiences and profoundly influences the response to illness. Cultures hold strong beliefs about cancer as an illness. Culture influences how one responds to the cancer diagnosis, as well as to all aspects of treatment and the cancer trajectory. Furthermore, the capacity for patients to give meaning to suffering and transcend it is intimately related to cultural beliefs and values (Chiu, 2000) (see Chapter 6).

Culture is bound in language and ritual. The simple word "cancer" has widely varied meanings across cultures. Understanding culturally held beliefs, customs, language, and rituals will enable nurses to view the suffering experience closely from their patients' perspectives. In assessing cultural influences on suffering, nurses may find it helpful to explore patients' past experiences with illness and ways of coping. Religion also is an important factor in cultural assessment because spirituality influences the personal interpretations of suffering, pain, and life after death (see Chapter 7).

Suffering in the Family

Oncology nursing has been family-centered since the inception of this specialty, and nurses have recognized that suffering often is more intense for the family caregivers who observe the illness than for patients with the cancer diagnosis. A diagnosis of cancer has been compared to a storm that blows through and burdens entire families with new responsibilities, limitations, and fears (Ferrell et al., 2003). Family caregivers often suffer from physical symptoms such as fatigue, which is an indication of the tremendous burden that caregivers carry in caring for their loved ones (Ferrell, Ervin, Smith, Marek, & Melancon, 2002). Psychological sources of suffering may include caregivers' sense of helplessness, lack of control, and feelings of inadequacy as a caregiver. Fears of recurrence and the lingering stress of the initial diagnosis may exacerbate this stress. As treatment begins, family caregivers express distress concerning the intensive and prolonged side effects of the cancer therapy that their loved ones were receiving (Ferrell et al., 2002).

Family caregivers often express spiritual distress in feeling abandoned by a God who would allow their loved one to die of this disease. Thus, they may feel a sense of abandonment from their faith that might otherwise have provided them support in the caregiving tasks (Coyle, 1996; Ferrell et al., 2002).

Just as peer support is important for patients, family caregivers may benefit from the support of other family caregivers. Support vehicles such as newsletters can allow caregivers to share helpful experiences and information regarding treatment and symptom management techniques (Ferrell et al., 2002). Caregivers have acknowledged the "community of suffering" that occurs late at night in the children's hospital when parents congregate in the waiting room and share their experiences of having a child diagnosed with cancer (Ferrell, Rhiner, Shapiro, & Dierkes, 1994). The parents acknowledge this as one of the most helpful means of maintaining their strength in what was perceived to be an unendurable situation. However, an impact of shifting from outpatient care to family care at home is the decreased opportunity for family caregivers to seek support from other caregivers. Family caregivers' suffering likely is intensified by the fact that they now suffer mostly in isolation (Borneman & Ferrell, 1996; Ferrell et al., 2002).

The suffering of family caregivers is closely related to their relationship with the patient. Those in different roles (e.g., daughter, mother, child, sister) experience suffering differently. Parents often have described their feelings of having a child diagnosed with cancer as a terrible injustice to have one's offspring face death before a parent (Ferrell, Taylor, Sattler, Fowler, & Cheyney, 1993).

Interventions

A discussion of nursing interventions for suffering should begin by acknowledging the unique nature of suffering and the goals of nursing. For many symptoms of cancer, such as pain or nausea, the ultimate goal is elimination of the problem. However, nurses should realize that the goal in regard to suffering is to support the sufferer through this process rather than to eliminate it. Nursing actions that attempt to stifle the voice of suffering, in fact, only intensify it. The nursing process, as applicable to suffering and care, begins with an assessment of the sources of suffering. Through careful assessment, nurses recognize that a patient on escalating doses of morphine is, in fact, experiencing profound suffering not amenable to any opioid dose. Exploration of patients' beliefs and concerns often will reveal sources of suffering, such as an unresolved relationship or feelings of abandonment by God (Kumasaka & Miles, 1996).

Careful diagnosis of the sources of suffering will help nurses to distinguish between those that should be eliminated and those that should be supported. Patients have difficulty dealing with issues of transcendence and life meaning if their basic needs of pain and symptom management are ignored. Exploring and diagnosing the sources of suffering will help nurses to determine the possible need for intervention by other professionals. Many sources of suffering are not attributable to the cancer diagnosis but rather result when the illness creates an urgency to resolve lifelong dilemmas.

Nursing intervention for suffering begins with simple presence, or "being with" the sufferer. Nurses frequently leave a home visit feeling frustrated that they have done little, only to be told by a patient how valuable their visit was. Nurses play a unique role through their presence and through active listening to patients' concerns. Their presence helps to intervene in the experience Reich (1989) referred to as mute suffering. In an interview, a Hispanic patient described a pivotal moment in her illness when she was gradually confined to a recliner in the living room because of her uncontrolled pain and increasing weakness. Her daughter and grandchildren came to visit, and the young granddaughter ran through the room eager to visit her grandmother. As the child ran into the room approaching the grandmother, she slipped and fell. For the patient, this was the first time in her life that she was not able to rise to offer comfort to her grandchild. The suffering associated with this pivotal moment was far more intense than any physical pain she had experienced. This suffering was intertwined with cultural beliefs about her role as a grandmother, with her sense of purpose, and with a clear awareness of this loss as one of many losses that would eventually lead to her death. One of the most important nursing interventions for this patient was to allow her to describe this experience and to give voice to this intense personal crisis that others might have viewed as a relatively insignificant event.

Spross (1996), an oncology nurse researcher, has explored the concept of suffering using the metaphor of the coach in supporting patients who are suffering. The role of the nurse as coach is to encourage and support and to provide direction and skills for the patient to meet this challenge of illness. Spross equated the nurse's role concerning suffering to other contexts, such as coaching during labor and delivery and coaching roles in other professions.

Battenfield (1984), Coyle (1996), and other nurse authors have emphasized the nursing role in suffering as active listening and being present. One of the major contributions to this area of nursing practice is the work of Kahn and Steeves (1994). Figure 10-1 summarizes the basic tenets of suffering as described by Kahn and Steeves (1996). They described the nurse as a witness and moral agent. A witness is a special kind of moral agent with an obligation to speak out about what is witnessed. The role of a witness may be viewed in four common ways, each of which provides an argument for the importance of speaking out and development of nursing's collective voice (Kahn & Steeves, 1994).

Figure 10-1. Tenets of Suffering

- Suffering is a private, lived experience of a whole person, unique to each individual.
- Suffering results when the most important aspects of a person's identity are threatened or lost.
- Because suffering is dependent on the meaning of an event or loss for the individual, it cannot be assumed present or absent in any given clinical condition.
- Suffering can be viewed as an experience of lost personal meaning.
- Possible sources of suffering are innumerable.
- We recognize certain kinds of experiences as forms of suffering; we acknowledge these forms as experiences that will lead to suffering for many who experience them.
- As a fundamental human experience, suffering has a basic structure.
- The experience of suffering involves the person in a larger process that includes the person's own coping with suffering and the caring of others.
- The caring environment in which the processes of suffering occur can influence a person's suffering positively and negatively.

Note. From "An Understanding of Suffering Grounded in Clinical Practice and Research" (pp. 3–27), by D.L. Kahn and R.H. Steeves in B.R. Ferrell (Ed.), *Suffering,* 1996, Sudbury, MA: Jones and Bartlett. Copyright 1996 by Jones and Bartlett. Reprinted with permission.

- **Firsthand observation:** Nurses are closest to the patient and have an opportunity to inform others of what was observed.
- **Ceremonial role:** Nurses reduce suffering by supporting or participating in rituals of transition or "rites of passage" that require witnesses to substantiate them.
- **Expert witness:** An expert witness is one who testifies or speaks in public forums about the special knowledge their expertise brings to a public issue. Oncology nurses have spoken out in their own institutions and, increasingly, in public forums about issues such as unrelieved pain, cancer survivorship, and breast cancer.
- **Visionary:** Nursing's collective vision develops as each nurse speaks out about the suffering he or she encounters, how to best respond to it, and the need for a future in which suffering is not ignored.

Nurses have emphasized that the process of finding meaning is a basic human endeavor (Dow et al., 1999; Ersek & Ferrell, 1994). Patients struggle with the questions "Why me?" and "Why now?" A patient with lung cancer may accept that the lung cancer is a result of smoking but then may struggle with guilt associated with the behavior that led to the disease. Research concerning suffering has led to nurses' understanding of the ways in which patients cope, such as the use of downward social comparison, in which patients compare themselves to others whose circumstances they believe are worse. Also, nurses now are speaking out about some of the burdens created by changes in the healthcare system. Figure 10-2 provides examples of nursing interventions for suffering and pain.

Suffering Among Professionals

Oncology nursing has both rewards and demands that add to the unique nature of the specialty. In the current changes in health care, nurses transitioning into oncology from other areas of acute care may experience a sense of helplessness in recognizing that suffering cannot be eliminated. The Oncology Nursing Society

---

Figure 10-2. Nursing Interventions to Facilitate the Search for Meaning in Cancer Pain

- Provide aggressive pharmacologic pain management to achieve optimum pain relief.
- Include nonpharmacologic interventions that enhance a sense of control.
- Assist patients to verbalize and understand the cause of their pain; clarify physiologic causes of pain.
- Explore with patients and family members their images of pain, including metaphors and visions.
- Overcome barriers, such as fear of addiction, to optimum use of analgesics.
- Distinguish between the feelings or meaning attributed to pain and beliefs about death.
- Empower patients to assume an active role in pain assessment and management.
- Explore the losses associated with the illness and pain.
- Facilitate discussion between patients and family caregivers to acquire a shared meaning of pain.
- Encourage comparison of patients' pain to pain experienced by others.
- Identify limits to pain that patients perceive to be necessary or deserved.
- Facilitate spiritual interventions, including spiritual counseling, rituals, and prayer.
- Explore pain as a sign of hopelessness, and foster altered hope consistent with advancing disease.

Note. From "The Meaning of Cancer Pain," by B.R. Ferrell and G. Dean, 1995, *Seminars in Oncology Nursing, 11,* p. 20. Copyright 1995 by W.B. Saunders. Reprinted with permission.

(ONS) supported a project designed to provide a better understanding of the unique role of oncology nurses and the meaning of their work. This project concluded that working with patients with cancer means "being there for people in their most private moments of suffering and responding to the heights and depths of their responses to this suffering" (Cohen & Sarter, 1992, p. 1485).

Fall-Dickson and Rose (1999) explored the meaning for oncology nurses of caring for patients with cancer who experience chemotherapy-induced side effects. The study showed that nurses derive a sense of self, forge relationships with patients and families under conditions of great stress, and are in constant search for successful management of treatment-related side effects. This search for a successful management plan was more difficult for some nurses who expressed strong frustration with the setting in which they practiced. Many were frustrated that the norms of practice did not recognize or promote nursing's role in the management of chemotherapy-induced side effects.

O'Connor (1996) studied ethical and moral experiences of oncology nurses. Seventy nurses from ONS wrote narratives about their experiences in a clinical situation in which they experienced ethical or moral dilemmas. Experiences reflected a care perspective focused on principles such as protecting patient autonomy and truth-telling. Moral themes included suffering, secrets, and struggle. These studies described the suffering not only of patients with cancer but also of nurses.

Smith (1996) observed that one of the greatest privileges of healthcare professionals is to be witness to suffering. He recommended that by participating in religion, art, literature, and other experiences, healthcare providers enhance their awareness of the depth of human experiences and thus strengthen their role.

Steeves, Cohen, and Wise (1994) used a phenomenologic approach to study 38 oncology nurses and their perceptions of the meaning of their work. Nurses described

---

three roles: maintaining the values of the organization through activities, such as monitoring the patients; participating in patients' experiences by being there for them, including during the dying process; and reconciling healthcare values and experiences of the patient through attempts such as maintaining truth-telling. Nurses in this study reported feeling isolated in their work and burdened by observing and experiencing suffering.

Nurses must receive support so that they can tend to their own suffering and do not feel helpless in their attempts to care for their patients. Nurses can derive great meaning from their work if they are able to grow from their interaction with patients and families in regard to suffering (Price, 1996).

Case Study

Mrs. Mendez is a 62-year-old woman with newly diagnosed breast cancer. She recently has completed surgery and is scheduled for chemotherapy and radiation therapy. The treatment has left her with many physical symptoms, including pain, extreme weight loss, and fatigue. Mrs. Mendez recently was forced to move in with her daughter and son-in-law. In a recent home visit, Mrs. Mendez asked the homecare nurse to communicate to her physician that she would prefer to cancel the chemotherapy and would rather let the cancer take its course and "die rather than prolong my suffering." On further assessment, the nurse identified many concerns and potential sources of suffering for Mrs. Mendez. The patient told the nurse that she cannot sleep at night because of the guilt and the anguish that she feels knowing that her three daughters are destined to have breast cancer and die. She also feels frustrated in her current living situation and has had conflicts with her son-in-law.

Mrs. Mendez always has relied on her cultural beliefs and traditional practices, including the use of a healer, herbal remedies, and many religious rituals to face illness. Her son-in-law, however, is not of Hispanic origin and has prohibited these practices in their home because he believes that they are "witchcraft" and he does not want his children exposed to such practices. Mrs. Mendez was divorced approximately 10 years ago and expresses her belief that this cancer is God's punishment because, as her family reminds her, divorce is unacceptable within their faith. Over the past two weeks, the home-health nurse has recognized an increased intensity in her suffering and that she has become more isolated over time. She asked the nurse to discontinue her pain medications because she does not feel comfortable having them in the home for fear that in her present state, she might consider suicide and believes that God would, in fact, further punish her for such an act. She tells the nurse, "I have gone from being the mother of seven children to now being the baby, dependent on my girls to care for me."

Discussion

Mrs. Mendez represents an individual described by Frankl (1963), Copp (1974), and others as experiencing a loss of integrity and meaning. The series of losses that she has encountered, including loss of function, health, role, and meaningful activity,

(Continued on next page)

Case Study *(Continued)*

has created extreme suffering, along with other physical problems. The forces that should sustain her through illness, such as her faith and cultural practices, have been removed because of the conflict with her son-in-law. The nursing care, in this case, should focus on recognition of the sources of suffering, allowing her expression of these sources, and identification of those issues that the nurse or other members of the healthcare team may improve.

Conclusion

Suffering is an inherent aspect of life-threatening illness and clearly is within the domain of nursing. Attending to suffering requires skills that are distinct from other clinical competencies. The challenge to "be with" the sufferer sharply contrasts the current emphasis on high-tech, aggressive care or "doing" in oncology. To achieve solidarity with the suffering patient means that nurses must have the courage to take off their protective armors and make themselves vulnerable to the feelings that opening up to people may give rise to. This is part of healthcare professionals' responsibilities if they are completely committed to every aspect of their patients' care (Penson et al., 2001). Kahn and Steeves (1994) stressed the importance of continuing to explore and value the role of nursing in suffering.

> One characteristic of nursing's development over the past decade is the discovery of its voice—the ability and willingness to express what nurses collectively know and understand about the nature of nursing practice. To continue the development of nursing's voice, it is crucial that we talk freely about what we know, including what we know about suffering. (p. 260)

References

Battenfield, B.L. (1984). Suffering: A conceptual description and content analysis of an operational schema. *Image: The Journal of Nursing Scholarship, 16,* 36–41.

Benedict, S. (1989). The suffering associated with lung cancer. *Cancer Nursing, 12,* 34–40.

Borneman, T., & Brown-Saltzman, K. (2001). Meaning in illness. In B.R. Ferrell & N. Coyle (Eds.), *Textbook of palliative nursing* (pp. 4–15). New York: Oxford University Press.

Borneman, T., & Ferrell, B.R. (1996). Ethical issues in pain management. *Clinics in Geriatric Medicine, 12,* 615–627.

Cassell, E.J. (1982). The nature of suffering and the goals of medicine. *New England Journal of Medicine, 306,* 639–645.

Cassell, E.J. (1999). Diagnosing suffering: A perspective. *Annals of Internal Medicine, 131,* 531–534.

Chiu, L. (2000). Transcending breast cancer, transcending death: A Taiwanese population. *Nursing Science Quarterly, 13*(1), 64–72.

Cohen, M.A., & Sarter, B. (1992). Love and work: Oncology nurses' view of the meaning of their work. *Oncology Nursing Forum, 19,* 1481–1486.

Copp, L.A. (1974). The spectrum of suffering. *Pain and Suffering, 74,* 491–495.

Copp, L.A. (1990a). The nature and prevention of suffering. *Journal of Professional Nursing, 6,* 247–249.

Copp, L.A. (1990b). Treatment, torture, suffering, and compassion. *Journal of Professional Nursing, 6,* 1–2.

Coyle, N. (1996). Suffering in the first person: Glimpses of suffering through patients' and family narratives. In B.R. Ferrell (Ed.), *Suffering* (pp. 29–64). Sudbury, MA: Jones and Bartlett.

Dow, K.H., Ferrell, B.R., & Annelo, C. (1997). Quality of life changes in patients with thyroid cancer after withdrawal of thyroid hormone therapy. *Thyroid, 7,* 613–619.

Dow, K.H., Ferrell, B.R., Haberman, M.R., & Eaton, L. (1999). The meaning of quality of life in cancer survivorship. *Oncology Nursing Forum, 26,* 519–528.

Dow, K.H., Ferrell, B.R., Leigh, S., Ly, J., & Gulasekaram, P. (1996). An evaluation of the quality of life among long-term survivors of breast cancer. *Breast Cancer Research and Treatment, 39,* 261–273.

Ersek, M., & Ferrell, B.R. (1994). Providing relief from cancer pain by assisting in the search for meaning. *Journal of Palliative Care, 10*(4), 15–22.

Ersek, M., Ferrell, B.R., Dow, K.H., & Melancon, C.H. (1997). Quality of life in women with ovarian cancer. *Western Journal of Nursing Research, 19,* 334–350.

Fall-Dickson, J.M., & Rose, L. (1999). Caring for patients who experience chemotherapy-induced side effects: The meaning for oncology nurses. *Oncology Nursing Forum, 26,* 901–907.

Ferrell, B., Smith, S., Cullinane, C., & Melancon, C. (2003a). Psychological well being and quality of life in ovarian cancer survivors. *Cancer, 98,* 1061–1071.

Ferrell, B., Smith, S., Cullinane, C., & Melancon, C. (2003b). Symptom concerns of women with ovarian cancer. *Journal of Pain and Symptom Management, 25,* 528–538.

Ferrell, B.R. (1993). To know suffering. *Oncology Nursing Forum, 20,* 1471–1477.

Ferrell, B.R. (1996). The quality of lives: 1,525 voices of cancer. *Oncology Nursing Forum, 23,* 907–916.

Ferrell, B.R., & Dean, G. (1995). The meaning of cancer pain. *Seminars in Oncology Nursing, 11,* 17–22.

Ferrell, B.R., Dow, K.H., Leigh, S., Ly, J., & Gulasekaram, P. (1995). Quality of life in long-term cancer survivors. *Oncology Nursing Forum, 22,* 915–922.

Ferrell, B.R., Ervin, K., Smith, S., Marek, T., & Melancon, C. (2002). Family perspectives of ovarian cancer. *Cancer Practice, 10,* 269–276.

Ferrell, B.R., Grant, M., Schmidt, G., Rhiner, M., Whitehead, C., Fonbuena, P., et al. (1992). The meaning of quality of life for bone marrow transplant survivors. Part I: The impact of bone marrow transplant on quality of life. *Cancer Nursing, 15,* 153–160.

Ferrell, B.R., Rhiner, M., Shapiro, B., & Dierkes, M. (1994). The experience of pediatric cancer pain. Part I: Impact of pain on the family. *Journal of Pediatric Nursing, 9,* 368–379.

Ferrell, B.R., Smith, S.L., Ervin, K.S., Itano, J., & Melancon, C. (2003). A qualitative analysis of social concerns of women with ovarian cancer. *Psycho-Oncology, 12,* 647–663.

Ferrell, B.R., Taylor, E.J., Sattler, G.R., Fowler, M., & Cheyney, B.L. (1993). Searching for the meaning of pain: Cancer patients', caregivers', and nurses' perspectives. *Cancer Practice, 1,* 185–194.

Ferrell, B.R., Wisdom, C., Wenzl, C., & Schneider, C. (1989). Quality of life as an outcome variable in pain research. *Cancer, 63,* 2321–2327.

Frankl, V. (1963). *Man's search for meaning: An introduction to logotherapy.* New York: Pocket Books.

Grant, M., Ferrell, B.R., Schmidt, G.M., Fonbuena, P., Niland, J.C., & Forman, S.J. (1992). Measurement of quality of life in bone marrow transplant survivors. *Quality of Life Research, 1,* 375–384.

Kahn, D.L., & Steeves, R.H. (1994). Witnesses to suffering: Nursing knowledge, voice, and vision. *Nursing Outlook, 42,* 260–264.

Kahn, D.L., & Steeves, R.H. (1996). An understanding of suffering grounded in clinical practice and research. In B.R. Ferrell (Ed.), *Suffering* (pp. 3–28). Sudbury, MA: Jones and Bartlett.

Kumasaka, L., & Miles, A. (1996). My pain is God's will. *American Journal of Nursing, 96*(6), 45–47.

Kuuppelomaki, M., & Sirkka, L. (1998). Cancer patients' reported experiences of suffering. *Cancer Nursing, 21,* 364–369.

Morse, J.M., Bottorff, J.L., & Hutchinson, S. (1995). The paradox of comfort. *Nursing Research, 44,* 14–19.

Morse, J.M., & Carter, B. (1996). The essence of enduring and expressions of suffering: The reformulation of self. *Scholarly Inquiry for Nursing Practice, 10*(1), 43–60.

O'Connor, K.F. (1996). Ethical/moral experiences of oncology nurses. *Oncology Nursing Forum, 23,* 787–794.

Padilla, G., Ferrell, B.R., Grant, M., & Rhiner, M. (1990). Defining the content domain of quality of life for cancer patients with pain. *Cancer Nursing, 13,* 108–115.

Penson, R.T., Yusuf, R.Z., Chabner, B.A., LaFrancesca, J.P., McElhinny, M., Axelrad, A.S., et al. (2001). Losing God. *Oncologist, 6,* 286–297.

Price, B. (1996). Illness careers: The chronic illness experience. *Journal of Advanced Nursing, 24,* 275–279.

Reich, W.T. (1987). Models of pain and suffering: Foundations for an ethic of compassion. *Acta Neurochirurgica Supplementum, 38,* 117–122.

Reich, W.T. (1989). Speaking of suffering: A moral account of compassion. *Soundings, 72*(1), 83–108.

Shapiro, B.S. (1996). The suffering of children and their families. In B.R. Ferrell (Ed.), *Suffering* (pp. 67–94). Sudbury, MA: Jones and Bartlett.

Smith, R. (1996). Theological perspectives. In B.R. Ferrell (Ed.), *Suffering* (pp. 159–172). Sudbury, MA: Jones and Bartlett.

Spross, J.A. (1996). Coaching and suffering: The role of the nurse in helping people facing illness. In B.R. Ferrell (Ed.), *Suffering* (pp. 173–208). Sudbury, MA: Jones and Bartlett.

Steeves, R.H., Cohen, M.Z., & Wise, C.T. (1994). An analysis of critical incidents describing the essence of oncology nursing. *Oncology Nursing Forum, 21*(Suppl. 8), 19–25.

Wolfe, J., Grier, H.E., Klar, N., Levin, S.B., Ellenbogen, J.M., Salem-Schatz, S., et al. (2000). Symptoms and suffering at the end of life in children with cancer. *New England Journal of Medicine, 342,* 326–333.

CHAPTER 11

Cancer-Related Fatigue

MADY C. STOVALL, RN, MSN, ONP, OCN®,
AND MERCEDES K. YOUNG, RN, MSN, ONP

Energy fuels our spirit.

—Anonymous

Fatigue is a universal experience of people with cancer. The experience of cancer-related fatigue (CRF) can negatively affect psychosocial well-being and quality of life (QOL). Fatigue may simply be a bothersome symptom for one patient, yet a completely debilitating symptom for another. The challenges faced by patients with CRF mandate oncology practitioners to address fatigue as a valid symptom, much like pain or anemia.

This chapter will describe the many facets of CRF. Studying fatigue is challenging because of its elusive nature and a general lack of consensus in defining the experience. Proposed CRF mechanisms will be reviewed, recognizing that the majority of anticancer treatments cause fatigue. Detailed assessment criteria will be outlined, including a review of established fatigue assessment tools. Finally, the impact of fatigue on patients and families will be discussed, followed by a review of management strategies. As the body of knowledge in respect to CRF continues to expand, oncology nurses can be better equipped to assist patients who must confront this often all-consuming symptom.

Defining Fatigue

CRF is the most commonly reported symptom among patients with cancer (Stasi, Abriani, Beccaglia, Terzoli, & Amadori, 2003). Patients report fatigue as the symptom that causes the most distress (Curt et al., 2000; Nail, 2002). Regardless of CRF prevalence, clinicians continue to overlook this symptom because of its prolonged nature, unlike acute symptoms related to disease and treatment (e.g., nausea, emesis, pain)

(Stasi et al.). Fatigue is a subjective symptom, which makes it difficult to quantify. Thus, the phenomenon has challenged clinicians, researchers, and patients for many years. Despite a growing body of research into CRF, a universally accepted definition remains problematic.

In the general population, fatigue is the natural response to energy expenditure and psychological stress (Tralongo, Respini, & Ferrau, 2003). It commonly is described as acute or chronic. Acute fatigue is identified as having a rapid onset with a short duration and is relieved by rest (Tralongo et al.). Most importantly, acute fatigue usually does not affect an individual's QOL (Tralongo et al.). Chronic fatigue most often is generalized. It is characterized as affecting one's physical and psychological state and having a prolonged duration, as well as indeterminate remission (Tralongo et al.). Acute fatigue also may occur in an individual experiencing chronic fatigue.

It is important to differentiate CRF from fatigue in a healthy population. General fatigue has been defined as a feeling of reduced energy, which may be associated with difficulty concentrating, decreased motivation, and decreased physical activity (Gelinas & Fillion, 2004). Research has established that CRF is qualitatively different from the fatigue experienced by the general population (Tralongo et al., 2003), with the following differentiating criteria: CRF occurs in the absence of physical exertion (Morrow, Andrews, Hickok, Roscoe, & Matteson, 2002), and the symptom develops over time and may result from the cumulative effects of treatment (e.g., chemotherapy, radiation, surgery). Additionally, CRF is perceived as being of greater magnitude, disproportionate to activity or exertion, and not completely relieved by rest—leaving the patient with an overwhelming and sustained sense of exhaustion (Ahlberg, Ekman, Gaston-Johansson, & Mock, 2003; Glaus, Crow, & Hammond, 1996). Of significance is that CRF may persist longer than the diagnosis and treatment of cancer itself (Stasi et al., 2003; Tralongo et al.).

The National Comprehensive Cancer Network (NCCN, 2004) has defined CRF as a "persistent, subjective sense of tiredness related to cancer or cancer treatment that interferes with usual functioning." NCCN has developed practice guidelines that include standards of care for both adult and pediatric patients, adding support for patients and practitioners dealing with CRF. Moreover, CRF has gained an overall awareness and acceptance, which thereby has resulted in the *International Classification of Diseases, Tenth Revision, Clinical Modification* including official criteria for the diagnosis of CRF (Manzullo & Escalante, 2002).

Conceptual Framework for Fatigue Assessment

The subjectivity and vagueness of CRF undoubtedly has resulted in obstacles in adequate reporting, diagnosis, and treatment (Dammacco, Castoldi, & Rodjer, 2001). Additional barriers include an overall lack of standardization for the assessment and treatment of this multidimensional symptom (Manzullo & Escalante, 2002). The National Institutes of Health (NIH, 2002) outlined factors contributing to the lack of consistency in estimating fatigue across clinical studies. These include (a) conceptualization and measurement; (b) heterogeneity of conditions or phenomena defined as fatigue; (c) lack of consensus on the criteria to define fatigue individually or in combination with other symptoms; and (d) a lack of consensus on the "best" measure in terms of validity and reliability for assessing fatigue alone or in combination with other symptoms. As researchers continue to study the subjective and objective nature of CRF, a conceptual framework for assessment can be derived by understanding the epidemiology, etiology, and treatment-related variables underlying CRF.

Epidemiology of Cancer-Related Fatigue

Fatigue has been the most common complaint in patients with cancer undergoing treatment (Stricker, Drake, Hoyer, & Mock, 2004), rated as being more distressing than nausea, hair loss, bowel disturbances, alterations in weight, or menopausal symptoms (Morrow et al., 2002). Research and clinical appreciation of the fatigue experience has yet to be as clearly defined as symptoms such as pain or nausea, despite mounting evidence that cancer survivors suffer lingering fatigue for months or years after treatment is completed (Loge, Abrahamsen, Ekeberg, & Kaasa, 2000; Okuyama et al., 2000; Stricker et al.).

NIH (2002) estimated that the prevalence of fatigue in people with cancer ranges from 4%–91%. The wide range reflects a lack of uniformity of measurement and methodology in fatigue research. NIH noted that published studies on fatigue, similar to those on pain and depression, are virtually restricted to prevalence data, with no reliable incidence studies carried out.

NCCN (2004) cited that 70%–100% of patients with cancer experience fatigue. Previous support for the prevalence of fatigue among patients with cancer was established with a population-based telephone survey conducted by the Fatigue Coalition, a multidisciplinary group of medical practitioners, researchers, and patient advocates created to study the incidence and functional impact of CRF and to develop diagnostic and treatment guidelines (Vogelzang et al., 1997). The survey represented a variety of cancer diagnoses (breast cancer represented 62% of respondents), and participants had received treatment with chemotherapy alone or in combination with other treatment modalities. Important data garnered from the coalition survey demonstrated that 78% of patients reported significant fatigue during the course of their disease and treatment, and the symptom adversely affected overall physical and social functioning in the majority of patients interviewed (Vogelzang et al.).

The experience of fatigue may be more severe for some patients, depending on the different type of cancer diagnosis and the treatment involved. In a self-administered survey evaluating the exercise and activity patterns of 219 patients with cancer and survivors, patients with leukemia, non-Hodgkin lymphoma, and testicular cancer reported more intense fatigue prior to treatment than patients with other diagnoses (Schwartz, 1998a). The type of treatment modality also influences the degree of CRF. In women who received a chemotherapy regimen with a doxorubicin-containing schedule versus cyclophosphamide, methotrexate, and 5-fluorouracil, variability existed in the CRF reported among the women in the different treatment groups (De Jong, Candel, Schouten, Abu-Saad, & Courtens, 2004). Women who received radiation in addition to chemotherapy experienced greater levels of fatigue than those receiving chemotherapy alone (De Jong et al.). Lastly, the surgical procedure affected the degree of fatigue in that women who underwent mastectomy reported greater fatigue than those having lumpectomy (De Jong et al.).

Fatigue has been reported as a side effect for patients undergoing high-dose cancer treatments for bone marrow transplantation (BMT) and peripheral blood stem cell transplantation (PBSCT) (El-Banna et al., 2004; Molassiotis, 1999). Patients undergoing BMT were observed to be more tired, anxious, and depressed than patients receiving maintenance chemotherapy for hematologic malignancies (Molassiotis), and patients undergoing PBSCT were found to experience a peak in fatigue and depression on day +7 into treatment (El-Banna et al.). BMT survivors have reported significant problems with social reintegration because of physical fatigue, psychological issues, and changing roles (Baker, Zabora, Polland, & Wingard, 1999). The impact and pattern of CRF may differ among patient populations because of the disease type, stage of illness, and the treatment modalities employed. The experience may be compounded by concurrent experiences such as depression and role changes.

Etiology of Cancer-Related Fatigue

Pathophysiology: Researchers have investigated the complexity of CRF, yet a definitive cause remains unknown. Proposed mechanisms include the production of cytokines, an abnormal accumulation of muscle metabolites, changes in neuromuscular functioning, abnormalities in adenosine triphosphate (ATP) synthesis, serotonin dysregulation, and vagal afferent activation (NCCN, 2004). These pathophysiologic changes can be disease-related, related to the side effects of treatment (e.g., anemia, anorexia, cachexia, vomiting), or a direct effect of the treatment itself (e.g., chemotherapy, radiation therapy, biologic therapy).

It has been postulated that CRF is a physiologic protective response whereby the cancer itself or the various treatment modalities elevate the levels of proinflammatory cytokines (Morrow et al., 2002). Research suggests that tumor necrosis factor (TNF), a proinflammatory cytokine, may alter central serotonin (5-HT, 5-hydroxytryptamine) through the increased neuronal release of serotonin and by the upregulation of 5-HT transporter. This dysregulation of the cytokine cascade, which results in the alteration of central serotonin, may thereby result in CRF (Morrow et al.). Conflicting data exist about this upregulation of proinflammatory cytokines correlating with CRF. One study with patients with breast cancer receiving radiotherapy failed to demonstrate a correlation with increasing levels of interleukin-1 beta (IL-1β), IL-6, or TNF-α to fatigue (Geinitz et al., 2001).

Other pathophysiologic changes that occur with cancer and its treatment may contribute to fatigue. Changes in the hypothalamic-pituitary-gonadal axis can cause hormonal changes affecting appetite and the response to stress (Gutstein, 2001). Cancer therapies can negatively affect neuroendocrine function, further contributing to hormonal imbalance and mood disturbances (e.g., depression), thus contributing to fatigue. It is evident that different disease processes and biochemical changes correlate with the presence of fatigue (Gutstein).

Impaired muscle function: Another relevant consideration for CRF is the effect of impaired muscular function occurring from changes in metabolism, prolonged disuse, muscle wasting, or treatment-related changes (i.e., radiation can alter cell membranes, affecting ion transportation). The relationship between neuromuscular function and fatigue was supported by Monga et al. (1997) when evaluating CRF in patients with prostate cancer undergoing radiotherapy. The reduced oxygen delivery to muscle cells and subsequent limitation in the availability of ATP to the mitochondria induced anaerobic metabolism and thus increased energy expenditure. Subsequently, neuromuscular output decreases with an ensuing accumulation of toxins. Therefore, the supply of oxygen to mitochondrial muscle fibers is a critical factor in the regulation of energy production, and a decreased supply may contribute to the pathogenesis of fatigue (Tralongo et al., 2003).

Anemia: It is well known that chemotherapy, radiotherapy, and other treatments can have a profound effect on blood and bone marrow, and the production of cytokines has been implicated in the suppression of erythrogenesis (Morrow et al., 2002). Anemia related to disease and treatment is a well-researched cause of fatigue. Data in multiple studies have consistently demonstrated a significant and positive relationship between hemoglobin rise and reduction in fatigue. In one growth-factor study, patients were randomized to receive darbepoetin, erythropoietin, or placebo, and those patients with a hemoglobin improvement of at least 2 g/dl over a period of 12 weeks reported significantly greater increases in the Functional Assessment of Cancer Therapy fatigue subscale (see Figure 11-1) scores relative to those who did not achieve this level of hemoglobin response (Cella, Kallich, McDermott, & Xu,

---

Figure 11-1. Multidimensional Fatigue Scales

- Piper Fatigue Scale (PFS)
  - PFS was the first validated multidimensional scale. It addresses the severity, distress, and impact of fatigue using a 40-item questionnaire (Iop et al., 2004).
  - The revised version of the PFS for patients with breast cancer consists of 22 items and 4 subscales: behavioral/severity (6 items), affective meaning (5 items), sensory (5 items), and cognitive/mood (6 items) (Piper et al., 1998).
- Schwartz Cancer Fatigue Scale (SCFS)
  - The 28-item SCFS has demonstrated reliability and content and construct validity using four subscales (physical, emotional, cognitive, and temporal) (Schwartz, 1998b). Lacking in this scale is an index of the impact of fatigue on various aspects of quality of life (e.g., ability to work or participate in social activities) (Hann et al., 2000).
- Fatigue Assessment Questionnaire (FAQ)
  - FAQ is a 20-item instrument that has demonstrated reliability and validity (Glaus, 1998; Glaus et al., 1996).
- Functional Assessment of Cancer Therapy—Anemia/Fatigue (FACT-F)
  - FACT-F is a 41-item scale made up of the FACT-General quality-of-life instrument (FACT-G) plus a fatigue subscale. It delineates physical and functional consequences of fatigue (Yellen et al., 1997).
  - The main disadvantage to FACT-F is the length, which may be challenging to patients lacking energy (Yellen et al.).
  - FACT-An is a 48-item scale made up of the FACT-G, the FACT-F, and questions specifically related to anemia in patients with cancer. FACT-F and FACT-An both exhibit consistency and reliability on test-retest (Yellen et al.).
- Brief Fatigue Inventory (BFI)
  - Based on the Brief Pain Inventory, the one-page BFI has only nine items, with the items measured on 0–10 numeric rating scales. Three items assess the severity of the fatigue in the past week, and then six interference items evaluate general activity, mood, walking ability, normal work, relations with other people, and enjoyment of life. BFI taps into a single dimension that can be thought of as the subjective report of fatigue severity. It is an internally stable instrument that is correlated with measures of performance status along with physiologic markers of anemia (hemoglobin) and nutritional status (albumin) known to be associated with fatigue, in addition to being easy to use. BFI does not capture the multiple dimensions that longer instruments were designed to measure, such as the cognitive, affective, and somatic components of fatigue (Mendoza et al., 1999).

(Continued on next page)

Figure 11-1. Multidimensional Fatigue Scales *(Continued)*

- Cancer Fatigue Scale (CFS)
  - CFS is a 15-item scale composed of three subscales (physical, affective, and cognitive), can be completed in approximately two minutes, and has demonstrated reliability and validity in patients with various types of cancer (Okuyama et al., 2000).
- Multidimensional Fatigue Symptom Inventory (MFSI)
  - MFSI measures four aspects: general and physical fatigue, reduced activity, reduced motivation, and mental fatigue. Reliability and validity are well supported in patients with cancer (Smets et al., 1995). MFSI evaluates global, somatic, affective, cognitive, and behavioral symptoms of fatigue with an 83-item questionnaire with demonstrated sensitivity (Iop et al., 2004). The length of this scale, however, may be problematic for use in clinical settings or in clinical trials as an outcome measure.

2004). Research studies have clearly demonstrated that exogenous stimulation of erythropoiesis can correct anemia and improve fatigue.

Cancer-related effects: Numerous disease processes can lead to a negative energy balance that may contribute to an associated component of fatigue (Gutstein, 2001). Although this seems easily apparent, it is not yet clear how a decreased energy supply could lead to the holistic experience of fatigue. The processes leading to energy imbalance from cancer are quite diverse. In addition to anemia, they include cachexia, infection, paraneoplastic syndromes, and metabolic disorders, all of which can occur along the continuum of disease and treatment (Gutstein). Research is ongoing to identify the pathophysiologic mechanisms behind CRF. Studies performed predominantly in rats have suggested an additional role—that of signaling information about peripheral pathogenic information to the brain—for abdominal vagal afferents, which may be relevant to the genesis of "sickness syndrome" (Morrow et al., 2002). If a vagal-somatic inhibitory reflex is identified in humans, it could have a role in the genesis of the lethargy, weakness, and fatigue associated with cancer and its treatment (Morrow et al.).

Cancer treatment effects: In a review of research on the side effects of cancer therapies, it is significant that 80%–96% of patients receiving chemotherapy experienced fatigue (Manzullo & Escalante, 2002; Stasi et al., 2003). Cyclic patterns have been reported in patients with breast cancer receiving adjuvant chemotherapy, with fatigue scores being higher during treatment and lower mid-chemotherapy cycle (Berger, 1998). In a second survey conducted by the Fatigue Coalition, the side effect reported to have the greatest negative impact after completion of chemotherapy was fatigue (Curt et al., 2000). Certain chemotherapy regimens are known for being more fatigue-inducing than others, especially when considering the dose intensity of the regimen. For example, patients receiving combination chemotherapy regimens and those with more advanced disease experience higher levels of fatigue (Schwartz, 1998a).

Radiotherapy has been reported to induce early fatigue (occurring during treatment or shortly after) in up to 80% of patients studied, and in approximately 30% of these cases, the fatigue lasted long after the completion of treatment (chronic fatigue) (Jereczek-Fossa, Marsiglia, & Orecchia, 2002). Levels of fatigue have been shown to be higher in women with breast cancer who have received a combination of chemotherapy and radiation as compared with women receiving chemotherapy alone (Woo, Dibble, Piper, Keating, & Weiss, 1998). Vice versa, women treated with radiation therapy alone have demonstrated lower levels of fatigue than those receiving chemotherapy alone or in combination with radiation. Early research on victims of accidental radiation exposure demonstrated that these patients suffer from fatigue similar to radiotherapy patients (Anno, Baum, Withers, & Young, 1989).

Severe fatigue is almost universal with the use of biologic response modifiers, including alpha interferon and the interleukins. Interferon has been reported to cause fatigue in 70% of cases, which is cited as interferon's most debilitating toxicity (Gutstein, 2001). In fact, fatigue often is a dose-limiting toxicity of biologic response modifier treatments (Hancock et al., 2004; Rosenthal & Oratz, 1998). Severe fatigue may influence the ability of study participants to maintain appropriate dosing because of decreasing physical performance. Participants may be unable to remain on-study because of the profound side effects of treatment.

Chronic fatigue in long-term cancer survivors has been reported in a variety of patient populations, such as Hodgkin disease or breast cancer survivors (Berglund, Bolund, Fornander, Rutqvist, & Sjoden, 1991; Fobair et al., 1986; Loge et al., 2000; Okuyama et al., 2000). Most survivor surveys link fatigue with complex phenomena related to impaired QOL, such as negative mood, diminished performance status, and sleep disturbances. In a study comparing the general population to breast cancer survivors, depression and pain surfaced as the strongest predictors of chronic fatigue (Bower et al., 2000).

Psychosocial Effects of Cancer-Related Fatigue

Fatigue is an obscure symptom that often is difficult to differentiate from other subjective symptoms, which can be challenging for patients, caregivers, healthcare personnel, and researchers (Manzullo & Escalante, 2002). Experienced by most patients as an extremely frustrating state of chronic energy depletion, fatigue leads to loss of productivity, which can reduce self-esteem (Cella, Peterman, Passik, Jacobsen, & Breitbart, 1998). The clinical and psychosocial impact of fatigue in patients with cancer is not clearly understood at this time. Significantly, the role of fatigue and QOL on overall survival is unknown (Stasi et al., 2003). A study of women receiving radiotherapy for breast cancer reported that those women high in catastrophizing had significantly greater fatigue than those low in catastrophizing, supporting the role of psychological factors on the symptom experience of patients (Jacobsen, Andrykowski, & Thors, 2004).

CRF can affect every aspect of patients' lives. Studies most often focus on the physical limitations, emotional consequences, and the psychological burden of fatigue as it relates to QOL. Fatigue, however, can affect anything from finances to emotional energy and sexual functioning to sleep. One theoretical framework proposed by Piper (1997) provided insight into the multidimensional facets of the fatigue experience for patients and can assist oncology nurses in understanding the psychosocial impact of this symptom (Ream & Richardson, 1999). The magnitude of CRF includes the timing of the experience (temporal dimension), the emotional meaning of fatigue (affective dimension), the physical and psychological symptoms of fatigue (sensory dimension), and the psychosocial impact of the experience (severity dimension) (Piper; Ream & Richardson). Nursing-oriented models of fatigue in the literature can be helpful for oncology nurses to identify patients' perceptions of CRF and guide interventions to screen, manage, and reduce this life-altering symptom (Ream & Richardson).

Predisposing factors: Dean and Anderson (2001) have outlined characteristics that have been found to predispose patients with cancer to fatigue. Research has indicated that younger patients with cancer report more fatigue than older patients, reflecting the possible importance of patients' developmental level in their response to the fatigue experience. For example, fatigue negatively affects the QOL of young adults who are balancing numerous roles and responsibilities, whereas older patients may attribute fatigue and change in health to advancing age (Dean & Anderson). Other predisposing factors that require more in-depth investigation include gender, culture, and ethnicity. A majority of fatigue research has focused upon women with breast cancer (Mock, 2001), but the experience of fatigue in men is less studied. Whether the patterns of CRF are similar is unknown; therefore, management strategies that have been found efficacious for women may not apply to men. Although fatigue research is expanding rapidly, no identified studies have investigated the role of culture and ethnicity on the perception and psychosocial impact of CRF. The meaning of strength and productivity, negatively affected by CRF, may be most central to certain patients' self-image, dependent upon their cultural belief system (Greenberg, 1998). Additional factors that influence the experience of fatigue that have not been studied in-depth include personal factors such as spirituality, income/insurance, unresolved family conflicts, unmet goals, and caregiver support (Dean & Anderson).

Emotional effects: As described earlier, psychological factors are known to influence CRF. Anxiety, fear, anger, sadness, and depressed mood comprise emotional distress contributing to fatigue (Gelinas & Fillion, 2004). Greenberg (1998) expressed the emotional impact of the fatigue experience for patients throughout the cancer journey. The anxiety and fear common at diagnosis can drain the patient's energy, contributing to fatigue. During treatment(s), the patient hopes that the loss of energy and endurance is a time-limited price that must be paid for cure. At other times, fatigue may raise fears that the cancer has recurred or will be victorious. Most distressing, fatigue may symbolize "progressive debility and waning of life" (Greenberg, p. 485). One study of patients with lung cancer found that an improvement in fatigue correlated with improvements in mood and a reduction in anxiety levels, pointing to a relationship between psychological distress and CRF (Tchekmedyian, Kallich, McDermott, Fayers, & Erder, 2003).

Sexual activity: Sexual activity may decrease in patients with cancer for a variety of reasons, including fatigue. Patients may experience a lack of interest or fear of performance failure directly related to decreased physical energy. Loss of sexual desire can result from other treatment-related conditions that compound the fatigue state, such as depression, the use of medications that affect energy and desire (e.g., opiates, antidepressants, antihypertensives, antiemetics), or the emotional grief related to loss of sexual function and body-image changes (Schover, 1998). One survey of patients with ovarian cancer cited lack of interest, physical limitation, and fatigue as the reasons for sexual inactivity (Taylor, Basen-Engquist, Shinn, & Bodurka, 2004).

Sleep patterns: Patients undergoing cancer treatment often report an alteration of normal sleep patterns. Circadian rhythm changes in patients with breast cancer undergoing chemotherapy have been shown to significantly correlate with increased fatigue, depression, and changes in mood (Roscoe et al., 2002). The literature has supported the relationship between CRF and sleep deprivation (Ancoli-Israel, Moore, & Jones, 2001). Sleep that is inadequate or "unrefreshing" not only influences the perception of fatigue but also negatively affects patients' QOL and tolerance to treatment. Illness-related symptoms, such as dyspnea and pain, interfere with sleep, as well as treatment-related symptoms, such as restless leg syndrome (akathisia) from dopamine-blocking antiemetics (Greenberg, 1998). Most significant is that lack of sleep and rest contributes to the development of mood disorders and clinical depression, further exacerbating patients' fatigue experience and decreasing QOL (Ancoli-Israel et al.).

Cognitive effects: Patients frequently report cognitive effects of CRF. Patients treated for cancer describe difficulty concentrating or attentional fatigue (Cimprich, 1992, 1993, 1995). This is experienced when the demands for directed attention exceed the person's capacity (Dean & Anderson, 2001), a very distressing symptom to patients who are employed in jobs that demand concentration and focus (e.g., accounting, engineering). Research has just begun to identify these changes often referred to as "chemo brain." Studies have documented these cognitive changes in breast cancer and lymphoma populations (Ream & Richardson, 1999), but continued research is needed because of the multifactorial etiology of cognitive deficits in patients with cancer. The degree of neurocognitive impairment related directly to CRF has yet to be delineated.

Pain, depression, anxiety, and fatigue: Pain and medications for pain management can contribute significantly to fatigue (Portenoy & Itri, 1999). Poorly controlled pain is a draining experience physically and psychologically. Furthermore, chronic pain is a constant stressor that can lead to alterations in the stress axis, thus predisposing a patient to depression (Gutstein, 2001). This "triad," chronic pain, chronic stress, and depression, could be extremely important in understanding the neural circuitry and neuroendocrine mechanisms contributing to chronic fatigue states (Gutstein). Hyperactivity of the hypothalamic-pituitary-adrenal axis can lead to depression, which enhances the sensation of fatigue (Gutstein).

The relationship between fatigue and depression is supported in the psychiatric disciplines; fatigue is a symptom of the diagnostic criteria *(DSM-IV-TR)* for depression (American Psychiatric Association, 2000), and major depressive disorder is the most common psychiatric diagnosis that causes fatigue in patients with cancer (Greenberg, 1998). However, the temporal relationship may not be clearly evident. Depression may develop as a result of being fatigued (Visser & Smets, 1998), or each diagnosis may coexist without a causal relationship. Another psychiatric syndrome that drains physical and emotional energy is anxiety (Greenberg). The anxiety related to diagnosis, the constant worries about treatment success or recurrence, and the fears related to the unknown can contribute to depression, fatigue, or both.

Economic/occupational impact: The economic and occupational impact of CRF affects both patients and their primary caregivers. The Fatigue Coalition's 1998 survey found that of patients who were actively employed at the time of a cancer diagnosis, 75% changed their employment status as a result of fatigue (Curt et al., 2000). Patients surveyed (N = 379) reported a need to push themselves to do things (77%), decreased motivation or interest (62%), and feelings of sadness, frustration, or irritability (53%) during their experiences with CRF. In addition, primary caregivers took more time off work, accepted fewer responsibilities, or reduced their working hours to help to meet the needs of the fatigued patient during treatment. A dearth of literature exists addressing the impact of fatigue on patients' ability to maintain employment and the subsequent financial impact on the patient and family if workdays are shortened or sick days are necessitated. Discussion of self-care strategies for the relief of fatigue rarely incorporate the employed patient. It is well understood that patients' overall well-being can be enhanced when they can achieve valued goals (Ream & Richardson, 1999), and for a majority of patients with cancer, these goals would include their job and financial stability.

Fatigue in survivors: Chronic fatigue after the completion of cancer therapy may be attributed to the long-term side effects of treatment(s) (Greenberg, 1998). This may include the loss of a bodily function that contributes to fatigue (e.g., chemotherapeutic-induced pulmonary fibrosis causing chronic dyspnea; cardiomyopathy from anthracycline therapy limiting activity tolerance; chronic graft-versus-host disease following BMT). Long-term side effects of fatigue and sleep disturbances have been reported in survivors of BMT, Hodgkin disease, and breast cancer (Greenberg).

Nursing Care of Patients Experiencing Cancer-Related Fatigue

Assessment

Oncology nurses play a vital role in identifying patients' experience of fatigue and its impact on their QOL both physically and psychologically. This begins with a thorough history to identify patients' perceptions of their disease, treatment(s), and concurrent symptoms, followed by a thorough physical exam to identify specific physical causes of fatigue. The history allows exploration of psychological fatigue contributors that may help to validate patients' emotional responses to the fatigue experience, such as mood disturbance or depression. Investigation into any possible physical causes (e.g., decreased activity tolerance, dyspnea) of fatigue helps to validate the physical fatigue experience of an individual patient. Assessment and screening of fatigue begin at initial diagnosis and persist throughout the cancer continuum from active treatment to survivorship.

Fatigue history: The history should include open-ended questions that encourage patients to describe their fatigue experience in their own words. Reflection and clarification of patient reports during the interview help to clarify the patients' fatigue experience and provide an opportunity to identify any associated symptoms (e.g., dyspnea, weakness, somnolence). CRF may be exacerbated by or contribute to other known causes of fatigue (see Figure 11-2). Fatigue, pain, and psychological distress are the most prevalent symptoms across varied cancer populations. Patients who report fatigue should be queried about the presence of concurrent symptoms and the degree to which each symptom predominates as a cause of emotional or physical distress (Portenoy & Itri, 1999).

A pertinent fatigue history should include evaluation of the onset (timing), duration (days versus weeks or months), characteristics (physical, mental, emotional, and spiritual), aggravating and alleviating factors (e.g., anxiety, rest), and treatments

Figure 11-2. Predisposing Factors/Possible Etiologies of Cancer-Related Fatigue

Cardiopulmonary
- Heart failure (congestive heart failure)
- Chronic obstructive pulmonary disease

Connective Tissue Disease
- Rheumatic disease

Endocrine or Metabolic Disorder
- Hypothyroidism/hyperthyroidism
- Diabetes mellitus
- Pituitary insufficiency
- Hypercalcemia
- Adrenal insufficiency
- Chronic renal failure
- Hepatic failure
- Malnutrition
- Menopausal symptoms

Infection
- Endocarditis
- Tuberculosis
- Mononucleosis
- Hepatitis
- Parasite infection
- HIV infection
- Cytomegalovirus
- Bacterial infection

Idiopathic (a diagnosis of exclusion)
- Idiopathic chronic fatigue
- Chronic fatigue syndrome

Psychological
- Depression
- Anxiety
- Somatization disorder
- Emotional distress
- Spiritual distress

Pharmacologic
- Hypnotics
- Antihypertensives
- Antidepressants
- Androgen deprivation
- Aromatase inhibitors
- Drug abuse and drug withdrawal

Sleep Disturbance
- Sleep apnea
- Gastroesophageal reflux disease
- Allergic rhinitis
- Psychological contributors (e.g., anxiety)

Oncologic
- Anemia (because of the neoplastic process or treatment)
- Occult malignancy
- Pain

Treatment
- Surgery
- Radiotherapy
- Chemotherapy
- Biologic response modifiers

Note. Based on information from Portenoy & Itri, 1999.

(e.g., exercise, medications) that the patients have experienced. It is very important to elicit the onset and duration of fatigue. Patients may be completely debilitated by the experience, reporting that fatigue interferes with work, family, and activities of daily living—leading to a complete lifestyle alteration. Other patients may report feeling fatigued but find that they are able to adapt and continue functioning, finding pleasure in their daily activities.

A comprehensive fatigue assessment includes a thorough review of systems, including evaluation of undiagnosed or unmanaged comorbidities (e.g., cardiac, pulmonary, renal, neurologic, endocrine diseases) and other possible contributing factors (e.g., medications, nutritional status, fluid, electrolyte and metabolic balance) (Mock, 2001). This is important to illuminate any associated symptoms such as nausea, vomiting, diarrhea, bleeding, pain, menopausal symptoms, or anorexia that compound the fatigue experience. Other complaints such as poor concentration or alteration in work or social routines should be documented as well to evaluate any associated cognitive changes. The history should assess quality and quantity of rest and sleep patterns to determine if rest and sleep are restorative. Inquiring about sleep aids and other medications (narcotics, anxiolytics, antiemetics) is important because medications within the treatment profile may contribute to or exacerbate CRF. Inquire about other pharmacologic agents as well, including alcohol, herbal remedies, and recreational drugs. The history must inquire about daily activities both in and out of the home, work, social involvement, and exercise. Over the course of treatment, other common causes of fatigue are inactivity and deconditioning that reduce the patients' normal tolerance for daily activities (Mock). Determine whether patients prioritize their activities each day and whether this intervention has been helpful. Lastly, explore any history of psychiatric illness. Depression, anxiety, substance abuse, somatization disorders, and other psychological conditions can contribute to the occurrence and perception of fatigue.

Evaluation tools: Fatigue inherently is subjective in nature. A variety of one-dimensional scales may be used to assess the severity of fatigue. If patients complain of fatigue during the initial history taking, it is important to quantify the presence of fatigue for future comparison and to evaluate the impact of treatments (Mock, 2001). In the busy clinical setting, a mild/moderate/severe, one-dimensional scale is used most frequently to assess fatigue. It has been reported that moderate levels of fatigue (i.e., 4–6) may signify a reduction in daily activity levels, whereas severe levels of fatigue (i.e., 7–10) have been associated with a marked decrease in physical functioning and stamina (Mock). Figure 11-3 outlines simple one-dimensional scales that can be incorporated in patients' initial assessment.

Measurement of CRF in clinical research relies on the use of valid and reliable assessment tools. Language comprehension, education level, and cultural norms are important considerations when using a standardized assessment tool for assessing and monitoring fatigue. Healthcare professionals should consider the readability,

---

Figure 11-3. One-Dimensional Fatigue Scales

- 4-point verbal rating scale
  - None, mild, moderate, severe
- 5-point verbal rating scale
  - None, mild, moderate, severe, very severe
- 11-point numeric rating scale
  - "On a scale of 0–10, with 0 being no fatigue and 10 being the worst imaginable fatigue, how would you rate your fatigue on average this past week?"
- 4-point numeric scale, such as the Common Toxicity Criteria of the National Cancer Institute
  - 0—None
  - 1—Increased fatigue over baseline but not altering normal activities
  - 2—Moderate (e.g., decrease in performance status by 1 level in the Eastern Cooperative Oncology Group [ECOG] scale or by 20% in the Karnofsky score) or causing difficulty performing some activities
  - 3—Severe (e.g., decrease in performance status by 2 ECOG levels or by 40% in the Karnofsky scale) or loss of ability to perform some activities
  - 4—Bedridden
- Linear analog scale assessment
  - Report on a scale from 0 (lowest value) to 100 (highest value)
- 10-cm visual analog scale
  - No fatigue |-----------------------------| Worst possible fatigue

Note. Based on information from Iop et al., 2004; National Institutes of Health, 2002.

---

length, age-appropriateness, and established reliability and validity for the specific population of interest. For clinical research, fatigue most often has been measured as part of a multidimensional symptom checklist. Multidimensional fatigue questionnaires may reveal more about the global experience of a person with CRF. The challenge of using multidimensional measures often lies in the completion of lengthy tools when patients already are physically, mentally, and/or emotionally fatigued. Multidimensional fatigue measures include those outlined in Figure 11-1.

Fatigue exam: A thorough physical examination is vital to establish a baseline for any patient, and ongoing physical evaluation will monitor changes in health status, including fatigue. Neurologic, cardiopulmonary, gastrointestinal, genitourinary, musculoskeletal, and integument assessment will provide clues to contributing or comorbid conditions that may need medical management (Mock, 2001). Laboratory tests should investigate possible physiologic causes of fatigue (e.g., hypothyroidism). A complete blood count with differential should be part of any initial workup to investigate any anemia or infectious processes. The erythrocyte sedimentation rate may indicate chronic infection or an inflammatory process. Order a comprehensive metabolic panel to investigate any liver or kidney disease or insufficiency. A chemistry panel to evaluate dehydration or electrolyte imbalance or as part of an initial nutrition evaluation also is prudent. Other tests, such as thyroid-stimulating hormone, calcium, or creatine kinase, may indicate other underlying metabolic problems that may be contributing to the fatigue experience. Mock asserted that the clinician should be attuned to five factors that have been highly correlated with CRF: pain, emotional distress, sleep disturbances, anemia, and hypothyroidism.

Management

Because the exact mechanisms of CRF are not yet clearly understood, management is focused on correction or control of comorbid conditions, managing associated symptoms, and providing emotional support. Clinical management should aim to correct anemia and other physiologic causes, improve nutrition, manage pain and depression, provide psychosocial support, and introduce an appropriate exercise or activity program. Portenoy and Itri's (1999) algorithm for the evaluation and management of CRF is a useful guide (see Figure 11-4). Symptomatic therapies may be nonpharmacologic or pharmacologic in approach, and any correctable causes of fatigue should promptly be addressed. No large, randomized quality-control studies have validated nonpharmacologic methods of managing fatigue; consequently, anecdotal reports provide most of the supportive evidence for the following interventions. It is important to utilize multiple nonpharmacologic modalities in combination for maximum benefit, although no recommendations or studies show which combinations are most appropriate. Nonpharmacologic interventions are aimed toward education and counseling, nutritional support, sleep and restorative therapy, and exercise (Mock, 2001).

Education: The primary intervention for fatigue always should be education. NCCN guidelines (2004) recommended educating all patients prior to beginning fatigue-inducing treatments about the expected pattern and duration of fatigue associated with their specific illness state and treatment(s). All patients receiving anticancer treatment should be informed that they may develop some degree of fatigue during therapy, and this symptom should not be interpreted as disease progression or failure

Figure 11-4. Algorithm for the Evaluation and Management of Cancer-Related Fatigue

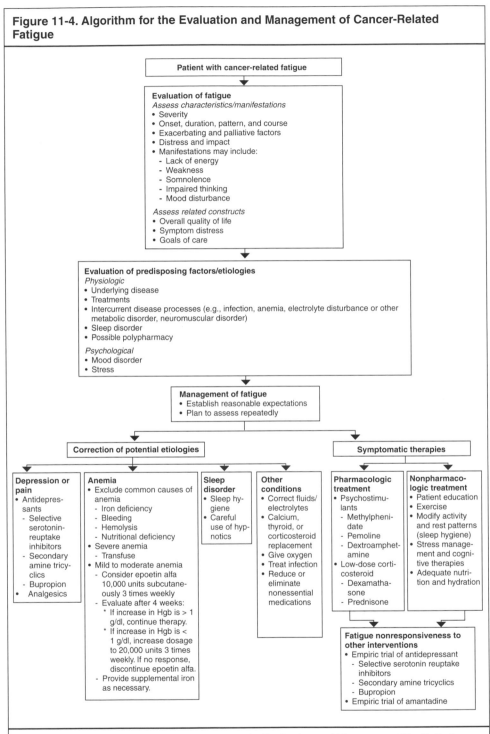

or inadequacy of treatment. Patients should be aware that fatigue is a real, multidimensional experience (NCCN; Valdres, Escalante, & Manzullo, 2001). Controlled clinical trials have demonstrated that patient education can improve outcomes (Fortin & Kirouac, 1976). If patients receive education and counseling regarding the patterns of fatigue that typically occur during specific treatment protocols, they are likely to be less stressed by the fatigue and better equipped to cope with it (Mock, 2001).

Correction of anemia: Anemia is a common and important clinical complication in patients with CRF. Oncology practitioners treating the anemia must investigate different causes such as bleeding, hematologic toxicity from cancer treatment, vitamin or mineral deficiencies, or anemia of chronic disease. A more accurate investigation requires a complete blood count and peripheral blood cytology, in addition to B_{12} assay, folate, iron, transferrin, ferritin and erythropoietin levels, Coombs direct and indirect test, and a bone marrow biopsy. Patients may need a blood transfusion, supplemental iron, recombinant human erythropoietin, or other management followed by regular (at least every fourth week) reevaluation of their anemia (Berger, 1998). If treatment of anemia does not resolve patients' experience of fatigue and no other physiologic cause can be identified (e.g., sleep deprivation), then nonpharmacologic behavioral interventions should be initiated (Mock, 2001).

NCCN (2004) has specific guidelines available online for the assessment and management of treatment-related anemia (www.nccn.org). Three large, prospective, nonrandomized, multicenter, community trials (combined N > 6,000) observed that patients treated with epoetin alfa who experienced a rise in hemoglobin reported significant improvements in energy level, activity level, functional status, and overall QOL (Demetri, Kris, Wade, Degos, & Cella, 1998; Gabrilove, 2000; Glaspy et al., 1997). The relationship between changes in hemoglobin level and QOL during chemotherapy treatment has gained research support (Crawford et al., 2002).

Nutritional evaluation: A full nutrition consultation and evaluation by a registered dietitian can improve overall nutritional status by offering strategies to manage deficiency states resulting from symptoms of anorexia, nausea, vomiting, diarrhea, or constipation. Strategies such as suggesting frequent small meals or drinks, proposing alternative eating times or places, encouraging healthy shopping and cooking habits, and providing education about high-protein supplements and other techniques may prove to be helpful. Good hydration and vitamin therapy, including supplemental iron and erythropoietin for anemic patients, also are recommended (Burks, 2001). Appetite stimulants may be indicated in some patients. Megestrol acetate (Megace®, Bristol-Myers Squibb, Princeton, NJ) and dronabinol (Marinol®, Unimed Pharmaceuticals, Marietta, GA) have different mechanisms of action with different physiologic effects. Megace inhibits the secretion of gonadotropin, releasing hormone from the pituitary gland, whereas Marinol acts on the central nervous system to stimulate hunger and relieve nausea. Megace should be administered with testosterone in men, should be avoided in people who are bed bound because of the risk of deep vein thrombosis, and should not be used for more than three months at a time (Morley, 2002). Megace should not be administered to patients who have hormone-responsive tumors. Marinol is indicated for primarily anorectic patients and may be used indefinitely (Morley).

Restorative therapy, energy conservation, and sleep hygiene: Restorative therapy has been described as activity that focuses on the sensory dimension of the fatigue experience and relates to preventing attentional fatigue, the inability to concentrate, focus attention, or problem solve (Mock, 2001). Relaxation activities, such as walking or sitting in a natural environment, tending plants, gardening, bird watching, or viewing trees, lawns, flowers, and water, can improve recovery and promote healing through tension and fatigue reduction (Cimprich, 1993, 1995; Cimprich & Ronis, 2003; Valdres et al., 2001). Similar activities such as listening to music, watching television, or reading also have been reported to be helpful in combating fatigue by providing relaxation and distraction (Mock).

Oncology nurses can educate and counsel patients on how to conserve their energy, especially during peak treatment times such as the first few days after chemotherapy or several weeks into radiation treatments. Energy conservation includes helping patients to prioritize their activities by scheduling high-priority activities at times when energy levels are highest (e.g., early morning) and scheduling rest and nap periods during the day when appropriate (Mock, 2001). Delegating high-energy responsibilities to others includes giving patients permission to ask for needed help and support from family members and friends. Sleep hygiene (e.g., avoidance of alcohol and caffeine) should be included as part of standardized teaching when patients report fatigue and/or sleep difficulties. Figure 11-5 outlines a plan for managing sleep. Implementation of other nonpharmacologic activities such as restorative therapy, relaxation techniques, and exercise has been shown to decrease stress and anxiety that can contribute to the insomnia that compounds the fatigue experience.

Figure 11-5. Management for Sleep and Rest

Good Sleep Hygiene
- During the Day
  - Exercise regularly. Even a 20-minute walk during the day can help you to relax. Do not exercise in the evening.
  - Limit naps if you can. If you must nap, limit your nap to 30 minutes.
- Before Bedtime
  - Avoid alcohol, caffeine, chocolate, and nicotine in the late afternoon and evening.
  - Limit liquids in the evening before going to bed.
  - Turn off the television one hour before bedtime. Listen to quiet music or take a warm bath.
  - If you worry or "can't turn your brain off" when you try to sleep, make a list of things you need to do before you go to bed and then stop thinking about them.
- At Bedtime
  - Go to bed and get up at the same time every day, even on weekends.
  - A bedtime snack of warm milk, turkey, or a banana may make you sleepy.
  - If you are a "clock watcher," turn the clock so that you cannot see its face.
  - To fall asleep, lie in the position that you normally find yourself in when you wake up.
  - Go to bed at the same time with your spouse.
- If You Cannot Fall Asleep
  - If you have not fallen asleep in 15 minutes, go to another room. Listen to quiet music. Avoid things that stimulate your mind (television, exciting books). Reading self-help books may help you to feel drowsy. Go back to bed when you feel sleepy. If you still cannot fall asleep, get up again and repeat as necessary.
- If You Wake Up During the Night
  - If you cannot get back to sleep, follow the procedure above (If You Cannot Fall Asleep).

Note. From "Fatigue: A Debilitating Symptom," by R. Valdres, C. Escalante, and E. Manzullo, 2001, *Nursing Clinics of North America, 36,* p. 693. Copyright 2001 by Elsevier. Reprinted with permission.

Exercise: Mock (2001) asserted that of all nonpharmacologic interventions for CRF, exercise has demonstrated the most benefit in decreasing fatigue for patients undergoing active treatment and for survivors who have completed treatment. The majority of studies evaluating the association between exercise and fatigue have investigated patients experiencing breast cancer. The studies have been experimental, but the results have been inarguably positive (Mock). The information from studies cannot always be extrapolated to other populations, yet this research provides a framework for interventions and future evaluation of outcomes.

Studies have demonstrated that exercise elevates mood, decreases the severity of chemotherapy side effects, and has positive effects on weight gain, insomnia, functional ability, and QOL (Mock, 2001; Schwartz, Mori, Gao, Nail, & King, 2001). Encouraging results from these studies have prompted other groups to begin examining the role of exercise in different populations of patients with cancer. Weight training for men with prostate cancer receiving androgen deprivation therapy recently was shown to have beneficial effects, decreasing fatigue and increasing strength (Segal et al., 2003). Individualize patients' exercise programs according to their physical capabilities, treatment protocols, and the comorbidities (e.g., bone metastases, neutropenia, thrombocytopenia) associated with their disease and treatment (Mock).

Most beneficial to patients may be the recommendation to remain active by carrying out their usual activities, such as household chores and walking, then tailoring an increase in their exercise based upon pretreatment levels, age, and interest (Ream & Richardson, 1999). To encourage patients to maintain an optimal level of physical activity during and following their treatment, assess patients' activity level at diagnosis, and, if necessary, refer them to physical therapy programs during treatment (Stricker et al., 2004).

Recognition and treatment of pain and depression: Clinically, depression contributes to both physical and emotional fatigue; therefore, it is vital for oncology nurses to assess separately, then together, the common signs and symptoms of both depression and CRF and the possible interface for each patient who presents with overlapping complaints (e.g., insomnia, anorexia, stress, anxiety). If clinical depression is suspected, then this underlying problem should be treated with continued evaluation of fatigue as the patient's mood lifts with supportive therapy. Greenberg (1998) provided a simple example to help to differentiate depression from CRF. If the patient states, "I'm too tired," then this implies that the patient has the desire but does not feel that he or she has the stamina required to carry out an activity. This is most likely related to fatigue versus a depressive state in which the patient lacks the desire because of dysphoria, loss of interest, and resultant fatigue.

Antidepressants may be effective in decreasing a depressed mood, which may increase energy. Studies need to evaluate the efficacy of these drugs as a primary therapy for fatigue and specifically determine outcome measures aimed at decreasing fatigue. Selective serotonin reuptake inhibitors (SSRIs), secondary amine tricyclics, and bupropion (Wellbutrin®, GlaxoSmithKline, Research Triangle Park, NC) may be administered with the goal of treating clinical depression, yet their efficacy to increase energy in nondepressed patients with fatigue still must be evaluated.

Portenoy and Itri's (1999) algorithm (see Figure 11-4) suggested using antidepressants and analgesic medications to manage depression or pain. Good pain management is essential to QOL. Analgesics should be used at the lowest dose necessary to achieve pain relief and to allow patients to carry out daily activities but as not to contribute to sedation. As noted earlier, chronic pain can lead to a cycle of depression and fatigue. Oncology nurses can recognize when referral to a pain specialist is needed. Ongoing treatment for clinical depression and pain is imperative to ensure that these conditions do not exacerbate CRF.

Emotional support: Fatigue has been reported to be associated with anxiety, depression, emotional distress, and anger in the majority of people with cancer (Ream & Richardson, 1999). Psychotherapy with a psychiatric clinical nurse specialist or psychiatrist may be helpful (Valdres et al., 2001). NCCN (2004) guidelines recommended counseling patients with cancer and referring them to available resources for the management of stress, depression, anxiety, and other emotions that can aggravate fatigue. Recommended resources include support groups, individual counseling, psychoeducational programs that teach coping strategies, stress management training, and tailored behavioral interventions (e.g., American Cancer Society's "I Can Cope" educational classes). The cause-and-effect interrelationships among fatigue, emotional distress, insomnia, depression, and anxiety are not clearly defined, yet the correlation between fatigue and emotional distress in patients with cancer is fairly positive (Mock, 2001). Participation in supportive group therapy or learning new coping strategies has been found to decrease the perception and experience of fatigue.

Pharmacologic interventions: Pharmacologic treatment for fatigue serves a specific role when a physiologic underpinning such as anemia, hypothyroidism, or clinical depression has been identified (Mock, 2001). Conversely, when no clear etiology for patients' fatigue exists, well-controlled clinical trials have not evaluated the efficacy of various pharmacologic agents in the management of CRF (Burks, 2001; Mock). Drugs used for the management of CRF include psychostimulants, antidepressants, and corticosteroids.

Psychostimulants increasingly are being used in the clinical setting for the management of daytime sleepiness and fatigue. Breitbart, Rosenfeld, Kaim, and Funesti-Esch (2001) conducted a randomized, placebo-controlled trial in which HIV-positive patients (N = 144) with fatigue were given methylphenidate hydrochloride (Ritalin®, Novartis, East Hanover, NJ), pemoline (Cylert®, Abbott Laboratories, Abbott Park, IL), and placebo. The results demonstrated that both the methylphenidate and pemoline groups experienced an improvement in fatigue. Methylphenidate and pemoline usually are administered to fatigued patients based solely on clinical observation of cognitive and physical fatigue symptoms. These drugs act upon the central nervous system and enhance patients' attention and alertness (Burks, 2001). Modafinil (Provigil®, Cephalon, West Chester, PA) is a newer psychostimulant approved for managing narcolepsy. It enhances wakefulness and vigilance. Some studies reported an improvement of fatigue in patients with multiple sclerosis using modafinil. Amantadine (Symmetrel®, Endo Pharmaceuticals, Chadds Ford, PA), an antiparkinsonian drug, has been used with some success in reducing fatigue in patients with multiple sclerosis who cannot tolerate or who fail modafinil. Modafinil is being used for the management of daytime fatigue in patients with cancer, and studies are needed to confirm the efficacy, relative safety, and a variety of other issues, including dose response and duration of effect. Important to note is the fact that psychostimulants also act as appetite suppressants, an adverse side effect when evaluated for use in the cancer population (Burks).

Another category of drugs that has been used to combat CRF is antidepressants, most often those classified as SSRIs. These drugs are most efficacious in treating patients with fatigue related to clinical depression because they have not proved to be effective in counteracting generalized fatigue, and they do not elevate mood in nondepressed patients (Burks, 2001). Another drawback is that SSRIs have a delayed onset of their therapeutic effect (Burks). An atypical antidepressant, bupropion has stimulant properties that may prove to be beneficial in the treatment of CRF. One study in 15 patients with cancer followed over a period of two years found that bupropion sustained-release (Wellbutrin SR) reduced fatigue in patients with a variety of tumor types (Cullum, Wojciechowski, Pelletier, & Simpson, 2004).

Lastly, the glucocorticoids (hydrocortisone, prednisone, or dexamethasone) have been theorized to improve fatigue states by enhancing mood (Burks, 2001). This classification of medications has been studied in patients with chronic fatigue syndrome, but research has not investigated their role in CRF. It is warned that the use of these drugs in the cancer population may be limited because of side effects related to adrenal insufficiency (i.e., the increased risk of infection in already immunosuppressed patients) (Burks). Future research may focus upon drugs that block the physiologic mechanisms that contribute to fatigue, such as cytokine release, IL-6, and TNF secretion.

Conclusion

CRF is gaining the appreciation it deserves as an all-encompassing symptom. Mock (2001) asserted that future research at the highest level of evidence needs to be carried out in the form of randomized clinical trials. Further fatigue studies are needed across different patient populations with diverse diagnoses, including different cancer treatment effects along the disease continuum from diagnosis to terminal illness (Mock). Refinement of fatigue evaluation tools can bring research to the clinical setting, and continued focus on this multidimensional symptom will provide further evidence-based practice in the management of CRF, strengthening the clinical practice guidelines set forth by NCCN (2004). The development of tighter fatigue nomenclature will enable researchers, clinicians, and patients to use much of the same language in their description and documentation of fatigue. This will provide progress in narrowing the wide range of descriptors and aid clinicians in assessing and managing fatigue, ultimately improving patients' QOL across the cancer continuum. Further investigations into the physiologic, biologic, pharmacologic, and neurochemical etiologies of fatigue also will lead to more effective and individualized approaches to clinical management, much like the symptom of pain is understood and treated today.

Special thanks to Anna L. Schwartz, PhD, CFNP, RN, who served as the author of this chapter in the first edition.

References

Ahlberg, K., Ekman, T., Gaston-Johansson, F., & Mock, V. (2003). Assessment and management of cancer-related fatigue in adults. *Lancet, 362,* 640–650.

American Psychiatric Association. (2000). *Diagnostic and statistical manual of mental disorders* (4th ed., text rev.). Washington, DC: Author.

Ancoli-Israel, S., Moore, P., & Jones, V. (2001). The relationship between fatigue and sleep in cancer patients: A review. *European Journal of Cancer Care, 10,* 245–255.

Anno, G., Baum, S., Withers, H., & Young, R. (1989). Symptomatology of acute radiation effects in humans after exposure to doses of 0.5–30 Gy. *Health Physics, 56,* 821–838.

Baker, F., Zabora, J., Polland, A., & Wingard, J. (1999). Reintegration after bone marrow transplantation. *Cancer Practice, 7,* 190–197.

Berger, A. (1998). Patterns of fatigue and activity and rest during adjuvant breast cancer chemotherapy. *Oncology Nursing Forum, 25,* 51–62.

Berglund, G., Bolund, C., Fornander, T., Rutqvist, L., & Sjoden, P. (1991). Late effects of adjuvant chemotherapy and postoperative radiotherapy on quality of life among breast cancer patients. *European Journal of Cancer, 27,* 1075–1081.

Bower, J., Ganz, P., Desmond, K., Rowland, J., Meyerowitz, B., & Belin, T. (2000). Fatigue in breast cancer survivors: Occurrence, correlates, and impact on quality of life. *Journal of Clinical Oncology, 18,* 743–753.

Breitbart, W., Rosenfeld, B., Kaim, M., & Funesti-Esch, J. (2001). A randomized, double-blind, placebo-controlled trial of psychostimulants for the treatment of fatigue in ambulatory patients with human immunodeficiency virus disease. *Archives of Internal Medicine, 161,* 411–420.

Burks, T.F. (2001). New agents for the treatment of cancer-related fatigue. *Cancer, 92*(6 Suppl.), 1714–1717.

Cella, D., Kallich, J., McDermott, A., & Xu, X. (2004). The longitudinal relationship of hemoglobin, fatigue and quality of life in anemic cancer patients: Results from five randomized clinical trials. *Annals of Oncology, 15,* 979–986.

Cella, D., Peterman, A., Passik, S., Jacobsen, P., & Breitbart, W. (1998). Progress toward guidelines for the management of fatigue. *Oncology, 12,* 369–377.

Cimprich, B. (1992). Attentional fatigue following breast cancer surgery. *Research in Nursing and Health, 15,* 199–207.

Cimprich, B. (1993). Development of an intervention to restore attention in cancer patients. *Cancer Nursing, 16,* 83–92.

Cimprich, B. (1995). Symptom management: Loss of concentration. *Seminars in Oncology Nursing, 11,* 279–288.

Cimprich, B., & Ronis, D. (2003). An environmental intervention to restore attention in women with newly diagnosed breast cancer. *Cancer Nursing, 26,* 284–294.

Crawford, J., Cella, D., Cleeland, C., Cremieux, P., Demetri, G., Sarokhan, B., et al. (2002). Relationship between changes in hemoglobin level and quality of life during chemotherapy in anemic cancer patients receiving epoetin alfa therapy. *Cancer, 95,* 888–895.

Cullum, J., Wojciechowski, A., Pelletier, G., & Simpson, J. (2004). Bupropion sustained release treatment reduces fatigue in cancer patients. *Canadian Journal of Psychiatry, 49,* 139–144.

Curt, G., Breitbart, W., Cella, D., Groopman, J., Horning, S., Itri, L., et al. (2000). Impact of cancer-related fatigue on lives of patients: New findings from the Fatigue Coalition. *Oncologist, 5,* 353–360.

Dammacco, F., Castoldi, G., & Rodjer, S. (2001). Efficacy of epoetin alfa in the treatment of anaemia of multiple myeloma. *British Journal of Haematology, 113,* 172–179.

Dean, G., & Anderson, P.R. (2001). Fatigue. In B.R. Ferrell & N. Coyle (Eds.), *Textbook of palliative nursing* (pp. 91–100). New York: Oxford University Press.

De Jong, N., Candel, M., Schouten, H., Abu-Saad, H., & Courtens, A. (2004). Prevalence and course of fatigue in breast cancer patients receiving adjuvant chemotherapy. *Annals of Oncology, 15,* 896–905.

Demetri, G., Kris, M., Wade, J., Degos, L., & Cella, D. (1998). Quality-of-life benefit in chemotherapy patients treated with epoetin alfa is independent of disease response or tumor type: Results from a prospective community oncology study. Procrit Study Group. *Journal of Clinical Oncology, 16,* 3412–3425.

El-Banna, M.M., Berger, A.M., Farr, L., Foxall, M.J., Friesth, B., & Schreiner, E. (2004). Fatigue and depression in patients with lymphoma undergoing autologous peripheral blood stem cell transplantation. *Oncology Nursing Forum, 31,* 937–944.

Fobair, P., Hoppe, R., Bloom, J., Cox, R., Varghese, A., & Spiegel, D. (1986). Psychosocial problems among survivors of Hodgkin's disease. *Journal of Clinical Oncology, 4,* 805–814.

Fortin, F., & Kirouac, S. (1976). A randomized controlled trial of preoperative patient education. *International Journal of Nursing Studies, 13,* 11–24.

Gabrilove, J. (2000). Overview: Erythropoiesis, anemia, and the impact of erythropoietin. *Seminars in Hematology, 37*(4 Suppl. 6), 1–3.

Geinitz, H., Zimmerman, F., Stoll, P., Thamm, R., Kaffenberger, W., Ansorg, K., et al. (2001). Fatigue, serum cytokine levels, and blood cell counts during radiotherapy of patients with breast cancer. *International Journal of Radiation Oncology, Biology, Physics, 51,* 691–698.

Gelinas, C., & Fillion, L. (2004). Factors related to persistent fatigue following completion of breast cancer treatment. *Oncology Nursing Forum, 31,* 269–278.

Glaspy, J., Bukowski, R., Steinberg, D., Taylor, C., Tchekmedyian, S., & Vadhan-Raj, S. (1997). Impact of therapy with epoetin alfa on clinical outcomes in patients with nonmyeloid malignancies during cancer chemotherapy in community oncology practice. Procrit Study Group. *Journal of Clinical Oncology, 15,* 1218–1234.

Glaus, A. (1998). Fatigue in patients with cancer. Analysis and assessment. *Recent Results in Cancer Research, 145,* I–XI, 1–172.

Glaus, A., Crow, R., & Hammond, S. (1996). A qualitative study to explore the concept of fatigue/tiredness in cancer patients and in healthy individuals. *Supportive Care in Cancer, 4,* 82–96.

Greenberg, D.B. (1998). Fatigue. In J.C. Holland (Ed.), *Psycho-oncology* (pp. 485–493). New York: Oxford University Press.

Gutstein, H. (2001). The biologic basis of fatigue. *Cancer, 92,* 1678–1683.

Hancock, B., Wheatley, K., Harris, S., Ives, N., Harrison, G., Horsman, J., et al. (2004). Adjuvant interferon in high-risk melanoma: The AIM HIGH Study—United Kingdom Coordinating Committee on Cancer Research randomized study of adjuvant low-dose extended-duration interferon alfa-2a in high-risk resected malignant melanoma. *Journal of Clinical Oncology, 22,* 53–61.

Hann, D., Denniston, M., & Baker, F. (2000). Measurement of fatigue in cancer patients: Further validation of the fatigue symptom inventory. *Quality of Life Research, 9,* 847–854.

Iop, A., Manfredi, A., & Bonura, S. (2004). Fatigue in cancer patients receiving chemotherapy: An analysis of published studies. *Annals of Oncology, 15,* 712–720.

Jacobsen, P., Andrykowski, M., & Thors, C. (2004). Relationship of catastrophizing to fatigue among women receiving treatment for breast cancer. *Journal of Consulting and Clinical Psychology, 72,* 355–361.

Jereczek-Fossa, B., Marsiglia, H., & Orecchia, R. (2002). Radiotherapy-related fatigue. *Critical Reviews in Oncology/Hematology, 41,* 317–325.

Loge, J., Abrahamsen, A., Ekeberg, O., & Kaasa, S. (2000). Fatigue and psychiatric morbidity among Hodgkin's disease survivors. *Journal of Pain and Symptom Management, 19,* 91–99.

Manzullo, E., & Escalante, C. (2002). Research into fatigue. *Hematology/Oncology Clinics of North America, 16,* 619–628.

Mendoza, T., Wang, X., Cleeland, C., Morrissey, M., Johnson, B., Wendt, J., et al. (1999). The rapid assessment of fatigue severity in cancer patients: Use of the Brief Fatigue Inventory. *Cancer, 85,* 1186–1196.

Mock, V. (2001). Fatigue management: Evidence and guidelines for practice. *Cancer, 92*(6 Suppl.), 1699–1707.

Molassiotis, A. (1999). A correlational evaluation of tiredness and lack of energy in survivors of haematological malignancies. *European Journal of Cancer Care, 8,* 19–25.

Monga, U., Jaweed, M., Kerrigan, A., Lawhon, L., Johnson, J., Vallbona, C., et al. (1997). Neuromuscular fatigue in prostate cancer patients undergoing radiation therapy. *Archives of Physical Medicine and Rehabilitation, 78,* 961–966.

Morley, J. (2002). Orexigenic and anabolic agents. *Clinics in Geriatric Medicine, 18,* 853–866.

Morrow, G., Andrews, P., Hickok, J., Roscoe, J., & Matteson, S. (2002). Fatigue associated with cancer and its treatment. *Supportive Care in Cancer, 10,* 389–398.

Nail, L. (2002). Fatigue in patients with cancer. *Oncology Nursing Forum, 29,* 537.

National Comprehensive Cancer Network. (2004). Cancer-related fatigue. *NCCN clinical practice guidelines in oncology v.1.2004.* Jenkintown, PA: Author. Retrieved March 10, 2005, from http://www.nccn.org/professionals/physician_gls/PDF/fatigue.pdf

National Institutes of Health. (2002). NIH State-of-the-Science Statement on symptom management in cancer: Pain, depression, and fatigue. *NIH Consensus and State-of-the-Science Statements, 19*(4), 1–30.

Okuyama, T., Akechi, T., Kugaya, A., Okamura, H., Imoto, S., Nakano, T., et al. (2000). Factors correlated with fatigue in disease-free breast cancer patients: Application of the Cancer Fatigue Scale. *Supportive Care in Cancer, 8,* 215–222.

Piper, B. (1997). Measuring fatigue. In M. Frank-Stromborg & S. Olsen (Eds.), *Instruments for clinical health-care research* (2nd ed., pp. 482–496). Sudbury, MA: Jones and Bartlett.

Piper, B., Dibble, S., Dodd, M., Weiss, M., Slaughter, R., & Paul, S. (1998). The revised Piper Fatigue Scale: Psychometric evaluation in women with breast cancer. *Oncology Nursing Forum, 25,* 677–684.

Portenoy, R., & Itri, L. (1999). Cancer-related fatigue: Guidelines for evaluation and management. *Oncologist, 4,* 1–10.

Ream, E., & Richardson, A. (1999). From theory to practice: Designing interventions to reduce fatigue in patients with cancer. *Oncology Nursing Forum, 26,* 1295–1303.

Roscoe, J., Morrow, G., Hickok, J., Bushunow, P., Matteson, S., Rakita, D., et al. (2002). Temporal interrelationships among fatigue, circadian rhythm and depression in breast cancer patients undergoing chemotherapy treatment. *Supportive Care in Cancer, 10,* 329–336.

Rosenthal, M., & Oratz, R. (1998). Phase II clinical trial of recombinant alpha 2b interferon and 13 cis retinoic acid in patients with metastatic melanoma. *American Journal of Clinical Oncology, 21,* 352–354.

Schover, L.R. (1998). Sexual dysfunction. In J.C. Holland (Ed.), *Psycho-oncology* (pp. 494–499). New York: Oxford University Press.

Schwartz, A. (1998a). Patterns of exercise and fatigue in physically active cancer survivors. *Oncology Nursing Forum, 25,* 485–491.

Schwartz, A. (1998b). The Schwartz Cancer Fatigue Scale: Testing reliability and validity. *Oncology Nursing Forum, 25,* 711–717.

Schwartz, A., Mori, M., Gao, R., Nail, L., & King, M. (2001). Exercise reduces daily fatigue in women with breast cancer receiving chemotherapy. *Medicine and Science in Sports and Exercise, 33,* 718–723.

Segal, R., Reid, R., Courneya, K., Malone, S., Parliament, M., Scott, C., et al. (2003). Resistance exercise in men receiving androgen deprivation therapy for prostate cancer. *Journal of Clinical Oncology, 21,* 1653–1659.

Smets, E., Garssen, B., Bonke, B., & de Haes, J. (1995). The Multidimensional Fatigue Inventory (MFI): Psychometric qualities of an instrument to assess fatigue. *Journal of Psychosomatic Research, 39,* 315–325.

Stasi, R., Abriani, L., Beccaglia, P., Terzoli, E., & Amadori, S. (2003). Cancer-related fatigue: Evolving concepts in evaluation and treatment. *Cancer, 98,* 1786–1801.

Stricker, C.T., Drake, D., Hoyer, K.A., & Mock, V. (2004). Evidence-based practice for fatigue management in adults with cancer: Exercise as an intervention. *Oncology Nursing Forum, 31,* 963–974.

Taylor, C., Basen-Engquist, K., Shinn, E., & Bodurka, D. (2004). Predictors of sexual functioning in ovarian cancer patients. *Journal of Clinical Oncology, 22,* 881–889.

Tchekmedyian, N., Kallich, J., McDermott, A., Fayers, P., & Erder, M. (2003). The relationship between psychologic distress and cancer-related fatigue. *Cancer, 98,* 198–203.

Tralongo, P., Respini, D., & Ferrau, F. (2003). Fatigue and aging. *Critical Reviews in Oncology/Hematology, 48*(Suppl.), S57–S67.

Valdres, R., Escalante, C., & Manzullo, E. (2001). Fatigue: A debilitating symptom. *Nursing Clinics of North America, 36,* 685–694.

Visser, M., & Smets, E. (1998). Fatigue, depression, and quality of life in cancer patients: How are they related? *Supportive Care in Cancer, 6,* 101–108.

Vogelzang, N., Breitbart, W., Cella, D., Curt, G., Groopman, J., Horning, S., et al. (1997). Patient, caregiver, and oncologist perceptions of cancer-related fatigue: Results of a tripart assessment survey. The Fatigue Coalition. *Seminars in Hematology, 34*(3 Suppl. 2), 4–12.

Woo, B., Dibble, S., Piper, B., Keating, S., & Weiss, M. (1998). Differences in fatigue by treatment methods in women with breast cancer. *Oncology Nursing Forum, 25,* 915–920.

Yellen, S., Cella, D., Webster, K., Blendowski, C., & Kaplan, E. (1997). Measuring fatigue and other anemia-related symptoms with the Functional Assessment of Cancer Therapy (FACT) measurement system. *Journal of Pain and Symptom Management, 13,* 63–74.

CHAPTER 12

Cognitive Impairment in Cancer

ESTHER MUSCARI, RN, MSN, APRN, BC

If one loves me for my judgment, memory, he does not love me, for I can lose these qualities without losing myself.

—Blaise Pascal

Cognitive functioning is the information handling aspect of behavior and involves the processes or domains of attention, concentration, learning and memory, psychomotor efficiency and manual dexterity, visuospatial ability, and general intelligence. Many of the processes or domains are highly interrelated and multidimensional. When any of the processes are affected, impairment is evident in a number of behaviors. For example, attention allows people to select information from the environment, concentrate on that information, exclude irrelevant information or simultaneous stimuli, and then sustain their attention on the specific selected information. Learning and memory are multidimensional and include short- and long-term memory. Memory is either contextual (information stored within the context of other information, such as being part of a greater story or memory) or noncontextual (information committed to memory without other information) (Bender, Kramer, & Miaskowski, 2002). Short-term memory involves everything associated with the present or recent hours or days. Long-term memory involves information storage that extends back years.

Cognitive impairments are perceived and described by patients as having difficulties with their ability to remember, think, find the right words, and concentrate. Patients may describe their difficulties as having "chemo brain" or "chemo clutter" (Brezden, Phillips, Abdolell, Bunston, & Tannock, 2000). The most frequently documented impairments to cognition in the oncology population are altered attention span, decreased concentration, and short-term memory loss. Other impairments that have been reported from alterations in cognitive domains include disorganization, difficulty with arithmetic skills, and altered language skills (Olin, 2001; Schagen et al., 1999; van Dam et al., 1998).

Cognitive impairment in people treated for cancer has only recently been gaining attention. The problem affects quality of life and, therefore, is an issue for cancer survivors (Dow, 2003). In fact, the National Coalition for Cancer Survivorship recognizes cognitive impairment as a challenge for people with cancer (Ferrell & Dow, 1997). Because cognitive impairment can last for years beyond treatment completion, cancer survivors need to find ways to incorporate deficits into their lives (Bowman, Deimling, Smerglia, Sage, & Kahana, 2002).

Contributing Factors

Factors contributing to cognitive impairment can be separated into direct/disease-related factors and indirect/treatment-related factors (Sjogren, 1997). Direct causes include primary or metastatic cancer and personal characteristics such as age and intelligence, whereas the list of indirect causes is extensive (see Figure 12-1).

Figure 12-1. Indirect/Treatment-Related Etiologies of Cognitive Impairment

- Antineoplastic therapies
- Infection/sepsis
- Nutritional deficiencies
- Hematologic abnormalities (e.g., anemia)
- Metabolic abnormalities (e.g., hypercalcemia, tumor lysis syndrome)
- Hyponatremia
- Endocrine abnormalities
- Hormonal imbalances
- Antiemetics
- Narcotics/analgesics
- Depression
- Anxiety
- Sleep disorders

Note. Based on information from Bender et al., 2002; Cherrier et al., 2001; Pickett et al., 1999; Schagen, Muller, Boogerd, Rosenbrand, et al., 2002; Schagen, Muller, Boogerd, & van Dam, 2002.

Personal Characteristics

Age influences cognitive functioning. As adults age, they often experience a progressive decline in cognitive function. Predictable changes occur in their performance on neuropsychological tests, with differences noted in short-term memory and the inability to learn new information (Life Extension Foundation, 2004; National Institute on Aging, 2005). This minimal cognitive impairment is normal age-associated mental impairment as opposed to a disease process such as dementia. Life expectancy is increasing in the United States, and the age group older than 85 is the fastest growing segment of the American population (Feinberg, 2000). By 2030, approximately 20% of the U.S. population is expected to be older than 65 (Ershler, 2003), increasing from 35 million people older than age 65 in 2000 to an expected

70 million by 2050 (U.S. Census Bureau, 2004). This demographic change will affect oncology care because the median age for all types and sites of cancer is 68 years, with the incidence of cancer greatly increasing with age (Yancik & Ries, 2000).

As the population ages, the incidence of dementia that people suffer from as they age is growing. Six percent to 10% of people older than the age of 65 suffer from dementia, with Alzheimer disease accounting for two-thirds of these cases (Hendrie, 1998). Interestingly, this 6%–10% prevalence is consistent with the findings of the control group rates in the breast cancer chemotherapy studies previously cited (Hendrie). Not all cognitive loss is dementia, and differentiating treatment-induced cognitive impairment, delirium, and depression will be critical in cancer care assessments. Cognitive impairment in older adults because of disease or treatment most likely will need to be subdivided into acute reversible and chronic irreversible forms. To support assessment, age adjustment and age-adjusted norms need to be incorporated into standardized neuropsychological testing (Ahles & Saykin, 2002).

Intelligence quotient (IQ) and education level need to be controlled within studies because of their influence on neuropsychological test scores. Additionally, having a higher IQ may reduce the negative impact of trauma to the brain, a concept known as cognitive reserve. "Cognitive reserve" refers to greater synaptic density associated with enriched cognitive stimulation that has developed over many years and has been examined in patients with Alzheimer disease (Ahles & Saykin, 2002). It has not been examined in the oncology population but most likely will be considered as the mechanisms of impairment are studied and researchers begin to consider why some patients develop cognitive impairment when others do not.

Indirect Factors

Chemotherapy: The majority of cognitive impairment research in patients with cancer has involved patients with breast cancer (Phillips & Bernhard, 2003). Van Dam et al. (1998) evaluated the prevalence of cognitive deficits in women randomized to receive high-dose or standard-dose chemotherapy plus tamoxifen. Investigators evaluated whether high-dose chemotherapy impaired cognition more than standard-dose chemotherapy. Patients' results were compared to a control group of stage I patients who had not received chemotherapy. All patients had received tamoxifen, and two years had passed since their last nonhormonal therapy. Patients treated with high-dose therapy had a 32% incidence of impairment compared to 17% of the patients treated with standard-dose therapy and 9% of the control patients. Patients treated with high-dose therapy had an 8.2 times higher risk of cognitive impairment than patients receiving standard doses. Although this was a hallmark study because it brought to the forefront the problem of cognitive impairment, limitations of the study included small sample sizes, the cross-sectional design, and the limited information about the potential mechanisms for the cognitive abnormalities (Ganz, 1998). The study used 13 neuropsychological tests plus patient interviews regarding their perceptions of impairments to test cognition.

Schagen et al. (1999) conducted a similar study in women with breast cancer treated with adjuvant cyclophosphamide, methotrexate, and 5-fluorouracil (CMF). These patients demonstrated a significantly higher risk of cognitive impairment (memory problems and difficulties with attention, visual memory, processing speed, mental flexibility, and motor functions) than those patients not treated with chemotherapy at two years after systemic chemotherapy. Twenty-eight percent of the patients who received CMF experienced cognitive impairment versus 12% in the control arm. Anxiety, depression, hormonal therapy, and fatigue did not contribute to the incidence of cognitive deficits.

Brezden et al. (2000) evaluated cognitive function and mood in 31 patients with breast cancer receiving adjuvant chemotherapy and compared them to 40 matched patients who had completed adjuvant chemotherapy a median of two years earlier and with 36 healthy individuals who served as the control group. Age, education level, and menopausal status were controlled in all groups. The treatment groups with moderate or severe cognitive impairment consisted of significantly more patients than the control group. Impairment was found in the memory and language domains in the patients in active treatment. In the patients who were two years out from treatment, language and visual motor skills were impaired when compared with the control group. The Profile of Mood States demonstrated no differences among the study groups.

In 2001, Schagen, Hamburger, Muller, Boogerd, and van Dam reported on the use of quantitative electroencephalography to study neurotoxicity in patients receiving adjuvant high-dose or standard-dose chemotherapy at two years postchemotherapy. Neurophysiologic testing showed that 7 of the 17 high-dose patients and 2 of the 16 standard-dose patients had asymmetry of the alpha rhythm on electroencephalograph. No asymmetry of the alpha rhythm was noted in the control group of stage I, nontreated patients. These results provided neurophysiologic support for cognitive dysfunction as a late complication of high-dose chemotherapy. Researchers observed cognitive improvement in both chemotherapy groups and noted a slight deterioration in the control group (Schagen, Muller, Boogerd, Rosenbrand, et al., 2002). A relatively high percentage of patients who were initially cognitively impaired dropped out because of disease progression.

Ahles et al. (2002) compared patients with lymphoma or breast cancer treated with systemic therapy to matching populations receiving local therapy only. Global cognitive deficits were associated with systemic chemotherapy, with significant differences in the specific domains of verbal memory and psychomotor functioning. Patients were, on average, 10 years out from chemotherapy, supporting the belief that deficits seen shortly after treatment or at two years can continue long-term. These findings set the stage for further study to define the extent of cognitive deficits, percentage of patients actually affected, and the factors that contribute to the risk of long-term cognitive deterioration.

Radiotherapy: Studies have examined the effects of radiotherapy on cognitive functioning in children and adults who received cranial radiotherapy (Langer et al., 2002; Lilja, Portin, Hamalainen, & Salminen, 2001; Senzer, 2002; Taylor et al., 1998). Findings were mixed, with deficits noted in children in the domains of attention, concentration, and the ability to sequence and process (Langer et al.). Lilja et al. found that adults treated with radiotherapy for brain tumors had cognitive deficits that were evident at baseline and were not the result of radiation effects. This raises the question of how to follow patients long-term because the effects of disease progression are difficult to differentiate from the effects of radiotherapy. Taylor et al. found that no clear decline in cognitive functioning could be distinguished from disease progression. These findings further raise the issue of what roles patients' overall condition and age play in cognitive performance.

The major limitation of this early literature is the use of cross-sectional, post-treatment-only designs. Pretreatment assessment is needed to accurately assess changes over time. The potential disadvantage of baseline assessment, although preferable, is that the anxiety and stresses associated with a new diagnosis and the impending onset of treatment could influence the assessment (Schagen, Muller, Boogerd, & van Dam, 2002). Within the study designs, the specifics of individual antineoplastic agents and disease site specifics need to be considered to identify which are more toxic to cognitive function and to what degree. Individual factors such as age, IQ, genetic factors, and estrogen levels predispose some patients to experience more significant cognitive deficits than others and will need to be considered when analyzing data (Ahles & Saykin, 2002). Preventive interventions that might minimize the impact of cognitive dysfunction after cancer treatment most likely will begin to be included in future trials (Phillips & Bernhard, 2003).

Hormonal influences: Estrogen deficits often are implicated as a causative factor in cognitive deficits (Barton & Loprinzi, 2002; Knobf, 2001). Reboussin, Greendale, and Espeland (1998) studied the effects of placebo, estrogen alone, or estrogen with a progesterone regimen on cognitive function. While controlling for vasomotor instability variables, the group receiving estrogen plus progesterone reported less forgetfulness and less distraction than those receiving estrogen alone. All treated groups had fewer deficits than the nontreated control group. This is clearly an area of influence that must be incorporated into further studies.

Within the male population, debate exists as to whether cognitive impairment results from reduced testosterone levels and whether increasing testosterone has an activational influence on cognitive function (Barrett-Connor, Goodman-Gruen, & Pray, 1999; Cherrier, Asthan, Plymate, & Baker, 2001; Green et al., 2002; Salminen et al., 2003). Changes, when observed, often occur in the initial period of testosterone therapy, but improvements are not sustained over time. Spatial performance (e.g., recall of a walking route) is the most common domain cited for improvement, with little, if any, effect on global measures of cognitive performance (Cherrier et al.; Green et al.)

Anemia: Anemia may exacerbate a decline in cognitive function. In a retrospective review, Beard, Kokmen, and O'Brien (1997) found an almost two-fold increase in the risk of new Alzheimer disease associated with hemoglobin levels less than 12 g/dl in women and 13 g/dl in men. Similar findings among patients undergoing regular dialysis have resulted in the use of recombinant human erythropoietin treatment with resulting improvement in brain and cognitive function (Pickett, Theberge, Brown, Schweitzer, & Nissenson, 1999). This area currently is under investigation in patients with breast cancer in an attempt to quantify any protective effect of elevated hemoglobin on cognitive function (O'Shaughnessy, 2002).

Assessment

When meeting with patients, first indications of cognitive impairment, if not volunteered by the patient, sometimes are reflected in conversation. Repeated questions, difficulty following directions, searching for a word, or inability to remember the sequence of past events since the last appointment may raise suspicions in the healthcare provider. Inquiring how patients arrived at the clinic, how they adapt when outside their home in an unfamiliar setting, or what recent decisions they have needed to make can indicate a need for more in-depth evaluation.

During the health history, pertinent questions, such as whether the onset was sudden or acute, can help in identifying an underlying acute medical condition (e.g., infection, trauma, small stroke). Patients often volunteer that they have experienced changes in cognitive function, such as short-term memory difficulty or trouble with word recall, and that can lead to further evaluation and possibly formal neuropsychological testing (Paraska & Bender, 2003). Delirium or confusion can be common in older adults who recently have been discharged from the hospital or who are recovering from an acute infection or surgery.

Patients or family members may volunteer that patients' participation in social activities has decreased. Patients often give up hobbies or avoid situations, people, or events that they previously enjoyed. Finances, housework, or meals may go unattended as patients become unable to carry out normal daily activities.

Agitation, paranoia, and irritability are indicators of possible cognitive impairment. Patients can become suspicious during the early stages of impairment because they have a subtle awareness of deficits or "changes" occurring within themselves. Healthcare providers should note patients' decreased ability to concentrate on the questioning, their emotional responses, and any unkempt outward appearance because these all are indications of problems.

The Mini-Mental State Examination (MMSE), developed from the more extensive cognitive mental status examination, offers clinicians a first-line assessment tool that can be used in any clinical setting (Folstein, Folstein, & McHugh, 1975). The MMSE separates patients with cognitive disturbances from those without such disturbances. It includes 11 questions, requires 10 minutes to administer, does not require the administrator to have special training, and therefore is very practical to use routinely and serially. It concentrates on the cognitive aspects of mental functions and excludes questions pertaining to mood, abnormal mental experiences, and the form of thinking. It tests patients' short-term memory, ability to spell forward and backward, ability to perform simple math equations, and the capacity to recall three unrelated words. Visuospatial skills are evaluated by asking the patient to draw the face of a clock. The MMSE has a maximum score of 30, with a score of 24 or less considered to be suggestive of cognitive impairment. The MMSE is not intended to diagnose but rather raise a flag of awareness that further testing is needed. MMSE failures on orientation, memory, reading, and writing have clear implications for patients with cancer who are trying to care for themselves, make decisions in their care, and move forward in their lives.

Neuropsychological testing examines the brain-behavior relationships. Assessment is standardized and crosses multiple domains. Assessment areas commonly tested are simple and complex attention, verbal and visual learning and memory, critical reasoning, complex problem solving, processing speed and mental efficiency, language comprehension and fluency, reaction time, motor dexterity, and sensory functioning (Freeman & Broshek, 2002). The testing aspect of assessment includes an array of tests that often are lengthy in nature (four to seven hours) and require a trained administrator. The assessment usually requires more than one test to capture all potentially impacted domains; therefore, these tests are not conducive to administration in the clinical oncology setting.

Neurocognitive testing addresses various thinking abilities, encompassing domains of attention and concentration, abstract reasoning, cognitive processing speed, language, visuospatial and visuoconstruction, executive functions, learning and memory, and sensorimotor functions. The necessary tests are different than those used for neuropsychological testing.

Figure 12-2 provides a list of commonly used neurocognitive and neuropsychological function assessment tools, most of which require a considerable amount of testing time. Traditional global measures sample a variety of neurocognitive and neuropsychological functions. These often serve as screening measures to indicate when additional assessment is necessary but also help to track changes in functioning over time.

Figure 12-2. Cognitive Function Testing and Domains Assessed

- Folstein Mini-Mental State Examination
- Hamburg-Wechsler Intelligence Scales for Children
  - Intellectual performance
- Wechsler Intelligence Scales for Adults
  - Conceptual knowledge
  - Semantic memory
  - Visual memory
  - Verbal memory
  - Attention
  - Concentration
  - Visuomotor speed
- Kaufman Factors
  - Verbal comprehension
  - Perceptual organization
  - Freedom from distractability
- Recurring Figures Test
  - Memory functioning
- Attention and Concentration Test
  - Speed and care in discriminating visual stimuli
  - Attention
  - Concentration
- Auditory Verbal Learning Test
  - Word recall
- Rey-Osterrieth Complex Figure Test
  - 30-minute delayed recall

- Stroop Test
  - Executive function
- Depression Anxiety Stress Scales
- CogniSpeed Program
  - Speed and accuracy of cognitive processing and attentional functioning
  - Well-learned and controlled attention
  - Automatic tasks
- Vigilance Test
  - Sustaining attention
- The High Sensitivity Cognitive Screen
  - Detects subtle cognitive impairment
  - Memory
  - Language
  - Visual-motor
  - Spatial
  - Attention and concentration
  - Self-regulation
  - Planning
  - Predicts overall qualitative results of formal neuropsychological testing
- California Learning Test
  - Verbal learning
- Continuous Performance Testing
  - Attention—vigilance and accuracy

Note. Based on information from Folstein et al., 1975; Freeman & Broshek, 2002; Langer et al., 2002; Phillips & Bernhard, 2003; Schagen et al., 2001.

Implications for Practice

Patients' abilities to care for themselves, recall daily responsibilities and events, and maintain their roles within their family and professional lives are dependent upon cognitive abilities. An alteration in any of these abilities potentially affects satisfaction with life and, ultimately, quality of life. As the research literature increases, a better understanding of the cognitive domains that are most often affected and by which treatment modalities will be a great asset to clinicians and can contribute to an appropriate neurocognitive assessment. As healthcare providers learn more about cognitive impairment, patients' risks for impairment and which potential domain will be affected can be determined before patients experience deficits. Patient and family education then can be tailored to specific risks (as determined by the cancer site, treatment modality, age, hormonal status, and education level).

Clinician awareness of the commonly affected domains can lead to appropriate tools to empower patients. Visual materials for home use can help patients to respond to short-term memory losses so that the deficits are not as debilitating. Maximizing patients' potential for optimal functioning can be achieved through frequent medication profile review, managing possible comorbid conditions, managing emotional/mood disorders, and maintaining normal hematology profiles. Causes of fatigue are numerous, and many are similar to those of cognitive disorders; therefore, addressing fatigue will complement any attempt at managing cognitive impairment (Meyers, 2000). Patients who are in pain must have their pain adequately managed because this contributes to deficits in attention and concentration, efficiency of thinking, and multitasking (Meyers). Additionally, cognitively impaired patients will need an appropriate and specialized assessment for healthcare providers to adequately capture patients' pain experiences (Soscia, 2003).

Consistent, frequent validation of patients' experiences is critical because a common fear is that their brain is not working well or that they are "losing their mind" (Breitbart, Gibson, & Tremblay, 2002). Knowing that cognitive deficits exist within specific domains and do not necessarily mean that all mental functions are altered can help patients to feel less vulnerable to changes.

Clinicians will need to be confident that patients experiencing cognitive impairment have given informed consent. This particularly is important in patients' decision-making capacity to provide consent for research (Casarett, Karlawish, & Hirschman, 2003). Patients might need more than one informative session, written materials, and assistance from a family member to learn about the clinical plan and to help them to adhere to the appointments.

Because the cognitive impairments experienced by most patients with cancer do not stop them from engaging in their daily activities, patients may respond well to cognitive rehabilitation. Cognitive rehabilitation is intended to improve patients' independence level, with vocational rehabilitation focused on improving productivity in their volunteer or professional efforts and daily activities. Cognitive rehabilitation begins with identifying and validating patients' deficits. Describing to patients how the cancer therapy causes cognitive impairment and affects their thinking is the first step. For example, a short attention span will increase the amount of time needed to learn a new task or possibly the time it takes to assist with a child's homework; spatial performance deficits will cause difficulty envisioning or describing the route between their home and work; short-term memory deficits will affect their appointments and responsibilities; word-recall problems will cause them to find themselves in the middle of a sentence struggling to say a word they have used many times; and number sequencing and math skills difficulties may decrease their ability to balance a checkbook. Once patients can see the specifics of how their cognition is impaired, they feel reassured that they are not "losing their mind" and can focus their attention on the identified areas to bolster and support themselves. For example, regular use of a daily electronic or paper calendar that has built-in alerts or reminders can assist with memory. Placing a small calculator in their checkbook can assist with arithmetic skills. Limiting activities to short, frequent periods, if energy levels allow, can lessen the difficulty with attention. Focusing on improving their independence level, performing daily activities, and engaging in vocational rehabilitation can empower cognitively impaired patients to function at their potential.

Conclusion

Cognitive impairment can be frightening to patients, families, and even caregivers because it is the ability to think, problem solve, follow directions, and make decisions that helps to define who we are as individuals. To have a person's cognition altered places a person in a position of vulnerability. Nurses are in an optimal position—by virtue of the many roles within oncology—to have an impact on patients and their family members who are at risk for or are actively experiencing cognitive impairment. Therefore, identifying risk factors, understanding, and differentiating the domains that process information allows for an assessment that produces interventions and assistance specific to the area of thinking that is affected. Rather than feeling vulnerable or overwhelmed with fear, patients and families can be encouraged and function at levels satisfying to their quality of life.

References

Ahles, T., & Saykin, A. (2002). Breast cancer chemotherapy-related cognitive dysfunction. *Clinical Breast Cancer, 3*(Suppl. 3), S84–S89.

Ahles, T., Saykin, A., Furstenberg, C., Cole, B., Mott, L., Skalla, K., et al. (2002). Neuropsychologic impact of standard-dose systemic chemotherapy in long-term survivors of breast cancer and lymphoma. *Journal of Clinical Oncology, 20,* 485–493.

Barrett-Connor, E., Goodman-Gruen, D., & Pray, B. (1999). Endogenous sex hormones and cognitive function in older men. *Journal of Clinical Endocrinology, 84,* 3681–3685.

Barton, D., & Loprinzi, C. (2002). Novel approaches to preventing chemotherapy-induced cognitive dysfunction in breast cancer: The art of the possible. *Clinical Breast Cancer, 3*(Suppl. 3), S121–S127.

Beard, C., Kokmen, E., & O'Brien, P. (1997). Risk of Alzheimer's disease among elderly patients with anemia: Population-based investigations in Olmsted County, Minnesota. *Annals of Epidemiology, 7,* 219–224.

Bender, C., Kramer, P., & Miaskowski, C. (2002). Processes involved in normal cognitive function. In *New directions in the management of cancer-related cognitive impairment, fatigue, and pain.* Bridgewater, NJ: Ortho Biotech.

Bowman, K., Deimling, G., Smerglia, V., Sage, P., & Kahana, B. (2002). Appraisal of the cancer experience by older long-term survivors. *Psycho-Oncology, 12,* 226–238.

Breitbart, W., Gibson, C., & Tremblay, A. (2002). The delirium experience: Delirium recall and delirium-related distress in hospitalized patients with cancer, their spouses/caregivers, and their nurses. *Psychosomatics, 43,* 183–194.

Brezden, C., Phillips, K., Abdolell, M., Bunston, T., & Tannock, I. (2000). Cognitive function in breast cancer patients receiving adjuvant chemotherapy. *Journal of Clinical Oncology, 18,* 2695–2701.

Casarett, D., Karlawish, J., & Hirschman, K. (2003). Identifying ambulatory cancer patients at risk of impaired capacity to consent to research. *Journal of Pain and Symptom Management, 26,* 615–622.

Cherrier, M.M., Asthan, S., Plymate, S., & Baker, L. (2001). Testosterone supplementation improves spatial and verbal memory in healthy older men. *Neurology, 57,* 80–88.

Dow, K.H. (2003). Challenges and opportunities in cancer survivorship research. *Oncology Nursing Forum, 30,* 455–469.

Ershler, W. (2003). Cancer: A disease of the elderly. *Journal of Supportive Oncology, 1*(4 Suppl. 2), 5–10.

Feinberg, A. (2000). *Cognitive impairment in the aged.* Medscape Coverage of American College of Physicians-American Society of Internal Medicine Annual Session 2000. Retrieved July 1, 2004, from http://www.medscape.com/viewarticle/420065

Ferrell, B.R., & Dow, K.H. (1997). Quality of life among long-term cancer survivors. *Oncology, 11,* 565–576.

Folstein, M., Folstein, S., & McHugh, P. (1975). "Mini-mental state": A practical method for grading the cognitive state of patients for the clinician. *Journal of Psychiatric Research, 12,* 189–198.

Freeman, J.R., & Broshek, D.K. (2002). Assessing cognitive dysfunction in breast cancer: What are the tools? *Clinical Breast Cancer, 3*(Suppl. 3), S91–S99.

Ganz, P. (1998). Cognitive dysfunction following adjuvant treatment of breast cancer: A new dose-limiting toxic effect? *Journal of the National Cancer Institute, 90,* 182–183.

Green, H., Pakenham, K., Headley, B., Yaxley, J., Nicol, P., Mactaggart, P., et al. (2002). Altered cognitive function in men treated for prostate cancer with luteinizing hormone-releasing hormone analogues and cyproterone acetate: A randomized controlled trial. *International Journal of Urology, 90,* 427–432.

Hendrie, H. (1998). Epidemiology of dementia and Alzheimer's disease. *American Journal of Geriatric Psychiatry, 6*(2 Suppl. 1), S3–S18.

Knobf, M. (2001). The menopausal symptom experience in young mid-life women with breast cancer. *Cancer Nursing, 24,* 201–209.

Langer, T., Martus, P., Ottensmeier, H., Hertzberg, H., Beck, J., & Meier, W. (2002). CNS late-effects after ALL therapy in childhood. Part III: Neuropsychological performance in long-term survivors of childhood ALL: Impairments of concentration, attention, and memory. *Medical and Pediatric Oncology, 38,* 320–328.

Life Extension Foundation. (2004, June). *Age-associated mental impairment.* Retrieved May 1, 2005, from http://www.lef.org/protocols/prtcl-003.shtml

Lilja, A., Portin, R., Hamalainen, P., & Salminen, E. (2001). Short-term effects of radiotherapy on attention and memory performances in patients with brain tumors. *Cancer, 91,* 2361–2368.

Meyers, C. (2000). Neurocognitive dysfunction in cancer patients. *Oncology, 14,* 75–81.

National Institute on Aging. (2005, February). *Subgoal 2: Maintain and enhance brain function, cognition and other behaviors.* Retrieved May 1, 2005, from http://www.nia.nih.gov/AboutNIA/StrategicPlan/ResearchGoalB/Subgoal2.htm

Olin, J. (2001). Cognitive function after systemic therapy for breast cancer. *Oncology, 15,* 613–624.

O'Shaughnessy, J. (2002). Effects of epoetin alfa on cognitive function, mood, asthenia, and quality of life in women with breast cancer undergoing adjuvant chemotherapy. *Clinical Breast Cancer, 3*(Suppl. 3), S116–S120.

Paraska, K., & Bender, C. (2003). Cognitive dysfunction following adjuvant chemotherapy for breast cancer: Two case studies. *Oncology Nursing Forum, 10,* 473–478.

Phillips, K., & Bernhard, J. (2003). Adjuvant breast cancer treatment and cognitive function: Current knowledge and research directions. *Journal of the National Cancer Institute, 95,* 190–195.

Pickett, J., Theberge, D., Brown, W., Schweitzer, S., & Nissenson, A. (1999). Normalizing hematocrit in dialysis patients improves brain function. *American Journal of Kidney Diseases, 33,* 1122–1130.

Reboussin, B., Greendale, G., & Espeland, M. (1998). Effect of hormone replacement therapy on self-reported cognitive symptoms: Results from the Postmenopausal Estrogen/Progestin Interventions (PEPI) trial. *Climacteric, 1,* 172–179.

Salminen, E., Portin, R., Korpela, J., Backman, H., Parvinen, L., Helenius, H., et al. (2003). Androgen deprivation and cognition in prostate cancer. *British Journal of Cancer, 89,* 971–976.

Schagen, S., Hamburger, H., Muller, M., Boogerd, W., & van Dam, F. (2001). Neurophysiological evaluation of late effects of adjuvant high-dose chemotherapy on cognitive function. *Journal of Neuro-Oncology, 51,* 159–165.

Schagen, S., Muller, M., Boogerd, W., Rosenbrand, R., van Rhijn, D., Rodenhuis, S., et al. (2002). Late effects of adjuvant chemotherapy on cognitive function: A follow-up study in breast cancer patients. *Annals of Oncology, 13,* 1387–1397.

Schagen, S., Muller, M., Boogerd, W., & van Dam, F. (2002). Cognitive dysfunction and chemotherapy: Neuropsychological findings in perspective. *Clinical Breast Cancer, 3*(Suppl. 3), S100–S108.

Schagen, S., van Dam, F., Muller, M., Boogerd, W., Lindeboom, J., & Bruning, P. (1999). Cognitive deficits after postoperative adjuvant chemotherapy for breast carcinoma. *Cancer, 85,* 640–650.

Senzer, N. (2002). Rationale for a phase III study of erythropoietin as a neurocognitive protectant in patients with lung cancer receiving prophylactic cranial radiation therapy. *Seminars in Oncology, 29*(Suppl. 19), 47–52.

Sjogren, P. (1997). Psychomotor and cognitive functioning in cancer patients. *Acta Anaesthesiologica Scandinavica, 41,* 159–161.

Soscia, J. (2003). Assessing pain in cognitively impaired older adults with cancer. *Clinical Journal of Oncology Nursing, 7,* 174–177.

Taylor, B., Buckner, J., Cascino, T., O'Fallon, J., Schaefer, P., Dinapoli, R., et al. (1998). Effects of radiation and chemotherapy on cognitive function in patients with high-grade glioma. *Journal of Clinical Oncology, 16,* 2195–2201.

U.S. Census Bureau. (2004). *U.S. interim projections by age, sex, race, and Hispanic origin.* Retrieved March 16, 2005, from http://www.census.gov/ipc/www/usinterimproj

van Dam, F., Schagen, S., Muller, M., Boogerd, W., Wall, E., Fortuyn, M., et al. (1998). Impairment of cognitive function in women receiving adjuvant treatment for high-risk breast cancer: High-dose versus standard-dose chemotherapy. *Journal of the National Cancer Institute, 90,* 210–218.

Yancik, R., & Ries, L. (2000). Aging and cancer in America: Demographic and epidemiologic perspectives. *Hematology/Oncology Clinics of North America, 14,* 17–23.

SECTION III

Specific Psychological/ Emotional Reactions

CHAPTER 13

Anxiety and the Cancer Experience

Nancy Jo Bush, RN, MN, MA, AOCN®

To venture causes anxiety, but not to venture is to lose one's self. And to venture in the highest sense is precisely to be conscious of one's self.

—Soren Kierkegaard

One of the most common psychological responses to the cancer experience is anxiety. Cancer is perceived as a threat to well-being, and responses to external and internal threats are defined in terms of fear and anxiety (Wolman, 1994). Feelings of fear and apprehension are normal when patients with cancer are confronted with possible losses and their own mortality. Normal anxiety reactions present at different points along the cancer continuum. An acute stress response often occurs at the time of initial diagnosis and at each transitional point of the illness (Pasacreta, Minarik, & Nield-Anderson, 2001). If uncontrolled anxiety develops, it can be disabling for the patient, interfering with both treatment response and psychosocial functioning. Of importance when working with patients with cancer are recognizing signs and symptoms of anxiety, differentiating between normal or expected anxiety responses, and intervening appropriately to prevent dysfunctional or abnormal reactions. A clear distinction does not always exist between the normal fears that cancer initiates and other anxiety reactions that are intense enough to meet the criteria for pathologic anxiety (Noyes, Holt, & Massie, 1998).

Important Principles Related to Anxiety

Threats to an individual's physical and psychological safety will cause fear and anxiety. Fear is an affective response to a *real* threat or danger, whereas anxiety is an affective response to a *perceived* threat or danger. Fear is the cognitive appraisal that an actual danger exists in a given situation, and anxiety involves the emotional response to that appraisal (Beck & Emery, 1985). Wolman (1994) further distinguished between fear and anxiety. Fear is a momentary, perceptual, and emotional response to pain, harm, or death. Anxiety is a continuous state of tension with the expectation of disaster. Fear leads to the stress response of "fight or flight" in contrast to anxiety, which reduces one's ability to act. Severe anxiety can cause individuals to feel emotionally paralyzed. It contributes to social isolation, intellectual impairment, and feelings of low self-esteem, irritability, and anger (Wolman). Anxiety also can cause psychosomatic symptoms. It is a state of arousal that can present as specific symptoms ranging from palpitations and shortness of breath (as in acute stress situations) to more diffuse symptoms, such as fatigue, insomnia, and restlessness (as with generalized anxiety disorders [GADs]). Therefore, fear and anxiety affect every system of the body—physiologic, cognitive, emotional, and behavioral (Beck & Emery). The somatic symptoms of anxiety overlap with many of the symptoms of cancer and side effects of treatment; therefore, healthcare professionals must recognize the psychological symptoms of anxiety to make an accurate diagnosis (Noyes et al., 1998).

Anxiety is experienced universally with both positive and negative ramifications (Stein, 2004). Normal anxiety often occurs when individuals face a new obstacle or challenge. For example, going off to college is an exciting yet anxiety-provoking experience. Normal or mild-to-moderate anxiety can motivate people by enhancing learning, problem solving, and attention. Normal anxiety may, therefore, serve an adaptive or "positive" function, preparing individuals physically and psychologically to meet challenges and avoid harm (Beck & Emery, 1985; Stein). As a transient arousal state, normal anxiety may signal coping responses to deal with any outside threat, for example, the diagnosis of cancer (Summerfeldt & Endler, 1996). Severe, sustained anxiety interferes with coping efforts by immobilizing individuals with associated symptoms. In fact, avoidance coping is considered to be a chief behavioral component of clinical anxiety—avoidance being the "negative" dimension of anxiety (Stein; Summerfeldt & Endler).

Although fear and anxiety are differentiated, often they are similar. Individuals experiencing anxiety usually describe a subjective feeling of fear that includes dread and apprehension (Massie, 1989) and impending doom (Noyes et al., 1998). Patients are especially anxious and fearful at the time of initial diagnosis and treatment (Pasacreta et al., 2001). Patients with cancer experience fear when they are confronted with real threats (e.g., a poor prognosis). Anxiety closely follows as patients face the perceived threats most often associated with cancer: pain, disfigurement, and multiple physical and psychosocial losses. Kunkel (1993) pointed out that despite many shared fears, each patient with cancer will experience different levels of anxiety. Anxiety may be a psychological response to the cancer, or the anxiety may be a chronic problem that is intensified by the disease or treatment. If a person has trait anxiety (a personality characteristic), he or she is predisposed to more frequent and intense reactions to stressful events (Gorman, Raines, & Sultan, 2002). In other words, normal anxieties experienced with cancer treatments may be exacerbated if the individual has preexisting trait anxiety. For example, research has shown that patients with trait anxiety are more prone to developing anticipatory nausea and vomiting prior to chemotherapy (Noyes et al.). These normal or expected anxious responses to cancer and treatment include feelings of apprehension, tension, nervousness, and worry. Heightened levels of arousal and anxiety proneness have been associated with the diagnosis of cancer. If individuals have a past coping history of generalized anxiety or a history of an anxiety disorder, such as panic attacks, they may experience more intense anxiety with a cancer diagnosis than the general population. The anxiety observed in patients with cancer has been associated with greater autonomic hyperactivity than those in the general population who suffer from generalized chronic anxiety (Noyes et al.).

Other factors such as prior coping history, emotional stability, social support, symptom distress, and sense of control also will influence how much anxiety individuals experience (Noyes et al., 1998; Pasacreta et al., 2001). In addition, anxiety often is associated with other psychiatric symptoms such as depression and may occur as a component of cancer pain, fatigue, treatment, or metabolic side effects. Severe anxiety reduces the threshold for patients' physical distress, especially pain (Noyes et al.). Finally, anxiety is an affective response to stress, and, according to Selye's (1956) stress theory, the symptoms of anxiety can put wear and tear on the body because of the physical and psychological energy required to support these symptoms. Most importantly, anxiety negatively affects coping (Summerfeldt & Endler, 1996) and may indirectly have a negative effect on immune function (Fawzy, Fawzy, Hyun, & Wheeler, 1997).

Cultural Influences on the Experience and Expression of Anxiety

The health- and illness-related responses and behaviors of patients with cancer develop through lifelong socialization (Helman, 2001). Nursing responses to a patient's expression of anxiety may seem judgmental or accusatory if they are not offered in the context of the individual's sociocultural background (Faysman & Oseguera, 2002). For example, members of the Russian culture generally are not told their diagnosis or prognosis by family members (Evanikoff, 1996). In this culture, by protecting their loved one from the truth, the family members believe that patients will be less burdened by worry, sparing their emotional energy for healing (Evanikoff). Therefore, the normal, expected anxious responses to cancer may be compounded and hidden if these patients are expected to be passive participants in their own care. In cases such as this, nurses must recognize that symptomatic complaints such as weakness, dizziness, palpitation, and tension may be masking an underlying anxiety disorder (Pasacreta et al., 2001).

Expressions of feelings such as anxiety also may go undetected because of communication barriers. Cancer is a very frightening experience, and anxiety may be intensified when patients find themselves unable to express their emotional distress to their caregivers. In addition, language barriers have been found to interfere with patients' ability to integrate the distressing experiences that cancer imposes (Die-Trill, 1998; Faysman & Oseguera, 2002). Emotional expressions of uncertainty, anxiety, and grief vary across cultures. For example, in some cultures, the display of intense emotions may be expected at times such as bereavement, whereas stoic reactions and the development of somatic symptoms may be more appropriate in other groups (Die-Trill). Stoic behavior serves to minimize discomfort and may reflect a cultural value learned and validated throughout one's lifetime (Pasacreta et al., 2001). Patients may feel anxious and worried but hesitate to share these feelings because of embarrassment or shame (Noyes et al., 1998). In contrast, some patients may appear overly angry and raged, intimidating and alienating those around them. Individuals' exaggerated emotional responses may not necessarily be indicative of abnormal behavior but, instead, a cultural norm (Pasacreta et al.). Therefore, emotional and coping responses (i.e., anxiety) must be assessed within the framework of patients' cultural values, attitudes, and normative behaviors. Assessment also should include prior coping history, social support, religious beliefs, and other life stressors. Providing a safe environment for patients to express anxiety within their own perspective of the cancer experience will ensure that they receive the appropriate help.

Classifications of Anxiety Disorders in Patients With Cancer

Adjustment Disorders

Anxiety disorders are the most prevalent group of psychiatric disorders in the United States and are found to be more common in women (Stein, 2004). Anxiety disorders often begin in childhood or adolescence and are characterized by significant comorbidity and chronicity; GAD alone is associated with increased medical-seeking behavior (Stein). The *Diagnostic and Statistical Manual of Mental Disorders (DSM-IV-TR)* (American Psychiatric Association [APA], 2000) contains a number of classifications of anxiety disorders. The most common anxiety disorder requiring psychiatric referral in the cancer population is reactive (situational) anxiety, which is classified in the *DSM-IV-TR* as *adjustment disorder with anxious mood* (Noyes et al., 1998). However, symptoms of anxiety in patients with cancer most often coexist with depression and other mixed states more commonly than anxiety existing alone (Noyes et al.). An adjustment disorder is defined as emotional or behavioral symptoms that occur in response to an identifiable stressor(s) (e.g., cancer, treatment) that develop within three months of the onset of the stressor(s) (APA). The predominant manifestations of anxiety are symptoms such as nervousness, worry, or jitteriness. Again, this diagnosis coexists with depressed mood. Therefore, adjustment disorder with mixed anxiety and depressed mood also encompasses depressive symptoms such as tearfulness and feelings of hopelessness.

The normal fears associated with cancer occur and change along the illness trajectory. Patients commonly feel overwhelmed at the time of diagnosis and at other transition points—onset of treatment, the end of treatment, recurrence, and terminal phases. Even during phases of remission, fears of cancer recurrence may overshadow individuals' psyche. The difference between these normal and expected fears and a diagnosis of adjustment disorder is based on the duration and intensity of symptoms, in addition to the functional impairment caused by the anxiety symptoms. An adjustment disorder has been defined as an intermediary psychological state that falls between normal coping under the stress of cancer and a major mental disorder (Strain, 1998). Clinical indicators for an adjustment disorder come under the realm of maladaptive responses affecting quality-of-life issues (e.g., interference with relationships, work, enjoyment of life's activities) (Strain). An enduring pattern of anxiety can lead to significant clinical distress, thus preventing adaptation, impairing problem solving and coping, and interfering with compliance with cancer treatment.

Preexisting Anxiety Disorders

Different than reactive or situational anxiety, preexisting anxiety disorders can recur and be exacerbated by the cancer diagnosis and treatment. Also, individuals with a history of anxiety (e.g., GAD, panic disorder) may be at a greater risk for appraising the stressor of cancer as more threatening and overwhelming than individuals without such a history (Noyes et al., 1998).

Generalized anxiety disorder: GAD is defined as excessive anxiety and worry regarding events or activities of daily life. Symptoms of GAD include restlessness, fatigue, difficulty concentrating, irritability, tension, and sleep disturbances (APA, 2000). Common to GAD and other preexisting anxiety disorders (e.g., panic disorder, phobias, post-traumatic stress disorder [PTSD]) is the extreme fear of losing control and of being overwhelmed and vulnerable to threatening experiences (Massie & Shakin, 1993). Genetics, temperament, and environment all may play a role in the development of GAD and other anxiety disorders (Hudson & Rapee, 2004). Most often, when asked, adult patients can confirm that anxious behaviors and emotions have been identifiable from an early age or earlier experience (Hudson & Rapee).

Panic disorder: Reactivation of preexisting anxiety disorders may interfere with cancer treatment and overwhelm the coping abilities of the individual. Panic disorder is the sudden and unpredictable attack of intense fear or discomfort, causing individuals to have an overwhelming urge to escape (Noyes et al., 1998). Panic attacks are associated with symptoms that range from trembling, palpitations, shortness of breath, and chest pain to fears of losing control, going crazy, or dying (APA, 2000). These terrifying feelings are abrupt, peak in approximately 10 minutes, and are followed by constant fears of recurring attacks (APA). Exposure to painful or frightening procedures (e.g., bone marrow biopsy) may cause the person to abruptly terminate treatments (Noyes et al.).

Panic disorder with phobia: Panic attacks may occur with agoraphobia (the fear of being in places or situations from which escape may be difficult) or claustrophobia (the fear of being in closed places) (APA, 2000). Agoraphobic patients may have difficulty being in strange hospital environments and treatment rooms; claustrophobic patients may have difficulty with magnetic resonance imaging (MRI) or radiation therapy (Noyes et al., 1998). A past history of phobias may complicate the care of patients with cancer because of the numerous medical procedures that patients must confront, such as receiving injections with a needle, seeing blood, or undergoing other invasive medical procedures. These specific phobias are described in the *DSM-IV-TR* and are termed "blood-injection-injury type" phobias (APA). This subtype is highly familial and is characterized by a strong vasovagal response (e.g., bradycardia, hypotension) to the feared object or treatment (Noyes et al.). Although the individuals recognize that the fear is unreasonable, avoidant behaviors, anxious anticipation, or distress becomes unavoidable (APA).

Post-traumatic stress disorder: PTSD may resurface during or may be a result of distressing or painful cancer treatments (Kunkel, 1993; Noyes et al., 1998). This response of intense fear or horror results from individuals witnessing (e.g., death of a loved one from cancer) or experiencing (e.g., personal injury from a previous cancer treatment) events that involved actual or threatened death or serious injury (APA, 2000). At risk for PTSD are patients with cancer who have survived traumatic experiences such as rape, war, the Holocaust, or natural disasters (Kunkel; Massie & Shakin, 1993). Massie (1989) discussed the possible risks of PTSD in children who have undergone long-term treatments for cancer. Children often face repeated painful procedures (e.g., venipunctures, lumbar punctures) that they experienced with fright or terror. These fears may reemerge if a different stressful event triggers a memory. As children with cancer survive into adulthood, as adults survive cancer, and as chronic illness becomes the norm, the risks of PTSD in these populations will need to be studied further.

Anxiety Disorders Caused by Medical Conditions

The *DSM-IV-TR* classifies anxiety disorders caused by medical factors associated with cancer or treatment separately (APA, 2000). Defined as "anxiety disorder due to a general medical condition," this classification of anxiety is a direct physiologic consequence of a medical disorder (APA). The most common medical problems that place patients with cancer at risk for anxiety include uncontrolled pain, cognitive deficits, central nervous system disorders, medication side effects, and metabolic abnormalities. The most common but preventable cause of anxiety related to cancer is uncontrolled pain (Noyes et al., 1998). Patients experiencing acute pain may exhibit symptoms associated with generalized anxiety (e.g., restlessness, irritability, muscle tension). Chronic pain may contribute to both chronic anxiety and depression. If the pain is unrelenting and severe, anxiety and agitation can lead to dissociative episodes or suicide ideation (Breitbart & Payne, 1998; Kunkel, 1993) (see Chapter 9).

Medications commonly used in the cancer setting also can contribute to symptoms of anxiety. Steroids (e.g., dexamethasone, prednisone) can place patients at risk for psychiatric symptoms that range from anxiousness, irritability, and agitation to psychosis. Steroid-induced anxiety often is difficult to differentiate from adjustment disorder with anxious mood; therefore, nurses must pay close attention to the onset of symptoms related to steroid treatment (Noyes et al., 1998). Antiemetics (e.g., metoclopramide, prochlorperazine) can contribute to motor restlessness (akathisia) several hours to days after chemotherapy treatment (Kunkel, 1993; Noyes et al.). Withdrawal symptoms will precipitate anxiety with the discontinuation of certain drugs such as alcohol, street drugs, narcotics, and anxiolytics. If alcohol is stopped abruptly for illness or hospitalization, some patients may exhibit severe anxiety within the first day (Noyes et al.). Prominent anxiety, panic attacks, obsessions, or compulsive behaviors can predominate this clinical picture of "substance-induced anxiety disorder" (APA, 2000).

Changes in metabolic, hormonal, or cognitive status can cause anxiety in patients with cancer. Abnormal metabolic states that cause anxiety include hypoxia, sepsis, hypoglycemia, hypocalcemia, and undetected bleeding. The most common metabolic change causing anxiety in patients with cancer is hypoxia (Noyes et al., 1998). Hypoxia is a very fearful experience for patients because of the frightening symptoms of restlessness, agitation, and the feeling of being smothered. Pulmonary embolism and coronary occlusion are examples of underlying medical problems that must be ruled out when anxiety appears with hypoxia and chest pain. Anxiety and restlessness often accompany the chills and fever associated with sepsis and may signal early delirium (Noyes et al.). Changes in electrolyte status resulting from endocrine abnormalities (e.g., hypoglycemia) or disease (e.g., metastatic hypercalcemia) cause anxiety, as well as hormone-secreting tumors (e.g., thyroid and parathyroid tumors). Paraneoplastic syndromes associated with certain malignancies (e.g., adrenocorticotropic-producing lung cancer) can cause anxiety, and pheochromocytoma (a rare tumor of the adrenal medulla) has been associated with panic symptoms (Noyes et al.). Patients with pancreatic cancer have been known to manifest symptoms of distress, anxiety, and depression that may be related to a false neurotransmitter released from the tumor (Massie, 1989).

The Response of Healthcare Professionals to Anxious Patients

Anxiety is a highly transferable emotion from patient to professional (Gorman et al., 2002; Pasacreta et al., 2001). Nurses may experience apprehension when caring for patients who are visibly anxious or experiencing panic attacks. If nurses have not had adequate training or experience in dealing with these intense reactions, feelings of inadequacy or fear may surface. Nurses also may experience frustration if constant reassurances and interventions do not appear to calm the patients. In these situations, nurses may have difficulty being consistent and supportive. If patients' anxiety is not controlled, the feelings most likely will surface and be exhibited by family members. Anxious patients and family members may appear to healthcare providers to be too demanding and unreasonable, adding further stress to an already difficult situation. Resentment and hostility may develop if nurses or physicians believe that a patient and his or her family members require more attention than the situation warrants. Finally, anxiety may not be recognized as a priority for nursing care, especially if nurses consider the anxiety to be a weakness or failure of patients to cope adequately. All of the aforementioned situations warrant further support for patients, as well as for the professionals involved in their care. A consultation with the psychiatric clinical nurse specialist could result in more in-depth assessment of patients' situations, in addition to supporting the nurses by helping them to understand and address their own concerns and frustrations.

Nursing Care of Patients Experiencing Anxiety

Assessment

Oncology nurses play a vital role in identifying patients' symptoms of anxiety and implementing appropriate interventions (see Figure 13-1). Assessment of anxiety has been defined as a standard of practice for oncology nursing (Zimberg, 1995). Assessing the "function" or role of anxiety for patients is important. Nurses must distinguish whether the vague, uneasy feelings described as anxiety are normal and expected or negative and disabling (Strain, 1998). The plan of care outlines criteria for assessment and intervention. Initially, patients should be evaluated for normal or expected anxiety symptoms at diagnosis and at stressful transition points along the disease continuum. Initial, early emotional reactions to the cancer experience have proved to be predictive of later adaptation, in addition to identifying patients at high-risk for future psychiatric disorders (Pasacreta et al., 2001). A thorough assessment will begin with patients' health history to determine any preexisting anxiety or related psychiatric disorders. A thorough physical examination must follow to determine whether any medical conditions (e.g., uncontrolled pain) are underlying the symptoms of anxiety. It is not possible to accurately evaluate anxiety unless medical symptoms such as pain have been addressed and controlled (Noyes et al., 1998). Nurses should assess all physical symptoms, emotions, cognitive changes, behavioral responses, and the stage of illness to determine the level of patients' anxiety to differentiate the contributing causes upon which to base interventions.

Physical symptoms: Anxiety affects every system of the body—most dramatically, the cardiovascular and gastrointestinal systems (Noyes et al., 1998). Cardiovascular effects include palpitations and chest pain combined with respiratory symptoms of hyperventilation and dyspnea. Patients experiencing anxiety may describe feelings of suffocation. Common gastrointestinal symptoms include anorexia, nausea, and diarrhea. Others include difficulty swallowing and heartburn. Patients may describe feelings of choking or may complain of vague stomach ailments. Dizziness, weakness, headaches, confusion, and fine tremors are common neurologic symptoms. Fears concerning genitourinary and gynecologic cancers may contribute to symptoms of dyspareunia, dysuria, frigidity, or impotence (Massie, 1989; Noyes et al.). The sympathetic "fight or flight" energy that anxiety demands leaves individuals physically and emotionally exhausted.

Emotional responses: Anxiety is known to intensify the physical symptoms associated with cancer, thereby negatively affecting quality of life (Schreier & Williams, 2004). High levels of anxiety have been found in women undergoing chemotherapy, and decreases in anxiety have not occurred over the course of treatment (Schreier & Williams). Patients experiencing anxiety appear to be tense and worried, and they may complain of feeling nervous. With anxiety disorders, patients' moods may be dominated by unrealistic worries, fears, and helplessness (Nesse, 1996). Patients have described this feeling as "anxious foreboding, or in more severe cases, a sense of impending doom" (Noyes et al., 1998, p. 552). Irritability and fatigue commonly occur and are related to the physiologic energy that anxiety consumes, in addition to difficulties with resting and sleeping. Impaired communication (e.g., rapid, pressured speech; repetitive questioning; silence and withdrawal) is another sign of anxiety (Zimberg, 1995).

Figure 13-1. Plan of Care

Assessment
- Recognize the signs and symptoms of anxiety.
- Validate patients' perceptions of the anxiety experience.
- Assess for anxiety at major transition points along the cancer continuum.
- Differentiate between normal or expected anxiety responses and abnormal responses.
- Assess for previous anxiety disorders (e.g., generalized anxiety disorder [GAD], panic, phobias, post-traumatic stress disorder [PTSD]).
- Assess for underlying medical conditions (e.g., pain, sepsis, medications, cognitive disruptions, metabolic imbalances, hormonal imbalances) that may be contributing to anxiety symptoms.
- Assess for concurrent symptoms of depression.

Nursing Diagnoses (NANDA International, 2005)
- Anxiety
- Ineffective coping
- Disturbed thought processes
- Impaired verbal communication
- Low self-esteem (chronic, situational)

DSM-IV-TR Diagnoses (American Psychiatric Association, 2000)
- Acute stress disorder
- GAD
- Adjustment disorder with anxiety
- Adjustment disorder with mixed anxiety and depressed mood
- Panic disorder (with or without agoraphobia)
- Specific phobia (blood-injection-injury type)
- PTSD
- Anxiety disorder because of general medical condition
- Substance-induced anxiety disorder

Expected Outcomes
- Patients will identify feelings associated with anxiety.
- Patients will identify causative factors for anxiety.
- Patients will problem solve and develop ways to recognize and control anxiety.
- Patients will participate in strategies to relieve anxiety (e.g., relaxation techniques) if appropriate.

Interventions
- Provide a safe, supportive environment.
- Reduce environmental stimuli.
- Educate patients regarding the disease and treatment.
- Inform patients of impending tests and procedures.
- Answer questions, and provide time for patients to reflect.
- Encourage verbalization of fears and anxieties.
- Normalize feelings for patients at each crisis point of the disease continuum.
- Assess present and past coping mechanisms.
- Assist patients to identify anxiety-provoking stimuli and the positive and negative ways to deal with it.
- Teach cognitive-behavioral techniques to decrease anxiety (e.g., relaxation exercises, cognitive reframing).
- Provide positive reinforcement for adaptive coping strategies.
- Administer anxiolytic medications, and educate patients about their purpose and effects.
- Refer patients for psychiatric evaluation, if necessary.
- Provide supportive resources for patients' coping (e.g., refer to support groups).
- Evaluate patients' outcomes, and revise plan of care, when appropriate.

Noncompliance with medical treatment may be another emotional response of anxiety and may cause patients to refuse tests, treatments, or procedures out of fear and apprehension. This warrants psychiatric evaluation (Massie & Shakin, 1993). Assessment for depressive symptoms is important because depression and anxiety commonly occur together in patients with cancer (Noyes et al., 1998; Pasacreta et al., 2001). A clinical indicator that distinguishes between the mood states of depression and anxiety is that depressed patients predominately feel hopeless, whereas anxious patients predominantly feel helpless (Nesse, 1996). Results of one study indicated that nurses' knowledge base of how to adequately assess these two psychosocial responses needs further investigation (Lampic, von Essen, Peterson, Larsson, & Sjoden, 1996). The results demonstrated that staff overestimated patient anxiety and showed limited ability to distinguish among the levels of anxiety and depression that patients were actually experiencing.

Cognitive changes: An anxious patient will have difficulty concentrating and maintaining attention (Zimberg, 1995). Memory may be affected, and the patient may be unable to focus on the conversation or task at hand. Problem-solving abilities may be impaired, which, in turn, may negatively affect coping. An adaptive response to stressful situations requires problem-solving activities to manage and solve the threat (Zeidner & Saklofske, 1996). Hyperactivity, hyper-vigilance, and "scanning" (i.e., jumping from task to task) are symptoms of GAD (Nesse, 1996; Noyes et al., 1998). Cognitive deficits from the disease or treatment also may contribute to anxiety and feelings of helplessness (Kunkel, 1993). Delirium must be ruled out because it can be accompanied by varying levels of anxiety. In fact, confusion and anxiety may be the first symptoms of delirium (Kunkel).

Behavioral responses: Patients experiencing anxiety will demonstrate changes in behaviors such as restlessness, pacing, wringing of hands, and nail biting. Anxiety can be immobilizing and can interfere with patients' ability to perform activities of daily living, solve problems, and interact with others (Zimberg, 1995). Other behavioral responses to the cancer experience may be linked to anxiety. Preexisting anxiety may be a causative factor in patients with anticipatory nausea and vomiting (Noyes et al., 1998). Evaluating other behaviors that may be linked to anxiety are important but often overlooked—risky behaviors and substance abuse are common when individuals try to mitigate the stressor and self-medicate (e.g., smoking, alcoholism, drug abuse). Again, anxious patients must be assessed for signs of withdrawal from these substances or other medications when treatment or hospitalization interferes with self-medication regimens (Kunkel, 1993).

Phase of illness: Different stages along the disease continuum require assessment of anxiety responses that are unique to the demands confronted at that phase of disease and treatment. The stage of diagnosis is one of shock and disbelief, and acute stress reactions are more common at this time. Reactivations of these same feelings have been reported at the time of recurrence, yet with more intensity (Fawzy et al., 1997; Howell, Fitch, & Deane, 2003). Women with ovarian cancer have expressed anticipatory fear and anxiety prior to follow-up appointments, anticipating recurrence (Howell et al.). During the terminal stages of cancer, anxiety is related to existential concerns and is complicated by symptoms such as pain, shortness of breath, and weakness (Massie, 1989; Pasacreta et al., 2001). Anxiety appears to increase with disease progression, and research has shown that overall mental health declines with advanced disease (Noyes et al., 1998). Lastly, anxiety has been described as interpersonally contagious (Pasacreta et al.); therefore, healthcare professionals should not overlook the anxiety experienced by family members. Family caregivers have demonstrated anxiety, uncertainty, and fear, before and after palliative surgery for their loved one with advanced disease (Borneman et al., 2003). If family caregivers do not possess the insight and abilities to meet the physical demands of patients, their levels of anxiety and frustration increase with the burden of care (Given, Given, & Kozachik, 2001).

Differential Diagnosis

In patients experiencing excessive anxiety, factors other than their psychological state must be ruled out first (Pasacreta & McCorkle, 1996). A differential diagnosis must address the possibility of underlying metabolic imbalances, pain, hypoxia, medications, or other medical states contributing to patients' anxious symptoms. The major challenge in diagnosing anxiety or coexisting depression is the overlap of somatic symptoms related to the cancer and treatment and those that are syndromes of these mental disorders (e.g., anorexia, weight loss, restlessness) (Pasacreta et al., 2001). Once nurses have ruled out medical conditions contributing to anxiety (e.g., pain is adequately controlled), then they must address direct psychosocial causes. If anxious behaviors are severe (e.g., patients are immobilized by fear) or interfere with treatment (e.g., noncompliance, avoidant coping), patients should be evaluated for underlying or preexisting anxiety disorders. Differentiating normal or expected anxiety responses from abnormal responses depends upon the intensity, extent, and duration of symptoms (Pasacreta et al.). If abnormal anxiety is suspected, patients must again be asked about a history of chronic fear, phobias, or panic attacks (Zimberg, 1995). Specific questions should address patients' subjective feelings and fears. Examples include, "What are the sensations you feel when you begin your chemotherapy treatment?" and "What particular situations in the past made you feel that the world was closing in on you?"

Interventions

The first step in the management of anxiety is to determine its exact cause. A thorough assessment can provide the necessary information for identifying causative factors, the duration and intensity of symptoms, and the resources needed to assist the patient. Interventions often are grouped into psychotherapeutic or pharmacologic but may be most effective when used simultaneously. If individuals are immobilized by anxiety, then pharmacologic intervention may be used to manage the physiologic symptoms, enabling patients to have the physical and emotional energy to focus on the beneficial psychotherapeutic interventions. For example, the use of anxiolytic medications may help to control ruminating thoughts and worries—enough to assist patients to work through fears and anxieties in psychotherapy, thus providing more permanent control over long-standing anxiety (Pasacreta & McCorkle, 1996). Different types of interventions may be beneficial at different transition points across the disease continuum. Psychoeducational approaches have proved to be beneficial at the time of diagnosis (Fawzy, Fawzy, Arndt, & Pasnau, 1995), and palliative, psychotherapeutic interventions are most beneficial at the end of life (Pasacreta et al., 2001). Nurses are in a key position to assess patients for anxiety, provide evidence-based interventions, and refer patients, if necessary, to the appropriate resource.

The primary physician should be notified if an underlying medical cause needs to be ruled out. If symptoms are severe enough to require psychotherapy or medication management, a psychiatric referral is warranted.

Psychotherapeutic interventions: The focus of a nondrug treatment of anxiety is providing cognitive and behavioral interventions intended to help patients to develop the skills needed to cope effectively with anxiety. The types of psychotherapeutic interventions studied have included behavioral training, education, individual psychotherapy, and group therapy support (Fawzy et al., 1995; Noyes et al., 1998), yet little research has addressed the influence of specific interventions and changes in anxiety levels (Noyes et al.). Danton, Altrocchi, Antonuccio, and Basta (1994) have created a framework outlining the components of psychotherapeutic interventions. Cognitive interventions begin with *cognitive restructuring* (Beck & Emery, 1985). This is the process of helping patients to understand how thought processes (e.g., constant worrying) can negatively influence mood. Interventions can teach patients how to take control over their worries. This includes initiating behaviors such as keeping a diary of daily concerns, setting aside a time each day to worry, and sharing concerns with supportive people for validation. These interventions will help patients to gain insight into the relationship between thinking and feeling. Working on changing negative thought patterns helps patients to regain a feeling of control over what is causing them anxiety and helps them to differentiate between realistic and unrealistic fears.

Another major component of psychotherapeutic interventions includes relaxation techniques—including progressive relaxation—breathing exercises, guided imagery, music, yoga, biofeedback, and meditation. The effectiveness of these distraction techniques in directly decreasing anxiety responses demands further study, but they have shown promise for managing procedural pain, chemotherapy-related nausea and vomiting, and specific phobias (Noyes et al., 1998). A regular exercise regimen can provide relaxation, stress reduction, and a time for cognitive restructuring. In severe cases of anxiety that involve phobias and panic, patients may find desensitization techniques to be useful. The goal is for patients to remain relaxed when confronted with the feared stimuli or thoughts of the feared stimuli (Danton et al., 1994). Finally, psychotherapy can be accomplished using a variety of methods: a short-term psychoeducational format (e.g., American Cancer Society's "I Can Cope" classes), support groups (e.g., Wellness Community®), and individual therapy of longer duration if patients have a past history of psychiatric problems or earlier trauma. Concurrent use of an anti-anxiety agent to support patients until cognitive and behavioral changes are learned may enhance any of these interventions.

Pharmacologic interventions: Short-acting anxiolytic medications are the drugs of choice for treating anxiety in patients with cancer. The most commonly used drugs are those of the benzodiazepine group, which includes alprazolam, lorazepam, and clonazepam. All are useful for treating short-term anxiety related to cancer treatment, as well as ongoing generalized anxiety and panic disorders. Because of their short half-life, alprazolam and lorazepam are the preferred drugs for older patients (Pasacreta & McCorkle, 1996). They also are useful for their sedative and muscle-relaxing effects and are effective in treating insomnia. The potentially beneficial side effect of transient amnesia with lorazepam has been a reason why this drug has been included to treat anxiety in prechemotherapy regimens or prior to anxiety-producing treatments (e.g., claustrophobia related to MRI). Lorazepam can help patients to forget other unpleasant experiences, such as nausea and vomiting, an important intervention for any patients with a prior history of trait anxiety (Noyes et al., 1998). Lorazepam has another benefit for anxious patients undergoing cancer treatment—it is available parenterally and patients can premedicate to mitigate apprehension prior to treatments. A cautionary side effect of these short-acting benzodiazepines is rebound anxiety between doses (Massie & Shakin, 1993). Patients who exhibit rebound anxiety may benefit from being switched to a longer-acting benzodiazepine (e.g., diazepam). Another caution with benzodiazepines is the possibility of respiratory depression. Patients with pulmonary disease or lung metastasis may benefit from an antihistamine instead (Massie & Lesko, 1989). The choice and dosage of anxiolytic medication must be made in accordance with patients' medical history (e.g., liver and cardiopulmonary function), age, symptoms, and goal of treatment.

Other classifications of drugs have been found to be clinically useful in treating anxiety. A drug that is beneficial in treating chronic anxiety and phobia is buspirone. Because of its nonaddictive quality, buspirone is beneficial for chronic anxiety, but it may take two to three weeks to become effective (Kunkel, 1993). Other advantages of buspirone include its lack of sedative effects, its limited effect on liver disease, and its lack of effect on cognition (Pasacreta et al., 2001). Tricyclic antidepressants have more sedative effects and have been used to treat anxiety-related insomnia and depression. A common example is amitriptyline. The antipsychotic drug chlorpromazine has more sedating effects. Antihistamines, such as diphenhydramine, have been used for their calming effects and to relieve the akathisia associated with phenothiazines used as antiemetics (Massie & Lesko, 1989). Combining a medication with sedative effects with the analgesic may relieve anxiety associated with painful procedures (Massie & Lesko). An example is hydroxyzine and fentanyl. For patients who present with mixed symptoms of anxiety and depression, an antidepressant with sedative effects may be the treatment of choice (Massie & Lesko). Many of the tricyclic antidepressants (e.g., imipramine) and the selective serotonin reuptake inhibitors (e.g., paroxetine) have sedative effects for treating the anxiety component of depression and appear to be well tolerated by patients (Noyes et al., 1998).

A major concern involved in pharmacologic management is using appropriate medication(s) to treat the correct symptom, and all agents must be monitored for effectiveness and side effects (Pasacreta et al., 2001). At times, patients with cancer may appear agitated or restless because of underlying medical problems, including pain, nausea, or dyspnea. Careful assessment is needed to ensure that the correct medication is being used to treat the appropriate symptom and that the underlying medical problem is being addressed. For example, if pain is controlled adequately with round-the-clock administration, anxiety symptoms should diminish if pain is the causative factor. In addition, pharmacologic management of anxiety often is underutilized or prescribed doses are too low because of fears of addiction. These fears generally are unwarranted in the cancer population, and patients most often discontinue the use of these medications when symptoms abate (Kunkel, 1993). Other concerns of pharmacologic treatment include unwanted side effects such as sedation and cognitive impairment, requiring cautionary use in older adults. Finally, when discontinued, these drugs must be tapered on a schedule to avoid withdrawal symptoms or rebound anxiety (Kunkel).

Case Study

Becky is a 38-year-old woman diagnosed with breast cancer two years prior to readmission to the hospital for evaluation of brain metastases. Originally, Becky had been treated with lumpectomy, chemotherapy, and radiation. She had enjoyed disease-free remission until one month ago, when she awoke one morning with partial paralysis of the left side of her face. Magnetic resonance imaging (MRI) revealed multiple metastatic foci throughout her cranium, and computerized axial tomography revealed spinal metastases in the lumbar area and one metastatic site in the left lung.

Prior to assessing the patient, the nurse took steps to review Becky's medical record to gain an understanding of her experiences with the illness. Until the day when she awoke with facial paralysis, Becky had coped relatively well with her surgery and treatments. Prior to her initial diagnosis, she had a history of generalized anxiety that had been treated with intermittent psychotherapy during stressful points in her life. At these times, she described feelings of anxiety when trying to juggle her career as a journalist with her two young children, husband, and housekeeping demands. During her chemotherapy and radiation treatments, Becky required anxiolytic medications to help to control symptoms of worry, insomnia, and irritability. When treatment ended, the symptoms abated, and medication support was discontinued without problems. Although Becky had never identified specific instances of panic attacks or phobias, she was claustrophobic and avoided closed-in spaces such as elevators. At the time of her initial workup and with the recent recurrence, lorazepam was administered prior to each MRI.

During this hospitalization, the nurse observed visual signs of anxiety. Becky appeared to be tense, worried, and somewhat tearful. As she sat on her hospital bed, she fidgeted and wrung her hands. As the nurse tried to take Becky's history, she noticed that Becky had difficulty concentrating and at times appeared to have fleeting thoughts. Assessment was complicated because Becky's speech was slurred slightly because of the brain metastases and subsequent cranial irradiation. The nurse was sensitive to Becky's anxious mood and intervened by communicating in a caring and supportive manner. The nursing assessment revealed that Becky had fears regarding the extent of metastatic disease and questioned whether treatment options were available to her. Her children were 8 and 10 years old, and she had feelings of guilt that her children and husband had to endure her illness. Becky's mother had died of breast cancer, so she related feelings of anguish and fear that her experiences would be similar. Becky's husband remained close to his wife during the examination and reassured her of his presence. After the examination, the nurse assisted Becky in getting comfortable in her room and closed the door for privacy. She explained to Becky that she would report the results of the history and examination to the physician and return with him on rounds within a half-hour.

Discussion

This case demonstrates the effectiveness of competent nursing assessment. The nurse recognized the signs of Becky's anxiety and immediately focused her

(Continued on next page)

Case Study *(Continued)*

interventions on reducing the patient's symptoms. She performed her assessment in an unhurried manner and validated the patient's perceptions of her experience and fears. Before leaving Becky, the nurse quieted the environment and gave her specific information on when she would return after speaking with the doctor. Prior to consulting with the primary physician, the nurse organized a plan of care for Becky to meet her specific needs as identified by her past medical history and her current status. First, the nurse was able to determine that this was a critical transition point along the cancer continuum for this patient. Normal anxiety responses are expected at transition points such as recurrence and terminal phases. Many fears surface, particularly existential issues, concerning prognosis and mortality. With Becky, these expected fears may be compounded by her past history of generalized anxiety and her painful experiences with her mother, who also died of breast cancer. The nurse's physical exam determined that cognitive changes caused by the brain metastases and radiation might have been affecting Becky's communication and thought patterns. The patient complained of pain in her lower back and left leg, which was another medical factor assessed by the nurse as influencing anxiety. The nursing diagnoses included anxiety related to the disease, the patient's perception of helplessness, and the possibility of ineffective individual coping.

Assessment and consultation with the physician confirmed the nurse's findings. A multidisciplinary treatment plan was set in motion. Becky would be started on an anxiolytic agent on a continuous basis, and additional medication support would be provided if treatments that may have heightened her anxiety were necessary (e.g., MRIs). Continued evaluation of Becky's anxiety would be necessary in addition to ongoing assessment for signs of depression. Pain medication and physical therapy were initiated to treat the symptoms of lower back and leg discomfort. The team recognized Becky's special emotional needs: two small children, a husband, career and household demands, and underlying fears related to the experience with her mother. The nursing staff responded to Becky's needs by creating a structured, safe environment and by providing emotional support and reassurance as part of their interventions. The psychiatric advanced practice nurse was contacted to teach Becky relaxation, breathing, and imagery techniques, and social service was contacted to provide additional support. The multidisciplinary team began to work on referrals that would be in place to help both Becky and her family as they faced the challenges ahead. The nurse's role proved to be pivotal in the ongoing assessment and treatment plan of this patient.

Conclusion

Anxiety is a normal response that appears at different transition points along the cancer trajectory. Although the experience of anxiety is a normal reaction to the threat of cancer, it is an uncomfortable and distressing emotion for most patients. For those patients at high-risk, anxiety can become overwhelming and disabling—even pathologic. Limited clinical research exists describing the anxiety response to cancer set apart from studies investigating overall psychological distress (Noyes et al., 1998). Therefore, interventions aimed at reducing patient anxiety generally have been grouped within programs for overall psychosocial support (Fawzy et al., 1995, 1997; Noyes et al.). The defining characteristics of anxiety disorders have been outlined in this chapter along with APA (2000) and NANDA International (2005) diagnostic criteria. Oncology nurses are in key positions to assess patients' anxiety, implement and test for evidence-based interventions, and evaluate effective outcomes. Validation of anxiety in patients with cancer and testing of interventions require future research to support evidence-based practice.

Intervention programs aimed at reducing levels of distress and anxiety and programs developed to support coping require further investigation in controlled clinical trials (Fawzy et al., 1997; Wells, McQuellon, Hinkle, & Cruz, 1995). Inherent in these programs are strategies for psychological support and education—major components of psychosocial oncology nursing. Standards of practice and outcome criteria exist to guide oncology nurses in the treatment of patient anxiety and call upon nursing to identify its role in providing effective anxiety interventions needed to enhance the coping and adaptation of patients with cancer.

References

American Psychiatric Association. (2000). *Diagnostic and statistical manual of mental disorders* (4th ed., text rev.). Washington, DC: Author.

Beck, A.T., & Emery, G. (1985). *Anxiety disorders and phobias: A cognitive perspective.* New York: Basic Books.

Borneman, T., Chu, D.Z.J., Wagman, L., Ferrell, B., Juarez, G., McCahill, L.E., et al. (2003). Concerns of family caregivers of patients with cancer facing palliative surgery for advanced malignancies. *Oncology Nursing Forum, 30,* 997–1005.

Breitbart, W., & Payne, D.K. (1998). Pain. In J.C. Holland (Ed.), *Psycho-oncology* (pp. 450–467). New York: Oxford University Press.

Danton, W.G., Altrocchi, J., Antonuccio, D., & Basta, R. (1994). Nondrug treatment of anxiety. *American Family Physician, 49*(10), 161–166.

Die-Trill, M. (1998). The patient from a different culture. In J.C. Holland (Ed.), *Psycho-oncology* (pp. 857–866). New York: Oxford University Press.

Evanikoff, L.J. (1996). Russians. In J.G. Lipson, S.L. Dibble, & P.A. Minarik (Eds.), *Culture and nursing care: A pocket guide* (pp. 239–249). San Francisco: University of California, San Francisco Nursing Press.

Fawzy, F.I., Fawzy, N.W., Arndt, L.A., & Pasnau, R.O. (1995). Critical review of psychosocial interventions in cancer care. *Archives of General Psychiatry, 52,* 100–112.

Fawzy, F.I., Fawzy, N.W., Hyun, C.S., & Wheeler, J.G. (1997). Brief, coping-oriented therapy for patients with malignant melanoma. In J.L. Spira (Ed.), *Group therapy for medically ill patients* (pp. 133–163). New York: Guilford Press.

Faysman, K., & Oseguera, D. (2002). Cultural dimensions of anxiety and truth telling. *Oncology Nursing Forum, 29,* 757–759.

Given, B.A., Given, C.W., & Kozachik, S. (2001). Family support in advanced cancer. *CA: A Cancer Journal for Clinicians, 51,* 213–231.

Gorman, L.M., Raines, M.L., & Sultan, D.F. (2002). *Psychosocial nursing for general patient care* (2nd ed.). Philadelphia: F.A. Davis.

Helman, C.G. (2001). *Culture, health and illness* (4th ed.). New York: Oxford University Press.

Howell, D., Fitch, M.I., & Deane, K.A. (2003). Women's experiences with recurrent ovarian cancer. *Cancer Nursing, 26,* 10–17.

Hudson, J.L., & Rapee, R.M. (2004). From anxious temperament to disorder. In R.G. Heimburg, C.L. Turk, & D.S. Mennin (Eds.), *Generalized anxiety disorder: Advances in research and practice* (pp. 51–74). New York: Guilford Press.

Kunkel, E.J. (1993). The assessment and management of anxiety in the patient with cancer. In T.L. Thompson (Ed.), *Medical-surgical psychiatry: Treating psychiatric aspects of physical disorders* (pp. 61–69). San Francisco: Jossey-Bass.

Lampic, C., von Essen, L., Peterson, V.W., Larsson, G., & Sjoden, P. (1996). Anxiety and depression in hospitalized patients with cancer: Agreement in patient-staff dyads. *Cancer Nursing, 19,* 419–428.

Massie, M.J. (1989). Anxiety, panic, and phobias. In J.C. Holland & J.H. Rowland (Eds.), *Handbook of psychooncology: Psychological care of the patient with cancer* (pp. 300–309). New York: Oxford University Press.

Massie, M.J., & Lesko, L.M. (1989). In J.C. Holland & J.H. Rowland (Eds.), *Handbook of psychooncology: Psychological care of the patient with cancer* (pp. 470–491). New York: Oxford University Press.

Massie, M.J., & Shakin, E.J. (1993). Management of depression and anxiety in cancer patients. In W. Breitbart & J.C. Holland (Eds.), *Psychiatric aspects of symptom management in cancer patients* (pp. 1–21). Washington, DC: American Psychiatric Press.

NANDA International. (2005). *NANDA nursing diagnoses: Definitions and classification, 2005–2006.* Philadelphia: Author.

Nesse, R.E. (1996). Feeling hopeless and helpless: When anxiety symptoms coexist with depressive disorder. *Postgraduate Medicine, 100*(2), 163–177.

Noyes, R., Holt, C.S., & Massie, M.J. (1998). Anxiety disorders. In J.C. Holland (Ed.), *Psycho-oncology* (pp. 548–563). New York: Oxford University Press.

Pasacreta, J., & McCorkle, R. (1996). Psychosocial aspects of cancer. In R. McCorkle, M. Grant, M. Frank-Stromborg, & S. Baird (Eds.), *Cancer nursing: A comprehensive textbook* (2nd ed., pp. 1074–1090). Philadelphia: Saunders.

Pasacreta, J.V., Minarik, P.A., & Nield-Anderson, L. (2001). Anxiety and depression. In B.R. Ferrell & N. Coyle (Eds.), *Textbook of palliative nursing* (pp. 269–289). New York: Oxford University Press.

Schreier, A.M., & Williams, S.A. (2004). Anxiety and quality of life of women who receive radiation or chemotherapy for breast cancer. *Oncology Nursing Forum, 31,* 127–130.

Selye, H. (1956). *The stress of life.* New York: McGraw-Hill.

Stein, D.J. (2004). *Clinical manual of anxiety disorders.* Washington, DC: American Psychiatric Publishing.

Strain, J.J. (1998). Adjustment disorders. In J.C. Holland (Ed.), *Psycho-oncology* (pp. 509–517). New York: Oxford University Press.

Summerfeldt, L.J., & Endler, N.S. (1996). Coping with emotion and psychopathology. In M. Zeidner & N.S. Endler (Eds.), *Handbook of coping: Theory, research, applications* (pp. 602–639). New York: John Wiley.

Wells, M.E., McQuellon, R.P., Hinkle, J.S., & Cruz, J.M. (1995). Reducing anxiety in newly diagnosed cancer patients. *Cancer Practice, 3,* 100–104.

Wolman, B.B. (1994). Defining anxiety. In B.B. Wolman & G. Stricker (Eds.), *Anxiety and related disorders: A handbook* (pp. 3–10). New York: John Wiley.

Zeidner, M., & Saklofske, D. (1996). Adaptive and maladaptive coping. In M. Zeidner & N.S. Endler (Eds.), *Handbook of coping: Theory, research, applications* (pp. 505–531). New York: John Wiley.

Zimberg, M. (1995). *Psychosocial standards of oncology nursing practice.* New York: Memorial Sloan-Kettering Cancer Center.

CHAPTER 14

Anger and Cancer

ASHBY C. WATSON, APRN, BC, OCN®

It is easy to fly into a passion—anybody can do that—but to be angry with the right person to the right extent and at the right time and with the right object and in the right way—that is not easy, and it is not everyone who can do it.

—Aristotle

Every human being has the capacity to feel and express anger. Anger can be viewed as an emotional response to provocation that has identifiable autonomic, central, and cognitive components. The emotion of anger often is confused with other constructs, particularly those of hostility and aggression, but each has its own distinct characteristics. Anger is "an emotion ranging in intensity from irritation to rage, usually in response to perceived mistreatment or provocation . . . and can be seen as both an emotional state and an enduring personality trait" (Smith, 1992, p. 139). Aggression is a behavioral construct and is an "attacking, destructive, or hurtful action" (Smith, p. 139). Hostility is "a set of negative attitudes, beliefs, and appraisals concerning others . . . and connotes a view of others as frequent and likely sources of mistreatment, frustration, and provocation" (Smith, p. 139). Anger also can be defined as "a strong, uncomfortable, emotional response to a provocation that is unwanted and incongruent with one's values, rights, or beliefs" (Thomas, 1998b, p. 61). The Chinese word for anger is *sheng ch'I*—also the word for energy.

Theories on Anger

Many theories exist about the nature of anger. These include psychoanalytic, behavioral, sociocultural, humanistic, and neurobiologic theories (Thomas, 1990).

Although many theories about anger and its management exist, few empirical studies have been done to support them.

Psychoanalytic Theory

According to psychoanalytic theory, anger is a powerful emotion or drive. Under the tenets of this theory, thwarting of drives is considered to be unhealthy. Therefore, to maintain psychological health, one should discharge angry feelings. It is thought that if anger is held in and turned inward toward the ego, feelings of guilt and depression and perhaps suicide may develop.

Behavioral Theory

Behavioral theorists believe that anger occurs when a goal is blocked (e.g., the frustration-aggression hypothesis). Classic behavioral learning theory holds that anger is a learned response to environmental stimuli. Social learning theorists have demonstrated that children can learn to be aggressive by imitating models and will repeat aggressive behaviors that bring them rewards. Novaco (1976, 1977), however, pointed out that frustration does not necessarily produce aggression. He emphasized the importance of cognitive appraisal as a central mediating factor in anger arousal. Others have stated that an individual's reaction depends on the nature of the provocation, the situational constraints, and the individual's preferred style of coping (Anderson-Malico, 1994). In other words, the same stimuli in different situations and under different conditions in different individuals could cause emotional reactions other than anger.

Cognitive behavioral therapists have suggested that anger, like all emotions, is created by the individual's cognition: "Before you can feel irritated by any event, you must first become aware of what is occurring and come to your own interpretation of it. Your feelings result from the meaning you give to the event, not from the event itself" (Burns, 1980, p. 140). Burns asserted that anger ultimately is caused by a belief that someone is acting unfairly or some event is unjust.

Sociocultural Theory

This perspective focuses on the context of anger, which includes the following variables: the interpersonal relationships between the parties, the level of perceived justice or injustice of the situation, social status and gender of the parties, the nature of the environment, and the specific values and beliefs of the sociocultural group. The nature of angry behavior must be studied within the context of the social event and cannot be separated from the cultural experience.

Humanistic Theory

This theory postulates that the discharge of one's affect, or overt emotion, becomes a motivational tool for interpersonal change. Anger is not learned, and it is not seen as an instinct or drive. When one does not discharge anger or other strong emotions, mental distress and perhaps mental illness can result. Therapists must facilitate individuals' expressions of feelings. More recently, practitioners have begun to actively emphasize the importance of experiencing emotion with a focus on the "here and now" (Goldfried, Raue, & Castonguay, 1998; Spira & Reed, 2003; Wiser & Goldfried, 1998). Limited empirical evidence exists on the effectiveness of this theory on the control of anger display.

Neurobiologic Theory

Evidence has shown that certain neurochemical and neurostructural abnormalities in the brain modulate impulsive aggression. The hippocampus is the brain's memory center, and the amygdala mediates basic drives of memory, emotion, and aggression. The frontal lobe of the brain, primarily the prefrontal cortex, modulates aggression. Research has implicated neurochemical and structural dysfunction of these structures and their neurotransmitters in impaired judgment, poor decision making, inappropriate conduct, personality changes, and aggressive outbursts (Linnoila & Charney, 1999).

Actual physical changes have been found in the brains of those who are impulsively aggressive. Neurochemical mediation of aggression is carried out by the neurotransmitters serotonin, dopamine, norepinephrine, Gamma-aminobutyric acid (GABA) and acetylcholine. Other substances are thought to influence aggressive behavior, including steroids, glucose, and neuropeptides. Increasingly, genetic factors are thought to play a role in aggression. Rapid advances in knowledge about the brain and its function likely will revolutionize future treatment approaches toward anger management.

Expression of Anger

Anger can be displayed on a continuum from mild annoyance to extreme rage. Physiologic arousal of the sympathetic division of the autonomic nervous system can lead to a number of bodily responses in those who are angry, including increased blood pressure, elevated pulse rate and body temperature, clenched jaw, tense muscles, gastrointestinal disturbances, and sweating. Patients with cancer may display anger in both overt and covert ways (see Figure 14-1).

Constructive and Destructive Anger in Those Experiencing Cancer

The expression of anger as a constructive mechanism can be helpful to patients with cancer. Those who act assertively may receive better medical care as a direct result of the behavior. Taking control can promote a feeling of empowerment, thus increasing a sense of personal control while reducing feelings of helplessness and hopelessness. Anger also can be expressed destructively, through various indirect expressions of anger (e.g., suppression, displacement, passive-aggression, denial, repression) and through expressions of anger that are not proportionate to the event. These behaviors may alienate others, further isolating patients and families from those who care for them (Tavris, 1989).

Handling anger appropriately is an interpersonal skill that can be developed. Being assertive, speaking out, setting boundaries, and standing up for one's rights

---

Figure 14-1. Expression of Anger

Overt Behavior	**Covert Behavior**
• Verbally abuses others	• Is silent, moody, withdrawn
• Criticizes; displays hostility	• Acts bitter, apathetic
• Explodes with little or no provocation	• Asks loaded questions
• Intimidates; threatens	• Attempts to control everything
• Curses; calls others names	• Refuses to see visitors, eat, or drink
• Strikes or throws objects	• Repeatedly breaks institutional rules
• Is sarcastic, demanding	• Is overly nice
• Is frequently irritated or annoyed	• Displays indecisiveness or ambivalence; procrastinates
• Has defensive/aggressive body language (tense, clenched fists)	• Detaches emotionally from others
	• "Forgets" to do important things

---

and needs without hurting others are constructive uses of anger (Fein, 1993). The question is not *whether* to express anger but *how* to use it as a resource. Expressing anger is not the same as acting aggressively. According to many experts, the healthiest solution to anger is to acknowledge its presence, experience the sensations in the body (e.g., tense muscles, warm feelings), and verbalize the feelings (Burns, 1980). A degree of anger that is directed toward achieving a goal may facilitate patients in dealing successfully with the complexity of cancer treatments, the pain of the disease, the loss of body image, and the disruption in their lives (Fein).

The Influence of Anger on Cancer

The effect of personality and stress on the development of cancer is unclear, but some studies have indicated that preexisting personality traits and the lack of emotional expression, particularly that of anger, may interact with biologic and environmental factors to promote the development of cancer, influence its progression, and affect survival outcomes.

At 10-year follow up in a Yugoslavian study that assessed anger, depression, anxiety, and emotionality in subjects, the researchers demonstrated a 78% success rate in predicting cancer based on "antiemotionality," which included denial of feelings and need for harmony. The incidence of cancer was 40 times greater among those scoring high on antiemotionality (Grossarth-Maticek, Bastiaans, & Kanazir, 1985).

In a classic study of medical students, those who later developed cancer had demonstrated the lowest anger, anxiety, and depression scores when compared with those who developed hypertension, heart attack, or mental illness or who committed suicide (Thomas, 1988). Researchers have described a "type C" personality characterized by passive coping, pleasant and self-sacrificing demeanor, and a marked inability to express emotion, especially fear and anger (Temoshok, 1985; Temoshok & Dreher, 1994). This behavior was labeled as a lifelong repressive coping style. In following subjects longitudinally, they found that people who lived longer were those who were in touch with their feelings and were able to express them.

Much of the psychosocial research in cancer has been carried out in the breast cancer population, where investigators have explored relationships among anger expression, coping styles, and survival outcomes. One study involving patients whose breast cancer had progressed indicated that individuals who experienced feelings of anger and used active coping styles survived longer than those who experienced feelings of helplessness and depression (Levy, 1984). Garrison (1995) performed a qualitative study of women with breast cancer and compared their responses to those of women with cardiovascular disease. The patients with cancer more often reported that they held in, hid, or "forgot" their anger, and its expression did not bring them relief. Also, women with breast cancer who were able to openly express their anger lived longer than those who did not (Derogatis, Abeloff, & Melisaratos, 1979).

Researchers were able to distinguish differences between benign and malignant breast disease in women according to how they handled their emotions (Greer & Morris, 1975; Morris, Greer, Pettingale, & Watson, 1981). Those women who suppressed their anger, the "extreme suppressors," had displayed anger only one or two times in their lives. The "extreme expressors" displayed frequent temper outbursts. Both groups had higher rates of diagnosed breast cancer than women with more moderate emotional behavior. They determined that a "fighting spirit" was important in taking control of one's life while experiencing cancer. Spiegel, Bloom, Kraemer, and Gottheil (1989) found that women with metastatic breast cancer who received supportive-expressive group therapy and who were able to express strong emotions lived twice as long as those in the control group. Survival rates were in direct proportion to the number of sessions attended.

Women with recurrent breast cancer who demonstrated low chronic anxiety scores and high emotional constraint scores experienced the highest mortality. Those women who demonstrated higher chronic anxiety scores, with or without higher constraint, also experienced earlier deaths (Weihs, Enright, Simmens, & Reiss, 2000). Lindop and Cannon (2001) studied the responses of women with breast cancer who identified self-assessed support needs and found that responses to statements of need varied among respondents. However, all respondents labeled coping with feelings of anger and dealing with the question "Why me?" as only moderately important to them. The authors surmised that either respondents had already moved on in their process of adaptation and these issues were no longer important to them or that taking a positive attitude toward one's illness would not allow one to dwell on negative emotions that might impede recovery. Harburg, Julius, Kaciroti, Gleiberman, and Schork (2003) noted that the number of stressful life events did not predict vulnerability to developing breast cancer or survival from it. Instead, the interaction among stress, the individual's personality, and available psychosocial support was the most important factor.

In a meta-analysis of 46 studies, McKenna, Zevon, Corn, and Rounds (1999) found only a modest association between specific psychosocial factors (anxiety-depression, denial/repression coping, childhood family environment, stressful life events, and separation/loss) and development of breast cancer. The most significant effects were found for denial/repression coping, separation/loss experiences, and stressful life events. They noted that only 10 of the 46 studies measured the expression of anger. They expressed concern about the generalizability of the data because a variety of anger measurement tools were used, some with little or no validity or reliability data. The authors concluded that stress and personality factors do not greatly influence the development of breast cancer.

Butow et al. (2000) reviewed empirical evidence for a relationship between psychosocial factors and breast cancer development. They found few well-designed studies that explored the association between life events and breast cancer. They found that anger suppression is a predictor of cancer risk, with the strongest evidence suggesting that younger women are at increased risk. Also, rationality/antiemotionality predicts cancer risk, but social support, chronic anxiety, and presence of depression do not affect breast cancer development. The authors concluded that emotional repression and severe life events were the strongest predictors in the development of breast cancer.

Butow, Coates, and Dunn (1999) found that patients with melanoma who exhibited greater levels of anger about their situation survived longer. In another study, women who suppressed anger in response to hypothetical unfair anger-provoking situations were more likely to experience early mortality from medical illnesses, including cardiovascular disease and cancer, when compared to nonsuppressors. However, men who expressed their anger were more likely to die earlier of cancer than suppressors (Harburg et al., 2003). Comparisons of patients with colorectal cancer with matched disease-free individuals found that patients with cancer had experienced significant childhood loss and unhappiness, avoided conflict, and did not express negative emotions (Kune, Kune, Watson, & Bahnson, 1991). Men with recurrent prostate cancer experienced greater difficulty than those without recurrent disease: twice as many men with recurrent disease experienced problems with anger (Fitch, Gray, Franssen, & Johnson, 2000). The authors suggested that nurses should target interventions toward this at-risk population.

Thomas et al. (2000) reviewed Profile of Mood States (POMS) scores of patients with cancer and compared them with scores for college students and outpatients with psychiatric disorders. The POMS is a widely used, reliable, and valid instrument in cancer populations. The researchers found that patients with cancer had lower anger scores than both control groups and indicated there was no explanation for low POMS anger scores in patients with cancer.

Recommendations for Future Research

Provocative evidence exists about the connection between anger and cancer. However, a dearth of reliable and valid studies on this topic. Future research on anger and cancer should focus on developing well-designed prospective qualitative and quantitative longitudinal studies that are undertaken in patients with a wide variety of cancer diagnoses. Anger assessment tools that can be easily used in the clinical environment need to be developed and tested. Individual anger management styles should be identified and correlated with outcomes. Anger should be studied in many cultural groups. Hispanic, African American, and Asian American populations currently are underrepresented in studies on anger. Study of the impact of support groups on patient outcomes should continue.

Anger as a Response to Cancer

Patients and family members may experience anger and distress at many points along the cancer continuum, and nurses should be prepared to assist families through these difficult times (Loscalzo & BrintzenhofeSzoc, 1998).

Integrating the Diagnosis

After the initial shock and disbelief, anger is the emotion that most patients exhibit at the time of diagnosis (Thomas et al., 2000). The diagnosis of cancer frequently disrupts one's belief in a fair and safe world, and people often express the subsequent disorientation and confusion as anger. Some people believe that if they have led a good life, behaved morally, and followed "the rules," they should be protected from the harm of life-threatening illness. Patients may strongly feel that it is unfair that they are sick. "Why me?" and "How did I get it?" are difficult questions to answer. Healthcare providers may attempt to answer these questions, but the existential issues of responsibility, guilt, punishment, and atonement need to be addressed at a deeper and more spiritual level. The values and beliefs of individuals and families about these issues can affect subsequent acceptance of the diagnosis and agreement to participate in the prescribed treatment program. Finding and integrating a new self-image that includes catastrophic illness is a task that patients with cancer must address.

Receiving a diagnosis of cancer is a trigger that may rekindle old feelings of sadness, loss, unfairness, and, sometimes, anger. Patients' perceptions of how they are being "mistreated" by healthcare professionals may parallel and reflect how they were mistreated as children (Kübler-Ross, 1969). Unresolved feelings of loss and unfairness may escalate into overt expressions of anger displaced onto people who are perceived as being healthy, including family members, friends, and coworkers. Feelings of unworthiness, guilt, or shame can lead to anger toward the self that manifests itself as depression. Holding on to feelings of unfairness may impede the process of mourning the losses associated with cancer. If these feelings are not resolved, they may manifest as ongoing dissatisfaction and anger with everything surrounding the illness, including the nursing care being received. If people involved with a patient do not understand the origin of the anger, they may react to it personally and begin to reject the patient even more, thus reinforcing the patient's experience of rejection and unfairness.

Preparing for and Facing Treatment

Patients newly diagnosed with cancer not only must come to terms with the loss of desired goals but also must focus on life-saving treatments rather than life-enhancing achievements. Patients and their families may find that old ways of coping are inadequate in helping them to deal with the physical and psychological pain associated with the illness (e.g., loss of health, mobility, independence). Major lifestyle changes that revolve around treatment schedules and doctors' visits can create major disruptions in the lives of family members. The presence of cancer in an individual's life immediately curtails or modifies the achievement of both short- and long-term goals. According to Fein (1993), "Achieving goals, not just perceiving them, is what reduces anger. People have to go out into the world and make things happen" (p. 56). When patients are involved in decisions concerning their illness, they can feel more empowered and less out-of-control. Frustration and anger decrease as more goal-directed behavior is manifested (Staples, Baruth, Jefferies, & Warder, 1994).

The combination of having a severe life-threatening illness, being identified as a "patient," and having to acquiesce to the demands of an impersonal hospital environment contributes significantly to patients' and family members' feelings of loss of control and competence (Simms, 1995). Prolonged waiting times for unfamiliar procedures, separation from family and friends, and disconnection from their world all contribute to patients' feelings of frustration and powerlessness. Hospital and clinic settings often are structured to be efficient rather than warm and inviting. Routines are designed to serve the masses, not necessarily to address the needs of individuals. Patients can feel unimportant, frightened, and neglected—feelings that may precede an outburst of anger.

In these situations, patients may express anger in a variety of ways. Patients and family members may direct abusive language or aggressive behavior at each other or toward others, express negative feelings about the hospital staff, or refuse to participate in the plan of care.

Anger as part of the mourning process often is felt most profoundly in those who experience disfiguring surgery, loss of body parts, and loss of control of the body (Simms, 1995). However, it is important to remember that it is the *perception* of the injury to patients' physical and emotional integrity that should guide the therapeutic response.

Those who face months or even years of intensive, life-threatening therapies (e.g., those undergoing treatment for leukemia) may be at greater risk for experiencing fear, isolation, alienation, and anger. Factors that can affect expression of these emotions during treatment include patients' and family members' need to "protect" one another from bad news, the pressure to think positive and not "jinx" treatment response, and not wanting to be a burden on others by admitting that one has negative thoughts or fears. In addition to treatment concerns, socioeconomic concerns may include worrying about keeping one's job and housing, gaining or maintaining health insurance, paying large out-of-pocket medical expenses, and taking care of other family members while participating in treatment. Some patients may respond to the experience by raging outwardly toward others using verbal threats and name calling, among other negative responses, to deal with their emotions. Others may turn their anger inward, seething quietly while cooperating with the designated protocol. Either way, patients' anger often is a mask for other feelings and is a coping mechanism for dealing with deeper, more frightening emotions.

Nurses can address the underlying feelings with reflective statements. A statement such as "Sounds like you are worried about the side effects of the chemotherapy; tell me what you know about it" will help patients to gain control and focus on the real issue. Provide factual information as needed, but continue to focus on the underlying feelings of anxiety, fear, and frustration.

When patients refuse to comply with a treatment protocol, nurses should try to ascertain the underlying reason. It is important to understand patients' and families' perceptions of the problem and other factors that are contributing to the refusal (e.g., physical limitations, family problems, environmental stressors). Explore alternatives and, in a nonintimidating manner, explain the possible consequences of not following medical advice. Educating patients about their condition empowers them to identify personal goals of care. Collaborating with patients and giving them the opportunity to participate in decisions about their care affirm their value and competence.

Becoming a Survivor and Returning to Normalcy

Survivors of cancer have several tasks to accomplish when treatment is complete. They must negotiate a return to normalcy that includes regaining previous family, occupational, and social roles. They must cope with and manage the anxiety associated with the possibility that the cancer may return. Through a constantly evolving process, they must integrate and find meaning in a new identity as a cancer survivor (see Chapter 2).

Survivors may experience difficulty in returning to old roles. Family members may have become comfortable in carrying out those roles and may not want to give them up. Survivors may not be willing to perform tasks that caregivers expect the now "healthy" individual to do. These are potential sources for conflict within the family. Some families will transition easily; others will have a more difficult time.

Survivors, with their lifeline to the treatment team newly cut, must learn to handle their fears of recurrence. For some, it is the first time during the experience that they have allowed themselves to deal with the full impact of cancer on their lives. They may feel many emotions—fear, relief, sadness, anxiety, and anger. Most will be able to manage these feelings without professional assistance. Others, especially those who find that their ability to function has been affected, may require further support and skills training to manage these difficult emotions.

Anger can be a demand for change or a passionate wish for things to be different. Survivors can channel their anger in positive ways, reestablishing important boundaries and asserting personal integrity in the face of body- and life-altering disease. Many survivors thus become active in cancer advocacy groups (e.g., National Coalition for Cancer Survivorship, American Cancer Society) that promote legislative, societal, and healthcare system changes to benefit those facing cancer.

Experiencing Progression or Recurrence and Making Difficult Decisions

Facing the real possibility that the cancer cannot be cured, only forestalled, may elicit strong negative emotions from patients and families. They often express disappointment and anger at this time. Patients and families may express dismay that the cancer has returned, insisting, "But they said they got it all." Perhaps physicians were not overtly direct in telling the family there was little likelihood of cure. Despite all efforts by professionals to communicate the gravity of the situation, patients and families may have not yet accepted that death is inevitable.

A major task that must be accomplished at this juncture is weighing the risks and benefits of further treatment while appraising the value of quality of life and what it means to the individual and family. At this time, patients and family members may wish to participate in clinical trials, some maintaining unrealistic hope for cure, others seeing this as the last chance to stay alive, and still others wishing to perform an altruistic act to benefit others. When the trial is unsuccessful or patients are found to be ineligible to participate in the trial, team members must be prepared to deal with the resulting anger, even rage, that patients and families may display (see Chapter 29).

Preparing for End of Life

It is most important at this time to put one's affairs in order, designate a proxy to make healthcare decisions, and begin the difficult process of letting go. Awareness of dying can precipitate expression of anger as individuals and family members mourn the loss of health, career, income, lifestyle, relationships, independence, and unattained goals. Individuals struggle to find meaning and purpose in life lived yet must face being deprived of a future while others live. Everyone and everything must be given up, and the short time remaining may be filled with emotional and physical pain. The bereaved and the dying patient may have difficulty acknowledging and accepting that anger is present. Writing a last will and testament or accepting hospice may be too painful because these are concrete indications that life is coming to a close. Terminally ill patients may vent anger at God, doctors, nurses, close family members, and others who are healthy; they also may direct anger at themselves. Kübler-Ross (1969) summed up the anger phase of the grieving process as the patient's last loud cry: "I am alive, don't forget that. You can hear my voice; I am not dead yet!" (p. 52).

When anger is present in the terminal stages of illness, patients have little energy to expend in angry outbursts. Silent bitterness, indifference, or apathy then may replace open anger and aggressive behavior (Kübler-Ross, 1969). Family members often become openly angry toward one another, particularly when there is disagreement about the loved one's treatment or end-of-life decisions. Family members may voice anger toward medical and nursing personnel as a reaction to overwhelming stress and feelings of helplessness, frustration, and the anticipatory loss of their loved one.

At Death

At the time of death, many families who have prepared for this moment are able to quietly accept the outcome and begin the process of preparation for family rituals of grief and bereavement. They easily accept nursing staff's offer of support and assistance. Some families, however, when facing the death of a loved one, may exhibit loud verbal or physical outbursts. Nursing staff need to be aware that in certain ethnic groups and cultures, overt displays of grief are accepted, even expected. These demonstrative behaviors include shouting, screaming, loud crying, rocking and wailing, "fainting" or "seizing," and self-flagellation (striking oneself). They may vent distress in a number of ways, including striking themselves, other objects (windows and furniture), or other people. Nursing staff should carefully assess the context of these situations. Nonintrusive nursing interventions should focus on promoting comfort, providing safety, and preventing self-harm, harm to others, or destruction of furniture or equipment during this difficult time. Further intervention may not be required. In very rare cases, nurses may need to set kind but firm limits on these behaviors. If ineffective, parties can be asked to leave the area to collect themselves. In rare instances, security personnel may need to be called.

Nurses' Responses to Anger

Nurses often become targets of patients' anger, and they may respond to this anger in a variety of ways. Although violence is difficult to predict, nurses can be better prepared if the potential for aggressive behavior has been fully assessed.

Assessment

Step 1: Look for factors that may elicit patients' and family members' anger (see Table 14-1). Anger is one of many normal human reactions to the diagnosis of

Table 14-1. Factors That Elicit Patients' Anger

Experience	Reaction
Physiologic/metabolic • Chemical imbalances • Metastatic disease • Treatment effects	Cognitive impairment Physical effects on body
Environmental/institutional • Powerlessness, vulnerability • External stimuli (noise, lights, loss of privacy, interruptions) • Frustrating people and situations • Loss of control	Unfamiliar treatments, tests and routines Long waiting periods Lack of control, competence, and decision making
Sociocultural/economic • Isolation, aloneness, abandonment • Humiliation, shame • Past anger, grief, unfairness	Feeling out of control, unable to manage emotions Asking "Why me?"
Psychological • Overwhelmed, confused • Unmet expectations • Fear, anxiety	Expression of vulnerability or little or no control Hypersensitive/overreactive

cancer. Nurses who feel threatened when patients become angry should remember that anger episodes do not always progress to physical aggression (Averill, 1982). However, when anger is too frequent, intense, or prolonged and adversely affects the patient's relationships with family and staff, then further assessment is required (Novaco, 1976). On a busy oncology unit, bedside nurses can perform a basic clinical interview with the patient and family: Is the patient easily angered or slow to anger? What situations trigger anger? Does he or she tend to hold anger in and then explode? How does the patient control anger or cool down? Has the patient hurt others or himself when angry? How do family members respond to the anger? What events have created anxiety and frustration during this and other hospitalizations? Is the patient experiencing pain (Glover, Dibble, Dodd, & Miaskowski, 1995; Sela, Bruera, Conner-Spady, Cumming, & Walker, 2002)? Is the family experiencing social and financial stressors (Cano & Vivian, 2003)? Has there been a history of alcohol abuse (Aviles, Earleywine, Pollock, Stratton, & Miller, 2005; Parrott & Zeichner, 2002) or psychiatric disorder (Thomas, 1998a)? The bedside nurse also may call on other resources to assess and intervene with angry patients and families, including advanced practice psychiatric nurses, social workers, chaplains, psychologists, and psychiatrists.

Step 2: Ask this question: "How do I feel about being with the patient?" Nurses' feelings of fear, anger, inadequacy, being manipulated, or desire to avoid the patient are signs that the therapeutic relationship needs to be examined more closely, and anger may be the problem.

Step 3: Continuing with further self-assessment, ask "How do I express and manage my own anger? Is it constructive in this case? Am I denying my angry feelings toward this patient? Is it helping the patient? Does it help me to achieve my desired goals, or does it defeat me? What kinds of patients are a problem for me? What situations push my buttons?" Self-awareness is an important component of assessment. Keeping an anger log can help nurses to identify themes and patterns and types of patients that provoke angry feelings.

Step 4: Identify early signs that indicate an escalation in anger. Increased frustration, a raised voice, rapid speech, agitated or rigid and tense body movements, demanding and aggressive statements, increased motor activity, and sudden silence are warning signs that anger is escalating. Understanding the progression of anger in both patients and family members helps nurses to assess and intervene early in the process to possibly defuse anger and to prevent aggression.

Interventions During an Angry Episode

Initially, interventions should be as supportive as possible (Zook, 1996). If not defused early, anger may escalate to aggression. When patients vent their anger verbally, wait until they have calmed down on their own. Becoming defensive or argumentative only worsens the situation. Define the situation, not the person, as the problem.

This appraisal of the event by nurses promotes collaborative problem solving rather than focusing blame on others. Once the angry display is completed, nurses should express to patients that they regret that the patients are feeling neglected, helpless, or hurt. Empathize and show understanding without being patronizing (e.g., "I know you feel discouraged that none of the treatments have made a difference so far. It must be really hard for you to continue").

Stay calm, and maintain eye contact with patients. Nurses should not set limits, argue, or try to intervene during the outburst because patients are not likely to hear them, nor are patients likely to benefit from what they say at this time. It may be helpful to take deep breaths, perform positive self-talk (e.g., "I can handle this"), count to 10 before responding, or remember words of wisdom from others (see Figure 14-2). This decreases the likelihood of responding angrily rather than therapeutically. Understanding why the patient's anger has escalated to this degree of frustration is most important. When patients have calmed down, acknowledge their feelings, express regret about the situation, and confirm, "Yes, having to wait 30 minutes for your pain medication is a problem." Understand that family members are acting as advocates for their loved ones. Use this knowledge to collaborate with patients and families on ways to address the problem. Do not justify the situation (e.g., "We are short-staffed today"). This only makes the situation worse. When possible, allow patients and families to consider the options and select the action they would like to take. In some cases, nurses may find it helpful to leave the situation to calm down first and then return to address patients' or families' concerns.

Nurses can manage their own responses, particularly anger (see Table 14-2), by taking advantage of "anger-busters," including talking to other nurse confidants; attending stress management, anger management, and conflict resolution classes; participating in assertiveness training; learning cognitive restructuring skills (e.g., reframing perceptions of an event to decrease anger, using cognitive self-control techniques); and by augmenting relaxation and focused breathing skills. Improving their self-control and problem-solving skills will help nurses to work with and

---

Figure 14-2. Words of Wisdom for Managing Anger

- Do not belittle: "When you act like a child, you get treated like a child."
- When you meet the needs of others, you become trustworthy.
- What is most important is not how you feel. It is how you behave.
- Practice what you preach.
- It is okay to have negative feelings toward patients with cancer. Acknowledge them and discharge them somewhere away from patients and families.
- Seek peer support. Other nurses know how you feel.
- Give yourself permission to rejuvenate away from patients for at least a few minutes each day.
- To reduce nurses' frustration and burnout, consider rotating nurses to take care of difficult and angry patients.
- Use case consultants and team conferences to discuss ways to handle the stress of caring for angry patients and families.

Note. Based on information from Thomas, 1998a.

Table 14-2. Patients' Anger and Nurses' Responses

Patients' Behavior as Interpreted by Nurse	Nurses' Feelings/Behavior
Insolent, entitled	Feels unappreciated, like a servant
Abusive, threatening	Feels fearful, anxious
Intimidating, hypercritical	Feels inadequate, defensive
Controlling	Feels manipulated, becomes controlling
Angry	Takes personally, becomes angry in return

Note. Based on information from Thomas, 1998a.

empower patients when they need to make decisions during potentially frustrating events (Thomas, 1998a).

When Violence Occurs

In very rare cases, patients or family members may lose control and become physically violent. Nurses must ensure the safety of themselves, others, and the violent patient or family member. Nurses should keep the room door open and position themselves so that they can leave quickly. Stay at least a few arm lengths away, with arms loosely folded, but maintain direct eye contact to anticipate aggressive movement and to exert some control. Maintain a quiet and confident voice, and tell the patient or family member that this behavior is unacceptable. Healthcare professionals should let the patient know that they will not allow anyone, including the patient, to get hurt. Nurses should maintain their composure to give the violent patient or family member less control over them and others. However, if violence or the threat of violence continues, retreat to safety, and call for adequate help. As a last resort, physical restraints or medication and intervention by appropriate personnel may be necessary to control the situation (see Figure 14-3).

Figure 14-3. Plan of Care

Assessment
- Identify presence of risk factors that could lead to violent behavior.
- Identify the patient who feels powerless.
- Recognize increasing signs of frustration, anger, and anxiety.
- Assist the patient to identify anger triggers.

Potential Nursing Diagnoses (NANDA International, 2005)
- Risk for other-directed violence
- Other relevant associated diagnoses: powerlessness, anxiety, fear, dysfunctional grieving, pain, chronic low self-esteem, social isolation

***DSM-IV-TR* Diagnosis** (American Psychiatric Association, 2000)
- Adjustment disorder with disturbance of conduct

Expected Outcomes
- Patients will acknowledge and express angry feelings appropriately.
- Patients will identify sources of frustration that trigger angry feelings.
- Patients will identify underlying feelings that contribute to angry outbursts.

Interventions: Patient
- Stay calm and quiet when the patient is expressing anger.
- Speak calmly, and do not argue with or threaten the patient.
- Make eye contact, call the patient by name, and do not cross arms or have hands on hips; do not touch the patient. Keep the exit open.
- Acknowledge the patient's feelings, express regret about the problem, and show empathy.
- Identify the patient's perception of the problem.
- Discern the triggering event and any underlying feelings.
- Provide factual information if the patient feels uninformed.

- Focus on the underlying feelings using reflective statements.
- If the patient is refusing a treatment or procedure, ascertain the reason for his or her refusal to comply with the medical regimen.
- Find ways to empower the patient that give him or her control over the situation.
- Advocate for the patient; discuss with the team possible options that allow for maximum patient control and accomplishment of treatment goals.
- Call for assistance if it appears that the patient may lose behavioral control. (A show of force may prevent further escalation.)
- Use chemical or physical restraints as a last resort.

Interventions: Family
- Share information with family members so that they are informed of treatment schedules and expected outcomes.
- Allow family members to vent feelings of anger over the potential or impending loss of their loved one.
- Recognize that some families will be strong advocates for their loved ones; avoid defensive responses.
- Address underlying feelings of anxiety, fear, grief, and guilt.
- Educate family members about the grieving process and the phases that they and the patient can expect to experience.
- If appropriate, refer family members for support group/individual grief counseling.

Case Study

Shelley is a 44-year-old woman who recently has been diagnosed with breast cancer. After a biopsy confirmed a malignancy, she was admitted to your unit for surgery. She has just had a lumpectomy. This is her first hospitalization.

Her husband of 12 years is still in shock about the sudden turn of events in his wife's life. Their children, an 8-year-old daughter and a 5-year-old son, know only that Mommy is sick and will be home soon. Shelley's mother is caring for the children while Shelley is hospitalized.

The oncologist recommends a course of radiation treatment that Shelley refuses. The oncologists tells her he will return later when she has had more time to think about her decision. She tells you, "The radiation will kill me before the cancer does, and I am not going to have that poison put into my body. They keep pressuring me to make a decision today and I can't." Her husband tries to intervene and convince her that the doctor knows best, but Shelley screams at him, "All you men are the same. You think you know what is best for women. Well, you don't. You don't understand. You don't understand!"

Later, after her husband leaves, you find Shelley lying in her bed, turned toward the wall with her lunch tray untouched. When you ask her what is going on, she says, "Leave me alone. I don't want to talk to anyone." You tell her, "You need to eat to regain your strength." Suddenly, Shelley sits up and pushes the tray off the nightstand onto the floor and screams, "That's what I think of your stupid hospital food. What do you know about anything? You don't know how I feel. Now get out of here. Leave me alone."

Her physical display of anger surprises you, and without thinking, you tell her, "That's no way to act." Shelley stiffens, glares at you, and shouts, "Don't tell me how I should act. Who do you think you are? What do you know about anything? You are just a nurse. Get out now!" As you walk away from her room, you can hear her crying.

You feel awful and decide to consult with the advanced practice nurse about Shelley. After you discuss the case, you summon up your courage to return to Shelley's room. You feel confident that you can handle her expression of anger because you have recognized that Shelley's outburst is not really about the hospital food or your competence as a nurse. Your goal is to help Shelley to identify and understand what her underlying feelings are and to assist her in determining how she can cope more effectively with her current situation.

Using reflective statements, empathy, and active listening, you learn that Shelley had been proud of her good health and often boasted that she never smoked, drank, or ate junk food. She loved giving advice to others on how to be healthy and was quite knowledgeable about nutrition and preventive health care. You begin to understand why she is so angry about her diagnosis.

Shelley insists that she will never consent to radiation "because the treatment is worse than the problem." You sense that she has strong feelings about the loss of her breast and the potential impact of radiation on the remaining breast tissue, and you gently validate this: "It must be really hard to face this loss." It is your expression of empathy that gives Shelley permission to cry softly, "I love wearing sexy nightgowns for my husband. What will I do now? It's just not fair. Why did this have to happen to me?" You continue to listen quietly until Shelley feels more calm.

(Continued on next page)

Case Study (Continued)

During the case conference, a plan of care is outlined that includes educating Shelley about the risks and benefits of radiation and the prognosis of her cancer without it. Another patient with breast cancer who has recovered successfully is invited to speak with her, and a referral is made to a support group. Shelley eventually consents to radiation treatments.

Discussion

Shelley never expected to have cancer. Her family had no history of cancer, and she had been extremely health conscious all of her life. The diagnosis and subsequent surgery were incomprehensible to Shelley. Her sense of power in the world centered on her ability to maintain excellent health. She had to come to terms with the helplessness of not being able to prevent breast cancer, and the radiation felt like a further assault to her once "pure" body.

Out of fear of experiencing this helplessness, she displaced anger onto her husband and the nurse and projected her sense of "not knowing" onto them. They became the "stupid" ones who did not understand, when, in fact, it was Shelley who could not understand. "Why me?" could not be answered because having cancer was not congruent with her belief that she could control her health through prudent health practices.

The feelings of unfairness and subsequent anger kept Shelley from experiencing her underlying fears and anxiety about her body image, her husband's response to her changed identity, and the gravity of the disease. Once these dilemmas became conscious and were expressed, she could begin the process of experiencing her feelings of loss, grief, fear, and helplessness and grappling with them in some meaningful way.

Conclusion

Nurses often are targets of patients' and families' anger. Oncology nurses who understand that patients' and families' anger often is a mask for more frightening underlying feelings of powerlessness, confusion, grief, anxiety, and fear will be most effective in providing important therapeutic support to others, helping them to defuse anger successfully, and assisting those experiencing cancer to deal constructively with their anger.

Special thanks to Mary Paquette, RN, MN, PhD, who served as the author of this chapter in the first edition.

References

American Psychiatric Association. (2000). *Diagnostic and statistical manual of mental disorders* (4th ed., text rev.). Washington, DC: Author.

Anderson-Malico, R. (1994). Anger management using cognitive group therapy. *Perspectives in Psychiatric Care, 30*(3), 17–20.

Averill, J.R. (1982). *Anger and aggression: An essay on emotion.* New York: Springer-Verlag.

Aviles, F., Earleywine, M., Pollock, V., Stratton, J., & Miller, N. (2005). Alcohol's effect on triggered displaced aggression. *Psychology of Addictive Behaviors, 19,* 108–111.

Burns, D. (1980). *Feeling good: The new mood therapy.* New York: New American Library.

Butow, P.N., Coates, A.S., & Dunn, S.M. (1999). Psychosocial predictors of survival in metastatic melanoma. *Journal of Clinical Oncology, 17,* 2256–2263.

Butow, P.N., Hiller, J.E., Price, M.A., Thackway, S.V., Kricker, A., & Tennant, C.A. (2000). Epidemiological evidence for a relationship between life events, coping style, and personality factors in the development of breast cancer. *Journal of Psychosomatic Research, 49,* 169–181.

Cano, A., & Vivian, D. (2003). Are life stressors associated with marital violence? *Journal of Family Psychology, 17,* 302–314.

Derogatis, L., Abeloff, M., & Melisaratos, N. (1979). Psychological coping mechanisms and survival time in metastatic breast cancer. *JAMA, 242,* 1504–1508.

Fein, M.L. (1993). *I.A.M.: A common sense guide to coping with anger.* Westport, CT: Praeger Press.

Fitch, M.I., Gray, R., Franssen, E., & Johnson, B. (2000). Men's perspectives on the impact of prostate cancer: Implications for oncology nurses. *Oncology Nursing Forum, 27,* 1255–1263.

Garrison, G.S. (1995). *A phenomenological study of the experience and expression of anger among women with cardiovascular disease and breast cancer.* Unpublished doctoral dissertation, University of Tennessee, Nashville.

Glover, J., Dibble, S.L., Dodd, M.J., & Miaskowski, C. (1995). Mood states of oncology outpatients: Does pain make a difference? *Journal of Pain and Symptom Management, 10,* 120–128.

Goldfried, M.R., Raue, P.J., & Castonguay, L.G. (1998). The therapeutic focus in significant sessions of master therapists: A comparison of cognitive-behavioral and psychodynamic-interpersonal interventions. *Journal of Consulting and Clinical Psychology, 66,* 803–810.

Greer, S., & Morris, T. (1975). Psychological attributes of women who develop breast cancer: A controlled study. *Journal of Psychosomatic Research, 19,* 147–153.

Grossarth-Maticek, R., Bastiaans, J., & Kanazir, D. (1985). Psychosocial factors as strong predictors of mortality from cancer, ischaemic heart disease and stroke: The Yugoslav prospective study. *Journal of Psychosomatic Research, 29,* 167–176.

Harburg, E., Julius, M., Kaciroti, N., Gleiberman, L., & Schork, M.A. (2003). Expressive/suppressive anger-coping responses, gender, and types of mortality: A 17-year follow-up (Tecumseh, Michigan, 1971–1988). *Psychosomatic Medicine, 65,* 588–597.

Kübler-Ross, E. (1969). *On death and dying.* New York: Macmillan.

Kune, G., Kune, S., Watson, L., & Bahnson, C. (1991). Personality as a risk factor in large bowel cancer: Data from the Melbourne Colorectal Cancer Study. *Psychological Medicine, 21,* 28–41.

Levy, S. (1984). Emotions and progression of cancer: A review. *Advances, 1*(1), 10–15.

Lindop, E., & Cannon, S. (2001). Evaluating the self-assessed support needs of women with breast cancer. *Journal of Advanced Nursing, 34,* 760–771.

Linnoila, M., & Charney, D.S. (1999). The neurobiology of aggression. In D.S. Charney, E.J. Nestler, & B.D. Bunney (Eds.), *Neurobiology of mental illness* (pp. 855–871). New York: Oxford University Press.

Loscalzo, M., & BrintzenhofeSzoc, K. (1998). Brief crisis counseling. In J.C. Holland (Ed.), *Psycho-oncology* (pp. 662–675). New York: Oxford University Press.

McKenna, M., Zevon, M.A., Corn, B., & Rounds, J. (1999). Psychosocial factors and the development of breast cancer: A meta-analysis. *Health Psychology, 18,* 520–531.

Morris, T., Greer, S., Pettingale, K., & Watson, M. (1981). Patterns of expression of anger and their psychological correlates in women with breast cancer. *Journal of Psychosomatic Research, 25,* 111–112.

NANDA International. (2005). *Nursing diagnoses: Definitions and classification, 2005–2006.* Philadelphia: Author.

Novaco, R.W. (1976). The functions and regulation of the arousal of anger. *American Journal of Psychiatry, 133,* 1124–1128.

Novaco, R.W. (1977). Stress inoculation: A cognitive therapy for anger and its application to a case of depression. *Journal of Consulting and Clinical Psychology, 45,* 600–608.

Parrott, D.J., & Zeichner, A. (2002). Effects of alcohol and trait anger on physical aggression in men. *Journal of Studies in Alcohol, 63,* 196–204.

Sela, R.A., Bruera, E., Conner-Spady, B., Cumming, C., & Walker, C. (2002). Sensory and affective dimensions of advanced cancer pain. *Psycho-Oncology, 11,* 23–34.

Simms, C. (1995). How to unmask the angry patient. *American Journal of Nursing, 95*(4), 36–40.

Smith, T.W. (1992). Hostility and health: Current status of a psychosomatic hypothesis. *Health Psychology, 11,* 139–150.

Spiegel, D.S., Bloom, J.R., Kraemer, H.C., & Gottheil, E. (1989). Effect of psychosocial treatment on survival of patients with metastatic breast cancer. *Lancet, 334,* 888–891.

Spira, J.L., & Reed, G.M. (2003). *Group psychotherapy for women with breast cancer.* Washington, DC: American Psychological Association.

Staples, P., Baruth, P., Jefferies, M., & Warder, L. (1994). Empowering the angry patient. *Canadian Nurse, 90*(4), 28–30.

Tavris, C. (1989). *Anger: The misunderstood emotion* (Rev. ed.). New York: Simon & Schuster.

Temoshok, L.R. (1985). Biopsychosocial studies on cutaneous malignant melanoma: Psychosocial factors associated with prognostic indicators, progression, psychophysiology, and tumor-host response. *Social Science and Medicine, 20,* 833–840.

Temoshok, L.R., & Dreher, H. (1994). Disconnects in understanding "the type C" connection. *Advances, 10*(2), 64–72.

Thomas, C.B. (1988). Cancer and the youthful mind: A forty-year perspective. *Advances, 5*(2), 42–58.

Thomas, S.P. (1990). Theoretical and empirical perspectives on anger. *Issues in Mental Health Nursing, 11,* 203–216.

Thomas, S.P. (1998a). Assessing and intervening with anger disorders. *Nursing Clinics of North America, 33,* 121–133.

Thomas, S.P. (1998b). *Transforming nurses' anger and pain: Steps toward healing.* New York: Springer.

Thomas, S.P., Greer, M., Davis, M., Droppleman, P., Mozingo, J., & Pierce, M. (2000). Anger and cancer: An analysis of the linkages. *Cancer Nursing, 23,* 344–349.

Weihs, K.L., Enright, T.M., Simmens, S.J., & Reiss, D. (2000). Negative affectivity, restriction of emotions, and site of metastases predict mortality in recurrent breast cancer. *Journal of Psychosomatic Research, 49,* 59–68.

Wiser, S., & Goldfried, M.R. (1998). Therapist interventions and client emotional experiencing in expert psychodynamic-interpersonal and cognitive-behavioral therapies. *Journal of Consulting and Clinical Psychology, 66,* 634–640.

Zook, R. (1996). Take action before anger builds up. *RN, 59*(4), 46–50.

CHAPTER 15

Depression and Suicide

Angela V. Albright, RN, APRN, BC, PhD, and
Sharon M. Valente, RN, APRN, BC, PhD, FAAN

Melancholy
Sits on me as a cloud along the sky
Which will not let the sunbeams through, nor yet
Descent in rain and end; but spreads itself
'Twixt heaven and earth, like envy between man
And man, and is an everlasting mist.

—Lord Byron

The sadness and dysphoric moods that patients with cancer experience upon receiving their diagnosis and while coping with treatment are not surprising. In addition to "normal" affective reactions, many cancer drugs, the disease process itself, or physical discomfort can induce depressive symptoms. At least 25% of patients with cancer suffer from levels of clinical depression that could be alleviated with proper treatment (Martin & Jackson, 2000). These depressions, however, often are overlooked and not treated when healthcare workers assume that depression is normal for the patient. Patients with cancer also are at higher risk for suicide (Valente & Saunders, 1997). Wishing to die might be confused with the desire for a "rational suicide" (i.e., the patient has understandable motives with unimpaired mental processes) and may not be evaluated properly (Valente & Trainor, 1998). Identifying and treating depression, therefore, are essential parts of the oncology nurse's role. Nurses are in a prime position to identify patients who are at risk and to carry out preventive and restorative measures.

Assessment of Depression

For an accurate diagnosis of a major depressive episode, according to the *Diagnostic and Statistical Manual of Mental Disorders (DSM-IV-TR)* (American Psychiatric

Association [APA], 2000), patients must have suffered from a depressed mood or loss of interest or pleasure in nearly all activities for at least two weeks. In addition, four of the following conditions must exist: (a) changes in appetite, weight, sleep, and psychomotor activity; (b) decreased energy; (c) feelings of worthlessness or guilt; (d) difficulty thinking, concentrating, or making decisions; and (e) recurrent thoughts of death or suicidal ideation, plans, or attempts. Certainly, physical symptoms such as loss of appetite, decreased energy, and insomnia could be related to the disease process or to treatment modalities such as medications. This makes the definitive diagnosis of depression a challenging process. Researchers have suggested that criteria for the diagnosis of depression in patients with cancer should exclude physical symptoms and focus only on psychological symptoms (Martin & Jackson, 2000). Others have argued that including the physical symptoms does not necessarily result in a false positive diagnosis. More risk may arise in not looking at all of the signs and symptoms (Holland, 2002; Valentine, 2003). These authors asserted that excluding the physical criteria for research purposes might be wise; however, for clinical purposes, the more inclusionary approach will protect against underdiagnosing depression. Akechi et al. (2003) found that diminished appetite and ability to think were more positively associated with depression in patients with cancer in a correlational study. Cavanaugh, Clark, and Gibbons (1983) identified feeling like a failure, loss of interest in people, feeling punished, suicidal ideation, dissatisfaction, difficulty with decisions, and crying as hallmark symptoms that were not confounded by medical illness or treatment measures. Crying and loss of interest indicated severe depression. In this study, depressed patients did not lose their interest in people and felt support and pleasure in their contacts.

Another category of diagnosis in the *DSM-IV-TR*, mood disorder due to a general medical condition, addresses depression that has a clear etiology in a medical illness (APA, 2000). This category would be used if a biologic condition existed that would induce depressive symptoms. Certain cancers (e.g., pancreatic [Holland, 2002], head and neck [Baile, Gilbertini, Scott, & Endicott, 1992]) seem to be more prone to association with depressive symptoms. Whether from a biologic condition directly causing symptoms, from treatment for a medical condition, or from a psychological process, depressed patients with cancer need intervention to help them to cope with or alleviate the depressive condition.

Nonpsychiatric clinicians often lack skill in detecting major depression. Studies have found that nurses underestimated the level of depressive symptoms in patients who were moderately or severely depressed (McDonald, Passik, Dugan, & Rosenfeld, 1999; Valente, in press-a). Nurses' diagnoses were most influenced by crying, depressed mood, and medical factors (e.g., anorexia, insomnia, constipation, fatigue), which are not reliable indicators of depression in a medically ill population. Most physicians and nurses only detected approximately 49% of depressed patients on a medical service, and only 10% of these patients received appropriate treatment for depression (Martin & Jackson, 2000). In a qualitative study, Williams and Payne (2003) found that nurses were more likely to focus on physical symptoms, were concerned with their lack of training in identifying psychiatric symptoms, and were frustrated in their inability to convince medical staff to seek further assessment or antidepressant medication for patients.

For screening purposes, the Hamilton Rating Scale, the Beck Depression Inventory, the Hospital Anxiety and Depression Scale (HADS), and the Zung Self-Rating Depression Scale have been used to identify patients with cancer with depressive symptoms who may need further evaluation and treatment (Carroll, Kathol, Noyes, Wald, & Clamon, 1993; Passik et al., 2002). The scores for depression, however, only have been determined for some medically ill populations. If anything, these rating tools would seem to render more false positives than false negatives (Patrick et al., 2003; Pignone et al., 2002). These self- and observer-rated scales can be useful tools for nurses because they can be administered quickly and efficiently (Valente, in press-b). Used as an adjunct to a thorough psychosocial history, these scales will help nurses to identify people in need of additional intervention.

Lampic, von Essen, Peterson, Larsson, and Sjoden (1996) found that staff members tend to estimate anxiety and depression at higher rates than patients, and identification of clinically significant depression with HADS was inaccurate. Lampic et al. hypothesized that staff members do this because they need to project how they would feel if they were in the patient's situation, or they need to see the patient's suffering to feel superior. This points out the need for nurses to use objective criteria in assessment as well as to be aware of their emotional issues so as not to confuse their own emotions with those of the patients'.

The incidence of depression in patients with cancer consistently has been significantly higher than that in the general population (Holland, 2002). Therefore, patients with cancer are at greater than average risk for depression. Carroll et al. (1993) found that among 809 inpatients and outpatients with cancer screened for depression and anxiety, nearly one-half had symptoms that warranted further evaluation. Caregivers need to acquire and maintain skill in accurate detection of depression (Valente, 2004).

Depression in Special Populations

The clinical features of major depressive episodes are more similar than different when compared among pediatric, adolescent, adult, and older patients; men and women; and ethnic groups (Lovejoy, Tabor, & Deloney, 2000; Lovejoy, Tabor, Matteis, & Lillis, 2000; Pignone et al., 2002). Because children may be unable to express their feelings, other signs may need to be analyzed (e.g., acting-out behaviors, not meeting developmental tasks, withdrawal, self-destructive behaviors). Depression can occur throughout childhood and adolescence. Clinically significant depressive symptoms affect older adults, especially if they are institutionalized or suffer from cognitive impairment (Hybels & Blazer, 2003). A medical illness such as cancer represents a poor prognostic sign and may mask the diagnosis. The clinical presentation is similar to that used for younger adults but may be more likely to include memory loss and poor concentration, which can be confused with dementia (Pignone et al.).

Depression can be undiagnosed or misdiagnosed in some cultural and ethnic groups because of healthcare professionals' stereotypes about the groups' expected behaviors, language barriers, and lack of access to mental health services (Mouton, 2000; Valente & Saunders, 2000). The *DSM-IV-TR* suggested that some cultures may differ in their judgments about the seriousness of depressive symptoms or may express depressive symptoms as "nerves" (Latino) or "imbalances" (Asian) (APA, 2000; Ersek, Kagawa-Singer, & Barnes, 1998; Mouton) (see Chapter 6).

Risk Factors for Depression

To assess for depression, nurses must identify factors that might contribute to depression. Several psychological and physical variables have been identified that may affect the level of distress that accompanies a cancer diagnosis.

Severity of Illness

Carroll et al. (1993) found that patients with active malignant disease scored highest of all inpatients and outpatients on depression subscales of HADS. One study revealed no difference in mean levels of depression between patients receiving chemotherapy at home or in a hospital (Schwartz, Lander, & Chochinov, 2002). The overall psychological distress was highest for those in the midst of treatment.

As severity of illness increases or, perhaps, *perception* of the severity increases, some patients might have an increased risk for depression. Nurses must find out what patients understand about their disease and their associated beliefs about what will happen next. At times, patients are not told about their prognosis, or it is discussed with them in an oblique way. Uncertainty is inevitable in the treatment of cancer; however, giving as much information as patients seem to need rather than ignoring or skirting the issues can minimize the anxiety caused by this uncertainty. Patients' perceptions of their illness are important for nurses to elicit and understand so that they can identify areas that need clarification (Chaturvedi & Maguire, 1998).

Stressful Life Events

A cancer diagnosis might be the "straw that broke the camel's back." Coping with the diagnosis of cancer is expected to be stressful. Nurses should not forget to find out what else might be happening in patients' lives. Because cancer often brings thoughts about one's mortality, nurses can increase patients' control by initiating a therapeutic discussion of the patients' wishes for end-of-life care and by considering their wishes for a surrogate decision maker or advance directive.

Experiencing recent losses is associated with depression. When a cancer diagnosis occurs, a loss of body image and self-concept following disfiguring surgery or the physical effects of chemotherapy may accompany it. Individuals might be considering the possibility of the loss of job, status, income, or relationships.

A cancer diagnosis might raise existential issues. Because it is associated with loss of life, the diagnosis might trigger a crisis of meaning. To the extent that a person has difficulty reconciling his or her condition within a belief system, the result could be a sense of futility. The belief system that always has worked for a person in the past might be challenged and found to be lacking.

History of Depression in Self or the Family

People who have experienced a major depressive episode are at risk for recurrent episodes of depression (APA, 2000). The risk of recurrence is 50% after one episode, 70% after two episodes, and 90% after three episodes (Pignone et al., 2002). Therefore, patients who have a past history of depression are considered to be at greater risk even if they have no medical diagnosis. Throughout the course of disease, healthcare professionals should carefully evaluate people with cancer who have had a depressive episode in the past. A previous suicide attempt greatly increases the risk for a subsequent attempt (Valente & Saunders, 1997).

A genetic predisposition to depression has been established. Therefore, a family history of depression might indicate that a person is at risk, even if he or she has not had a previous episode, but especially if the family member's depression is recurrent.

Medications

Many chemotherapeutic agents that are used to fight cancer as well as other commonly used drugs have side effects that include depression (see Figure 15-1). If depression is severe, the drug's benefits should be weighed against the risks and suffering of the depression, and modifications in dose or drug selection should be made accordingly. One study suggested that pretreatment with antidepressants can prevent medication-induced depression in patients with cancer (Musselman et al., 2001).

Figure 15-1. Examples of Drugs That May Cause Depressive Side Effects

- Methyldopa
- Reserpine
- Hydralazine
- Digoxin
- Clonidine
- Levodopa
- Estrogens/oral contraceptives
- Corticosteroids
- Beta blockers/calcium channel blockers
- Diuretics
- Benzodiazepines/sedatives/hypnotics

Socioeconomic Pressures

Fear of or actual inability to hold a job or position that provides income because of the illness can be overwhelming, depending on individuals and their financial situation. Losing a job also might result in loss of social status.

A Tendency Toward Pessimism

People who have developed a pessimistic outlook on life are more prone to depression (Beck, Rush, Shaw, & Emery, 1979; Weishaar & Beck, 1992). With the added stress of a cancer diagnosis, the pessimism might seem additionally validated and may reinforce a negative world view. According to cognitive therapy principles, depression arises primarily from negative distortions in cognitive processes of thinking, knowing, and perceiving. The person believes that he or she is worthless, the world is barren, and the future is bleak. Degner (2003), in a cross-sectional and follow-up study, found that most women with breast cancer described the meaning of cancer as a "challenge" or "value." However, those who described it as an "enemy," "loss," or "punishment" were more likely to have depression, as well as anxiety and poorer quality of life. Bishop and Warr (2003) found that patients with cancer who catastrophized their illness had greater emotional distress. These distortions and irrational pessimistic beliefs automatically guide thoughts and shape emotional responses, but these thinking patterns can be changed.

Differential Diagnosis

Symptoms of depression may coexist with other major psychological diagnoses (e.g., anxiety) (see Chapter 13). Uncontrolled symptoms related to disease and treatment also may contribute to or exacerbate depression (e.g., fatigue). Metabolic status (e.g., electrolyte imbalances) that increase the risk of confusional states (e.g., psychosis, delirium) need to be differentiated from depressive symptoms.

Depression may be an outcome of chronic alcohol intake as well as alcohol and substance abuse (Cassem, 1995). Another possibility is that people who use alcohol or other substances as regular coping mechanisms have not developed more positive, affirming methods of coping.

Investigations into the relationship between cancer pain and depression have suggested that depression enhances pain, and pain and its treatment can contribute to depression (Patrick et al., 2003). Despite advances in the assessment and treatment of pain, undertreatment occurs because of a lack of knowledge, the fear of addiction, and the failure of the healthcare system to facilitate delivery of proper pain management care (Patrick et al.).

Interventions for Depression

Oncology nurses need to be aware of the importance of their relationship with patients in case finding, intervening directly, and making proper referrals. Nurses must know what resources and treatment modalities are available to assist depressed patients with cancer.

Psychiatric consultation is necessary for patients with severe depression and suicidal thoughts. Medications to treat depression have been found to be effective, and meta-analyses have shown a modest benefit of cognitive, behavioral, and/or psychosocial interventions (Patrick et al., 2003). These analyses, however, have been criticized as underestimating the interventions' effects because of methodologic problems (Bredart, Cayrou, & Dolbreault, 2002). Other treatments for depression include education and, in recalcitrant cases, electroconvulsive therapy. Unfortunately, treatment for children, older adults, and special populations is not sufficiently supported with evidence at this time, nor are uses of complementary and alternative approaches (Patrick et al.).

Psychotherapy for depression provides an opportunity for patients to explore issues that arise (e.g., existential questions of the meaning of life, death, and loss of control; impact on relationships; vulnerable feelings). Management of affect and behavior is possible with cognitive behavioral approaches that teach patients to recognize the triggers for nonproductive and self-defeating thinking. Once the pattern is recognized, patients are assisted in developing new thought patterns that lead to more positive behaviors and outcomes. Oncology nurses can take an active role in helping patients to identify self-defeating behaviors. Nurses who have formed a therapeutic relationship with patients can coach them to have positive thoughts and behaviors.

Relaxation skills can help to prevent aggravating anxiety and tension. Patients can learn simple, progressive muscle relaxation as a form of self-regulation. Visualization exercises also are effective and can be conducted easily. Relaxation to counter anxiety and tension is effective in reducing pain. Pain always should be addressed, and every avenue of relief should be pursued.

Family therapy can provide a forum where family members can identify and address unresolved conflicts. The therapist can help family members to voice their sense of the strain brought on by the disease. This can be crucial because the depression that exists might be a shared one (Given et al., 1993). Family caregivers may feel resentful and guilty about those feelings. The patient feels the resentment and also feels guilty. A chance to discuss the circular effects that family members and patients have on one another could bring increased understanding and relief. Who to include in the therapy should be explored carefully; the significant others who make up the support system should be identified and included. Oncology nurses are encouraged to make the effort to include family members in care planning meetings to solicit their support and give them a chance to identify needs that arise while caring for a loved one.

Group counseling is an excellent modality that provides patients with a chance to improve their outlook via sharing their experiences with others and gaining feedback in an accepting atmosphere. Educational programs (e.g., American Cancer Society's "I Can Cope") can clarify misconceptions about the disease and its treatment and contribute to an awareness of patients' ability to engage in self-care and improve their sense of control and mastery over their situation. Other psychoeducational programs have been shown to increase survival times and compliance with medical treatment and to reduce mood disturbance (Martin & Jackson, 2000).

Antidepressants

Antidepressant medications can be a very useful adjunct to psychotherapy by improving mood and increasing energy that, in turn, can be channeled into productive activity that increases self-esteem. Researchers have suggested that these therapies should be used in conjunction with one another because the medication will make individuals more amenable to the work of psychotherapy. When depression is severe, recurrent, or experienced in conjunction with psychotic symptoms, medication is indicated before psychotherapy (Pignone et al., 2002).

The antidepressant medication chosen should be determined by assessing what side effects might be most beneficial or least antagonizing (see Table 15-1). For example, some have sedative side effects that might assist in reducing insomnia. Others have properties that contribute to blocking neuropathic pain.

Tricyclic antidepressants, selective serotonin reuptake inhibitors, and monoamine oxidase inhibitors (MAOIs) are the major groups of antidepressants. Each has advantages and disadvantages that must be considered before prescribing. Tricyclic antidepressants take four to six weeks to take effect. The side effects, however, can begin shortly after patients begin taking them. Serotonin inhibitors are a newer category of antidepressants that seem to be well tolerated and have short-lived initial side effects. MAOIs must be used with caution because of strict dietary restrictions (e.g., foods with tyramine [beer, wine, chocolate, cheese, broad beans] can cause a fatal hypertensive crisis). However, these drugs can be useful with long-term depression that has been resistant to other types of antidepressants.

Another class of medications that is useful in treating depression is the psychostimulants (e.g., methylphenidate). This treatment has not been researched as

Table 15-1. Side Effect Profiles of Antidepressants

Drug Category	Anticholinergic Effects[a]	CNS Drowsiness	CNS Agitation/Insomnia	Cardiac Orthostatic Hypotension	Cardiac Dysrhythmia	Gastrointestinal[b]	Weight Gain
SSRIs							
Fluoxetine	1	0	3	0	0	2	2
Sertraline	1	1	1	0	0	3	2
Paroxetine	2	2	1	0	0	2	2
Citalopram	1	1	1	0	0	2	2
Fluvoxamine	1	2	0	0	0	2	2
Escitalopram	1	0	0	0	0	1–2	2
Tricyclics[c]							
Amitriptyline	4	4	0	4	3	0	4
Desipramine	1	1	1	2	2	0	1
Doxepin	3	4	0	2	2	0	3
Imipramine	3	3	1	4	3	1	3
Nortriptyline	1	2	1	2	2	0	2

Potential for side effects is rated on a 0–4 scale: 0 = none; 1 = rare; 2 = low; 3 = moderate; 4 = high

[a] Dry mouth, blurred vision, urinary hesitancy, constipation
[b] Nausea, vomiting, diarrhea
[c] If the patient is likely to plan suicide with an overdose, clinicians are advised to dispense limited amounts of MAOIs or tricyclic antidepressants and monitor the patient closely before ordering refills. When the patient has a high risk of suicide, SSRIs are typically preferred because an overdose is not lethal. *Note.* No one antidepressant medication is clearly more effective than another. Selection of a specific medication depends on various factors (e.g., short- and long-term side effects, potential interactions with other medications and disorders, prior response to antidepressants).

CNS—central nervous system; MAOI—monoamine oxidase inhibitor; SSRI—selective serotonin reuptake inhibitor

(Continued on next page)

Table 15-1. Side Effect Profiles of Antidepressants (Continued)

Drug Category	Anticholinergic Effects[a]	CNS		Cardiac		Gastrointestinal[b]	Weight Gain
		Drowsiness	Agitation/Insomnia	Orthostatic Hypotension	Dysrhythmia		
Heterocyclics							
Amoxapine	2	2	3	0	1	1	1
Bupropion	0–1	0	1	1	0	2	1
Maprotiline	0–4	0	1	0	2	1	1
Trazodone	0–1	1	1	1	1	1	1
MAOIs							
Phenelzine	1	1	2	2	0	1	2
Tranylcypromine	1	1	2	2	0	1	2
Other							
Mirtazapine	1	4	1	1	1	1	2
Venlafaxine	2	1	1	1	1	1	1
Nefazodone	1	2	1	2	1	2	2
Duloxetine	2	1	2	1	1	2	2

Potential for side effects is rated on a 0–4 scale: 0 = none; 1 = rare; 2 = low; 3 = moderate; 4 = high

[a] Dry mouth, blurred vision, urinary hesitancy, constipation
[b] Nausea, vomiting, diarrhea
[c] If the patient is likely to plan suicide with an overdose, clinicians are advised to dispense limited amounts of MAOIs or tricyclic antidepressants and monitor the patient closely before ordering refills. When the patient has a high risk of suicide, SSRIs are typically preferred because an overdose is not lethal.
Note. No one antidepressant medication is clearly more effective than another. Selection of a specific medication depends on various factors (e.g., short- and long-term side effects, potential interactions with other medications and disorders, prior response to antidepressants).

CNS—central nervous system; MAOI—monoamine oxidase inhibitor; SSRI—selective serotonin reuptake inhibitor

Note. From "Diagnosis and Treatment of Major Depression Among People With Cancer," by S.M. Valente and J.M. Saunders, 1997, Cancer Nursing, 20, p. 173. Copyright 1997 by Lippincott Williams & Wilkins. Adapted with permission.

thoroughly as antidepressants, but small studies indicate its usefulness for rapidly reducing symptoms and increasing appetite, which could be very important in a severely inhibiting depression (Breitbart, Rosenfeld, Kaim, & Funesti-Esch, 2001).

All antidepressants need to be prescribed in adequate dosages and administered over the proper amount of time required for them to take effect. Depressed people might need encouragement to comply with the treatment regimen if they are feeling excessively hopeless and helpless. One guideline is that a medication should be reconsidered or augmented if no improvement has occurred after 12 weeks (Pignone et al., 2002). Physicians who are not educated in psychopharmacology risk undertreating patients who are depressed. With psychotherapy and psychopharmacologic interventions, evaluation of the efficacy of treatment should be continuous.

Oncology nurses who are in frequent contact with their patients are in a prime position to identify emotional issues, support positive behaviors, assist in mobilizing support systems, and restore hope. A treatment plan should include not only the establishment of a trusting and caring relationship but also the facilitation of additional help when it is needed.

Assessment and Intervention for Suicide

The topic of suicide is one that nurses often are reluctant to address, partially because of cultural taboos about the topic and also because of lack of confidence in exploring such an emotionally charged topic. Table 15-2 summarizes nurses' difficulties in responding to suicidal patients. Screening tools can help clinicians to demonstrate concern about another person's behavior and exercise diligence to foresee and prevent suicide (Sheeran & Zimmerman, 2002). Clinicians meet the standard of care by showing adherence to the assessment, screening, treatment, and management strategies that a reasonably prudent clinician would exercise under similar circumstances (Bongar et al., 1998). Commonly used screening tools include the Hopelessness Scale (Beck, Weissman, Lester, & Trexler, 1974), the Index of Potential Suicide (Zung, 1974), the Reasons for Living Inventory, the Suicide Probability Scale (Cull & Gill, 1982), and the Suicide Risk Measure (Plutchik, van Praag, Conte, & Picard, 1989).

Clues that a patient is thinking of suicide may be written or spoken. In the words of one patient, "I don't know; I am so tired of all this; I should just jump out of this window!" Other clues may be more subtle, such as jokes or offhand remarks that indicate giving up, lack of hope, or feelings of worthlessness. In an assessment, nurses must ask directly about suicidal thoughts (e.g., "Have you been thinking at all about wanting to kill yourself?"). If the patient responds affirmatively, nurses should use follow-up questions to determine the immediacy and lethality of the plans, as well as to offer the patient a chance to vent about what is going on that would cause such desperation (e.g., "What has been going on that has made you feel like that is a good alternative?"; "Have you thought about how you would do it?"). If the patient has a specific method in mind, the nurse needs to find out how realistic that plan is for follow-through. For example, if the patient imagines shooting him- or herself, nurses should determine whether the patient has access to a gun. If the patient is considering taking pills, their availability should be elicited (e.g., "Have prescriptions for antidepressants or pain

Table 15-2. Nurses' Difficulties in Responding to Suicidal Patients

Category	Nurses' Comments	Implications for Practice
Religious, spiritual, or other values about suicide	Religious beliefs are antisuicide. Topic is taboo in society. Religious convictions—suicide is wrong, a mortal sin. "It's a coward's way out."	Seek consultation. Clarify and discuss your values/feelings; examine your professional role versus personal values. Provide unbiased care; find ways to evaluate risk and act. Distinguish personal values from professional duty.
Uncomfortable feelings or fears (e.g., failure to prevent suicide)	Fear of failure: "If the patient commits suicide, did I do enough?" Fear of feeling helpless Fear of inadequate response Fear of not being able to care for the patient's needs that are not being met	Recognize that fear is a common response. Know that as part of a team, your duty is to detect, evaluate, take action, get help, and notify the healthcare team. Do not let fears prevent assessment. Provide high-quality care, but recognize that not every suicide will be prevented.
Inadequate skills, knowledge, and experience	Do not want to say the wrong thing Unsure of ability to help Uncertainty of own skill/knowledge to assess risk Frustration with inability to convince patient that he or she is needed and loved Failure—"I may not be able to fix things. I'm not a psychiatrist, and I don't have skills to deal with this." Do not know what to say "How can I impact one who is so troubled?"	Recognize feelings. Do not avoid assessment. Improve knowledge/skills. Use consultation. Acknowledge that your task is not to "fix things" or be the expert. Say to patient, "I care about your pain and distress and want to make sure you get the treatment you need. We need to talk about this, make sure you are safe, and consult with our team of experts."
Personal experiences with a loved one's suicide	"Because of a chronic illness, my parent committed suicide when I was young." "My young brother impulsively committed suicide."	Seek consultation to help to resolve your painful loss. Detect risk and get support and consultation for the patient.
Weight of professional responsibility	Not wanting to get involved but knowing that you already are Fear of not having the best response Feeling responsible for patient's reaction Tension in medical, legal, and ethical duties	Seek consultation or case consultation to discuss duties and to plan care. Clarify duty and roles. (You are not responsible for the patient's action. Your duty is to detect, assess, monitor risk, take action, and notify the healthcare team.)

Note. From "Management of Suicidal Patients" (p. 563), by S.M. Valente in A.W. Burgess (Ed.), *Psychiatric Nursing: Promoting Mental Health,* 1997, Stamford, CT: Appleton and Lange. Copyright 1997 by Appleton and Lange. Adapted with permission.

medications been filled?"). If the patient describes a clear method, the nurse should continue to find out how intent the patient is on following through with the plan. If a lethal plan is in place with high intent and availability of the method, a psychiatric consultation should be obtained immediately. Nurses can make a contract with the patient to not follow through with the plan or to seek professional help if feelings reach an overwhelming point. Although research does not show the benefit of a contract in reducing suicide risk, it may be useful in assessment. Within the context of a trusting and caring relationship, the existence of a contract may keep a person from self-harm. No guarantee exists, however, and clinicians must use their judgment to determine the person's ability to keep a contract. Manipulative or angry patients might not be able to follow through with a stated plan and may need more intensive precautions, such as a suicide watch. Inpatient psychiatric treatment might be indicated. No nurse should feel entirely responsible for a suicidal patient. The nurse should seek agency resources and develop a care plan with a team of caregivers (professionals and significant others).

Interventions should include assisting patients in mobilizing their own support systems that might be unused because of feelings of "being stuck" or an unwillingness to ask for help. Assisting patients to take action of any kind is immensely helpful in restoring a sense of control and mastery of the situation. A suicide hot line number or a list of people to call must be available to patients. Clinicians should explain clearly that suicide cannot be an automatic solution to the problem, and interventions to improve symptom relief, quality of life, and depression should be considered. A danger lies in patients assuming that no solution exists and that the request to die is rational. Patients' hopelessness can spread to the caregivers unless they understand that the depression is not inevitable and can be lessened. See Figure 15-2 for a summary of clinical guidelines for suicide.

A significant number of patients with cancer who decide to attempt suicide base their decision on a lack of relief from unrelenting physical symptoms (Foley, 1991). The risk of suicide in patients with pancreatic, head and neck, and gastrointestinal cancers is higher than that of patients with other cancers (Holland, 2002). In Oregon, terminally ill patients have had the right to hasten death by physician-assisted suicide (PAS) since 1997 (Oregon Department of Human Services, 2003). In 2003, 42 deaths resulted from PAS (up from 38 in 2002). A total of 171 deaths occurred from 1997–2003. The most frequent underlying disease has been end-stage amyotrophic lateral sclerosis. In 2003, the most frequent motivations for PAS requests were loss of autonomy (93%), decreasing ability to participate in activities that make life enjoyable (93%), and loss of dignity (82%). Ninety-three percent of these patients were enrolled in hospice programs. The prescribing physician was present at the death in 29% of the cases (Oregon Department of Human Services).

Major assessment and treatment of patients considering suicide must focus on relief of physical symptoms so that the quality of life can improve. Referrals can be made to pain specialists, oncologists, palliative care, and hospice organizations.

Suicide might appear to be a good option when a person fears becoming a burden to others, especially if caregivers, loved ones, and even nurses have subtly or inadvertently communicated their tiredness and impatience. Sometimes called a "duty to die," patients may interpret the behavior of others to mean "everyone would be better off if I were dead." Patients must address their feelings of being a burden. Family members might be in relationships that make clearly stating one's thoughts and feelings difficult. Providing emotional support, recommending resources for

Figure 15-2. Clinical Practice Guidelines for Suicide

Assessment

- Perform close nonjudgmental monitoring of all suicidal cognitions and emotions (e.g., thought, hopelessness, depression).
- Monitor with objective measures (e.g., Beck Depression, Beck Hopelessness Scale).
- Complete a detailed history of prescribed and other medications, drugs, and alcohol consumption.
- Determine whether the patient can cope with current distress or crisis without hospitalization.
- Understand why the person is feeling suicidal now and what has increased the risk.

Specific indicators of significant suicidal risk

1. High suicide level/intent or significant acute risk
   - Specificity of method
   - Plan for actual attempt
   - Low impulse control
   - Desire to attempt
   - Absence of deterrents
   - Absence of environmental support or pressure/antagonism from significant others
   - New, pronounced life stressors
   - Overt verbalizations of above
2. Sudden increase/recurrence of significant suicidal ideas
3. Evidence of recent attempts or indications of imminence
4. Strong positive history of attempts; appears increasingly depressed (or elated) when experiencing unusual external stress

Management

- Ask directly and fully about suicidal issues; evaluate frequently and regularly.
- Evaluate rationality of choices.
- Recommend consultation or referral to psychiatric consultant.
- Discuss the situation with psychiatric liaison consultant.
- Ensure that treatment (e.g., antidepressant drugs, doses, length of time on drug) follows standards of care for treatment of depression.
- Detect signs that suicidal impulses are becoming more intense.
- Intervene to support the patient's power, control, sense of esteem, and coping strategies.
- Treat and reduce symptom distress, pain, depression, or dementia.
- Challenge sense of hopelessness, and improve resources.
- Expand social network, reduce isolation, and involve significant others.
- Reduce powerlessness and hopelessness.
- Advocate for increased pain and symptom management.

For imminent suicidal emergency

- Focus on the immediate perceptions of the patient and the goal of the suicidal behavior.
- Institute suicide precautions, and improve safety: Consider hospitalization for acute crisis when choice is not rational or provide supervision at home, and reduce access to suicide methods (e.g., have medications supervised, remove other methods).
- Seek consultation regarding management and bioethical dilemmas.
- Document thorough neurobehavioral, mental status, and suicide assessment.
- Document rationale for treatment decisions.

Note. From "Suicide and HIV Disease" (p. 277), by S.M. Valente and J.M. Saunders in W. van Gorp and S. Buckingham (Eds.), *Practitioner's Guide to the Neuropsychiatry Complications of HIV/AIDS,* 1998, New York: Guilford Press. Copyright 1998 by Guilford Press. Adapted with permission.

help at home, or addressing financial constraints can create much-needed relief for caregivers.

Rational Suicide

It might be assumed that verbalizing a wish to die represents a request for a "rational" suicide. However, Valente and Trainor (1998) referred to suicide as rational when it is carried out by someone with a realistic assessment of the situation, unimpaired mental processes, and an understandable motive. Figure 15-3 summarizes suggestions for evaluation of rational suicide. These questions can help oncology nurses to begin the sensitive dialogue to determine what is behind a desire to die. Today's trend toward societal acceptance of suicide as a choice for the terminally ill also may be a factor (Suarez-Almazor, 2002; Valente & Saunders, 1997). What is important to remember is that most suicides involving patients with cancer are associated with undiagnosed and untreated depression or confusional states and poorly managed

---

Figure 15-3. Questions That Help Clinicians to Evaluate Rational Suicide

1. Is the patient making a request for help? Is it a request for help in committing suicide—either in obtaining the means for suicide or in carrying out the act? Is it a request for help in justifying the suicide to others? Is it a request for help in avoiding a suicide one has already decided to commit?
2. Why is the patient consulting a health professional?
3. What has kept the patient from attempting or committing suicide so far? Is it fear of death or fear of violent means of death that discourages such action?
4. Is the request for help in suicide a request for someone else to decide?
5. How stable and consistent with the patient's values is the request?
6. How far in the future would the suicide take place?
7. Are the medical and nonmedical facts cited in the request accurate? Specifically, is the diagnosis accurate? What confirmation of the diagnosis does he or she have? What about the prognosis? How secure is it? Has an independent second or third opinion been obtained? Does the patient accurately understand treatment options for future stages of terminal illness (e.g., pain control in terminal cancer)?
8. Is the suicide plan financially motivated?
9. Has the patient considered the effects of suicide on other people? Has the patient considered possible emotional trauma to survivors? What about the stigma associated with suicide?
10. Does the patient fear becoming a burden?
11. What cultural influences are shaping the patient's choice?
12. Are the patient's affairs in order?
13. Has the patient picked a method of committing suicide?
14. Would the patient be willing to tell others about the suicide plan? Would he or she be willing to confide the plan to friends?
15. Does the patient see suicide as the only way out? Does he or she have an alternative plan for coping with terminal illness, and, if so, how realistic is this plan?
16. Does the patient have a hopeless condition?
17. Has the patient made the decision to commit suicide without coercion from others?
18. Has the person demonstrated the use of a sound decision-making process (e.g., mentally competent, nonimpulsive consideration of alternatives, congruence between suicide and personal values, consideration of impact on others, consultation with significant others)?

Note. From "Rational Suicide: How Can We Respond to a Request for Help?" by M.P. Battin, 1991, *Crisis, 12*(2), pp. 74–77. Copyright 1991 by Hogrefe and Huber Publishers. Reprinted with permission.

---

pain (Breitbart, 1993; Meier, Emmons, Litke, Wallenstein, & Morrison, 2003). Suicide might be one of several options patients consider in an attempt to gain control of a seemingly uncontrollable situation (Valente & Saunders, 1997).

Avoiding countertransference responses is important for professional caregivers. These responses occur when healthcare professionals' personal beliefs impede caregiving. Nurses have reported that countertransference responses can impede their assessments of, interventions for, and relationships with patients. For example, oncology nurses have reported that feelings about their own loved one's suicide make it difficult for them to care for patients who are suicidal. Other nurses reported difficulty evaluating suicidal patients because of personal values that forbid suicide (Valente & Saunders, 1997). Such responses might manifest in overidentifying with a suicidal patient (Rudestam, 1993) and then reacting to the patient as one did in the personal experience. Nurses should be able to reflect on their personal reactions and make a clear boundary between that experience and that of the patient. With separateness, yet empathy for the patient's experience, nurses can keep a line of communication open and encourage patients to say what *they* are thinking and share what *they* are feeling (Valente & Saunders, 1997).

Evidence-Based Practice

Depression has been studied extensively. Twenty-five percent of patients with cancer suffer from depression (Martin & Jackson, 2000). Because evidence suggests that people with depression have poorer outcomes from their physical illness than their counterparts who are not depressed, effective assessment and treatment are essential (Devine & Westlake, 1995). Because physicians and nurses may not always detect depression, objectives tools such as the HADS, the Beck Depression Inventory, and the Hamilton Rating Scale should be incorporated into the assessment process (Martin & Jackson; Passik et al., 2002). Studies have shown that a history of depression increases the risk for recurrent depression (APA, 2000; Pignone et al., 2002). Likewise, a history of a suicide attempt greatly increases the risk for subsequent attempts (Valente & Saunders, 1997). This information is key for professionals to incorporate into a thorough psychosocial history and assessment as part of the cancer care treatment plan (see Figure 15-4).

Figure 15-4. Plan of Care

Assessment
- Identify presence of risk factors for depression and suicide.
- Determine previous coping methods.
- Identify the meaning of the illness to the patient.
- Consider confounding factors (e.g., illness, medications).
- Identify physical and emotional symptoms of depression.
- Explore degree and duration of symptoms.

(Continued on next page)

Figure 15-4. Plan of Care *(Continued)*

Nursing Diagnoses (NANDA International, 2005)
- Powerlessness
- Ineffective coping
- Dysfunctional grieving
- Spiritual distress
- Risk for self-directed violence
- Disturbed thought processes

***DSM-IV-TR* Diagnoses** (American Psychiatric Association, 2000)
- Major depressive disorder
- Mood disorder due to a general medical condition
- Cognitive mental disorder due to a general medical condition

Expected Outcomes
- Patients will experience an increased sense of control and self-efficacy.
- Patients will verbalize hope about quality of life and current relationships.
- Patients will name at least three sources of support for emotional and physical needs.
- Patients will replace automatic negative thoughts and distortions with two or three alternative explanations.

Interventions
- Correct cognitive distortions by discussing irrational thoughts and automatic and negative thinking patterns.
- Offer support.
- Assist in setting attainable goals.
- Encourage maximum possible participation in self-care activities.
- Mobilize support systems, including family, friends, professionals, and spiritual leaders.
- Alleviate physical suffering and physical symptoms that impede the quality of life.
- Use a therapeutic relationship to facilitate dialogue, venting, and exploration of feelings and thoughts.
- In moderate to severe cases of depression or cases of attempted suicide, refer for psychiatric consultation for psychotherapy or pharmacologic interventions.
- Refer for pain management, social support, pastoral counseling, or hospice care as appropriate.
- Create and monitor no-suicide contracts as needed.
- Refer for music or other adjunctive therapies (e.g., self-hypnosis, positive thinking, problem solving).

Case Study

Mr. Lin, a divorced, 53-year-old lawyer, was diagnosed with a high-grade non-Hodgkin lymphoma. His treatment began with a course of combination chemotherapy. Initially, he read literature, participated in treatments, asked questions, and explored alternative treatments. He focused his energy on getting through the treatments. He had no previous psychiatric or substance abuse history. Mr. Lin was not in contact with his three children or members of his immediate family. In the past, Mr. Lin enjoyed tennis, kickboxing, and running and said this was how he had relieved tension. He occasionally had a glass of wine and very rarely took diazepam. He denied having any religious beliefs or spiritual values.

(Continued on next page)

Case Study *(Continued)*

After starting chemotherapy with methotrexate, doxorubicin, cyclophosphamide, vincristine, and high-dose prednisone, he complained of increasing fatigue, nausea, anorexia, insomnia, and headaches. He became more inactive and indecisive. He hated the uncertainty and worried about treatment failure. Mr. Lin stated, "Being a patient on chemotherapy outweighs the rest of my life. I am afraid it will not work." He complained of restlessness, irritability, and trouble concentrating and remembering things. "I wake up terrified and in tears. My sense of humor is gone. I'm not one to talk about myself, so I don't tell people I have cancer. I do not want to burden them or my family." He shared that he felt worthless and guilty about his divorce. He wondered if death was the only escape from his misery. After the nurse asked if he was considering suicide, he admitted that he had thought of jumping from his fourth-floor window.

During one course of chemotherapy, the nurse inquired about depressive symptoms and feelings, social support, and stress management. Mr. Lin responded, "Asians don't complain. I've avoided family for years after my shameful divorce." Further inquiry revealed that most of his depressive symptoms (e.g., sadness, anhedonia, slowed behavior, thoughts of death, insomnia, suicidal impulses) began two months ago after the initiation of two new chemotherapy agents and prednisone. The accompanying fatigue prevented his participation in competitive sports. He said, "I feel terrible; I'll probably stop chemo; it is no use."

The nurse suspected a major depressive episode and suicidal impulses caused by chemotherapy and prednisone. Initial goals were to prevent suicide and reduce depressive symptoms by having Mr. Lin express his depressive feelings and thoughts, begin antidepressant therapy, reduce negative thinking patterns, increase social support, reduce powerlessness, improve knowledge of treatment, increase his control/participation in treatment, and improve stress management. After requesting a psychiatric consultation and antidepressants, the nurse taught Mr. Lin about depression, lymphoma, treatment goals, and plans. She emphasized that depression is treatable, may be precipitated by cancer drugs, and may lessen after at least three to four weeks of antidepressants. She gave him literature about reducing depression by cognitive (reducing negative thinking) and emotional strategies. Although Mr. Lin was not religious and did not want psychotherapy, he agreed to meet once with an Asian counselor/chaplain and to tell the nurse about his feelings of worthlessness, suicide, guilt, and depression. Mr. Lin made a no-suicide contract but refused to participate in a cancer support group or take advantage of other resources. He likes music, however, and agreed to talk with the music therapist and possibly explore meditation or hypnosis for stress. Mr. Lin refused to discuss contacting his immediate family but agreed to contact a cousin and one old law school friend.

Discussion

Initial goals were met as Mr. Lin expressed his feelings, remained free of suicidal acts, learned about depression, and participated in treatment. Music therapy, the Asian counselor, and the literature on cognitive strategies helped to reduce

(Continued on next page)

Case Study *(Continued)*

his fears, guilt, and stress. After four weeks of antidepressant therapy, Mr. Lin's depressive symptoms, negativity, and hopelessness were lessened, and his sense of humor was reappearing. Writing a journal about his experiences and using meditation have been very helpful. His suicidal impulses have faded.

The nurse's invitation to talk about himself gave Mr. Lin permission to share his concerns and to reveal possible sources of support. Because Mr. Lin identified himself as stoic ("Asians don't complain"), the nurse might have been tempted to support his avoidance and not attempt to encourage him to talk about his experience. However, the nurse did probe, and, in the course of the development of the relationship, Mr. Lin was able to discuss the things that were important to him. The nurse's acknowledgment of how that might not be easy to do conveyed a sense of empathy that was crucial to Mr. Lin, who otherwise was cut off from close contact with others. Mr. Lin's willingness to explore new coping mechanisms was crucial and required that he felt he was being heard and that someone was concerned for his safety. As the level of trust between Mr. Lin and the nurse increased, he became open to the nurse's suggestions about counseling, the use of music therapy and medications, and contacting a chaplain, a cousin, and an old friend. Ongoing evaluation of each of these approaches was made jointly by Mr. Lin and the nurse. Empowering Mr. Lin with choices, respecting his desire to be self-sufficient, and increasing his understanding of his treatments were actions of the nurse that led to a desirable outcome.

Conclusion

Patients with cancer are more likely than the general population to become depressed and suicidal. Depression often is undetected or undertreated because of the assumption that it is normal following a diagnosis of cancer or that, to some healthcare professionals and loved ones, suicide might be a rational choice. Interventions, including psychotherapy, medications, education, and self-care skill attainment, can relieve clinical depression in patients with cancer. Oncology nurses need to become adept in accurately identifying patients at risk for depression and suicide. They need to be aware of their own attitudes about suicide and depression so that they can be effective in listening, interviewing, supporting, and planning care.

References

Akechi, T., Nakano, T., Akizuki, N., Okamura, M., Sakuma, K., Nakanishi, T., et al. (2003). Somatic symptoms for diagnosing major depression in cancer patients. *Psychosomatics, 44,* 244–248.

American Psychiatric Association. (2000). *Diagnostic and statistical manual of mental disorders* (4th ed., text rev.). Washington, DC: Author.

Baile, W.F., Gilbertini, M., Scott, L., & Endicott, J. (1992). Depression and tumor stage in cancer of the head and neck. *Psycho-Oncology, 1,* 15–24.

Beck, A.T., Rush, A.J., Shaw, B.F., & Emery, G. (1979). *Cognitive therapy of depression*. New York: Guilford Press.

Beck, A.T., Weissman, A., Lester, D., & Trexler, L. (1974). The measurement of pessimism: The Hopelessness Scale. *Journal of Consulting and Clinical Psychology, 42,* 861–865.

Bishop, S.R., & Warr, D. (2003). Coping, catastrophizing and chronic pain in breast cancer. *Journal of Behavioral Medicine, 26,* 265–281.

Bongar, B., Berman, A.L., Maris, R.W., Silverman, M.M., Harris, E.A., & Packman, W.L. (1998). *Risk management with suicidal patients*. New York: Guilford Press.

Bredart, A., Cayrou, S., & Dolbreault, S. (2002). Re: Systematic review of psychological therapies for cancer patients: Overview and recommendations for future research. *Journal of the National Cancer Institute, 94,* 1810–1811.

Breitbart, W. (1993). Suicide risk and pain in cancer and AIDS patients. In C.R. Chapman & K.M. Foley (Eds.), *Current and emerging issues in cancer pain research and practice: The Bristol-Myers Squibb Symposium on Pain Research* (pp. 49–65). New York: Raven Press.

Breitbart, W., Rosenfeld, B., Kaim, M., & Funesti-Esch, J. (2001). A randomized, double-blind, placebo-controlled trial of psychostimulants for the treatment of fatigue in ambulatory patients with human immunodeficiency virus disease. *Archives of Internal Medicine, 161,* 411–420.

Carroll, B.T., Kathol, R.G., Noyes, R., Jr., Wald, T.G., & Clamon, G.H. (1993). Screening for depression and anxiety in cancer patients using the hospital anxiety and depression scale. *General Hospital Psychiatry, 15,* 69–74.

Cassem, E.H. (1995). Depressive disorders in the medically ill: An overview. *Psychosomatics, 36*(2), S2–S10.

Cavanaugh, S., Clark, D.C., & Gibbons, R.D. (1983). Diagnosing depression in the hospitalized medically ill. *Psychosomatics, 24,* 809–815.

Chaturvedi, S.K., & Maguire, G.P. (1998). Persistent somatization in cancer: A controlled follow-up study. *Journal of Psychosomatic Research, 45,* 249–256.

Cull, J.G., & Gill, W.S. (1982). *Suicide Probability Scale manual*. Los Angeles: Western Psychological Services.

Degner, L.F. (2003). A new approach to eliciting the meaning in the context of breast cancer. *Cancer Nursing, 26,* 169–178.

Devine, E.C., & Westlake, S.K. (1995). The effects of psychoeducational care provided to adults with cancer: Meta-analysis of 116 studies. *Oncology Nursing Forum, 22,* 1369–1381.

Ersek, M., Kagawa-Singer, M., & Barnes, D. (1998). Multicultural considerations in the use of advance directives. *Oncology Nursing Forum, 25,* 1683–1690.

Foley, K.M. (1991). The relationship of pain and symptom management to patient requests for physician assisted suicide. *Journal of Pain and Symptom Management, 6,* 289–297.

Given, C.W., Stommel, M., Given, B., Osuch, J., Kurtz, M.E., & Kurtz, J.C. (1993). The influence of cancer patients' symptoms and functional states on patients' depression and family caregivers' reaction and depression. *Health Psychology, 12,* 277–285.

Holland, J.C. (2002). History of psycho-oncology: Overcoming attitudinal and conceptual barriers. *Psychosomatic Medicine, 64,* 206–221.

Hybels, C.F., & Blazer, D.G. (2003). Epidemiology of late-life disorders. *Clinics in Geriatric Medicine, 19,* 663–696.

Lampic, C., von Essen, L., Peterson, V.W., Larsson, G., & Sjoden, P. (1996). Anxiety and depression in hospitalized patients with cancer: Agreement in patient-staff dyads. *Cancer Nursing, 19,* 419–428.

Lovejoy, N.C., Tabor, D., & Deloney, P. (2000). Cancer-related depression: Part II—Neurologic alterations and evolving approaches to psychopharmacology. *Oncology Nursing Forum, 27,* 795–808.

Lovejoy, N.C., Tabor, D., Matteis, M., & Lillis, P. (2000). Cancer-related depression: Part I—Neurologic alterations and cognitive-behavioral therapy. *Oncology Nursing Forum, 27,* 667–678.

Martin, A.C., & Jackson, K.C. (2000). Depression in palliative care patients. *Journal of Pharmaceutical Care in Pain and Symptom Control, 7,* 71–89.

McDonald, M., Passik, S.D., Dugan, W., & Rosenfeld, B. (1999). RN recognition of depression in patients with cancer. *Oncology Nursing Forum, 21,* 493–499.

Meier, D.E., Emmons, C., Litke, A., Wallenstein, S., & Morrison, R.S. (2003). Characteristics of patients requesting and receiving physician-assisted death. *Archives of Internal Medicine, 163,* 1537–1542.

Mouton, C.P. (2000). Cultural and religious issues. In K.L. Braun, J.H. Pietsch, & P.L. Blanchette (Eds.), *Cultural issues in end-of-life decision making* (pp. 71–82). Thousand Oaks, CA: Sage.

Musselman, D.L., Lawson, D.H., Gummick, J.F., Manatunga, A.K., Penna, S., Gondkin, R.S., et al. (2001). Paroxetine for the prevention of depression induced by high-dose interferon-alfa. *New England Journal of Medicine, 344,* 961–966.

NANDA International. (2005). *Nursing diagnoses: Definitions and classification, 2005–2006.* Philadelphia: Author.

Oregon Department of Human Services. (2003). *Death with Dignity annual report, 2003.* Retrieved May 3, 2004, from http://www.dhs.state.or.us/publichealth/chs/pas/ar-index.cfm

Passik, S.D., Kirsh, K.L., Theobald, D., Donaghy, K., Holtsclaw, E., Edgerton, S., et al. (2002). Use of a depression screening tool and a fluoxetine-based algorithm to improve the recognition and treatment of depression in cancer patients: A demonstration project. *Journal of Pain and Symptom Management, 24,* 318–327.

Patrick, D.L., Ferketich, S.L., Frame, P.S., Harris, J.J., Hendricks, C.B., Levin, B., et al. (2003). National Institutes of Health State-of-the-Science Conference Statement: Symptom management in cancer: Pain, depression, and fatigue. *Journal of the National Cancer Institute, 95,* 1110–1117.

Pignone, M., Gaynes, B.N., Rushton, J.L., Mulrow, C.D., Orleans, C.T., Whitener, B.L., et al. (2002). *Screening for depression. Systematic evidence review No. 6* (Prepared by the Research Triangle Institute—University of North Carolina Evidence-Based Practice Center under contract no. 290-97-0011). AHRQ Publication No. 02-S002. Rockville, MD: Agency for Healthcare Research and Quality.

Plutchik, R., van Praag, H.M., Conte, H.R., & Picard, S. (1989). Correlates of suicide and violence risk. 1: The Suicide Risk Measure. *Comprehensive Psychiatry, 30,* 296–302.

Rudestam, K. (1993). Comment of the case consultation Nicole: Suicide and terminal illness. *Suicide and Life-Threatening Behavior, 23,* 76–82.

Schwartz, L., Lander, M., & Chochinov, H.M. (2002). Current management of depression in cancer patients: Article review. *Oncology, 16,* 1110, 1114–1115.

Sheeran, T., & Zimmerman, M. (2002). Case identification of depression with self-report questionnaires. *Psychiatry Research, 109,* 51–59.

Suarez-Almazor, M.E. (2002). Attitudes of terminally ill cancer patients about euthanasia and assisted suicide: Predominance of psychosocial determinants and beliefs over symptom distress and subsequent survival. *Journal of Clinical Oncology, 20,* 2134–2141.

Valente, S.M. (2004). End-of-life challenges: Honoring autonomy. *Cancer Nursing, 27,* 314–319.

Valente, S.M. (in press-a). Oncology nurses teaching and support for suicidal patients. *Journal of Psychosocial Oncology.*

Valente, S.M. (in press-b). Self-rating instruments for depression and suicide. *Journal of Psychosocial and Mental Health Nursing.*

Valente, S.M., & Saunders, J.M. (1997). Diagnosis and treatment of major depression among people with cancer. *Cancer Nursing, 20,* 168–177.

Valente, S.M., & Saunders, J.M. (2000). Oncology nurses' difficulties with suicide. *Medicine and Law, 19,* 793–814.

Valente, S.M., & Trainor, D. (1998). Rational suicide among terminally ill patients. *Association of Operating Room Nurses Journal, 68*(2), 1–10.

Valentine, A.D. (2003). Cancer pain and depression: Management of the dual-diagnosed patient. *Current Pain and Headache Reports, 7,* 262–269.

Weishaar, M.E., & Beck, A.T. (1992). Clinical and cognitive predictors of suicide. In R.W. Maris, A.L. Berman, J.T. Maltsberger, & R. Yufit (Eds.), *Assessment and prediction of suicide* (pp. 457–484). New York: Guilford Press.

Williams, M.L., & Payne, S. (2003). A qualitative study of clinical nurse specialists' views on depression in palliative care patients. *Palliative Medicine, 17,* 334–338.

Zung, W. (1974). Index of Potential Suicide (IPS): A rating scale for suicide prevention. In A.T. Beck, H.L.P. Resnick, & D.J. Lettieri (Eds.), *The prediction of suicide* (pp. 221–249). Bowie, MD: Charles Press.

CHAPTER 16

Denial

Linda M. Gorman, RN, MN, APRN, BC, OCN®, CHPN

A great deal of intelligence can be invested in ignorance when the need for illusion is deep.

—Saul Bellow

Faced with a diagnosis of cancer, people initially may react with numb disbelief and an inability to make a decision about a treatment plan. At the time of diagnosis of metastasis, a family member may try to persuade the patient to refuse therapy because of the belief that the patient really does not have cancer. A patient who is dying may refuse home hospice care because he or she plans to "beat this thing." All of these scenarios exemplify varying degrees of denial. Although extensive literature related to this subject exists, the concept of denial remains confusing and elusive. Denial sometimes is called "hope," "wisdom," "confusion," "avoidance," "escape," and "misinformation" (Kreitler, 1999).

Strictly speaking, denial is a form of self-deception. It is a defense against anxiety because of a threat. Individuals minimize or disavow thoughts or feelings related to this threat to protect themselves from intolerable ideas, wishes, deeds, feelings, and situations (Levine, Rudy, & Kerns, 1994). Rousseau (2000) defined denial as an unconscious mechanism aimed at negating a disease-oriented threat to the integrity of personhood and daily life. Psychoanalysts have identified denial as a primitive defense that is basically pathologic. Freud (1952) extended the concept of denial, which she viewed as a characteristic and normal defense of childhood, and suggested that its use may not always be pathologic in adults. Today, it is well accepted that denial may be pathologic, but it is more often a useful and healthy initial response to a crisis.

Denial is a diverse and complex set of mental processes, cognitions, and behaviors. Kreitler (1999) reported that denial is basically a cognitive strategy that is applied in a partial or selective manner and constitutes a part of the overall coping effort. In psychiatric literature, denial traditionally has been described as an unconscious defense mechanism in which the individual disavows threatening aspects of reality as a way to reduce anxiety (Sadock, 2005). In recent years, mental health professionals have expanded the concept of denial and no longer consider it to always be an unconscious process (Greer, 1992). However, Greer noted that in clinical practice, the important factor is not whether denial is conscious or unconscious but, rather, the degree of denial the person shows and its consequences.

Vachon (1998) differentiated between denial and avoidance. Denial is unconscious in her view, whereas avoidance is a conscious defense mechanism reflecting an effort to shun circumstances that bring up stressful material.

At times, individuals' cultural beliefs or language barriers can mimic denial. Some cultures may have taboos against mentioning a certain disease, so patients may appear to be in denial when, in reality, they simply do not believe in acknowledging the condition verbally. Many cultures (e.g., Asian, Middle Eastern, Eastern European) have certain taboos, particularly about acknowledging cancer. Also, if a person has not been given a diagnosis in a way he or she can understand, his or her reaction may be wrongly assessed as denial (Vachon, 1998) (see Chapter 6).

Families may go to great lengths to avoid letting the patient hear the word "cancer," and this easily could be misidentified as denial. If a language barrier exists, patients could act as if they understood the information when, in reality, they did not comprehend the implications. Patients might not react as expected and then could be mistakenly labeled as being in denial.

Important Principles About Denial

Denial as an initial response to bad news is considered to be a normal and adaptive response to any loss (Kreitler, 1999; Stephenson, 2004). Hearing that a breast lump is malignant or that a loved one suddenly has died may represent such overwhelming stress to individuals that blocking it out becomes a protective mechanism. In this way, denial protects the integrity of self-concept by distorting reality in a self-enhancing way. It promotes a sense of mastery and control that, in turn, leads to lowered anxiety, which may enhance decision making under stress (Russell, 1993). Using the examples stated earlier, patients may demonstrate denial by refusing to believe what the doctor is saying, showing no emotional reaction, or disavowing knowledge of what the doctor has told them. Denial functions as a positive reaction because, initially, the person's coping resources are insufficient to adequately deal with the stress. Minutes, hours, or days later, when the individual has had an opportunity to develop some coping resources, he or she usually will begin to face the meaning of the information. During this time, individuals can gain a sense of control that can inhibit the very distressing feelings of powerlessness. Denial can be intermittent as individuals have brief periods of awareness of a painful reality and then a short time later deny its existence. Clinically, it has been documented that at least transient denial is common in individuals facing a life-threatening illness (Rousseau, 2000).

Continuation of denial over a long period of time usually is considered to be maladaptive because the psychic energy required to maintain the defense becomes a physical and emotional drain that can have a negative impact on individuals (Kreitler, 1999). Individuals who maintain a strong denial defense over months or even years most likely are exhibiting a pathologic process because they never are able to attain a sense of mastery over the loss. Nevertheless, for some, ongoing denial may be the only way to maintain functioning.

The circumstances under which people use denial will determine its positive or negative value. For example, avoiding treatment for a skin lesion or breast lump for months could be life-threatening. In these situations, denial not only shields the person from facing the possible meaning of the lesion but also becomes destructive because treatment is delayed. In contrast, refusing to believe a terminal prognosis may allow the patient to maintain hope and feel less anxious. Appearing cheerful or emotionally detached but still pursuing cancer treatment would not have life-threatening implications and may help the person to cope.

Denial related to illness exist in two forms (Minarek, 1996). **Affective** denial is when individuals deny anxiety or other painful feelings about the illness. With **cognitive** (or factual) denial, individuals deny specific information about the nature or severity of the illness. See Table 16-1 for examples of affective and cognitive denial.

Table 16-1. Examples of Affective and Cognitive Denial

Type of Denial	Examples	Mechanism
Affective	"I'm not scared." "I know the cancer is spreading, but I'm not upset about it."	Individual acknowledges threat but disavows anxiety and anger.
Cognitive	"I've always been healthy, so I don't need to quit smoking."	Individual acknowledges threat but denies that it applies to himself or herself.
	"I can wait six months to see a doctor for this lump."	Individual acknowledges threat but convinces himself or herself that it is not an immediate personal threat.
	"I don't need to follow up with the doctor's office. They'll call me if there's a problem."	Individual projects responsibility onto others as a way to avoid dealing with the threat.
	"A lot of people have cancer, and they don't die. Neither will I."	Individual acknowledges information but disavows threat.
	"The doctor said I have a lump but not cancer."	Individual is unable to acknowledge any information, so he or she is able to completely block out what the doctor said.

Denial and Illness

Much of the early clinical research related to denial has been conducted on patients with cardiac disease (Hackett, Cassem, & Wishnie, 1968; Levine et al., 1987; Lowery, 1991). Denial was found to keep a patient's heart rate and blood pressure lower following myocardial infarction; patients who are flooded with fear of the implications of their condition have a higher heart rate and blood pressure. "Deniers" were identified as individuals who were able to admit having had a heart attack but described little awareness of fear. At the other extreme, however, were patients who did not seek treatment for chest pain (calling it indigestion) or who were found doing push-ups in the coronary care unit. The initial research by Hackett et al. (1968) revealed that denial reduces distress following a heart attack, deniers resumed work and sexual activity sooner than nondeniers, and denial may be associated with lower mortality following a heart attack. Although these results have never been replicated, they have stimulated interest in this topic related to other illnesses, including cancer. More recent studies (McKinley, Moser, & Dracup, 2000; Zerwic & Ryan, 2004) continue to find that denial in the presence of cardiac symptoms is common. Carney, Fitzsimons, and Dempster (2002) found that previous experience with heart disease was not a predictor of seeking help within 60 minutes of symptoms.

Denial and Cancer

Because cancer represents many people's worst fear, overwhelming anxiety caused by a symptom that could indicate cancer or the idea of facing cancer treatment certainly is understandable. Specific fears include that cancer represents terrible pain and suffering and then death; disfigurement; loss of role, financial security, or job; separation or rejection by loved ones; or tremendous threat to self-concept, especially in individuals who associate cancer with guilt and punishment for past "sins" (e.g., promiscuity, drug use) (Holland, 2003).

Studies have examined denial and its impact on the diagnosis of cancer. Mor, Allen, Goldberg, Guadagnoli, and Wool (1990) found that 25% of patients delayed seeking medical treatment for cancer symptoms by more than three months. In one of the earliest studies by Hackett, Cassem, and Raker (1973), 39% of patients waited longer than three months to seek medical attention, and 8% became incapacitated, requiring others to persuade them to seek medical care. Kreitler (1999) reported that denial remains a key factor in people delaying diagnostic testing and avoiding exposure to information for early detection of cancer.

The incidence of denial tends to increase at the time of diagnosis, recurrence, and terminal stages when individuals are facing new threats (Kreitler, 1999). Extreme denial at the time that symptoms appear leads to late diagnosis and contributes to the need for more aggressive treatment when the disease is more advanced. Unfortunately, because of the intense fear some people have about cancer, oncology professionals often see denial of cancer symptoms. A patient with a fungating chest wound from an undiagnosed breast cancer who avoided seeking medical attention for years demonstrates the power of denial. Individuals can go to such lengths as wearing loose clothing, using pads to absorb drainage, and applying generous amounts of perfume to cover up the odor from the draining tumor but still be unable to acknowledge the need for medical attention. Whether this denial protects people from awareness of suffering and pain caused by the disease symptoms is open for debate. Little research has been done on these patients because they are often at the end stage of disease when they finally seek care.

Denial in regard to cancer treatment also can manifest itself as noncompliance with treatment when patients fail to complete a course of chemotherapy or radiation.

Facing the reality of treatment and side effects may force patients to face the threat of cancer for the first time. Patients may be so overwhelmed that the only way to deal with the threat is to refuse more treatment. Patients in denial probably are less likely to attend support groups or educational programs because they have convinced themselves that the information would not apply to them. No one knows how much suffering is created by advanced symptoms of pain, bowel obstructions, or pathologic fractures because patients with cancer who are in denial are unable to acknowledge symptoms and do not seek treatment. Denial may be a factor for individuals who pursue unproven therapy in place of traditional treatment. Patients in denial may be more prone to accept claims of practitioners of unproven methods who reinforce their denial by devaluing what oncology professionals offer. However, not everyone who pursues alternative therapies is in denial (Cousins, 1982). These alternatives can be important parts of the treatment plan for some patients.

With advanced disease, some patients are able to maintain an upbeat, hopeful outlook that may be denial. This response can give patients energy to keep trying new therapies or can lessen anxiety and depression, which affect not only patients but also those around them. However, denial may prevent individuals from making end-of-life decisions and financial arrangements (e.g., writing a will) and result in isolation from family and friends who are fearful of saying the "wrong thing" around the patients. They are being prevented from saying goodbye. One should remember that not all patients with an upbeat, hopeful attitude with advanced disease are in denial. This may be patients' normal personality or the result of true acceptance.

Denial and Death

Although death is an inevitability that all people must face, trying to imagine one's own nonexistence is nearly impossible. This, combined with the taboo of discussing and facing death in Western culture, adds to the prevalent use of denial at the end of life. Death is a reminder of a person's ultimate powerlessness, and denial often is used when facing death because the idea of nonexistence is so threatening. In American society, end-of-life care often takes place in the hospital (National Hospice and Palliative Care Organization, 2004). Family members may have little experience being with someone who is close to death. This contributes to intense fears that may eventually be dealt with through denial.

In his classic book *On Dying and Denying*, Weisman (1972) identified three levels of denial related to illness and death. **First-order denial** is based on how patients perceive the primary facts of the illness. **Second-order denial** involves the inferences that patients draw or fail to draw about the extensions and implications of the illness (e.g., What does metastasis mean? Does a new symptom mean the disease has spread?). **Third-order denial** is concerned with the image of death itself and represents denial of one's own extinction. This level of denial is exemplified by an inability to believe that the illness will result in death. Weisman noted that although individuals can face a diagnosis and the implications of the diagnosis, facing death is another matter that presents a struggle for most individuals. The amount of distress created by facing death will determine the need for denial to control the anxiety. Spiritual beliefs will contribute to some patients' ability to face the anxiety of terminal illness.

Some terminally ill individuals may maintain denial until the very end, even in the face of advanced disease. For these individuals, denial represents the ultimate control in an uncontrollable situation. Professionals must closely examine the patient's use of denial at the end of life to determine whether it needs to be "fixed," what will happen if the patient maintains strong denial until the end, and whether intervention is needed. Evaluating all the implications of denial for the patient and family is essential before intervening.

Copp and Field (2002) conducted a qualitative study of a small group of hospice patients on coping. They found that patients fluctuated between denial and acceptance. They proposed that denial preserves self-esteem, maintains relationships, and prevents disintegration and chaos.

Connor (2000) pointed out that denial may be a key factor in anticipatory mourning. It may explain why anticipatory mourning does not necessarily increase as the loss gets closer.

Some ethicists and palliative care professionals now are concerned that American society's denial of death is contributing to the increased acceptance and even demand for physician-assisted suicide and euthanasia. Scott (1994) commented that if healthcare professionals cannot promise immediate and complete cessation of suffering during a terminal illness and full personal autonomy in dying, physician-assisted suicide and euthanasia will be viewed as justified. Controlling exactly how and when one will die may be a way of attaining mastery and therefore denying the inevitable because death is ultimately a loss of control. Physician-assisted suicide and euthanasia could be used to ensure that death is quick, and the emotions faced during terminal illness are avoided.

Healthcare Professionals' Responses to Denial

Often, healthcare professionals react with concern when faced with patients in denial. Nurses may feel that patients are not coping effectively and need intervention. Denial can inhibit the therapeutic relationship when patients are unable to talk about their emotional response to an illness or may not be able to tolerate needed teaching about chemotherapy because of the inability to believe treatment is needed. Copp and Field's (2002) study pointed out the need for nurses to be skilled at recognizing the adaptive role of denial yet also to know when further intervention is needed.

Ross, Peteet, Medeiros, Walsh-Burke, and Rieker (1992) noted in a study comparing physicians' and nurses' responses to patients' denial that physicians were less concerned with denial and saw it more as a temporary phase. Nurses were concerned that patients would suffer more because they were not participating in end-of-life decisions. Nurses expressed more concern about the need for honesty and were uncomfortable around patients who were experiencing adverse effects of treatment and were not facing treatment issues. Differences in the two groups' responses may be explained by their differing views of their roles. Nurses focus on comfort and safety rather than being empowered to offer hope by giving the diagnosis and treatment information as the physician usually does. Rousseau (2000) pointed out that physicians even may collude with patients in fostering denial to avoid addressing difficult topics.

Healthcare professionals need to be aware of their own use of denial. Are they offering treatment to a patient because of their own inability to face the inevitable or their lack of skill in giving bad news? Are side effects minimized and unrealistic hopes reinforced with a favorite patient or one who reminds them of themselves? All oncology professionals must ask themselves these questions. A factor that may contribute to professionals' use of denial may be personal experience with cancer. A personal history of cancer or a close family member with cancer may reinforce professionals' need to reduce the threat associated with the patient's diagnosis. Individuals may identify with certain patients (e.g., young women, mothers, nurses who have cancer). Professionals may feel that they, too, are vulnerable. Using denial will reduce the threat but may be unfair in terms of what is communicated to patients. Professionals must be aware that having strong feelings about a patient may signify a personal emotional link that could contribute to denial or other personal reactions to patients (Gorman, Raines, & Sultan, 2002). In a study of 437 ambulance drivers, Wastell (2002) found that the more people used emotional suppression to deal with stress, the more physical and psychological stress symptoms they experienced.

Healthcare professionals' use of denial may be seen at the end of life. The healthcare system in the United States often uses its technology to the extreme in keeping people alive who clearly are dying. Using healthcare resources to prolong life may create more suffering by instituting aggressive treatments that are futile. Offering futile treatment may represent denial on the part of professionals, patients, and families rather than acceptance of the role of palliative care. It also may be a factor in late referrals to hospice care.

Evidence-Based Practice

Weisman (1972) remains the seminal work on the use of denial in patients with cancer. This study is based on multiple interviews with people in different stages of illness. His work became the basis for much future research. Recent research on this topic is limited, and the results are conflicting (Rousseau, 2000).

Filipp (1992) found that the use of denial was highest before a biopsy or diagnosis and did not decrease until two years after diagnosis. Stanton and Snider (1993) found that women with a cancer diagnosis who used more denial had greater levels of distress after diagnosis and surgery. Carver et al. (1993) reported that denial related positively to distress (and negatively to optimism) from presurgery to one-year postsurgery. Kreitler, Chaitchik, Rapoport, and Algor (1995) studied patients with head and neck cancer. These researchers found that the high deniers had less anxiety and were more well-adjusted at work, and low deniers were more anxious but better able to ask for help.

Copp and Field (2002) studied the experiences of 12 hospice patients and their nurses. They found that denial and acceptance of dying among patients fluctuated during the period of dying, even in the presence of open awareness about prognosis, and appeared to form an important aspect of their coping process.

The effects of denial on coping vary with the phase of the disease and tend to fluctuate with time. In general, a potential benefit to denial exists in early and terminal stages of cancer (Kreitler, 1999).

Nursing Care of Patients in Denial

Assessment

Nurses need to be alert to the many different forms denial can take. Often, the first sign is when a patient denies awareness of information the nurse knows he or she has received. For example, after the doctor has told the patient about a new metastasis, the patient tells the nurse he just heard everything is going well. Other signs might include not asking questions when questions normally are expected, absence of signs of an expected normal emotional response to bad news just given, or inappropriate emotions such as laughing and joking. More subtle signs might include changing the subject when the illness is discussed, avoiding use of the word "cancer," or minimizing or hiding symptoms in an effort to maintain the denial (e.g., referring to respiratory distress from a pleural effusion as a cold, refusing to acknowledge pain).

Once nurses determine that the patient is using denial, they should try to identify factors that may contribute to the patient's need to use this defense. Collecting information on the patient's current stresses and past coping style may provide that information.

More extreme maladaptive behaviors may include refusing to see the physician or follow through with treatment. Patients may be unable to acknowledge even obvious complications (e.g., a pathologic fracture, bleeding). Denial also could be a factor when patients pursue unconventional therapy. A particular concern is when very ill patients refuse conventional therapy and seek unproven methods, including special diets or unusual drugs that may be promoted by unscrupulous providers.

A family that is using denial may exhibit the same types of behaviors as patients, such as going to great lengths to dismiss new symptoms, encouraging the patient not to listen to healthcare professionals, becoming angry if the nurse talks about cancer or chemotherapy, or exhibiting a lack of expected emotions regarding the patient's illness.

Differential Diagnosis

Differentiating adaptive and normal denial from denial with deleterious effects is an important part of the assessment (see Figure 16-1). Although both forms protect individuals emotionally, maladaptive denial can be dangerous because the disease can progress when treatment is avoided. In addition, emotional sequelae of maladaptive denial includes isolation of family members from the patient because they fear saying the wrong thing around the patient, inhibition of emotional growth when the individual never deals with a major loss, and the risk of future emotional problems.

Psychotic thought processes, dementia, delirium, or other psychiatric disorders could be labeled incorrectly as denial. If patients refuse to believe a diagnosis because of confusion or delusional thoughts, denial is not the mechanism. Further psychiatric evaluation must be provided. In addition, neurologic impairments (e.g., stroke, brain tumor) can mimic denial if they cause a neglect syndrome in which patients disavow a symptom or even a part of the body.

Figure 16-1. Characteristics of Adaptive and Maladaptive Denial

Adaptive denial
- Temporary, short-lived
- Intermittent
- Allows time to develop coping mechanisms
- Does not influence major decisions
- Others rally around the person until he or she can cope.

Maladaptive denial
- Lasts much longer than expected
- Persistent use of denial even in the face of obvious truth
- No indication of use or new development of more adaptive coping skills
- Influences major decisions
- Denial may isolate the person from others.

Note. Based on information from Rousseau, 2000; Stephenson, 2004.

Interventions

A nonintrusive, supportive approach should be the initial intervention with patients in denial. Incorporate statements and questions such as, "Tell me what the doctor told you about your condition," "What adjustments have you had to make with your illness?" and "What are you concerned about?" into the nursing assessment. Answers to these questions will provide information about the patient's perspective. Reassessment using these same questions will help to establish how firm the denial is.

When approaching a patient who has a history of or is suspected of using denial, nurses must ensure that they know what the patient has been told and in what words. Be aware of discrepancies between what the patient says and what the professionals have told the patient. Initially, use the same words the patient uses to describe the condition in an effort to establish rapport. For example, if the patient uses the word "growth" or "lump" to describe the disease, initially use this word, too.

Nurses should not confront an individual with information they believe he or she should have; rather, they should recognize the need that denial serves and consider the patient's fears, the issues that need to be addressed, and the role that teaching and support play in addressing the denial. Spend time listening to the person and provide support to build a trusting relationship. Confronting the patient with the truth may lead to extreme reactions of anger, anxiety, and distress. Patients may react with more denial and be able to ignore the information. Nurses risk isolating the patient further because the patient could feel that the staff is cruel, harsh, or negative and untrustworthy.

Providing information to patients in small amounts is important. Provide some information about side effects or the treatment plan, and observe the response. Reinforce the information, and ask patients to repeat what they understand. Presenting information in small amounts produces much less anxiety than presenting the whole picture at one time.

If patients focus on unrealistic goals or hopes, listen to them but avoid agreeing with or reinforcing them. Focus instead on specific, potentially achievable goals. For example, if the patient is bed bound, do not focus on being able to play tennis soon but rather direct the discussion to identify ways to increase muscle strength. Sometimes, developing a backup plan for patients can help. For example, if a patient refuses home care because he or she believes help is unnecessary, arrange a one-time evaluation visit "just in case."

For patients who demonstrate denial and will not accept any teaching or assistance, give family members information on what to expect. Work with them to establish a plan of action if the patient's condition deteriorates. Ensure that they know how to set up home care, have keys to the patient's home, and have the doctor's telephone number. Educate them regarding signs of pain or other indications of deterioration. Provide support to family members about how difficult the current situation is but review with them the reasons the patient needs this defense.

If family members are using extensive denial, try to encourage them to participate in the patient's care to increase their understanding of the extent of the patient's illness or disability. Engage family members in a discussion about observations regarding the patient's condition and needs. Assist them in identifying their fears about the patient's illness.

If patients are using denial that has life-threatening implications, the healthcare team may consider a psychiatric consultation. The consultant may be able to determine if a psychiatric disorder is inhibiting patients' acceptance of the illness. If patients do not have a psychiatric disorder and have the capacity to make medical decisions, they have the right to refuse medical treatment. As difficult as this can be for the families and healthcare professionals, patients have the right to use denial to protect themselves from the information and cannot be forced into treatment (see Figure 16-2).

Figure 16-2. Plan of Care

Assessment
- Recognize the various forms denial can take.
- Reassess the patient's response at different points of the disease or hospital stay.
- Consider variables that may be causing the patient to use denial.
- Determine adaptive and maladaptive effects of the use of denial.
- Identify possible differential diagnoses.

Nursing Diagnoses (NANDA International, 2005)
- Ineffective coping
- Ineffective denial

***DSM-IV-TR* Diagnoses** (American Psychiatric Association, 2000)
- Adjustment disorder with anxiety
- Adjustment disorder with depressed mood

Differential Diagnoses
- Neurologic impairment
- Psychosis
- Depression

Expected Outcomes
- Patients will seek and follow through with medical interventions.
- Patients will accurately describe implications of the illness.
- Patients will acknowledge emotional responses to the diagnosis.
- Patients will verbalize realistic expectations of the illness.

(Continued on next page)

Figure 16-2. Plan of Care *(Continued)*

Interventions: Patient
- Determine the degree of denial and effectiveness of denial as a coping strategy.
- Observe patients' responses to information given by the healthcare team.
- Give patients information about their condition in small amounts without being threatening.
- Avoid confronting patients' denial directly.
- Take time to encourage a trusting, supportive relationship.
- Recognize patients' need for extra support.
- Reinforce possible positive outcomes of treatment.
- Consider psychiatric consultation if the denial has life-threatening implications.

Interventions: Family
- Include family members in patients' care so they can see the extent of the disease.
- Identify which family members can tolerate even a little information about the patients.
- Help families to establish an action plan if the patients' condition deteriorates.

Case Study

A 47-year-old Asian man, Mr. A, is admitted to the hospital with a bowel obstruction from end-stage colon cancer. Mr. A is married and has two sons, ages 12 and 15. Mr. A is an executive with a local insurance company. He was diagnosed three years ago and has undergone surgery and chemotherapy. Liver metastasis was diagnosed one year ago. The patient has been treated with chemotherapy until the present time. For several months, the oncologist has recommended that Mr. A stop chemotherapy because it is not helping, and the severe side effects are causing many complications. Mr. A has repeatedly demanded more treatment. He speaks of waiting to hear from cancer programs around the world that he has contacted with hopes of finding a new treatment program. He now has a bowel obstruction and a nasogastric tube in place. A consulting surgeon told Mr. A that surgery is not an option because of the extent of disease in his abdomen.

The patient's wife and sons visit frequently, and it has become clear to the staff that neither Mrs. A nor her sons are aware of the patient's very poor prognosis. Mrs. A speaks animatedly of how happy she will be when Mr. A is discharged and that he will return to work soon. Further discussion reveals that no plan has been made regarding what will happen after Mr. A dies. Mrs. A is a housewife. Mr. A makes all decisions about finances and other major areas. He has no will.

Mr. A's oncologist spoke with him on several occasions to discuss his prognosis. The patient refuses to look at the doctor, barely speaks, and gives very little indication of his feelings. The doctor encourages the patient to talk to his wife and sons. The patient responds with "everything will be all right as soon as I get home. Then I will get stronger."

After attempting to talk with Mr. A several times, the oncologist and clinical nurse specialist discuss the situation and decide to tell Mr. A that they plan to talk with Mrs. A about their concerns. Mr. A voices no objection.

(Continued on next page)

Case Study *(Continued)*

This information is given to the patient's wife and, after some expression of emotion, she is able to admit that she has suspected this. With the help of the interdisciplinary team, Mrs. A contacts an attorney and develops a strategy for the family's financial planning. After she speaks with her sons, the unit social worker meets with them to provide emotional support. Mrs. A makes several attempts to talk with her husband, but he becomes increasingly uncommunicative and angry, telling her he will get better very soon. The patient dies in the hospital several days later. He was found dead, and resuscitation was not instituted.

In talking with Mrs. A after her husband's death, she indicates her gratitude to the team for preparing her and her sons for what to expect. She realizes that Mr. A had been completely unable to accept his prognosis and, although she is very sorry that he did not allow the family to fully share his final weeks, she realizes it was too threatening for him. The sons remain devoted to their mother but are very sad at the loss of their father. They will continue with counseling for several more months.

Discussion

The staff in this case realized the extent of the patient's denial and, after making several attempts to address the problems with the patient, changed the focus of the treatment plan. Realizing that the wife was the one most at risk, interventions focused on preparing the family for the patient's death. For this patient, acknowledging his terminal illness was too great a threat. The denial allowed him to maintain his self-image and not face feelings of powerlessness and intense sadness.

The wife felt totally isolated from her husband. She was able to share with the interdisciplinary team how important maintaining a sense of control and dignity was for him and that demonstrating any emotion was a sign of weakness. This pattern continued to the end of his life.

With time and support from others, the team hopes that Mrs. A will come to understand that her effort to maintain her husband's dignity at the end was the most meaningful thing she could do for him.

Conclusion

Denial tends to occur frequently at times of stress during the cancer experience. It is particularly evident at the onset of cancer symptoms, diagnosis, metastasis/recurrence, and end-stage disease. The initial appearance of denial symptoms should be considered to be normal, adaptive behavior. Denial indicates that the person is overwhelmed with the emotional impact of this stress and, at least initially, does not have adequate coping mechanisms to deal with the anxiety. Denial provides protection from an overwhelming threat. If denial behavior persists, healthcare professionals must evaluate whether the denial is adaptive or maladaptive. Maladaptive denial may require more intensive assessment and intervention but should never be approached in a harsh manner as something that must be "fixed." The impact of maladaptive denial may include late diagnosis, incomplete treatment, and isolation from family and healthcare professionals. Whatever the extent of the denial, healthcare professionals must continue to support patients without reinforcing the maladaptive aspects of the denial.

References

American Psychiatric Association. (2000). *Diagnostic and statistical manual of mental disorders* (4th ed., text rev.). Washington, DC: Author.

Carney, R., Fitzsimons, D., & Dempster, M. (2002). Why people experiencing acute myocardial infarction delay seeking medical assistance. *European Journal of Cardiovascular Nursing, 1,* 237–242.

Carver, C.S., Pozo, C., Harris, S.D., Noriega, V., Scheier, M.F., Robinson, D.S., et al. (1993). How coping mediates the effect of optimism on distress: A study of women with early stage breast cancer. *Journal of Personality and Social Psychology, 65,* 375–390.

Connor, S.R. (2000). Denial and the limits of anticipatory mourning. In T.A. Rando (Ed.), *Clinical dimensions of anticipatory mourning: Theory and practice in working with the dying, their loved ones, and their caregivers* (pp. 253–265). Champaign, IL: Research Press.

Copp, G., & Field, D. (2002). Open awareness and dying: The use of denial and acceptance as coping strategies by hospice patients. *NT Research, 7,* 118–127.

Cousins, N. (1982). Denial: Are sharper definitions needed? *JAMA, 248,* 210–212.

Filipp, S.H. (1992). Could it be worse? The diagnosis of cancer as a prototype of traumatic life events. In L. Montada, S.H. Filipp, & M.J. Lerner (Eds.), *Life crises and experiences of loss in adulthood* (pp. 23–56). Hillsdale, NJ: L. Erlbaum Associates.

Freud, A. (1952). The mutual influence in development of ego and id. *Psychoanalytic Studies in Children, 7,* 42–50.

Gorman, L.M., Raines, M., & Sultan, D.F. (2002). *Psychosocial nursing for general patient care* (2nd ed.). Philadelphia: F.A. Davis.

Greer, S. (1992). Management of denial in cancer patients. *Oncology, 6*(12), 33–39.

Hackett, T.P., Cassem, N.H., & Raker, J.W. (1973). Patient delay in cancer. *New England Journal of Medicine, 289,* 14–20.

Hackett, T.P., Cassem, N.H., & Wishnie, H.A. (1968). The coronary care unit: An appraisal of its psychologic hazards. *New England Journal of Medicine, 279,* 1365–1370.

Holland, J.C. (2003). American Cancer Society Award lecture. Psychological care of patients: Psycho oncology's contribution. *Journal of Clinical Oncology, 21*(Suppl. 23), 253s–265s.

Kreitler, S. (1999). Denial in cancer patients. *Cancer Investigation, 17,* 514–534.

Kreitler, S., Chaitchik, S., Rapoport, Y., & Algor, R. (1995). Psychosocial effects of level of information and severity of disease on head-and-neck cancer patients. *Journal of Cancer Education, 10,* 144–154.

Levine, J., Rudy, T., & Kerns, R. (1994). A two-factor model of denial of illness: A confirmatory factor analysis. *Journal of Psychosomatic Research, 38,* 99–110.

Levine, J., Warrenburg, S., Kerns, R., Schwartz, E.G., Delaney, R., Fontana, A., et al. (1987). The relationship of denial to the course of recovery in coronary heart disease. *Psychosomatic Medicine, 49,* 109–117.

Lowery, B.J. (1991). Psychological stress, denial and myocardial infarction outcomes. *Image: The Journal of Nursing Scholarship, 23,* 51–55.

McKinley, S., Moser, D.K., & Dracup, K. (2000). Treatment-seeking behavior for acute myocardial infarction symptoms in North America and Australia. *Heart and Lung, 29,* 237–247.

Minarek, P. (1996). Psychosocial interventions with ineffective coping responses to physical illness: Anxiety-related. In P. Barry (Ed.), *Psychosocial nursing: Care of physically ill patients and their families* (3rd ed., pp. 301–324). Philadelphia: Lippincott.

Mor, V., Allen, S.M., Goldberg, R., Guadagnoli, E., & Wool, M.S. (1990). Prediagnostic symptom recognition and help-seeking among cancer patients. *Journal of Community Health, 15,* 253–266.

NANDA International. (2005). *Nursing diagnoses: Definitions and classification, 2005–2006.* Philadelphia: Author.

National Hospice and Palliative Care Organization. (2002). *2002 hospice statistics*. Retrieved May 4, 2004, from http://nhpco.org

Ross, D.M., Peteet, F.R., Medeiros, C., Walsh-Burke, K., & Rieker, P. (1992). Differences between nurses' and physicians' approach to denial in oncology. *Cancer Nursing, 15*, 422–428.

Rousseau, P. (2000). Death denial. *Journal of Clinical Oncology, 18*, 3998–3999.

Russell, G.C. (1993). The role of denial in clinical practice. *Journal of Advanced Nursing, 18*, 938–940.

Sadock, B.J. (2005). Signs and symptoms in psychiatry. In B.J. Sadock & V.A. Sadock (Eds.), *Kaplan and Sadock's comprehensive textbook of psychiatry* (8th ed., pp. 847–859). Philadelphia: Lippincott Williams & Wilkins.

Scott, J.F. (1994). More money for palliative care? The economics of denial. *Journal of Palliative Care, 10*(3), 14–20.

Stanton, A.L., & Snider, P.R. (1993). Coping with a breast cancer diagnosis: A prospective study. *Health Psychology, 12*, 16–23.

Stephenson, P.S. (2004). Understanding denial. *Oncology Nursing Forum, 31*, 985–988.

Vachon, M.L.S. (1998). The emotional problems of the patient. In D. Doyle, G. Hanks, & N. MacDonald (Eds.), *The Oxford textbook of palliative medicine* (2nd ed., pp. 883–907). New York: Oxford University Press.

Wastell, C.A. (2002). Exposure to trauma: The long-term effects of suppressing emotional reactions. *Journal of Nervous and Mental Disorders, 190*, 839–845.

Weisman, A.D. (1972). *On dying and denying*. New York: Behavioral Publications.

Zerwic, J.J., & Ryan, C.J. (2004). Delays in seeking MI treatment: Chances of survival increase if symptoms are treated within two hours of onset. *American Journal of Nursing, 104*(1), 81–83.

CHAPTER 17

Body Image Disturbance

JUDITH A. SHELL, PHD, LMFT, RN, AOCN®, AND
CAROL CAMPBELL-NORRIS, BA, MS

The rift in the chest of a mountain,
The twist in the trunk of a tree,
The water-cut cave in the hollow,
The rough, rocky rim of the sea—

Each one has a scar of distortion,
Yet each has this sermon to sing,
"The presence of what would deface me,
Has made me a beautiful thing."

—Frank H. Keith

Body image involves an individual's perception of his or her body. It is derived from a combination of physical, psychological, interpersonal, and social experiences and is influenced by a person's parents, caregivers, and peers (Olivo & Woolverton, 2001). Furthermore, a positive body image is associated with sexual satisfaction (Schover, 2000, 2001a, 2001b). Body image, which is subject to constant change resulting from personal, physical, cultural, social, and biologic experiences, begins to develop in infancy. As people mature through early childhood and adolescence and into adulthood, self-image grows and diversifies and can be influenced by several factors (see Table 17-1). Because body image is determined in a personal manner, people constantly reexamine themselves, and their perceptions easily can influence or distort what they see and how satisfied they are with their bodies. They tend not to believe objective opinion, especially from a close friend or a spouse.

Cusumano and Thompson (1997) proposed that the need to conform to certain standards related to body image and shape comes pragmatically from social pressure.

Table 17-1. The Development of Body Image

Developmental Stage	Influences
Infancy	Separation of self from mother and father is a first step in formation of body boundaries.
Young childhood (2–4 years old)	Mastery of physical/motor tasks becomes the foundation for feelings of control of self and environments and toward positive feelings of self.
Early childhood (5–10 years old)	Child begins to recognize maleness and femaleness without any real recognition of physical attributes of the sexes. Sex differentiation must develop prior to further boundary expansion.
Adolescence: Onset of puberty	Body image constantly is changing. Interactions with peers often are more important than with parents. Adolescents are aware of changes in their own bodies and in friends/peers. Adolescents may feel threatened with feelings of insecurity or fear as they compare their bodies to others. Peer acceptance heavily influences self-acceptance.
Adulthood	Body image becomes more stable but is never fully constant or formed. As maturity increases, the adult faces recognition of physiologic adaptation in the body caused by aging. Changes perceived as less than attractive will affect perception of worth.

Note. Based on information from Stern, 1990.

Film, television, and the printed word, particularly advertising, endorse the "ideal" body. Because the "ideal" usually is impossible to achieve, this pressure often is associated with body image disturbance that can evolve into eating disorders and other ailments, such as depressive, anxiety, and somatoform disorders.

One of the most important aspects of body image is physical attractiveness. In American culture, the standard of physical attractiveness often is based on youth and vitality. Men frequently place great importance on the physical attractiveness of a possible mate, which relates to the "objectification" of women more often than men (Wiederman & Hurst, 1998).

> The popular media sorely lack images that accurately reflect the diversity and range of shapes, sizes, colors, contours, and appearances that represent the physical realities of most middle-aged women. As such, it is difficult for women not to feel that they have somehow failed themselves, and others, when the images they see in the mirror do not resemble those celluloid images that they are bombarded with from television screens and newsstands on a daily basis. (Daniluk, 1998, p. 297)

On a more positive note, Pollin (1995) revealed that "thanks to patient advocacy, new legislation, sensitive media attention, enabling medical devices, and other factors, people with impairments are now increasingly active and visible . . . and society's concept of 'normal' appearance and behavior is widening and social stigma is a less-powerful constraint" (p. 70). Although illness and deformity hold less stigma today, a natural human tendency still exists to label or avoid people who are different or vulnerable and weak. Therefore, people with chronic conditions or illnesses, especially those that cause visible symptoms, must be prepared to develop ways to deal with stigmas such as avoidance, discrimination, hostility, fear, disgust, condescension, and simple curiosity (Pollin).

Important Principles About Body Image

Several concepts are central to developing an understanding of body image. As people mature, they begin to assimilate individual, unique qualities into their personality. People's own definitive talents and abilities make them distinct from others. Individuals are more likely to value their self-image if they see themselves as worthy and exclusive.

Stern (1990) indicated that one of the most critical features of body image is the element of control. People generally value the ability to be in control, whether it is to control normal bodily functions or their daily schedules. Correctly assessing one's ability to be in control enhances self-perception, which supports a more positive body image.

The concept of body boundary also is important to the understanding of body image. Body boundary includes the entire physical appearance, which varies in importance to each individual. Men or women who choose to wear certain clothing, jewelry, hairstyles, or make-up are portraying their own perceived body image to all observers. A person's outward appearance dictates how well defined his or her body boundaries are; that is, an immaculate outward image depicts body control and well-defined body boundaries.

Van der Velde (1985) proposed the concept of multiple body images that exist simultaneously based on several premises.

1. Multiple and innumerable body images are present because humans are not able to view the entire self at any one time.
2. Body images incorporate one's interpretations of others' appraisals and evaluations, as well as their reactions to one's appearance.
3. The formation of body image includes perceptions of the physical appearances of others.
4. Body image is important in its necessity for the interaction with others. Any contact with other people, whether verbal, tactile, or physical, requires an image of self to be projected.

Trauma, major illness or injury, or other physical conditions can cause an alteration in body image. Stern (1990) described stages of adaptation that enable people to adjust to this alteration: impact, retreat, acknowledgment, and reconstruction (see Table 17-2). Successful adaptation depends on age and performance status of the individual, nature of the illness/condition, the individual's perception of the alteration, how long the alteration will last, and the person's previous coping abilities.

Table 17-2. Stages of Adaptation

Stage	Descriptors
Impact Patient experiences initial encounter with illness or injury.	Awareness of change in body or its functions develops. Patient enters a state of shock as irreversibility becomes evident (sudden alterations create longer impact). Anxiety becomes dominant expression. Sense of depersonalization may be assumed. Patient becomes self-centered, owing to situational loss of personal control. Developmental regression may occur. Patient may feel a sense of failure in own body.
Retreat Patient attempts to return to stable feelings of self that existed before the critical event.	Patient may indulge in wishful thinking and avoid reality through fantasy. Process of reorganization and strengthening begins. Patient begins to sort and reorganize the shattered self-image.
Acknowledgment Patient actively mourns his or her loss and experiences a sense of hopelessness.	Patient experiences a sensation of "self-not-self." A new body is forcibly recognized. Patient clings to a strong image of the old body. Patient begins to resolve conflicts resulting from newly formed or altered self. Patient continues to be self-centered, focusing on the needs of the self. Patient may feel that relationships are threatened and may feel abandonment. Family may feel grief for the patient's lost body image.
Reconstruction Patient replaces the need to mourn with the decision to try new approaches to living.	Patient reintegrates positive life experiences. Patient reintegrates altered body image, reorganizes social values, and adjusts to technical devices or procedures.

Note. Based on information from Stern, 1990.

Body Image and Illness

Responses to body image disturbance caused by illness may be subtle. Morse, Bottorff, and Hutchinson (1995) characterized four different types of reactions.

1. The deceiving body: Some patients have reported a sadness because their body has deceived them. It acted normal, with no symptoms, and then disease was discovered during a routine examination. Trust in their body is lost.

2. The vulnerable body: Because of the violation of disease and treatment, some patients report feeling vulnerable and fear future experiences. Patients wage a constant vigil to watch for signs of impending pain or discomfort. They feel fragile and move cautiously and hesitantly to protect the self that is left.

3. The violated body: Boundaries often are violated, not only through the indignity of exposing intimate and private parts to strangers but also when

caregivers enter a room without knocking or ask patients whether their bowels have moved today. Although patients experience anger, embarrassment, and a loss of personhood, they passively participate in diagnostic or treatment procedures as if they have no choice, believing this simply is part of their care.

4. The betraying body: Patients often feel that their body has betrayed them. They have taken good care of themselves, eaten all the right foods, exercised, and had regular medical checkups, but they still have become ill. The once strong, beautiful, and healthy self-image can vanish as treatment or disease progresses.

One of the first comments made by the woman in the case study at the end of this chapter was in relation to how her "body had betrayed her." She was very angry because she had treated her body well, had adhered to frequent doctor visits, and still had to endure the violation of mastectomy and reconstruction that left her with an unfamiliar body.

Reports in the literature, as well as scientific studies, have demonstrated the relationship between body image dysfunction and chronic illness. Patients with diabetes who must endure daily insulin injections, patients with impaired memories following cerebral hemorrhage, patients with complete spinal cord injury, and patients with hypertension or epilepsy receiving daily medication that can affect libido and other sexual function are but a few examples of people who have had to make major changes in their lifestyles, including a change in how they perceive their own bodies (Leiblum & Segraves, 2000; Moreno et al., 1995; Schover, 2000). A self-image that integrates the illness is necessary for the individual's adjustment, and this transition is easier if self-image and ego are strong before the illness (Dropkin, 1999). Patients who have a poor self-image and a limited ego prior to a major change in life or body integrity may not be as open and flexible during the adaptation process because they will have fewer personal resources.

When people experience chronic illness, they can explore several avenues in relation to self-evaluation and how others evaluate them, including internal or personal sensations, experiences with a partner, and interactions with society. Other factors that may influence an individual's body image include when the changes occur (e.g., adulthood is more difficult than childhood) and how rapidly they occur (e.g., rapid change is more difficult to assimilate than slow change). It may seem like a Herculean task to relinquish an image of oneself as healthy, invulnerable, or quick-witted and replace it with something equally acceptable, yet this is just what happens when sudden or unexpected physiologic changes create a need to generate a new body image from one that has taken a lifetime to create.

Concerns about body image are not always related to changes in physical appearance. Even if a change is not visible, people still may feel damaged and stigmatized and must learn to cope with the fact that they will never be quite the same, physically or psychologically (Carver et al., 1998). Laken (Laken & Laken, 2002) explained how his feelings of emasculinization and incompetence were validated when the doctor reminded him "that a large part of a man's identity is entwined with his ability to perform, [and] he stated that it's 'natural and normal' to feel inadequate when that is taken away [and that] it would take a lot of determination and hard work to regain his confidence and reframe his self-perception" (p. 122). A visible change, however, can be more devastating than imperceptible changes, particularly if the person places emphasis on physical attributes or beauty. Difficulty arises if a loss of uniqueness of the self accompanies the change. Even though a body normally undergoes continual change, a crisis can occur if a person experiences a change in some characteristic that he or she attributes to his or her uniqueness and individuality (Laken & Laken). Illness breeds uncertainty, and whether dealing with an unexpected improvement in or worsening of a condition, the person must adapt. When a person's health changes frequently or extensively, the sense of integration among past, present, and future images of oneself may be lost (Schover, 2000).

Changes in the patient's health will affect the family's and partner's perceptions of the individual, and their reactions will have an impact on the patient's body image. Family members may suffer feelings of loss, disorientation, aversion, and fear that, in turn, may evoke sensations of rejection and undesirability on the part of the person who has changed. Does the spouse continue to reach out with an affectionate touch or hold hands in public? Are family members willing to participate in rehabilitation efforts?

Pollin (1995) explained that self-image addresses a person's sense of self, whereas stigma results from other people's attitudes toward the person. Feelings of acceptance and attractiveness certainly will be negatively influenced if friends, coworkers, or strangers avert their gaze, look with pity, or use too much kindness when interacting with the affected person.

Body Image and Cancer

Katz, Rodin, and Devins (1995), in their literature review, asserted that impaired body self-esteem (their descriptor for what commonly is referred to as body image) in patients with disfiguring cancer treatments was one of the most consistent empirical findings. Patients with cancer not only experience a most-feared diagnosis, but many endure months of (or even permanent) insult to their bodies and body image (Green et al., 2000; Hart et al., 1999).

Temporary or permanent disfigurement, wounds and scars, and prostheses and appliances cause a level of distress that many patients hesitate to admit. Less severe alterations (e.g., hair loss, weight loss or gain, skin changes) can be just as devastating (Lin, 1996). Alopecia, which can include the loss of all body hair, including pubic hair, can be embarrassing and cause feelings of unattractiveness (McGarvey, Baum, Pinkerton, & Rogers, 2001; Williams, Wood, & Cunningham-Warburton, 1999). Hair loss also indicates to others that the person is most likely someone with cancer.

Chemotherapy has been associated with weight changes (loss and gain) and pallor that can negatively influence body image. Cancer cachexia is often a principal source of distress and anxiety because it is a common sign of disease progression. It impairs the sense of adequacy and self-esteem, and the image of an emaciated body will affect feelings of femininity or masculinity, worthiness, and competence (Shell, 2001).

Schover et al. (1995) revealed that chemotherapy was associated with a poorer body image and long-term problems with sexual function. With the use of adjuvant chemotherapy, especially in younger women, long-term impact on quality of life may include changes in reproductive status caused by premature menopause (Schover et al.). Changes in perceived sexual attractiveness may occur as a result of loss of sexual desire, vaginal dryness, and dyspareunia. Recurrent urinary tract or vaginal monilial infections triggered by sexual intercourse, the presence of whitish plaques on the vulva, and exacerbations of genital herpes or human papillomavirus because of chemotherapy-related immunosuppression can further contribute to diminished body image.

Many investigators have studied women with breast cancer and the psychological effects they experience throughout treatment (Arora et al., 2001; Fobair et al., 2002; Girotto, Schreiber, & Nahabedian, 2003; Schover et al., 1995). Mastectomy may affect the concept of body image more than breast-conserving treatment in relation to disfigurement and loss of femininity (Arora et al.; Schover et al.). Kraus (1999) addressed the issue of women who believed their breasts were important to their feelings of femininity and attractiveness. These women had more problems with body image after breast cancer treatment than those women who had strong identities and were less concerned with physical appearance. Women with good self-concepts were satisfied with their body image and were less concerned with physical presentation after treatment for breast cancer.

Another note of importance is that the public is beginning to question the medical community regarding its notions about what is "right" and for whom information related to treatment options for breast cancer is provided. Carter (2003) explained that the American Cancer Society does not address the lesbian female, the man with breast cancer, or single females in its video *A Significant Journey: Breast Cancer Survivors and the Men Who Love Them.*

Three studies using data from questionnaires examined various other surgical outcomes in relation to self-perception and body image. Dropkin (1999) affirmed that body image reintegration is critical to subsequent quality of life after disfiguring head and neck cancer surgery. Andersen, Woods, and Copeland (1997) designed a questionnaire to ascertain the patients' views of themselves as sexual beings following gynecologic cancer. Women with a negative self-schema (picture themselves as less feminine) were less sexually responsive.

Men with prostate cancer also encounter troubling problems with body image (Bostwick, MacLennan, & Larson, 1999; Schover, 1997). Radical prostatectomy may cause problems with urinary incontinence, and social activities may be severely curtailed because incontinence is difficult to conceal or is associated with uncleanliness. Inability to achieve or maintain an erection can be devastating to a man's body image and self-esteem. Although nerve-sparing surgery often prevents this side effect, preservation or recovery of erectile function declines with age and increased tumor volume (Fossa et al., 1997; Talcott et al., 1998). If prostate cancer recurs, hormonal manipulation is the treatment of choice, which may involve bilateral orchiectomy or testosterone-depleting medication. Using estrogen or luteinizing hormone-releasing hormone antagonists such as leuprolide may cause hot flashes, mood swings, and thinning hair, all of which may have a negative influence on masculine body image.

The loss of a testicle may affect male identity. Incrocci, Bosch, and Slob (1999) reported in their retrospective questionnaire study of testicular seminoma patients (N = 22) who had undergone surgery and radiation therapy that 52% of the subjects sustained a change in their body image. Furthermore, the loss of a testicle can create feelings of embarrassment with a partner or if they happen to undress in the presence of other men during sports activities. Those who had problems with sexual contacts or who had concerns about undressing in front of others had not had a testicular prosthesis placed. Only 50% of the subjects had been informed by their urologist that testicular implants were available. Incrocci, Hop, Wijnmaalen, and Slob (2002) demonstrated that implantation of testicular prostheses is virtually without complications and has provided many patients with improved body image.

Although breast and prostate cancer have been studied more extensively than most other types of cancer in relation to body image, sexuality, and psychosocial concerns, patients with any cancer most likely suffer from some form of body image dysfunction because of the extensive surgery often needed to eradicate disease or the adjuvant chemotherapy needed to prevent disease recurrence. Table 17-3 presents special issues that may affect body image related to various cancers. Researchers must

Table 17-3. Site-Specific Body Image and Sexual Concerns

Site	Issues
Breast	Affects large number of patients Emotional and sexual significance of breast Appearance concerns (scar, prosthesis, reconstruction) Surgical treatment (loss of breast) Chemotherapy (loss of ovarian function, alopecia) Young patients (childbearing possible after treatment)
Gynecologic	Affects patients of all ages Emotional, sexual, and reproductive significance of gynecologic organs Surgical treatment (loss of uterus, ovaries, vagina, external genitals) Chemotherapy (loss of ovarian function, appearance concerns) Radiation therapy (fibrosis and scarring of vagina) Sexual dysfunction (fear of pain with intercourse, other concerns) Loss of childbearing capacity
Testicular	Affects young men Emotional, sexual, and reproductive significance of testes Appearance concerns (prosthesis, alopecia) Treatment (surgery, chemotherapy) may cause sterility and changes in ejaculation. Sperm banking is an option.
Bladder and prostate	Affects middle-aged or older men (experiencing the effects of aging on erection) Surgical treatment (high incidence of impotence) Impact of ostomy, even temporary
Colon and rectal	Affects middle-aged or older patients Surgical treatment (high incidence of impotence) Impact of ostomy, even temporary
Lymphoma and leukemia	Affects young patients Long, stressful treatment Alopecia Treatment (chemotherapy, radiation) can cause sterility and loss of ovarian function.

Note. From "Sexual Dysfunction in Cancer Patients: Issues in Evaluation and Treatment" (p. 391), by S. Auchincloss in J.C. Holland (Ed.), *Psycho-Oncology*, 1998, New York: Oxford University Press. Copyright 1998 by Oxford University Press. Reprinted with permission.

begin to explore patients with other cancers, such as lung, esophagus, pancreas, and brain, to ensure optimal attention to body-image concerns for all patients.

Nursing Care of Patients With Body Image Disturbance

Assessment

Because body image disturbances may adversely affect a patient's recovery from illness and relationships with others, nurses have a responsibility to assess and identify adverse changes in body image and begin appropriate interventions. Body image is discussed often as it relates to patients with cancer and the effects of cancer treatments and clearly is an important end point in quality-of-life evaluation. Hopwood, Fletcher, Lee, and Al Ghazal (2001) created (in collaboration with the European Organization for Research and Treatment of Cancer Quality of Life Study Group) a 10-item body image scale. The scale was first tested in a heterogeneous sample of 276 British patients with cancer and then underwent psychometric testing in 682 patients with breast cancer. The scale has high reliability and good clinical validity and is suitable for use in clinical trials. Another body image scale (Polivy, 1977) uses a 27-item Likert-type scale to measure individuals' satisfaction with various body parts. This scale has demonstrated good internal consistency and criterion-related, convergent, and construct validity (Bohrnstedt, 1977).

White (2000) noted that cancer and its treatments have a negative impact on "appearance-related" variables and suggested using a cognitive behavioral model to assess for body-image disturbance in patients with cancer.

Many other body image scales have been developed, some specific to a particular age group (e.g., Body Image Instrument developed for young people with cancer) or disease site (e.g., breast cancer, hematologic malignancies) (Kopel, Eiser, Cool, Grimer, & Carter, 1998; Lasry, Margolese, & Poisson, 1987; Weber et al., 2001; Zarcone, Classen, Smithline, & Spiegel, 1993).

Nurses must approach the issue of body image with warmth and sensitivity. A cool, overly professional demeanor does little to allay patients' concerns, but an overly familiar or joking stance is equally inappropriate. Healthcare professionals must consider various elements when assessing for a loss of identity that can lead to body image disturbances (see Table 17-4). Nurses often feel a decided discomfort in discussing personal or intimate details with their patients; however, with a little time and practice, these fears subside.

Differential Diagnosis

Body image disturbance may only be a symptom of a much broader group of issues. These may include
- The ability to learn to use the maximum amount of self-reliance to problem solve
- The ability to accept a certain level of physical dependence
- The ability to develop certain social skills to deal with society's stigmas and attitudes toward individuals with an altered physical appearance.

Table 17-4. Assessment Parameters Related to Body Image Disturbance

Loss of Identity	Interpretation
Treatment-related issues	Chronic illness progresses; patient feels defined by it and becomes "a cancer patient." Changes in sexuality and role changes deprive patients of identity.
Meaning of illness	Hospital anxieties: regression, separation, loss of privacy Surgery: loss of function, disfigurement, castration Chemotherapy: powerful side effects Radiation: feared as unknown, possible harmful force
Fear of death	Patients attribute meanings to illness and how/why they became ill. Meanings amplify suffering; patient loses control of body.
Disrupted self-esteem	Self-esteem is disrupted because of unaccomplished goals. Completing everyday life tasks may be difficult.

Note. Based on information from Postone, 1998.

Body image disturbance may involve more serious psychiatric diagnoses, including mood disorders (e.g., depression), anxiety disorders (e.g., panic attacks), somatoform disorders (e.g., body dysmorphic disorders), or sexual and gender-identity disorders (e.g., sexual aversion disorders) (American Psychiatric Association, 2000).

An individual's response to a body alteration will be determined, in part, by the meaning of the change for the person, which may include loss of control, change in appearance, altered sexual functioning, or a change in self-esteem and self-identity. Finally, body image problems can masquerade as denial, depression, shame, or casual indifference (Carpenito, 2002).

Interventions

Because the impact of disease upon body image is closely bound to psychological symptoms and the physical effects of the illness and its treatment, nurses must be able to address body-image dysfunction with timely interventions. Several interventions may be appropriate.
1. Provide opportunities to discuss body changes, what they mean to the patients, and how they will compensate for the loss.
2. Acknowledge patients' loss, normalize feelings of grief and anger, and encourage their expression.
3. Maintain modesty and privacy so patients can look at or think about the altered body part and begin to integrate these changes into an altered body image.
4. Assist with/provide meticulous personal care.
5. Provide realistic compliments about the patients' appearance to focus attention on positive personal characteristics.
6. Accept patients' altered body or changes in function, and serve as a role model for family and friends by accepting the changes (e.g., changing a dressing without expressions of aversion or disgust).
7. Assist partners to accept the change by encouraging expression of feelings and dispelling myths about the disease (Schover, 2000).

8. Help patients to learn that they have not lost everything (i.e., not all positive attributes are undermined by the cancer) and to strengthen and integrate the newly reorganized sense of self.

9. Make patients aware of possible surgical procedures (e.g., testicular and penile prostheses, breast reconstruction) that can enhance their sense of body image (Shell, 2001).

Nurses may ask particular questions or make statements when providing supportive interventions. For example, nurses may begin a conversation with a comment such as, "It's a rough surgery or treatment that you have been through," and then respond to the patient's concerns to encourage him or her to keep talking. Use of reflective techniques, open-ended statements, and validation of responses encourages patients to express feelings and promotes open communication. Schover (2000) encouraged nurses to ask questions related to how sexually attractive the patient feels even though physical changes have occurred. Some of the questions may include, "Has your illness or the sexual problem changed how attractive you feel?" or perhaps, "How do you feel about your own sexual attractiveness?" (p. 412).

Nurses who have extra time to devote to patients or who are interested in providing more in-depth intervention can begin a conversation asking the patients what their life was like before the illness. This can lead to an exploration of the meaning and importance of the losses experienced during the current treatment regimen.

Asking patients to detail their losses in writing is another strategy. Patients may wish to write a list of the losses according to whether the lost characteristic(s) can be recovered (Daniluk, 1998; Pollin, 1995). More specifically, Rancour and Brauer (2003) gave patients a homework assignment and encouraged them to write a letter to the affected body part, describing their reactions to its impending loss. Enabling patients to focus on their strengths, which will include the qualities that will be recovered, is encouraging and helps them to grieve for those abilities that will be lost forever. Nurses can help to normalize feelings of sadness and anger by restating patients' frustrations, which can help patients through this difficult process.

Other approaches to counseling patients about body image include conducting a joint session with patients and their partners to discuss the changes and the effect of those changes on the relationship. Unmarried patients may need to plan how to meet new dating partners and if or when to disclose the diagnosis (Schover, 2001a, 2001b). These patients may benefit from participating in a support group or an intervention group specifically designed to address patients' concerns such as body image (Fobair et al., 2002; Roberts, Piper, Denny, & Cuddeback, 1997). As patients begin to feel accepted as worthy, loved, and wanted as individuals, the threat to body image begins to decrease. Sometimes, brief counseling is not enough, and formal therapy may be more beneficial if specific individual, couple, or family issues are addressed.

Evidence-Based Practice

All studies discussed previously have been retrospective or prospective, nonexperimental, correlational, or descriptive studies done to prove that body image dysfunction exists or how body image is affected during treatment. Rutledge and Grant (2002) considered this type of evidence-based research to be moderately strong evidence. No strong research-based studies exist relative to interventions to promote healthy body image in patients with cancer, although many nonrandomized studies have documented a problem with body-image disturbance in the cancer population. The strongest research-based evidence regarding the recommendations for interventions includes three nonexperimental studies: two group therapy interventions and one surgical procedure.

The two group therapy studies involved 14 and 20 subjects, respectively. The first study (Roberts et al., 1997) used psychoeducational strategies and group therapy techniques, and the second study (Fobair et al., 2002) used supportive-expressive group therapy techniques. Both concluded that positive changes occurred, and the group process helped patients to adjust to their diagnoses. However, neither study was specific to body image alone, and both included several medical-related psychosocial end points (e.g., coping with diagnosis, illness, and treatment) The third study looked at the impact of a testicular prosthesis relative to body image, and after reviewing 22 subjects' questionnaires, researchers concluded that almost all patients reported an improved body image with the testicular implant (Incrocci et al., 1999).

Evidence-based clinical practice guidelines do not exist per se for body image disturbance. Both the National Guideline Clearinghouse (www.guideline.gov) and the National Comprehensive Cancer Network (www.nccn.org) have guidelines that indirectly may affect body image, and the reader is encouraged to contact these resources if further information is desired.

Most of the interventions currently in use stem from non–research-based evidence and include case studies and opinions of experts. In a case study, Rancour and Brauer (2003) reported on the use of letter writing as a technique to help patients to integrate an altered body image into their sense of self during and after cancer treatment. They concluded that this technique was effective in helping patients to adjust to the reconstruction of a lost breast. Other interventions come from several expert opinion resources, and although this is valuable information, it is the weakest type of evidence to be used to make practice recommendations. However, it is the current practice within the field of oncology nursing. Quality practice only can be realized with experimental, well-controlled, randomized clinical trials that address body image (see Figure 17-1).

Figure 17-1. Plan of Care

Assessment
- Recognize that body image includes more than the physical body alone.
- Consider the variables that may have an impact on body image (e.g., loss of a body part, change or loss of function, immediate versus prolonged change).
- Use one of the body-image tools available to assess the extent of possible concern or dysfunction.
- Identify the following.
    - Feelings of anger, sadness, frustration, and guilt
    - The nature of the threat
    - The patient's age
    - The degree of support from family

(Continued on next page)

Figure 17-1. Plan of Care *(Continued)*

- Continue to reassess the patient's responses at all stages (e.g., diagnosis, treatment, recovery).
- Evaluate the need for more extensive assessment and in-depth counseling.

Nursing Diagnoses (NANDA International, 2005)
- Disturbed body image
- Disturbed personal identity

***DSM-IV-TR* Diagnoses** (American Psychiatric Association, 2000)
- Adjustment disorder
- Major depressive disorder

Expected Outcomes
- Patients/partners will accept help or care.
- Patients/partners will acknowledge and discuss body loss/changes.
- Patients/partners will look at the affected area.
- Patients/partners will reject feelings of being dirty or defiled and contaminated.
- Patients/partners will resume sexual activity as appropriate.

Interventions
- Acknowledge loss.
- Provide opportunity for discussion of body changes.
- Maintain modesty and privacy to show patients that they are valued.
- Demonstrate acceptance of altered body and change in functions.
- Provide/assist with meticulous personal care.
- Offer realistic compliments.
- Assist partners to accept change.
- Assist patients to strengthen newly reorganized sense of self.
- Help patients to view and touch changed area as appropriate.
- Provide necessary strategies (e.g., wig, prosthesis) for dealing with anticipated changes.
- Provide access to specific group therapy resources, support groups, and other services (e.g., Reach to Recovery, Look Good . . . Feel Better, Y-Me).

Case Study

Mrs. H, a 43-year-old, white, married woman with two children, was diagnosed with breast cancer and underwent a mastectomy. She had 10 of 18 lymph nodes test positive for cancer. Mrs. H was a homemaker who had previously worked as an executive secretary. She was attractive, was of average height and weight, and had wavy, brown hair. She explained to the nurse that it was her choice to have a mastectomy with immediate reconstruction. She felt more comfortable having the breast with cancer completely removed rather than having a lumpectomy. She stated that she and her husband discussed the decision, and he was very supportive. The reason she decided on immediate reconstruction was because she did not want to have to bother with a prosthesis and thought reconstruction would feel more natural. When she awoke from surgery, it was as if no mastectomy had been performed; she had a breast mound, and this pleased her. At that point, she was very satisfied with her body image because she could wear all of her usual clothing

(Continued on next page)

Case Study *(Continued)*

and still outwardly look the same. She stated that she felt somewhat self-conscious and embarrassed appearing naked in front of her husband, although she never was a person who felt completely comfortable with being naked. Her husband was very gentle with her because of the acute surgical discomfort she experienced. As Mrs. H's wound and reconstruction healed, her husband remained reluctant to touch the reconstructed breast, even though she encouraged him to do so. This did not distress her because she knew he loved her and thought he still may be afraid that he would hurt her. She had a very positive concept of her body image and had decided not to have nipple reconstruction because she was so satisfied with her results. The reconstruction had accomplished exactly what she had hoped for—that she appear "normal" to anyone who saw her and that she feel "normal" if anyone felt or bumped into her.

Eleven months after surgery, Mrs. H comes into the hospital for her high-dose induction treatment prior to stem cell transplant. She reports having several body-image concerns. The reconstructed breast is still satisfactory to her; however, she avoids looking at her naked body in the mirror because it makes her sad and angry. She feels betrayed by her body and also feels vulnerable. She says she did not realize how fragile the human body could be and now will have a difficult time trusting her body. The chemotherapy she has received has caused her to lose all of her hair, including her eyebrows and eyelashes, and this has been more devastating to her than losing the hair on her head. She can wear a wig to cover her bald head, but she feels less comfortable with penciled-on eyebrows and fake eyelashes. She states that eyebrows and lashes are what frame her face, and now she feels like "an alien" when she looks into the mirror. She acknowledges that her husband remains supportive and loving to her, but she wonders if she is still attractive to the opposite sex because she feels she is a changed person, with low confidence.

Discussion

The clinical nurse specialist's (CNS's) assessment of Mrs. H was that she was experiencing some body-image dysfunction. However, Mrs. H was willing to express these concerns and ask for help. The CNS was able to intervene with Mrs. H by encouraging and allowing her to verbalize and grieve over her losses and acknowledge her pain. This validated Mrs. H's feelings. The CNS encouraged Mrs. H by complimenting her on her ability to apply makeup skillfully. She also encouraged Mrs. H's continued communication with her spouse about her fears and concerns regarding the changes in her body. She had no problems with menopausal symptoms (e.g., vaginal dryness during intercourse) but still is self-conscious when appearing naked in front of her husband. The CNS suggested that Mrs. H wear a fancy camisole or sleeveless pajama top during intercourse to increase Mrs. H's comfort with her nakedness. The CNS concluded that Mrs. H did not need in-depth counseling at this time but that it is important for her to continue to feel comfortable discussing these issues with the CNS and with her husband.

Conclusion

Body image is how people think about themselves and their bodies, along with the way people experience themselves in the mirror and how their bodies smell, work, and appear to others. A chronic physical illness such as cancer can create a complex array of internal and external experiences that translate into changes and distortions in body image. These changes will vary depending on the cancer site and treatment and will be affected by the patient's age, sex, life experience, and usual or preillness coping mechanisms.

Research is needed to describe the impact of cancer and its treatment on body image specific to all cancer sites. Investigators must describe and test specific interventions related to body image and assess their ability to help to improve body self-esteem and image. Through continued efforts encompassing assessment and intervention guided by evidence-based practice, nurses will be able to be more sensitive to the ways in which patients maintain or restore their orientation to their bodies and body function. These patients then may be able to look forward with realistic hope to the whole range of individual relationships with themselves, as well as richer human interrelationships (including parent, child, sibling, partner, community participant, and career person), with a revised and renewed body image.

References

American Psychiatric Association. (2000). *Diagnostic and statistical manual of mental disorders* (4th ed., text rev.). Washington, DC: Author.

Andersen, B.L., Woods, X.A., & Copeland, L.J. (1997). Sexual self-schema and sexual morbidity among gynecologic cancer survivors. *Journal of Consulting and Clinical Psychology, 65*, 221–229.

Arora, N.K., Gustafson, D.H., Hawkins, R.P., McTavish, F., Cella, D.F., Pingree, S., et al. (2001). Impact of surgery and chemotherapy on the quality of life of younger women with breast carcinoma: A prospective study. *Cancer, 92*, 1288–1298.

Bohrnstedt, G.W. (1977). *On measuring body satisfaction.* Bloomington, IN: University Press.

Bostwick, D.G., MacLennan, G.T., & Larson, T.R. (1999). *Prostate cancer: What every man—and his family—needs to know* (Rev. ed.). New York: Villard Books.

Carpenito, L. (Ed.). (2002). *Nursing diagnosis: Application to clinical practice* (9th ed.). Philadelphia: Lippincott.

Carter, T. (2003). Body count: Autobiographies by women living with breast cancer. *Journal of Popular Culture, 36*, 653–664.

Carver, C.S., Pozo-Kaderman, C., Price, A.A., Noriega, V., Harris, S.D., Derhagopian, R.P., et al. (1998). Concern about aspects of body image and adjustment to early stage breast cancer. *Psychosomatic Medicine, 60*, 168–174.

Cusumano, D.L., & Thompson, J.K. (1997). Body image and body shape ideals in magazines: Exposure, awareness, and internalization. *Sex Roles, 37*, 701–722.

Daniluk, J. (1998). *Women's sexuality across the life span: Challenging myths, creating meanings.* New York: Guilford Press.

Dropkin, M.J. (1999). Body image and quality of life after head and neck cancer surgery. *Cancer Practice, 7*, 309–313.

Fobair, P., Kloopman, C., Dimiceli, S., O'Hanlan, K., Butler, L.D., Classen, C., et al. (2002). Psychosocial intervention for lesbians with primary breast cancer. *Psycho-Oncology, 11*, 427–438.

Fossa, S.D., Woehre, H., Kurth, K.H., Hetherington, J., Bakker, H., Rustad, D.A., et al. (1997). Influence of urological morbidity on quality of life in patients with prostate cancer. *European Urology, 31*(Suppl. 3), 3–8.

Girotto, J.A., Schreiber, J., & Nahabedian, M.Y. (2003). Breast reconstruction in the elderly: Preserving excellent quality of life. *Annals of Plastic Surgery, 50,* 572–578.

Green, M.S., Naumann, R.W., Elliot, M., Hall, J.B., Higgins, R.V., & Grigsby, J.H. (2000). Sexual dysfunction following vulvectomy. *Gynecologic Oncology, 77,* 73–77.

Hart, S., Skinner, E.C., Meyerowitz, B.E., Boyd, S., Lieskovsky, G., & Skinner, D.G. (1999). Quality of life after radical cystectomy for bladder cancer in patients with an ileal conduit, cutaneous or urethral kock pouch. *Journal of Urology, 62,* 77–81.

Hopwood, P., Fletcher, I., Lee, A., & Al Ghazal, S. (2001). A body image scale for use with cancer patients. *European Journal of Cancer, 37,* 189–197.

Incrocci, L., Bosch, J.L., & Slob, A.K. (1999). Testicular prosthesis: Body image and sexual functioning. *British Journal of Urology International, 84,* 1043–1045.

Incrocci, L., Hop, W.C., Wijnmaalen, A., & Slob, A.K. (2002). Treatment outcome, body image, and sexual functioning after orchiectomy and radiotherapy for stage I–II testicular seminoma. *International Journal of Radiation Oncology, Biology, Physics, 53,* 1165–1173.

Katz, M., Rodin, G., & Devins, G. (1995). Self-esteem and cancer: Theory and research. *Canadian Journal of Psychiatry, 40,* 608–615.

Kopel, S.J., Eiser, C., Cool, P., Grimer, R.J., & Carter, S.J. (1998). Brief report: Assessment of body image in survivors of childhood cancer. *Journal of Pediatric Psychiatry, 23,* 141–147.

Kraus, P.L. (1999). Body image, decision making, and breast cancer treatment. *Cancer Nursing, 22,* 421–427.

Laken, V., & Laken, K. (2002). *Making love again.* East Sandwich, MA: North Star Publications/Ant Hill Press.

Lasry, J.M., Margolese, R.G., & Poisson, R. (1987). Depression and body image following mastectomy and lumpectomy. *Journal of Chronic Disease, 40,* 529–534.

Leiblum, S.R., & Segraves, R.T. (2000). Sex therapy with aging adults. In S.R. Leiblum & R.C. Rosen (Eds.), *Principles and practice of sex therapy* (3rd ed., pp. 423–448). New York: Guilford Press.

Lin, E.M. (1996). Coping with altered body image. In C.M. Hogan & R. Wickham (Eds.), *Issues in managing the oncology patient* (pp. 8–16). New York: Philips Healthcare Communications.

McGarvey, E.L., Baum, L.D., Pinkerton, R.C., & Rogers, L.M. (2001). Psychological sequelae and alopecia among women with cancer. *Cancer Practice, 9,* 283–289.

Moreno, J., Chancellor, M., Karasick, S., King, S., Abdill, C., & Rivas, D. (1995). Improved quality of life and sexuality with continent urinary diversion in quadriplegic women with umbilical stoma. *Archives of Physical Medicine and Rehabilitation, 76,* 758–761.

Morse, J.M., Bottorff, J.L., & Hutchinson, S. (1995). The paradox of comfort. *Nursing Research, 44,* 14–19.

NANDA International. (2005). *Nursing diagnoses: Definitions and classification, 2005–2006.* Philadelphia: Author.

Olivo, E.L., & Woolverton, K. (2001). Surviving childhood cancer: Disruptions in the developmental building blocks of sexuality. *Journal of Sex Education and Therapy, 26,* 172–181.

Polivy, J. (1977). Psychological effects of mastectomy on a woman's feminine self-concept. *Journal of Nervous Mental Disorders, 164,* 77–87.

Pollin, I. (with Kanaan, S.). (1995). *Medical crisis counseling: Short-term therapy for long-term illness.* New York: Norton.

Postone, N. (1998). Psychotherapy with cancer patients. *American Journal of Psychotherapy, 52,* 412–424.

Rancour, P., & Brauer, K. (2003). Use of letter writing as a means of integrating an altered body image: A case study. *Oncology Nursing Forum, 30,* 841–846.

Roberts, C.S., Piper, L., Denny, J., & Cuddeback, G. (1997). A support group intervention to facilitate young adults' adjustment to cancer. *Health and Social Work, 22,* 133–141.

Rutledge, D.N., & Grant, M. (2002). Evidence-based practice in cancer nursing: Introduction. *Seminars in Oncology Nursing, 18,* 1–2.

Schover, L., Yetman, R., Tuason, L., Meisler, E., Esselstyn, C., Hermann, R., et al. (1995). Comparison of partial mastectomy with breast reconstruction on psychosocial adjustment, body image, and sexuality. *Cancer, 75,* 54–64.

Schover, L.R. (1997). *Sexuality and fertility after cancer.* New York: John Wiley.

Schover, L.R. (2000). Sexual problems in chronic illness. In S.R. Leiblum & R.C. Rosen (Eds.), *Principles and practice of sex therapy* (3rd ed., pp. 398–422). New York: Guilford Press.

Schover, L.R. (2001a). *Sexuality and cancer: For the man who has cancer, and his partner.* Atlanta, GA: American Cancer Society.

Schover, L.R. (2001b). *Sexuality and cancer: For the woman who has cancer, and her partner.* Atlanta, GA: American Cancer Society.

Shell, J. (2001). Impact of cancer on sexuality. In S. Otto (Ed.), *Oncology nursing* (4th ed., pp. 973–999). St. Louis, MO: Mosby.

Stern, C. (1990). Body image concerns, surgical conditions, and sexuality. In C. Fogel & D. Lauver (Eds.), *Sexual health promotion* (pp. 498–516). Philadelphia: Saunders.

Talcott, J.A., Rieker, P., Clark, J.A., Propert, K.J., Weeks, J.C., Beard, C.J., et al. (1998). Patient-reported symptoms after primary therapy for early prostate cancer: Results of a prospective cohort study. *Journal of Clinical Oncology, 16,* 275–283.

Van der Velde, C.D. (1985). Body images of one's self and of others: Developmental and clinical significance. *American Journal of Psychiatry, 142,* 527–537.

Weber, C., Bronner, E., Their, P., Schoeneich, F., Walter, O., Klapp, B.F., et al. (2001). Body experience and mental representation of body image in patients with haematological malignancies and cancer as assessed with the body grid. *British Journal of Medical Psychology, 74,* 507–521.

White, C.A. (2000). Body image dimensions and cancer: A heuristic cognitive behavioural model. *Psycho-Oncology, 9,* 183–192.

Wiederman, M.W., & Hurst, S.R. (1998). Body size, physical attractiveness, and body image among young adult women: Relationships to sexual experience and sexual esteem. *Journal of Sex Research, 35,* 272–282.

Williams, J., Wood, C., & Cunningham-Warburton, P. (1999). A narrative study of chemotherapy-induced alopecia. *Oncology Nursing Forum, 26,* 1463–1468.

Zarcone, J., Classen, C., Smithline, R., & Spiegel, D. (1993). The Body Image and Sexuality Scale for women with breast cancer (BISS). Unpublished scale.

CHAPTER 18

Transforming the Grief Experience

KATHERINE BROWN-SALTZMAN, RN, MA

Give sorrow words; the grief that does not speak
Whispers the o'er-fraught heart, and bids it break.

—William Shakespeare

Mrs. Rivers, a 50-year-old woman diagnosed with acute myelogenous leukemia, had failed traditional therapy and had undergone a bone marrow transplant. She had a normal course with manageable complications (an infection and significant pain from mouth sores). She coped well with minimal supportive therapy from the social worker and daily visits from her family. Because she recovered quickly, discharge was timely, and preparations were made for her homecoming. She remained at home for only four days and was readmitted with severe nausea and dehydration. Her spouse reported that just two days after her return home, their eldest grandchild had been killed in an accidental shooting. In the hospital, Mrs. Rivers became more despondent. She experienced increased nausea, refused food, and began to vomit. She became weak and did not leave her hospital bed except to use the commode. Mr. Rivers was fearful of the change he was witnessing in his normally strong wife. He reported that she occasionally was tearful, yet she expressed the wish not to talk about her grandson's death and seemed to become progressively more withdrawn. He felt helpless and expressed concern that she would not be able to "fight" and become well. A research nurse who knew the patient well referred her to the clinical nurse specialist for support after observing the increasing depression.

Bereavement and Grief

To be bereaved is to be deprived of something (especially hope or joy) ruthlessly or to become desolate through loss. The etymology of the word comes from the Old English roots "be" and "reafian," meaning "be-robbed" (Barnhart, 1962, p. 115). In personal terms, that translates to being robbed of a loved one and of all the future hopes and plans for and with that loved one. Does the bereaved person even recognize how grief-filled he or she has become? Bereaved children lose not only a family member but also their surviving parent or parents, who are changed by sorrow and may become emotionally inaccessible. The patient who is dying experiences many losses, and anticipatory grief evokes the loss of oneself and all that one knows and loves. Bereavement often is seen as the process of grief, most often related to loss through death or, as Lindemann (1944) noted, the threat of death. Grief is simply the reaction to loss (Corr & Doka, 1994). In oncology, healthcare professionals are familiar with losses that may occur throughout the trajectory of illness: amputation, colostomy, infertility, loss of hair, loss of appetite and normal sense of taste, loss of energy, and loss of sexual intimacy.

As patients come to know nurses, they may share stories of other losses, including the significant other who left after the diagnosis, the marriage that fell apart because of the added pressures of illness, the old wounds from a long-ago divorce that now are intensified, or the job or school left, even if only temporarily. Losing a sense of normalcy and innocence ("I will never be worry-free again. I will always wonder if it is coming back.") may have the greatest impact on a person. Nurses' roles in working with the bereaved are to develop a basic understanding of the grief process, to acquire assessment skills that enable them to delineate normal and complicated grief, and to discover potential interventions and referrals.

Grief may cause healthcare professionals to feel helpless and uncomfortable. Remaining present in the face of such sorrow is not easy. Nurses may wonder about saying the right thing or worry that somehow patients' feelings of grief were accentuated through a clumsy comment. By gaining knowledge about the grief process, nurses become more competent to care for patients with cancer and their families. This also assists nurses in understanding their own (and other healthcare team members') responses to patients' deaths.

Freud (1961) established that the task of grieving is a process of disconnecting from the one who has died; essentially, it is a process of decathexis and then a gradual reattachment to another. Most theories of grief are based on this premise. In the 1940s, Lindemann (1944) studied the survivors of the Coconut Grove nightclub fire in Boston, MA, and described grief reactions that lasted six to eight weeks. As a result of this work, a crisis intervention model of caring for the bereaved emerged. Subsequently, researchers recognized that the normal length of the grief process may, in fact, last one year and perhaps as long as four years (Gerber, Rusalem, Hannon, Battin, & Arkin, 1975). Some have described grief as a lifelong process in which adjustments occur on anniversaries and during major life events. Edelman (1994) described a woman's lifetime grief over the death of her mother: "The intervals between grief responses lengthen over time, but the longing never disappears. It always hovers at the edge of your awareness, prepared to surface at any time . . ." (p. 24). The Committee for the Study of Health Consequences of the Stress of Bereavement, formed by the Institute of Medicine to study the impact of grief on health, found that a normal grief process may be lengthy for some individuals (Osterweis, Solomon, & Green, 1984). They noted that it is not the length of time per se that distinguishes normal from abnormal grief but the quality and quantity of reactions over time. Clearly, people have come to understand another dimension of grief since the events of September 11. The issues of complicated and traumatic grief have been powerful, not only for the bereaved families and the survivors but also for the whole country as it went from disbelief, to anger, to despair and depression, and then finally attempting to find meaning and healing.

Theoretical Tasks of Grief

Kübler-Ross (1969) was one of the early professionals to articulate the process of death and dying. Her concept of stages of dying established the expectation that a grieving person moved from denial, to anger, to bargaining, to depression, and, finally, to acceptance. This work opened doors to understanding the process, but it is now understood in a less rigid context. Patients can skip a stage or pass in and out of stages. Whether it is the work of the dying or grief work of the living, each goes through an individual journey as they attempt to come to terms with death.

Based on his studies of widows, Parkes (1987) described five aspects of grief. **Alarm** reflects the physiologic response. This is a state of high arousal with components of the fight or flight mechanism and irritability. In the area of research on stress responses, a growing body of literature exists related to the neurochemical and immune responses to bereavement. **Searching** involves spontaneous "pangs" of grief that come over the bereaved. The pangs are described as episodes of severe anxiety and psychological pain and most often are expressed with sighing and weeping. These episodes are most intense in the first 5–14 days and then gradually lessen. Memories of the loss stimulate these episodes. Pining, a persistent and obtrusive wish for the person who is gone, also occurs. Parkes interpreted this as the need to search for the lost person. Searching contraindicates one's rational knowledge of death and can include restless movement, thoughts preoccupied by the deceased, a preconscious recognition that "sets" the bereaved to anticipate and "see" the dead person, actual scanning of the environment for the person, and a loss of concentration. At times, the bereaved may describe seeing, hearing, or calling out to the deceased. **Mitigation** is another aspect of the process. Behaviors used to lessen the pain include feeling comfort in sensing the presence of the dead person, talking or praying (either while awake or asleep) to the dead person with the belief that he or she hears, denying the loss, and turning away from thoughts about the dead person. Increasing activity, returning to work, putting away the deceased person's possessions, and leaving the area or home for a period of time are other ways of mitigating. An attempt is made to make sense of the loss; Parkes saw this as a way of restoring what is lost by fitting its absence into some fundamental pattern.

Anger and guilt also are components of the bereavement process. Parkes (1987) found that anger was greatest in the first month and almost always occurred sometime during the first year. People may focus anger and aggression at the dead person for "leaving," at God, or at the healthcare team for not saving the deceased. At times, the grieving direct their anger and irritability at those most near, even themselves. Those with the greatest anger became the most socially isolated. Guilt over some aspect of their relationship with the deceased was associated with complicated grief. The bereaved had difficulty relinquishing the deceased.

Finally, Parkes (1987) described **gaining a new identity.** An example of this is a widow in his study describing a sense of waking up and living again a year after her husband's death. The Committee for the Study of Health Consequences of the Stress of Bereavement described the culmination of a healthy bereavement process as including recovery of lost functions (including investment in current life, hopefulness, and the capacity to experience gratification), adaptation to new roles and status, and completion of acute grieving (Osterweis et al., 1984). Figure 18-1 presents a summary of additional grief theorists.

Figure 18-1. Additional Theoretical Perspectives of Grief		
Bowlby's Phases	**Worden's Tasks**	**Rando's Processes for Complicated Mourning**
1. Begins with numbing with potential disturbances or anguish/anger 2. One of searching and longing for the deceased person 3. Disorganization and despair 4. Reorganization	1. Accept the reality of the loss. 2. Experience the pain of the grief. 3. Adjust to an environment in which the deceased is missing. 4. Withdraw emotional energy from the deceased, and reinvest it in another relationship.	1. Recognize the loss; acknowledge and understand the death. 2. React to, experience, and express the separation and pain; be aware of and grieve secondary losses. 3. Recollect thoughts about the deceased, remember him or her realistically, and revive feelings for him or her. 4. Relinquish old attachments to the deceased. 5. Readjust and adapt to new ways of being without the deceased while maintaining memories, and form a new identity. 6. Reinvest.
Note. Based on information from Bowlby, 1980; Rando, 1993; Worden, 1991.		

Children and Bereavement

When they must help children to face death, nurses may feel stretched beyond their capabilities. In addition to feeling intimidated by the developmental issues, nurses may experience a heightened sense of loss and bereavement resulting from witnessing children's grief. Still, nurses often will be the ones at the bedside when a crisis occurs and the "specialists" are not available. In the United States, more than two million children younger than the age of 18 have lost a parent (Christ, Siegel, & Christ, 2002). Nurses who normally care for adults may be called upon to help with the patient's child or grandchild.

In a classic study, Nagy (1948) interviewed hundreds of Hungarian children and found that, prior to age five, they viewed death as a separation that was reversible. Between the ages of five and nine, the children personified death (i.e., something that could be outrun). By the time the children had reached age 10, they had developed a mature, cognitive concept of death as something final and universal.

American researchers have not been able to replicate these findings in regard to personification of death. They attribute this to cultural differences. In fact, Koocher (1974) found that children avoided abstraction when describing death and relied on specific details. He attributed this to an attempt to "control" death. In questioning children, Koocher found that those in the preoperational stage (seven years of age and younger) described death as being reversible.

Children's initial reaction to death is often shock and sadness, but they quickly return to seemingly inappropriate laughter or activity. In reality, their suffering may take many forms. Bowlby (1969) showed that mourning begins at six months as the infant separates from the mother. Furman (1964) determined that two- to three-year-olds are capable of comprehending the meaning of death. Like adults, children can somatize grief reactions with headaches and stomach pains and by imitating symptoms of the family member who has died. For children to regress and develop enuresis, separation anxieties, and phobias is not uncommon. As children grow and face new developmental challenges, they may reexperience the loss in new ways.

Helping a child to cope with death is a complex process. A good approach is to begin early and give the child some warning about the impending death. Nurses can make suggestions to help parents know how and what to tell a child and can offer guidelines on what the child can do in the hospital room. Regardless of the child's age, he or she should be prepared for how the family member will look or act. This will help the child to anticipate and cope. If a visit is not possible because of distance or the child's fear, the parent can suggest that the child send drawings, letters, video/audiotapes, or simple gifts. This can help the child to be present and say goodbye, even from afar. The child will long remember these offerings or a chance to talk. Allowing a child to help with the patient's care, when appropriate, also can ease some anxiety. Suggesting that the parent break up the visit with a special trip to the hospital cafeteria, museum, or a nearby park can make the experience more tolerable for the child. The institution's resources, such as child-life specialists or pediatric unit nurses, also can be called on for help. Resources for children often are available at bereavement centers and hospices, and the Internet has exploded with bereavement information. The American Cancer Society's "I Count, Too" is a support program for children and adolescents that assists them in dealing with the impact of the disease and sometimes aids in bereavement. Such a program may be available in the community. Being available to answer questions and respond to children's fears as well as helping them to understand the normalcy of family members' tears, anger, or sadness are important interventions. Nurses can consider writing a memory letter for a child. If a nurse has worked closely with the family member who has died, documenting the relationship, the characteristics of the person, and things he or she might have said about the child can provide a keepsake to be cherished later. See Figure 18-2 for additional suggestions.

Cultural Issues

Although guidelines and manuals are helpful in assisting healthcare professionals to understand death and grief practices, one cannot possibly know all the beliefs, customs, and nuances of individual families and sects. Asking for more information

---

Figure 18-2. Ways to Help Children to Cope With Grief

- Use simple and truthful answers and questions.
- Use direct language; use the words "death" and "died."
- Discuss religious and spiritual beliefs in simple terms, but avoid omnipresent language, such as "God took your uncle to heaven to be with Him." This could create fear for the child of being taken. Although it may be comforting to envision a family member who has died now in heaven, endowing that person with the ability to see all the child does may leave the child feeling shadowed. This could be frightening and create guilt for the child when he or she does something wrong.
- Do not compare death to sleep, which also can create fears and sleep disturbances.
- Help the child to understand adult responses to loss.
- Give the child the whole picture—that people heal and are not always engulfed by grief.
- Assess the child's belief that she or he is in some way responsible for the death and provide reassurance.
- Prepare the child for what he or she will see during the dying process, the funeral, or other rituals. Encourage the child's participation if appropriate.
- Consider creating a memory book that allows the child to express emotions and document memories using drawings, pictures, collages, poems, etc.
- Encourage referrals for additional support.

from the family and patient will help to unlock cultural complexities. Setting aside value judgments and acknowledging that the world can be viewed from many perspectives are important (Brown-Saltzman, 1995). The following story demonstrates the difficulty of sorting out the larger cultural issues and the individual interpretation and experience of those issues. A young Filipino woman with a brain tumor died after a long and difficult course of chemotherapy and radiation. The family had not been able to acknowledge her impending death until the very last moment, believing that a miracle would save her. Moments after the patient's death, the grandmother, who had remained at her bedside throughout the illness, asked to be left alone with the body. When the nurse returned, she found that the young girl's wrist had been slashed. Shocked by the sight and the blood, she ran from the room to call a security guard. After a great deal of confusion, they asked the grandmother what she had done. Through an interpreter, she shared that she had cut her granddaughter to let the blood flow out so that she could be sure that the patient was dead. The grandmother was afraid that her granddaughter would be buried alive and suffer as a friend of the family had. What appeared to be a bizarre act at first was, in fact, a last desperate act of love. Still, the staff viewed it as a desecration of the body. Although this is not a Filipino death tradition, the grandmother's past experience in her homeland left her wary of healthcare professionals' abilities to accurately determine death. Had the healthcare team been able to reassure the grandmother that they had reliable ways to determine death (e.g., a heart monitor, electroencephalogram), this incident might have been avoided. Although no one shared this woman's concerns, showing understanding and compassion for her in that moment and acknowledging her fears and concerns while withholding judgment facilitated healing.

Another aspect to consider in working with other cultures is the experience of immigration. Often, immigrants have come from war-torn countries and may have experienced the deaths of family and friends or, possibly worse, have family members who are missing. They may have experienced torture and abuse. Even if they emigrated from a peaceful country out of a desire for an improved life or simply for adventure, many immigrants have endured multiple losses along the way (e.g., loss of daily contact with family and friends, traditions, and language, changes in way of life or profession). Experiencing a new loss may awaken past losses and increase the sadness and isolation as well as complicate the grief process.

Lastly, one might look at ageism from a cultural perspective. Older adults may be at greater risk when it comes to bereavement, although the research is conflicting (Stroebe & Schut, 2001; Traylor, Hayslip, Kaminski, & York, 2003). One must avoid ageist stereotyping but at the same time be cognizant of the factors affecting bereaved older adults, especially multiple losses. For example, those entering residential care experience the potential losses of identity, control, spontaneity, and the right to take risks (Thompson, 2002). Older adults are at risk for disenfranchised grief. Disenfranchised grief occurs when there is a loss that cannot be acknowledged or publicly shared. The many losses in aging can be considered to be "normal" and therefore lose their significance.

Within the healthcare environment, professionals must take on the responsibility of honoring other cultures. Witnessing the suffering of grief reactions stirs discomfort in all people and is barely tolerable even when it is familiar to one's culture. When observing a reaction that is foreign to one's experience, professional fear and anxiety may increase. Clements et al. (2003) encouraged professionals to honor adaptive coping of individual cultures so that patients and families have permission to express grief according to their cultural norm. The challenge is to discover that norm for the many cultures and individuals.

Completion of Case Study

To reflect on the case of Mrs. Rivers that began this chapter, one sees that this patient was in a state of numbness and more than likely was still experiencing alarm. She, in fact, had not allowed herself to cry or express emotion over her grandson's death. This reaction may be in keeping with her personality, but it also may reflect her extreme vulnerability and fragility because of all that she had been through. Her own health is still precarious. It takes emotional, physical, and spiritual energy to grieve, and sometimes the grief process is halted because of extreme situations (e.g., too many losses in a relatively short period of time).

During the initial interview with the clinical nurse specialist, Mrs. Rivers appeared drawn and exhibited little energy. She responded to questions with simple answers. Her affect was flat and distant. When her grandson's death was acknowledged, she fought back tears and became shaky, and her mouth trembled. The magnitude of the grief was acknowledged. Gently, the nurse used reflective statements to describe a grief response. "You have been through a terrible loss, an overwhelming loss. I can see the pain of it in you, the sorrow." With the grief recognized, tears began to fall; Mrs. Rivers could not answer with words but only nodded. The nurse took her hand, and Mrs. Rivers responded by holding tightly. The nurse continued, "It makes no sense. He was so young. We cannot make sense of such an accident, and yet we ask why, over and over again." These words and the nurse's empathy touched the deep hurt, and the patient began to sob. As the tears flowed, she fought to maintain some control; the sobs caught in her throat. The nurse acknowledged how overwhelming grief would feel when it spilled seemingly out of control and assured her that it would not become uncontrollable. The patient seemed reassured, and when the nurse offered to hold her, the sobs came without restraint. After being held and crying for some time, she began to talk and verbalize the grief thus far contained. In between sighs, she described the feeling that she was going crazy, spiraling out of control. Now she could tell the story, how no one even told her the first day that he died because relatives were fearful that it would be too much for her. She had been too ill to attend the funeral, and she talked about how unreal the death seemed and how she woke each morning to the horror and knowledge, "He's dead!" When asked what had helped to get her through hard things in her life, she shook her head and responded, "I've always been strong. I just put one foot in front of another—had a stiff upper lip. My family has always depended upon me. I have never fallen apart." "And now you are feeling like you are falling apart?" "Yes! Yes! I am very frightened." The nurse reflected, "You have been through so much. Losing your grandson has been the last straw. You came to this news already having lost so much." The tears began to fall again. The nurse continued, "First, you found out you had leukemia, and you felt you lost your health and sense of well-being, the normalcy of life. You underwent treatment, hoping for a remission and cure, yet relapse brought another loss. Then you came in for a bone marrow transplant and, even though you gained this new life, it is as though you had to die first. You became incredibly vulnerable."

The patient nodded as the tears continued and now began to acknowledge the many losses. "Look at my skin. I look like an old woman. I never dreamed I would be so ill. I lost all of my strength. I am not the woman I was. I wonder over and over why I did this to myself." The nurse responded, "All of this, and now you lose your grandson. Of course you have fallen apart. How could it be otherwise? And sometimes you must wonder, 'Why him, why did he die, why not me?' Now, the unmentionable has been said. Mrs. Rivers' eyes met the nurse's gaze, and she nodded over and over. The tears poured out again. "I begged God to go back and take me instead. I feel guilty that my life was spared and his taken." The nurse held her hands and offered silent comfort. At last the nurse spoke, "I do not understand why. I am only grateful that you have been able to share these tears today. It is the only way that I know of that your grief will heal: to share it with another."

The nurse then asked about spiritual beliefs. With downcast eyes, Mrs. Rivers replied that she was a Christian. Asked if she felt that God had abandoned her, she once again began to cry and confirmed the feeling. "I keep wondering over and over what I did to be punished so much." "Was there anything you could have done that would deserve such suffering?" the nurse asked. "No, no," Mrs. Rivers replied. She then summarized her worst sins in life: divorcing a husband who had been unfaithful and taking life for granted. She affirmed to herself that these were not worthy of such punishment. "Then sometimes I think I am being tested, and I think, 'God, I can not take anymore.'" "Do you pray? Do you talk to God?" the nurse questioned. "I haven't been able to since my grandson died" was her reply. The nurse then shared, "Lots of people are unable to pray when they are so burdened or so angry. Sometimes, it helps to have another pray for you." "I am angry, but how can I be angry at God?" The nurse shared a past experience. "A child taught me once that if God was as great as we thought He was, then He could handle our anger. I sometimes think that all God asks of us is to be in relationship with Him, and sometimes that means letting

Him know when we've had it." "Yes, yes," she affirmed. The nurse then offered to pray for Mrs. Rivers, and she replied appreciatively, "Please." The nurse placed her hands on the patient's shoulders, and a silent prayer was offered, ending with an audible prayer that the patient be brought comfort and the grandson be blessed. The heaviness in the room changed; the sorrow, of course, was immense, but having been shared, it now was altered.

The nurse continued to see the patient daily for support. On the next visit, Mrs. Rivers told the nurse, "You saved my life yesterday. I was on the edge, and you helped me beyond words."

Care of the Grieving Individual

Assessment

The grief assessment is integrated into the conversation with the patient and is never simply a checklist. A nurse who sits with a form hurriedly checking off the answers will come away with a very different picture of a patient than one who gathers the information through conversation with the patient over time. If the patient is hospitalized and severely ill, issues such as sleep disturbance, appetite, and depression will be difficult to sort out in terms of what is a physical complication and what is caused by grief.

Each response to assessment questions brings the building of trust, a potential for teaching, and the therapeutic response and intervention. The family or patient is asked to tell what happened. So often, they have abbreviated or edited the story to accommodate what family or friends can tolerate, but the nurse's openness allows for the outpouring of details and difficult aspects.

The assessment includes not only what is relayed verbally by the patient but also other cues (e.g., trembling of the mouth, change in breathing, sighing, tightening of the face as the individual attempts to contain the emotion). Nurses should conduct the assessment gently without probing questions. The assessment is part of the process of building a trusting relationship. Imagine the difference if the nurse in the case study had entered the room saying, "Mrs. Rivers, I understand you lost your grandson while you were home. I am sorry. How did he die? Did you attend the funeral? How do you feel about this? Are you sleeping at night? How is your appetite?" Rather, the assessment should be intertwined with nurturing and comforting actions, soothing touch, a gentle voice, the impression that one has all the time in the world, and an intense sense of presence and compassion. Awareness of how the bereaved individual is caring for him- or herself physically is important. Research has begun to demonstrate a change in the immune response during periods of grief (e.g., lymphocyte reduction, lower natural killer cell activity) (Calabrese, Kling, & Gold, 1987; Irwin, Daniels, Risch, Bloom, & Weiner, 1988). Social support and relaxation training appear to abate some of this impairment in the immune function (Houldin, McCorkle, & Lowery, 1993). In one study, bereaved individuals participated in disclosure writing (writing that facilitates emotional disclosure). Those who found heightened meaning over the course of the intervention showed increases in natural killer cell cytotoxicity (Bower, Kemeny, Taylor, & Fahey, 2003).

Red flags, such as the passing comment "I sometimes wish I were dead," need direct and immediate assessment. Although this response is not uncommon, the patient's tendency toward suicide needs to be assessed. Szanto, Prigerson, Houck, Ehrenpreis, and Reynolds (1997) found that grieving older adults with high levels of complicated grief symptoms and depression were more likely to express suicidal ideation. In addition, those bereaved who had a history of suicide attempts tended to express more suicidal thoughts than other bereaved older adults. This research may well be transferable to other age groups. If the nurse has established a relationship, simply asking, "Have you ever considered taking your own life?" will provide a good first step. If the response is positive, assess whether the patient has thought through a plan, and have a strategy for intervention.

Differential Diagnosis

Grief sometimes can be confused with depression, especially when the mourning period seems to extend beyond expected time frames. The *Diagnostic and Statistical Manual of Mental Disorders (DSM-IV-TR)* categorizes a major depressive disorder when the symptoms continue two months after the loss (American Psychiatric Association, 2000). Rather than focusing on length of time, differentiating the individual's symptoms that indicate depression may be more useful, whether it occurs sooner than the two months or later. Depression is characterized by feelings of worthlessness and low self-esteem. With grief, the individual's sadness is related more to the death and loss, and the symptoms tend to vary in intensity. Individuals with a history of depression who have lost a loved one may be more at risk for depression overlaying the grief (Zisook, Paulus, Shuchter, & Judd, 1997). Zisook, Shuchter, Sledge, Paulus, and Judd (1994) found that only 24% of those diagnosed with depression following the death of a spouse were being treated pharmacologically, demonstrating real concerns about minimizing the potential consequences of depression such as chronicity, suicide, and social isolation.

Interventions

Just as assessment is ongoing, interventions begin with the first contact with the individual and continue with each interaction. The telling of the story begins the healing. Being sensitive to what the person is expressing is essential. Teaching about normal grief occurs throughout the interaction. Again, handing the patient a list of normal grief reactions would not have the same effect. The important thing is the reassurance that someone understands an experience that the individual may be unable to put into words. This is not as simple as saying to a patient or family, "I know how you feel." When the nurse in the case study says, "It makes no sense. He was so young. We cannot make sense of such an accident, and yet we ask why, over and over again," she may be intuitively in touch with the patient's feelings and the experience of listening to many grieving families over time. Or, she may be completely wrong, and the patient could respond, "No, I don't feel that way. I trust in God. He knows what He is doing." This is the risk nurses take in being genuine with the patients, of learning from each new situation and letting it evolve, knowing that sometimes they will take the wrong fork in the road and will have to retrace their steps back to the patients. Nevertheless, nurses still can educate patients about normal grief and relieve and reassure them. By giving the person permission to grieve, nurses may be contradicting the cultural "voice" that calls the bereaved to be strong. Nurses encourage the patients to voice their feelings. Interactions should allow the patients to "come up for air" after a particularly intense moment or when there are tears by providing quiet time and a slower pace. Periodically, nurses can ask less weighted questions and even use humor appropriately at times. This helps the patients to feel a sense of containment. This subtle change in the therapeutic flow teaches the patients that one can tap into what seems overwhelming and remain in control and secure. Nurses also can pace themselves. They are able to scan their own bodies and wonder if they are taking in too much of the patients' pain. Where are they holding the tension: in the shoulders, the face, the back? Are they feeling pity or compassion? A deep breath at the appropriate moment will model for patients a helpful coping mechanism. See Figure 18-3 for a summary of interventions used in the case study.

Figure 18-3. Specific Interventions Used With Mrs. Rivers

- Assisted the patient in writing a letter to her grandson, reflecting all she wished she had been able to tell him
- Provided the patient with a period of time when the healthcare team and family did not push her to fight, allowing her to grieve and "lick her own wounds"
- Prayed with the patient and referred her to chaplaincy for additional support
- Assisted her in calling her younger sister, the bone marrow donor, to tell her about the grandson's death (she had refused to have the family call the sister, as she did not want to burden her with yet another sadness). During this call, Mrs. Rivers came to realize how much she had missed her sister's support and that she had underestimated her baby sister's strength.
- Elicited a life review, both of her own and her grandson's (photographs helped with this process)
- Encouraged the playing of music as a way of bringing life into the sterile hospital room and decreasing the sense of isolation
- Planned and anticipated her needs for when she returned home some type of memorial service or death ritual, a visit to the gravesite, and ongoing support

---

Rabow, Hauser, and Adams (2004) encouraged physicians to become aware not only of caregiver burdens at the end of life (e.g., mental and physical health risks, financial and emotional weights) but also to become skilled in communications, empathic support, and understanding of grief that will help to influence the adjustment of the bereaved. Research has demonstrated that supportive follow-up phone calls by nurses to the bereaved make an impact (Kaunonen, Aalto, Tarkka, & Paunonen, 2000).

Complicated Grief

The Committee for the Study of Health Consequences of the Stress of Bereavement (Osterweis et al., 1984) reviewed a number of grief theories, beginning with Freud's psychoanalytic model, and described the factors contributing to complicated grief. This model incorporates interpersonal dynamics and examines (a) the role of the preexisting personality (those who are psychologically healthy will do better; they will not experience less pain, but they have the coping skills to process psychic pain),

(b) the activation of latent negative self-images (these dormant negative thoughts of oneself are resurrected with the death and lead individuals to view themselves as bad or incompetent and, in turn, complicate the grieving process), (c) ambivalent relationships (in which conflict has been high and feelings of affection conflict with hostility; in turn, the hostility may awaken after a death and leave the mourner with feelings of guilt), and (d) dependent relationships (in which the adult experiences intense anxiety and fear with separation; these feelings are based on a perceived lack of protection during separation in childhood).

Complicated grief occurs more frequently with particular types of deaths and with certain characteristics of the bereaved (see Figure 18-4). One might think the chance for traumatic death in oncology would be limited, but this is not always the case. Death of a patient by hemorrhage or extensive side effects that distort the person beyond recognition (e.g., graft-versus-host disease) might easily be categorized as traumatic. A related bone marrow donor whose family member dies is at particular risk for feeling a sense of responsibility for the death and deserves special attention.

Figure 18-4. Situations With Potential for Complicated Grief

Form of death	Characteristics of the bereaved
• Traumatic death	• Ambivalent or dependent relationship
• Sudden death	• Multiple losses
• Death of an organ or bone marrow transplant recipient	• History of depression or mental illness
• Death by suicide or homicide	• History of drug or alcohol abuse
• Prolonged illness	
• Death of a child	

Examples of complicated grief include prolonged grief, absent grief (i.e., no obvious reaction), depression, and the use of self-destructive behaviors (e.g., suicide, alcohol or drug abuse). Excessive guilt, feelings of worthlessness, and unusual or protracted functional impairment also would be of concern. Post-traumatic stress disorder can occur in response to a traumatic death or multiple traumas.

Osterweis et al. (1984) noted that bereavement might exacerbate a pattern of negative thoughts that could intensify or prolong grief in individuals with a premorbid tendency to see themselves and the world in a negative light. These individuals are at risk for avoiding the painful experience of grief because any thought of the deceased leads to heightened anxiety.

The family caregiver experiences a double loss after the death of the loved one. He or she may have been so absorbed in the patient's care that a more intense attachment developed. After caring for a dying spouse, a widow described a different kind of intimacy: "You know, I never knew so much about his body before." After death, the time-consuming role of physical and supportive caring is lost. Without immediate pressing responsibilities, the caregiver wakes up in the morning with a loss of purpose. This may leave him or her feeling more empty and alone.

At the other extreme is premature detachment. In a prolonged dying process, the family may no longer be able to maintain the intense involvement with the patient.

Exhausted by the caring and the suffering, they already have grieved and now find themselves wishing that death would come. Often, this will create feelings of guilt either immediately or after the death. Helping families to understand that these feelings are normal and exploring ways for them to care for themselves and still maintain contact with the patient is important. Rando (1993) suggested that anything that the family can do to support the patient's coping, assist with life review, and maintain the balance of the patient's autonomy in the face of increasing dependency will, in turn, support healthy grieving.

Anticipatory Grief

Rando (1997, 2000) has extensively researched and written about anticipatory grief, which, in a sense, might be called "preventive grief." Although her definition is expansive, it is worth quoting as it encapsulates the process so well. Anticipatory grief is "the process of mourning, coping, interaction, planning, and psychosocial reorganization that is stimulated and begun, in part, in response to the awareness of the impending loss of a loved one and the recognition of associated losses in the past, present, and future" (Rando, 1997, p. 35). Rando (1997) goes on to define the therapeutic aspects of this anticipation in which the family must "balance among the mutually conflicting demands of simultaneously holding on to, letting go of, and drawing closer to the dying patient" (p. 35). The patient, too, goes through this process in facing death. Nurses might have the greatest impact in this area in terms of preventive work because during this time, they can help patients and families to resolve some issues that, if left unresolved, might later produce complicated mourning. One enters into an anticipatory phase when the realization of death has been reinforced by the progression of the illness, and an awareness gradually surfaces. The patient who enters hospice, makes decisions about code status, or takes care of financial and legal issues is more likely to be in this process. Rarely, however, are all of the family members and the patient at the same place in the process. Some members, particularly those who are coping long distance, may need special or additional support. Each family member may be at a different point in the grief process.

Healthcare professionals, too, may have difficulty with anticipatory grief. For example, when physicians and nurses focus on an aggressive treatment plan for a patient who will die without a bone marrow transplant, balancing the anticipatory work with fighting for the patient's survival becomes very difficult. If a patient develops complications from the treatment and begins to deteriorate, everyone has difficulty shifting the focus. If the disease is cured, how can the patient be allowed to die from the treatment? Sometimes, patients or family members realize that death is near before the healthcare team. Nurses may perceive its nearness before the physician. One begins anticipating death while the other remains focused on the cure. As multiorgan system failure occurs, the family may receive conflicting information from different members of the healthcare team. A consulting physician may indicate that the patient's liver or kidney function is improving, but the whole picture still represents impending death. The family and patient are left in crisis, and the benefits of anticipatory grieving may be lost.

Evidence-Based Practice

Although the literature is rich in topics related to bereavement, actual research that can affect practice is more limited. A need clearly exists for further research in this area, especially in the arena of nursing assessment and interventions. One such recent study done by a sociologist gives the nursing community powerful data that may alter outcomes for the bereaved. A large prospective study of 250 widowed older adults assessed the elements of death that altered bereavement symptoms. Perception of a painful death correlated with increased levels of yearning, anxiety, and intrusive thoughts in the bereaved. At the same time, an increased positive interaction with the spouse near the time of death or being present at the time of death decreased anger and intrusive thoughts during bereavement (Carr, 2003). Two interventions that nurses could integrate into preventive bereavement care are (a) improved pain management and (b) increased interaction prior to death between the patient and spouse (e.g., privacy, increased support) and amplified efforts to have the spouse present when possible at the time of death.

Traylor et al.'s (2003) study, although primarily focused on parental loss, looked at the relationship between grief and family systems. Three characteristics within families demonstrated less intense grief over time: affect (the ability to express emotions), communication of those feelings, and cohesion, which provides social support and refocused attachments. This study could enhance nurses' assessment of families at risk for more problematic grief reactions and those in need of additional support.

Christakis and Iwashyna's (2003) study encouraged nurses to think of referrals to hospice not only for the dying patient but also in terms of reducing the death risk of the bereaved spouse. This large retrospective study looked at bereavement survival in older adults and found that those who had hospice care provided for their spouse had lower death rates following the loss. This was particularly true in females, where the statistical significance was nearly equivalent to other health benefits, such as diet and exercise.

Another study of bereaved husbands and daughters of patients with breast cancer found that older individuals experienced less grief (Bernard & Guarnaccia, 2003). The daughters in this study experienced more symptoms of depression and anxiety than the husbands. Careful assessment of families as a whole may help to reveal the different aspects of stress that a family death can cause and its ensuing effect on bereavement.

Nurses might consider a study by Warner, Metcalfe, and King (2001) regarding the use of benzodiazepines. This double-blind study demonstrated that the appropriate use of diazepam had no negative or positive effect on bereavement distress. Although a small study, it reminded nurses that grief is not a pathology that needs to be pharmacologically treated. Further research needs to be done in this area.

Although not easily translatable at this time, Gundel, O'Connor, Littrell, Fort, and Lane (2003) attempted to use magnetic resonance imaging to determine the neuroanatomy of grief. It is interesting to note that the activation of the grief response in the brain was greatest when a picture of the deceased was used in conjunction with grief-related words. Moderate responses occurred when the stimulants were used individually. The work may help researchers to find the underlying neuroanatomy of Bowlby's (1969) "attachment behavioral system." During this research, the caudate nucleus was one of the areas activated, similar to other studies researching the neural responses to romantic love. This work demonstrated that the grief response is truly physiologic and in the future may provide further insights into bereavement.

When Death Approaches

As death approaches, the nurse's role becomes focused on providing comfort to patients and families, preparing the families for what to expect, and anticipating and dealing with conflicts and crises (see Figure 18-5).

Figure 18-5. Interventions for Patients Who Are Close to Death

- Determine what the patient's and family's wishes are, and encourage their fulfillment where possible (e.g., a pet visit, funeral plans).
- Assess cultural or religious traditions, and provide for a flexible environment.
- Educate family members about physiologic aspects of death to increase their comfort (many may never have been present at a death).
- Encourage family participation in providing comfort measures to assist in alleviating their sense of helplessness (e.g., the family that is assisting the patient to eat can be encouraged to use teaspoons of diluted juice and ultimately to just give mouth care).
- Offer gestures of comfort (e.g., a cup of tea, a private phone).
- Explore symbolic language and the use of music.

When death appears to be near but is being prolonged by some unfinished business or because the patient believes the family is not ready, it is common to coach families to grant permission for the dying person to "let go." This permission granting, however, can be confused with "pushing" the patients. When working with families, a key role is to help them to understand that death, like birth, has its own timetable. The nurse can be a role model for appropriate behavior.

Symbolic language from the patient, the family, and the professionals can be used to facilitate communication during this transition from life to death. Callanan and Kelley (1992) wrote about how dying patients often use special communication with themes that include travel or a need for change. Their words may seem like confusion to some but actually may be an attempt to communicate on a different level. Family and caregivers may be more comfortable using less direct language as a way to filter their pain. The metaphor is a way of speaking indirectly; its gentle nature allows one to hear the meaning and understand it. For example, the patient who is dying may speak of taking a trip or going home rather than speaking directly about death. The use of guided imagery can be a way to use metaphor and can be most helpful for patients during the transition of dying. An example of this follows.

The nurse spoke softly to the dying patient and began to describe the image of a flowing river, using a vivid description of the water. The river was depicted as coming to an obstacle that forced it to split and now create two paths. The imagery continued, describing the choice of the journey whether to go against the current or to allow the flow of the river to carry one, to trust the flow. The nurse used symbolic language to help the patient to visualize alternatives and achieve some peace in whatever choice was made.

Unusual Experiences

Unusual experiences of the bereaved in which individuals feel they have contact with the deceased often are discounted as dreams or a form of hallucinations (Rosenblatt, 1983). LaGrand (1997) coined the phrase "after-death communication" as spontaneous contact by the deceased loved one or the mourner's experiencing of the deceased. The literature is only now addressing this phenomenon. The actual incidence of these occurrences is not certain; however, they probably occur more frequently than some might think. Therapeutic effects of these experiences include affirmation of the death, completion of unfinished business, a sense that the dead person is all right, or a reduction in the bereaved person's suffering.

When bereaved people are asked directly about the topic, it is remarkable how often they will acknowledge strange experiences or coincidences. The following are accounts of unusual experiences.

- A nurse awoke suddenly in the night. She looked at the clock and felt her mother's presence. The phone rang, and she was told that her mother had died unexpectedly, at the exact time that she awakened.
- After her husband's death, one woman reported being so burdened that she kept forgetting to purchase birdseed, a task her husband had always taken care of. Each time she thought of it, she felt the need to continue the practice as he would have, but each day, distracted, she returned, forgetting the seed. One day, she came home to find the counter where they kept messages and bills disheveled. Puzzled, she looked around, wondering if someone had been there. Her eye then caught sight of a miniature decorative birdcage that normally hung in the window but was now under the counter. A pen was wrapped around the wire hanger. Amazed, the woman believed her husband had found a way to communicate with her. She bought the birdseed and felt very comforted by this event.
- A nurse awoke one morning aware that she had had a strange dream that she could not remember. Later that day, a memory of the dream spontaneously returned. In the dream, she was at work and passed a deceased patient wearing a lab coat. She was startled and confused that he was alive. He smiled radiantly at her, and she asked, "Robert, how are you?" He replied, "I'm well," again with a tremendous smile. The nurse had had only two brief interactions with this very sick patient before he died. In one conversation, the patient was so ill that he only shared a few words and never smiled; the other was the day he died when he was barely responsive. She had entered the room, supported the wife, spoken with him about the dignity he carried and how he would carry that even as he died, and then prayed with the patient and his wife. Within moments, the patient died. The day of the dream, the nurse was scheduled to have a bereavement visit with the wife, and she dismissed it as unconscious processing for the anticipated visit. During the bereavement meeting, the wife mentioned that she thought about bringing a picture of her deceased husband and said, "I just wanted you to see his smile." The mention of the smile stirred the memory of the dream, and the nurse felt

compelled to share it with the wife. The wife, moved by the dream, stated, "That is exactly how Robert would have responded to your question; that is what he always answered." When the nurse commented about being puzzled about the lab coat, the wife responded, "He was a researcher; he lived in a white lab coat!" This became a great comfort to the wife, who took it as a message from her husband that he was all right, something she had repeatedly hoped for but had feared was not true.

These experiences can be dismissed easily but may warrant continued exploration.

Morse's (1990, 1994) research on near-death experiences with children led to unusual and unexplainable scenarios in which children were able to describe events in other areas of the hospital or in their own homes while they were being resuscitated in the hospital. Morse suggested that sharing this near-death research might help other families to cope with anticipatory grieving and, ultimately, bereavement. Families are reluctant to share these unusual stories for fear of being labeled crazy, especially given the feelings of loss of control related to the grief process. More research needs to be conducted in this area. Nurses should encourage the sharing of unusual events, without passing judgment, dismissing them, or labeling them as hallucinations.

Professional Grief

Oncology nurses, in whatever setting they work, frequently establish powerful and intimate bonds with patients. When a patient dies, nurses face the difficult task of mourning that loss regardless of the nature of the relationship (e.g., close, ambivalent, hostile) or the number of times they have experienced a death. Oncology nurses do not become immune to grief over time. Occasionally, the death of a particularly close patient results in an expression of grief that has been "saved up" from many deaths.

Slaby (1988) addressed the issue of dealing with death when he described the caregiver's task. "Those who care for patients with cancer must either directly confront their own mortality or expend psychic energy to mollify the intensity of the reality to allow for some reconciliation with the idea of death" (p. 139). As often is the case, oncology nurses reflect on the gifts the work brings. Living on the edge with others enhances one's appreciation of life. Still, the emotional work and grief and its ensuing emotions need attention.

Saunders and Valente (1994) surveyed nurses attending bereavement workshops. They found that nurses reported coping well with "good" deaths. They defined those as deaths in which symptoms were managed, the nurse felt he or she gave the best care possible, the patient came to some resolution, and the death did not violate a natural order (i.e., the patient was not a child or young adult). Conversely, when the death was not considered "good" or the nurse was not present at the time of death, nurses characterized the grief as painful, complicated, distressing, or difficult.

In Western culture, anger is an emotion that is poorly tolerated; yet, anger is not an uncommon response to ongoing exposure to death and grief (Rueth & Hall, 1999). Slaby (1988) described anger in caregivers as a natural response to many demands that become increasingly difficult to fill and, if sustained, a contributing factor in burnout. The anger can be magnified if one feels responsible for not curing the patient, not eliminating symptoms, or even worsening the symptoms because of the side effects of treatment. Anger can be passed back and forth between the patient/family and the healthcare team. Nurses working with patients with advanced cancer may hold themselves in the role of the "good" nurse, who never had "bad" feelings. This can lead to a tremendous sense of isolation (Vachon, Lyall, & Freeman, 1978). Simply acknowledging anger can go a long way in helping to understand the secondary depression and guilt that it can create. Hill (1989) described the burdens aptly.

> Will this be the time when I am truly depleted . . . that I must make a change because I can no longer care for my patients and can barely care for myself . . . when I barely managed to restrain myself from snapping at people who were trying to make appropriate referrals and when I used all my resources to walk through hospital room doors to see sick, sorrowful people one more time. (p. 146)

Feldstein and Gemma (1995) studied 50 professional oncology nurses using the Grief Experience Inventory to assess differences between those who remained in their positions and those who left. Both groups had high scores for despair, social isolation, and somatization. Those nurses who remained had lower scores on loss of control and death anxiety, whereas those who left had low levels of anger/hostility, loss of control, and death anxiety. Of even greater interest was the high percentage who had experienced a death in their immediate family within the last year (31% of those who stayed and 37% of those who left). In both groups, the nurses used spouses and close friends more frequently than colleagues for support. More studies like these are needed to give a greater insight into the complexity of professional grief and its impact.

Self-Care

No single correct way exists to care for oneself. Support groups can help, and any way of reducing the isolation of feelings will make a difference. A monthly self-assessment regarding how many deaths have occurred and the toll taken can be useful. Addressing other areas of stress in one's life (e.g., lack of sleep or exercise, too many commitments) is helpful. The cumulative effect may have the greatest impact, generating grief overload (Vachon, 1998). Acknowledge limitations, and learn and use appropriate boundaries about how involved to become. The literature has become rich in the significance of pairing engagement with detachment in this work (Carmack, 1997; Rittman, Rivera, Sutphin, & Godown, 1997). Be aware of signs when colleagues are stepping beyond their role as professionals. Assess participation in life-affirming beliefs and actions (e.g., sexuality, spirituality, laughter, play, creativity). Clinics and units might consider ceremonies and programs that serve to acknowledge and discharge the cumulative grief of families and professionals (Burke & Gerraughty, 1994; Coolican & Pearce, 1995; Lewis, 1999). Follow-up programs as simple as sending a bereavement card or as complex as telephone contact can be helpful for the families as well as the staff (Kaunonen et al., 2000). Some institutions have a remembrance service for those who have died; this is very common in hospice. Staff members at times resist attending such programs, not wanting to face the full measure of grief during an annual remembrance. Yet, these programs can function as catharses that allow nurses to begin again. Self-care, which is demanded by all aspects of nursing, is especially important for those who care for the dying (Wakefield, 2000; Zerbe & Steinberg, 2000). Whatever action is taken, the key is to initiate some action on individual, managerial, and institutional levels to acknowledge and cope with the grief (see Figure 18-6).

Figure 18-6. Plan of Care

Assessment
- Description of the death in the patient's or family's own words (e.g., "Tell me what happened.")
- Concurrent stressors and past losses, both deaths and other losses, and reaction to anniversaries
- Affective responses (e.g., anger, sadness, hopelessness, guilt, self-reproach, inability to concentrate, fear, anxiety)
- Somatic responses (e.g., sleep disturbances, poor appetite, pain, weakness, symptoms similar to those of the person who died)
- Support systems (e.g., family, community)
- Financial concerns
- Past history of coping mechanisms and psychiatric history, particularly depression
- Suicidal tendencies
- Alcohol or drug abuse; increased use of tobacco
- Spiritual beliefs
- Cultural traditions
- Unusual experiences since the death

Nursing Diagnoses (NANDA International, 2005)
- Anticipatory grieving
- Ineffective coping
- Dysfunctional grieving
- Impaired adjustment
- Death anxiety

***DSM-IV-TR* Diagnoses** (American Psychiatric Association, 2000)
- Bereavement
- Major depressive disorder
- Post-traumatic stress disorder

Expected Outcomes
- Patients/families will begin the grief process within their cultural norms and family traditions
- Patients/families will describe the grief reaction and its impact on daily life.
- Patients/families will seek support as needed.
- Patients/families will engage, over time, in life and other relationships.

Interventions
- Provide ongoing supportive listening.
- Elicit a life review when appropriate; photographs, journals, music, and art may be helpful.
- Provide patients/families with privacy.
- Encourage assessment of unfinished business, and assist patients/families in achieving intentions.
- Respect and encourage use of cultural practices.
- Offer spiritual support and referrals as appropriate.
- Describe the normal grief process and what to expect.

(Continued on next page)

Figure 18-6. Plan of Care *(Continued)*

- Integrate touch, holding, and presence as appropriate.
- Recognize when silent presence is most important.
- Teach relaxation techniques, particularly breathing exercises, to reduce tension.
- Use guided imagery to create a safe haven or time out.
- Refer for appropriate support groups or psychiatric/psychological assistance as needed.
- Encourage social support and increased contact and connection.
- Encourage healthy coping mechanisms such as exercise, proper nutrition, and rest.

Conclusion

Everyone can master grief, but he who has it.

—William Shakespeare

In a culture that traditionally has been phobic about death, best-sellers have embraced the subject, and hospices have been mainstreamed. Still, many families have never been at a bedside during the dying process. Bereavement care does not begin after the death, but in a preventive sense, in the many events leading up to the death. Nurses have an obligation to care for the bereaved, whether it is making sure that a child's needs are attended to, listening to a dying patient's grief, assisting families in communication, teaching families about the physiologic aspects of the dying process, or facilitating a bereavement support group. Nurses hold the opportunity to transform. The word "transform" comes from the Latin *trans*, meaning "across and beyond." When nurses take on the challenge of helping to heal grief, they affect not only the individual but also all who are touched by the experience. Nurses change the bereaved by helping them across the suffering, first and foremost by hearing the words, the moans, the ache, the breaking of the heart. This act of compassion begins the long journey back to wellness, when bittersweet memories bring the tears and the joy of who the person was and always will be in the lives of the bereaved.

References

American Psychiatric Association. (2000). *Diagnostic and statistical manual of mental disorders* (4th ed., text rev.). Washington, DC: Author.

Barnhart, C.L. (Ed.). (1962). *The American college dictionary.* New York: Random House.

Bernard, L.L., & Guarnaccia, C.A. (2003). Two models of caregiver strain and bereavement adjustment: A comparison of husband and daughter caregivers of breast cancer hospice patients. *Gerontologist, 43,* 808–816.

Bower, J.E., Kemeny, M.E., Taylor, S.E., & Fahey, J.L. (2003). Finding positive meaning and its association with natural killer cell cytotoxicity among participants in a bereavement-related disclosure intervention. *Annals of Behavioral Medicine, 25,* 146–155.

Bowlby, J. (1969). Childhood mourning and its implications for psychiatry. *American Journal of Psychiatry, 118,* 481–498.

Bowlby, J. (1980). *Attachment and loss.* New York: Basic Books.

Brown-Saltzman, K.A. (1995). Multicultural perspectives in palliative care. *Quality of Life: A Nursing Challenge, 3*(3), 41–47.

Burke, C., & Gerraughty, S.M. (1994). An oncology unit's initiation of a bereavement support program. *Oncology Nursing Forum, 21,* 1675–1680.

Calabrese, J.R., Kling, M.A., & Gold, P.W. (1987). Alterations in immunocompetence during stress, bereavement, and depression: Focus on neuroendocrine regulation. *American Journal of Psychiatry, 144,* 1123–1134.

Callanan, M., & Kelley, P. (1992). *Final gifts: Understanding the special awareness, needs, and communications of the dying.* New York: Poseidon Press.

Carmack, B. (1997). Balancing engagement and detachment in caregiving. *Image: The Journal of Nursing Scholarship, 29,* 139–144.

Carr, D. (2003). A "good death" for whom? Quality of spouse's death and psychological distress among older widowed persons. *Journal of Health and Social Behavior, 44,* 215–232.

Christ, G.H., Siegel, K., & Christ, A.E. (2002). Adolescent grief: "It never really hit me . . . until it actually happened." *JAMA, 288,* 1269–1278.

Christakis, N.A., & Iwashyna, T.J. (2003). The health impact of health care on families: A matched cohort study of hospice use by decedents and mortality outcomes in surviving, widowed spouses. *Social Science and Medicine, 57,* 465–475.

Clements, P.T., Vigil, G.T., Manno, M.S., Henry, G.C., Wilks, J., Das, S., et al. (2003). Cultural perspectives of death, grief, and bereavement. *Journal of Psychosocial Nursing and Mental Health Services, 41*(7), 18–26.

Coolican, M.B., & Pearce, T. (1995). Aftercare bereavement program. *Critical Care Nursing Clinics of North America, 7,* 519–527.

Corr, C.A., & Doka, K.J. (1994). Current models of death, dying, and bereavement. *Critical Care Nursing Clinics of North America, 6,* 545–552.

Edelman, H. (1994). *Motherless daughters: The legacy of loss.* Reading, MA: Addison-Wesley.

Feldstein, M.A., & Gemma, P.B. (1995). Oncology nurses and chronic compounded grief. *Cancer Nursing, 18,* 228–236.

Freud, S. (1961). The future of an illusion (W.D. Robson-Scott, Trans.). In J. Strachey (Ed.), *The standard edition of the complete psychological works of Sigmund Freud* (Vol. 21). London: Hogarth Press.

Furman, R. (1964). Death and the young child. *Psychoanalytic Study of the Child, 19,* 321–333.

Gerber, I., Rusalem, P., Hannon, N., Battin, D., & Arkin, A. (1975). Anticipatory grief and aged widows and widowers. *Journal of Gerontology, 30,* 225–229.

Gundel, H., O'Connor, M., Littrell, L., Fort, C., & Lane, R.D. (2003). Functional neuroanatomy of grief: An FMRI study. *American Journal of Psychiatry, 160,* 1946–1953.

Hill, H.L. (1989). To fill a heart: Oncology over the long haul. *Journal of Psychosocial Oncology, 7,* 145–152.

Houldin, A.D., McCorkle, R., & Lowery, B.J. (1993). Relaxation training and psychoimmunological status of bereaved spouses: A pilot study. *Cancer Nursing, 16,* 47–52.

Irwin, M., Daniels, M., Risch, S.C., Bloom, E., & Weiner, H. (1988). Plasma cortisol and natural killer cell activity during bereavement. *Biological Psychiatry, 24,* 173–178.

Kaunonen, M., Aalto, P., Tarkka, M.T., & Paunonen, M. (2000). Oncology ward nurses' perspectives of family grief and a supportive telephone call after the death of a significant other. *Cancer Nursing, 23,* 314–324.

Koocher, G. (1974). Talking with children about death. *American Journal of Orthopsychiatry, 44,* 404–411.

Kübler-Ross, E. (1969). *On death and dying.* New York: Macmillan.

LaGrand, L.E. (1997, June). *Understanding after-death communication in the lives of the bereaved.* Paper presented at the International Conference on Grief and Bereavement in Contemporary Society, Washington, DC.

Lewis, A.E. (1999). Reducing burnout: Development of an oncology staff bereavement program. *Oncology Nursing Forum, 26,* 1065–1069.

Lindemann, E. (1944). Symptomatology and management of acute grief. *American Journal of Psychiatry, 101,* 141–148.

Morse, M. (with Perry, P.). (1990). *Closer to the light: Learning from the near-death experiences of children.* New York: Ivy Books.

Morse, M. (with Perry, P.). (1994). *Parting visions: Uses and meanings of pre-death, psychic, and spiritual experiences.* New York: Villard Books.

Nagy, M. (1948). The child's theories concerning death. *Journal of Genetic Psychology, 73,* 3–27.

NANDA International. (2005). *Nursing diagnoses: Definitions and classification, 2005–2006.* Philadelphia: Author.

Osterweis, M., Solomon, F., & Green, M. (Eds.). (1984). *Bereavement reactions, consequences, and care.* Washington, DC: National Academies Press.

Parkes, C.M. (1987). *Bereavement: Studies of grief in adult life.* Madison, CT: International Universities Press.

Rabow, J.W., Hauser, J.M., & Adams, J. (2004). Supporting family caregivers at the end of life. *JAMA, 291,* 483–491.

Rando, T.A. (1993). *Treatment of complicated mourning.* Champaign, IL: Research Press.

Rando, T.A. (1997). Living and learning the reality of a loved one's dying: Traumatic stress and cognitive process in anticipatory grief. In K.J. Doka & J. Davidson (Eds.), *Living with grief when illness is prolonged* (pp. 33–50). Washington, DC: Hospice Foundation of America.

Rando, T.A. (2000). Anticipatory mourning: A review and critique of the literature. In T.A. Rando (Ed.), *Clinical dimensions of anticipatory mourning: Theory and practice in working with the dying, their loved ones, and their caregivers* (pp. 17–50). Champaign, IL: Research Press.

Rittman, M., Rivera, J., Sutphin, L., & Godown, I. (1997). Phenomenological study of nurses caring for dying patients. *Cancer Nursing, 20,* 115–119.

Rosenblatt, P.C. (1983). *Bitter, bitter tears: Nineteenth-century diarists and twentieth-century grief theories.* Minneapolis, MN: University of Minnesota Press.

Rueth, T.W., & Hall, S.E. (1999). Dealing with the anger and hostility of those who grieve. *American Journal of Hospice and Palliative Care, 16,* 743–746.

Saunders, J.M., & Valente, S.M. (1994). Nurse's grief. *Cancer Nursing, 17,* 318–325.

Slaby, A.E. (1988). Cancer's impact on caregivers. *Advances in Psychosomatic Medicine, 18,* 135–153.

Stroebe, W., & Schut, H. (2001). Risk factors in bereavement outcome: A methodological and empirical review. In M.S. Stroebe, R.O. Hansson, W. Stroebe, & H. Schut (Eds.), *Handbook of bereavement research: Consequences, coping and care* (pp. 349–371). Washington, DC: American Psychological Association.

Szanto, K., Prigerson, H., Houck, P., Ehrenpreis, L., & Reynolds, C.F. (1997). Suicidal ideation in elderly bereaved: The role of complicated grief. *Suicide and Life-Threatening Behavior, 27,* 194–207.

Thompson, S. (2002). Older people. In N. Thompson (Ed.), *Loss and grief: A guide for human services practitioners* (pp. 162–173). New York: Palgrave.

Traylor, E.S., Hayslip, B., Kaminski, P.L., & York, C. (2003). Relationships between grief and family system characteristics: A cross lagged longitudinal analysis. *Death Studies, 27,* 575–601.

Vachon, M. (1998). Caring for the caregiver in oncology and palliative care. *Seminars in Oncology Nursing, 14,* 152–157.

Vachon, M.L., Lyall, W.A., & Freeman, S.J. (1978). Measurement and management of stress in health professionals working with advanced cancer patients. *Death Education, 1,* 365–375.

Wakefield, A. (2000). Nurses' responses to death and dying: A need for relentless self-care. *International Journal of Palliative Nursing, 6,* 245–251.

Warner, J., Metcalfe, C., & King, M. (2001). Evaluating the use of benzodiazepines following recent bereavement. *British Journal of Psychiatry, 178,* 36–41.

Worden, J.W. (1991). *Grief counseling and grief therapy: A handbook for the mental health practitioner.* New York: Springer.

Zerbe, K.J., & Steinberg, D.L. (2000). Coming to terms with grief and loss. Can skills for dealing with bereavement be learned? *Postgraduate Medicine, 108,* 97–98, 101–104, 106.

Zisook, S., Paulus, M., Shuchter, S.R., & Judd, L.L. (1997). The many faces of depression following spousal bereavement. *Journal of Affective Disorders, 45,* 85–95.

Zisook, S., Shuchter, S.R., Sledge, P.A., Paulus, M., & Judd, L.L. (1994). The spectrum of depressive phenomena after spousal bereavement. *Journal of Clinical Psychiatry, 55*(Suppl.), 29–36.

CHAPTER 19

Guilt

Phyllis Gorney Cooper, RN, MN

The pangs of conscience are better than floggings.
—The Talmud

Guilt is defined as the "painful feeling of self-reproach resulting from a belief that one has done something wrong" (Guralink, 1984, p. 622). It is a feeling that usually involves self-criticism and results from an internal conflict with one's conscience. One's conscience creates a sense of what is right and wrong and a compulsion to do that which is right. The teachings of childhood, which are influenced by religious, cultural, and social norms, usually determine the boundaries of an individual's conscience. Mothers frequently have been accused of using guilt to manipulate their children. A request for correct behavior is accompanied by a statement geared toward generating guilt (e.g., "You know how much I worry when you . . .", "After all I have done for you, the least you could do is . . ."). The guilt can be intended as punishment for past digressions as well as an inducement for future correct behavior. Often, these efforts at controlling behavior through guilt are done at a semiconscious level. The parent may say the words out of habit or experience and may not realize what is being said.

Guilt has been a component of many of the world's religions in an effort to control behavior. Feelings of guilt are so unpleasant that many will not commit a prohibited behavior, or if they do, they will feel so overwhelmed by guilt that they will never do so again. As a shaper of filial, moral, and ethical behavior, guilt arguably may have value. However, the role of guilt in relation to cancer often is counterproductive.

Because of the wonders of modern medicine, dealing with a life-threatening yet often chronic disease is a unique experience for most people. Many individuals do not know what is expected or accepted behavior in this situation and, therefore, believe that certain behaviors might not be "correct." If the "incorrect" somehow occurs, guilt frequently follows. The problem is that, in most cases, no absolute right or wrong exists. If the purpose of guilt is to prevent the occurrence of "wrong" behavior and promote "right" behavior, the resulting feelings of guilt experienced by patients with cancer, their families, and healthcare professionals often are entirely unwarranted. This guilt then becomes an additional yet unnecessary source of emotional stress in an already highly stressful situation.

The Nature of Guilt in Cancer

The seriousness of a cancer diagnosis and its ramifications naturally cause patients and families to question "why?" and to examine personal behaviors and circumstances in an effort to find an answer to that question. Potential sources of patients' guilt are almost limitless and include beliefs that they caused their cancer, delayed the diagnosis, chose the wrong treatment, were noncompliant with their treatment plan, or survived when others have not. Researchers have found that levels of self-blame and guilt at the time of diagnosis, although unrelated to concurrent psychological distress, were significantly predictive of psychological distress four months later (Malcarne, Compas, Epping-Jordan, & Howell, 1995). Based on such research, as well as on clinical observation, it is not difficult to conclude that self-blame and guilt can be ongoing and significant sources of distress for people dealing with cancer. The guilt can take many forms (see Figure 19-1). The goal of cancer care providers is to assist those dealing with cancer to understand and eliminate their feelings of guilt whenever possible.

Sources of Guilt

Hero Myth

Perhaps the most pervasive and insidious source of guilt in patients with cancer stems from what Gray and Doan (1990) characterized as the "Hero Myth." This

---

Figure 19-1. Glossary of Terms

Conscience: The consciousness of the right or wrong of one's own actions or motives.
Guilt: A painful feeling of self-reproach resulting from a belief that one has done something wrong
Hero Myth: A popular cultural belief that patients have the power and ability to both cause their cancer and to cure themselves using psychological interventions.
Justified guilt: Feelings of guilt that arise when an incorrect behavior has led to a forewarned result (e.g., smoking and lung cancer). The patient/family and healthcare personnel may believe that the guilt is warranted.
Positive attitude: The belief that one or more options are available to deal with a problem and that at least one of these options will be successful. Positive attitude often is incorrectly interpreted as the absence of negative feelings.
Self-blame: To hold oneself responsible for something. Although sometimes used interchangeably with guilt, self-blame may or may not be accompanied by feelings of guilt.
Survivor guilt: The ironic feelings of guilt held by some patients who survive their cancer when others they know have died.

---

notion compares an individual's battle with cancer to the mythical warrior hero who overcomes the devouring monster after a series of trials and immense suffering. According to popular belief, the Hero Myth involves beating cancer through a psychological transformation that includes becoming a more effective, more expressive, more loving, more positive, and more courageous person. Popular books such as *Getting Well Again* (Simonton, Matthews-Simonton, & Creighton, 1978) and *Love, Medicine, and Miracles* (Siegel, 1986) have expounded on the Hero Myth. Two basic assumptions underlie this myth in dealing with cancer: (a) Cancer is caused at least partly by psychological factors, and (b) progression of the disease is affected by these same factors. The implication is that controlling or fixing these problems can lead to a cure.

Many patients with cancer feel guilty for psychological problems, such as having a "cancer personality," having too much stress in their lives, and also for more tangible reasons, including having spent too much time in the sun or eating a poor diet. One or more of these psychological and behavioral factors may play a role in the development of the cancer. However, to be guilty, a person has to know for a fact that this activity was contributory and then proceed to do it anyway. This is not the case for most people. Scientists only recently have identified the association of sunburns suffered as children to malignant melanoma later in life, the relation of high-fat diets to breast cancer, and the link between low-fiber diets and colon cancer. The degree to which these actions contribute to cancer is only partially known. The relationship of stress to cancer is more evident and is based on scientists' current understanding of psychoneuroimmunology and body energy systems (Mate, 2003), but research has yet to explain why some people experience severe stress and yet do not develop cancer.

Psychoanalytic theories that cancer occurs or spreads because of some deep-seated desire for self-punishment or feeling of unworthiness have never been supported or substantiated. These issues should be explained logically and carefully to patients who admit to feeling guilt for causing their cancer and to family members who may be blaming patients for developing cancer.

The second assumption of the Hero Myth states that controlling contributing factors can influence the course of the disease, even to a cure (Malcarne et al., 1995). Common sense and current research indicate that patients can do certain things to improve the odds, such as eating a better diet, managing stress, enhancing coping abilities, and balancing the body's energy centers (Chopra, 2003). Documented cases of spontaneous remission have occurred after patients have embarked on these positive lifestyle changes and began showing and sharing their emotions.

Patients who assume more personal responsibility for their health and well-being after a diagnosis of cancer may experience benefits; however, it is important not to assume that changes in diet, stress, and coping alone, no matter how dramatic, are sufficient to cure cancer. Some comprehensive treatment models encourage such positive changes as an important adjunct (i.e., additional things that can be done) that may enhance the ability to respond to or endure standard medical treatment (e.g., surgery, chemotherapy, radiation therapy). Encouraging patients to take personal responsibility is a two-edged sword. Such tasks may give patients a sense of control and hopefulness. Conversely, patients may feel tremendous pressure to comply and may feel guilty when unable to do so on a regular basis. If the disease progresses or recurs, they may feel additional self-blame and guilt. Offering these as options but with no guarantees, encouraging slow but steady lifestyle changes, and permitting occasional guilt-free lapses in the regimen might result in beneficial changes without the ensuing guilt (Fawzy et al., 1990). Making sure the patients learn to recognize and experience emotions and communicate emotional needs and issues can lead to biopsychosocial/spiritual support of cancer prevention and treatment.

Some researchers have focused on the importance of feelings and their relationship to overall health (Lewis, O'Sullivan, & Barraclough, 1994; Mate, 2003). A positive attitude consists of believing that options are available to address their problems and that one or more of those options will be successful. Having a positive attitude does not mean that one will never feel or express a negative emotion. The diagnosis and treatment of cancer bring a whole range of painful emotions, such as anxiety, depression, anger, sadness, hopelessness, helplessness, lack of control, and guilt. When patients try to be "emotionally up" and happy all the time (i.e., what they view as having a positive attitude) or maintain a repressive, nonemotional stance, failure is almost inevitable, and guilt ensues.

Patients who first acknowledge that they have these negative emotions, accept them as normal given the situation, and then express them appropriately seem to have much better quality of life, and, in some cases, their reactions may positively influence the course of their disease (Classen, Hermanson, & Spiegel, 1994; Fawzy et al., 1993; Mate, 2003; Spiegel, Bloom, Kraemer, & Gottheil, 1989).

People generally accept that thoughts and feelings kept bottled up inside will serve as major stressors that can affect emotional state and may, in turn, negatively affect the immune system and health outcomes (Chopra, 1990; Dienstfrey, 1993; Dossey, Keegan, Guzzetta, & Kolkmeier, 1995). Expressing these same thoughts and feelings will "put them on the outside" where they can no longer hurt as much. Having negative feelings toward cancer and finding ways of appropriately expressing them should never be a source of guilt for patients. Oncology healthcare professionals can do a great deal to help patients with cancer and their families to understand this.

Justified Guilt

One notable exception related to self-blame and guilt may be the smoker who develops lung cancer. Smoking has been known for at least 30 years to cause cancer. Those who choose to smoke and subsequently develop lung cancer may be consumed with guilt that actually is justified. Because the wrong behavior (i.e., smoking) already has led to dire consequences (i.e., cancer), interventions for this population should be geared toward fostering self-forgiveness and moving beyond guilt. Interestingly, in cases where such a patient continues to smoke, the guiding philosophy of interventions to get the patient to cease this harmful behavior often relies on guilt. For instance, asking patients, "How can you possibly keep smoking when you can hardly breathe? You know that you are just making things worse, and all that passive smoke is harming your family" may not be the appropriate approach.

Diagnosis and Treatment

Patients who express guilt over delaying diagnosis, not initiating treatment soon enough, or not complying with treatment require special assessment to uncover the reasons for their behavior. These may include knowledge deficits, lack of understanding, an avoidant coping style, fear, denial, or something as practical as the inability to pay for medical care. If patients fail to understand their behavior, helping them to gain insight is the first step of intervention. Addressing the specific issue is the next step. Letting go of the guilt and moving on to a more health-promoting behavior is the final goal.

One particularly sensitive issue is guilt over having chosen the wrong treatment if the cancer recurs. If the treatment was a standard medical option, reviewing any valid reasons for making the original choice, as well as current options, may be helpful. Reiterating that no cancer treatment comes with a guarantee also may help to alleviate guilt. If an alternative treatment was selected in place of standard therapy, the patient may need help in reviewing why he or she chose that option in the first place. Education about standard treatments that are now available may need to be repeated, and the patient may need to be encouraged to try standard therapy in conjunction with other options. Disparaging remarks about the alternative therapy and any manner of "I told you so" will only foster more guilt and might drive the patient away again. As stated earlier, the goal is to remove the feelings of guilt and to move on. This process is accomplished either by helping the patient to understand that the guilt is unwarranted or by fostering self-forgiveness.

Survivor Guilt

Although not a common theme among patients with cancer, the issue of survivor guilt exists. It has been reported among survivors of childhood cancers (Shanfield, 1980), as well as among adults (Hill, 1991). In essence, survivor guilt refers to those patients who are cured but are having difficulty understanding why they were spared when similar patients died. Exploring patients' feelings of self-esteem and pointing out their value and worth may be helpful. Ironically, these individuals may find themselves asking the question "Why me?" both when they got the cancer and when they survived. In both instances, the only answer may be "Why not me?"

Transmission Guilt

One of the most confusing sources of guilt relates to cancer inheritance. Researchers have found that a number of cancers, including breast, colon, and ovarian, occur in families. Some patients with no family history of cancer develop the disease in their later years after having children. They then feel guilty for potentially passing on their cancer genes to their offspring. Lerman, Croyle, Tercyak, and Hamann (2002) noted that as scientists begin to determine the genes associated with inherited disease, healthcare providers more frequently will encounter the complex psychological issues faced by individuals at risk for these diseases. Prenatal genetic counseling in these individuals should include counseling about transmission guilt and ways to deal with feelings and issues both short- and long-term. Being prepared to address these healthcare issues can assist a family to grow in a healthy yet watchful manner.

Researchers have found that mothers who took the drug diethylstilbestrol (DES) between 1943 and 1971 to prevent miscarriages have an increased lifetime risk of breast cancer (Saunders, 1988). Further, their daughters have been found to have, among other anatomic and functional reproductive tract problems, an increased risk of clear-cell adenocarcinoma, a rare form of vaginal and cervical cancer. Male offspring of DES mothers also have reproductive problems and may have an increased risk of testicular cancer. Many of these mothers feel a sense of guilt for having caused these potentially life-threatening problems for their children. They need to be reminded that the reason they took DES was to preserve life and bring it into this world. If this issue has impaired the relationship between a mother and her daughter or son, referral to family therapy is indicated.

Family Member Guilt

Children

Siblings of children with cancer face a set of unique problems that can generate guilt. The healthy children in the family may experience difficult role changes, such as becoming baby-sitters or caretakers for the ill child or even cooks and housekeepers. They may find themselves shifted from place to place while their parents attend to the sick child during hospitalization. Plans often cannot be made or frequently are changed because of the uncertainty of the illness. Discipline and affection may be erratically and unevenly meted out between the sick child and the siblings. The healthy children may feel neglected, lonely, and unsupported while simultaneously feeling overprotected by parents who are now oversensitive and fearful for the safety of all their children (Bluebond-Langner, 1989). The healthy children may love the sick child, but the emergence of feelings of anger, resentment, and jealousy is understandable. Unfortunately, these feelings then may lead to feelings of guilt (Gogan, Koocher, Foster, & O'Malley, 1977). In addition, healthy children have an almost universal fantasy about having caused the sick child's illness, perhaps having wished the sick child ill or inflicted some injury during play or a fight. Finally, these children often feel guilty for surviving when their sibling has died. In some tragic cases, the parent who has lost a favorite child may foster this feeling. These feelings of guilt may persist well into adulthood and, for some, until their own deaths (Adams-Greenly, Shiminsky-Maher, McGown, & Meyer, 1987).

Children, both healthy and sick, rarely receive the full information about the ill sibling's condition and, in an effort by the parents to protect them in some way, may receive misinformation. Rather than being helpful, this approach of nondisclosure often exacerbates a bad situation. The sick child, while dealing with all of the other emotions inherent in fighting a life-threatening disease, may feel anger at the healthy children who do not have to go through this experience and then subsequently feel guilty for thinking bad things about the siblings (Adams-Greenly et al., 1987). A sense of guilt may develop if the sick child thinks that the illness is punishment for some previous bad deed, real or imagined (Shanfield, 1980; Silberfarb & Greer, 1982).

Most children in a family triad have a much better grasp of the seriousness of what is going on than adults believe. Children may gather information by listening on phone extensions, intentionally eavesdropping behind closed doors, inadvertently overhearing snippets of conversation, picking up on "emotional vibes" of the adults around them, or hearing rumors from their peers. This behavior in itself may generate guilt. Parents rarely sense all of the issues, juggle all of their responsibilities, and fully attend to the needs of both their sick and healthy children. The healthcare team can foster an atmosphere of openness and communication among all family members, providing them with accurate information and emotional support. Counseling may be warranted to assist all parties to understand, accept, and deal with these complex situations.

Adults

Some family members are quick to label any concern about their own stress as self-pity and feel guilty about not being focused entirely on the patient. In contrast to this self-generated guilt, some patients induce guilt to get family members to stay with them and focus on their needs to the exclusion of the rest of the family (Vess, Moreland, Schwebel, & Kraut, 1988). Both patients and family members may need help in gaining insight into their behavior. Everyone should understand and acknowledge that numerous needs exist in this situation. Although the patient requires attention and support, the family caregivers must attend to their own needs as well as to those of the rest of the family to keep the family unit as intact as possible during this difficult time.

Parents are as subject to feelings of guilt as children. They may feel guilty about not being available enough for both the healthy siblings and the ill child. They may feel guilty that they could not save the ill child. They may feel guilty for having passed on a genetic predisposition to the cancer (Miller, Bauman, Friedman, & DeCosse, 1986). Both the patient and family members may think that the patient's illness is a burden and then feel guilty about having these thoughts. They may view this burden as financial, physical, and emotional. Recognizing that the patient did not deliberately develop cancer and is powerless to change the situation does little to lessen these guilty feelings. Again, the way to overcome this guilt is for both patients and family members to acknowledge these emotions, accept them as normal and commonplace, and then work toward minimizing the effects of the illness on the family. Family members need to keep life as routine as possible and continue to participate in pleasurable activities. In most cases, both patients and family members feel less burden and guilt when family members attend to their own needs (Vess et al., 1988).

Family members may feel guilty for not having insisted that the adult patient be diagnosed earlier or for not getting a second opinion. Guilt may stem from anger at the patient for not following these suggestions or from the belief that the patient caused the cancer (e.g., smoked for years). Healthcare professionals can help tremendously by pointing out that these kinds of feelings serve no beneficial purpose and by encouraging family members to let them go (Welch-McCaffrey, 1988).

Family members who are struggling to care for a dying member may feel tremendous guilt if the patient is in pain. Healthcare professionals need to do everything possible to help the patient to achieve a level of comfort while being particularly cognizant of family members' levels of frustration and fear. Planned respites from the caregiving experience can help to rejuvenate exhausted caregivers and mitigate the burden of continuous care and high levels of negative emotions.

Family members often feel a sense of relief after a patient has died. This feeling is particularly common when the illness has been prolonged and difficult. Although it is a completely natural and understandable feeling, many family members subsequently feel guilty. Nurses should reassure these individuals that being glad that the ordeal is over does not mean that they are glad the patient is gone from their lives. Whatever kind and caring behaviors they displayed while the patient was alive should be enumerated and praised. Reassuring the family that the deceased is now free from pain and that he or she was grateful for the care the family provided can support families experiencing these feelings.

Staff Member Guilt

Staff members working with patients with cancer have their own unique sources of guilt. Many healthcare professionals, especially nurses, often feel guilty for subjecting patients to painful, intrusive, and debilitating treatments. These guilty feelings intensify when the likelihood of the treatment resulting in cure is very low. Finally, the most intense feelings of guilt occur when patients die despite the best efforts of the healthcare team. Frequently, staff member guilt is related to denial of feelings of loss when treatment does not turn out as planned. Remen (1996) cautioned healthcare practitioners that it is not possible to be immersed in suffering and loss daily and not be touched by it. She related denial of these feelings to burnout (see Chapter 35).

Staff members need to remember that they did not cause the cancer, and their care may have offered patients and family members some hope and a fighting chance. Staff members also need to recognize that they are not omnipotent, and no one expects them to be all-powerful. Setting appropriate goals for each patient is helpful in preventing a sense of failure and guilt from developing. When a patient's remaining time clearly is very limited, switching the goal from cure or prolongation of life to assisting in a calm death is critical. This process may involve symptom control (including good pain management) and helping the patient and family to finish all of their instrumental business (e.g., wills, funeral preferences) as well as their emotional business (e.g., resolution of family conflicts). Allowing the patient the opportunity for verbal exploration of existential issues such as beliefs in God and an afterlife, and the meaning of one's life is the final step in facilitating a calm death. Any nurse who has done all this for the patient will still feel sadness and loss but also a sense of satisfaction in a job well done that leaves no room for guilt (Koocher, 1980) (see Figure 19-2).

Figure 19-2. Plan of Care

Assessment
- Determine presence and degree of guilt.
- Systematically evaluate for the presence of guilt in every patient with cancer (e.g., "What do you think caused your cancer? Do you think that you did anything to contribute to the development of your cancer? Do you feel you are to blame for causing your cancer?").
- Recognize spontaneous phrases that might indicate guilt (e.g., "This is my fault," "I caused my cancer," "I think this is why I got cancer").
- Differentiate between the patients' beliefs that contributing factors for cancer development existed and their actual feelings of guilt.

(Continued on next page)

Figure 19-2. Plan of Care *(Continued)*

- Determine the knowledge level of patients and family members regarding technical and social issues that might lead to the development of guilt (e.g., cancer development, Hero Myth, positive attitude).
- Discuss with patients and family members religious and cultural beliefs that might be influencing their feelings of guilt; determine how congruent their beliefs are with the stated belief or culture.
- Determine the impact of the guilt on patients' overall affective state and treatment compliance.

Nursing Diagnoses (NANDA International, 2005**)**
- Ineffective coping
- Anxiety
- Deficient knowledge

***DSM-IV-TR* Diagnoses** (American Psychiatric Association, 2000)
- Adjustment disorder
- Major depression

Expected Outcomes
- Patients and family members will describe accurate technical knowledge about the relevant issues.
- Patients and family members will demonstrate understanding of the role of contributing social factors to the development of guilt.
- Patients and family members will have a greater understanding of the role of their religious and cultural beliefs in the development of guilt.
- Patients and family members will express relief from feelings of guilt.

Interventions
- Provide appropriate information about whatever issue is related to guilt (e.g., cancer recurrence, genetics).
- Provide information about social factors contributing to guilt (e.g., Hero Myth, positive attitude).
- Discuss the effect of patients' belief systems (i.e., religious and cultural factors) in the development of guilt; use insight, education, and reframing to assuage feelings of guilt without disparaging patients' beliefs.
- Consider psychiatric consultation for psychotherapy and pharmacologic management for patients whose guilt is seriously affecting their emotional state or interfering with treatment compliance.
- Include family members in educational sessions and discussions whenever possible.
- Have separate discussions with family members, if necessary, to help them to understand the role that they may be playing in the development of guilt; provide reassurance that they should not feel guilt for their behavior if it was based on their level of knowledge and best intentions at the time

---

Case Study

Judy, a 48-year-old widow, underwent a mastectomy for node-negative invasive lobular carcinoma six years ago. She recently underwent a segmental mastectomy (i.e., lumpectomy) for a second primary, 0.8 cm, contralateral breast cancer. She was scheduled for radiation therapy, and chemotherapy was recommended. Before her first chemotherapy session, Judy began crying and stated, "This is all my fault. I can't put my children through this again. I don't want to do this chemotherapy.

(Continued on next page)

Case Study *(Continued)*

Maybe it would be better if I just died now." Discussions with Judy regarding these statements revealed that she believed she had gotten her first cancer as a result of the stress of her husband's death. She knew that having a positive attitude about life was important but had found that doing so was impossible after suddenly losing her spouse of 23 years. She related how depressed she had been at the time and how six months later she was diagnosed with breast cancer. Judy stated that her three children provided a great deal of emotional support at the time of her first surgery. Afterward, they gave her many self-help books on how to survive cancer. They told her that they already had lost a father and that they simply could not stand losing a mother as well.

After the first surgery, Judy dutifully read everything that had been given to her and embarked on a course of self-improvement. She began eating a low-fat diet, started walking every day, lost weight, and began performing daily meditation with positive affirmations. Judy stated that she had kept this regimen up fairly well for about three years and then became more lax. Six months earlier, her twin sister died. Judy was devastated by this second major loss and again was unable to maintain a positive attitude. She now believes that her cancer has come back because she failed to stay on her health regimen and because of her inability to think positively. She feels especially bad for putting her children through this all again.

Over the next two cycles of chemotherapy, staff members discussed with Judy the concepts involved in having a positive attitude and the Hero Myth. She began to understand that she was not responsible for causing either of her cancers. Judy was assured that the feelings of sadness and grief she experienced over the deaths of her husband and sister were part of a normal course of bereavement and had nothing to do with lacking a positive attitude.

At one point, Judy reported that she had been unable to convey this information clearly to her children. She felt that they still believed she was responsible for her cancer's return and were upset when she talked about it. Again, Judy stated how guilty she felt about upsetting her children. During the family conference, her three children were very receptive to the information presented and were horrified to realize that they had inadvertently been contributing to their mother's sense of guilt and overall stress. They assured her that they were not blaming her and were just trying to do everything they could to ensure her survival and to feel as if they were doing something to help. They told her that they were grateful that they could return some of the care and attention she had lavished on them for so many years. The staff reassured the children that they should not feel guilty for their behavior. They agreed to attend a psychoeducational support group as a family to learn more about these issues.

Discussion

The staff realized that Judy's belief system and subsequent guilt were seriously influencing her emotional or affective state. There was an indication that this

(Continued on next page)

Case Study *(Continued)*

might affect her treatment compliance and, more seriously, contribute to suicidal ideation. Her strong support system had become a source of additional distress because of misinformation and miscommunication. Her depression and desire not to upset them inhibited her ability to understand and communicate information to her family members. A family session was necessary to relay factual information to all concerned and to foster better communication and understanding between Judy and her children. This session was considered to be very successful, but the staff realized that lifelong patterns of communication and belief systems could not be changed easily. The family, therefore, was referred to a psychoeducational support group offered by the hospital that would provide additional opportunities to gather information and reinforce their effective coping skills.

Conclusion

Guilt is a negative emotion stemming from the belief that one has done something wrong. In relation to cancer, feelings of guilt rarely, if ever, serve a useful purpose and frequently are a source of additional emotional stress in an already stressful situation. Patients, families, and the healthcare staff may feel guilt. Children and adults may suffer equally. The causes of guilt surrounding cancer may include things that were done or not done, thoughts or feelings that have occurred or the absence of these thoughts or feelings, and things said or left unspoken. These causes of guilt may be real or imagined. Healthcare professionals need to assess the presence of guilt in their patients and explore its sources. If reasons for guilt are unwarranted, misconceptions and misunderstandings need to be clarified. If the source of guilt seems real and justified, patients need help in letting go and moving on to a more effective coping behavior. For staff members who are suffering from guilt, the administration needs to provide whatever support and therapeutic assistance necessary to help them to cope.

Special thanks to Daniel L. Cooper, MS, for his assistance with the preparation of this chapter, and to Nancy W. Fawzy, RN, DNSc, who served as the author of this chapter in the first edition.

References

Adams-Greenly, M., Shiminsky-Maher, T., McGown, N., & Meyer, P.A. (1987). A group program for helping siblings of children with cancer. *Journal of Psychosocial Oncology, 4*(4), 55–67.

American Psychiatric Association. (2000). *Diagnostic and statistical manual of mental disorders* (4th ed., text rev.). Washington, DC: Author.

Bluebond-Langner, M. (1989). Worlds of dying children and their well siblings. *Death Studies, 13*, 1–16.

Chopra, D. (1990). *Quantum healing.* New York: Bantam Books.

Chopra, D. (2003, December 8). *The soul of healing* [Television broadcast]. Los Angeles: KOCE-TV.

Classen, C., Hermanson, K.S., & Spiegel, D. (1994). Psychotherapy, stress, and survival in breast cancer. In C.E. Lewis, C. O'Sullivan, & J. Barraclough (Eds.), *The psychoimmunology of cancer: Mind and body in the fight for survival* (pp. 123–162). New York: Oxford University Press.

Dienstfrey, H. (1993). A review of Lydia Temoshok's and Henry Dreher's the type C connection: The behavioral links to cancer and your health. *Advances, 9*(4), 99–107.

Dossey, B.M., Keegan, L., Guzzetta, C., & Kolkmeier, L.G. (1995). *Holistic nursing* (2nd ed.). Gaithersburg, MD: Aspen.

Fawzy, F.I., Cousins, N., Fawzy, N.W., Kemeny, M.E., Elashoff, R., & Morton, D.L. (1990). A structured psychiatric intervention for cancer patients: I. Changes over time in methods of coping and affective distress. *Archives of General Psychiatry, 47*, 720–725.

Fawzy, F.I., Fawzy, N.W., Hyun, C.S., Elashoff, R., Guthrie, D., Fahey, J.L., et al. (1993). Malignant melanoma: Effects of an early structured psychiatric intervention, coping, and affective state on recurrence and survival 6 years later. *Archives of General Psychiatry, 50*, 681–689.

Gogan, J.L., Koocher, J.P., Foster, D.J., & O'Malley, J.E. (1977). Impact of childhood cancer on siblings. *Health and Social Work, 2*(1), 41–57.

Gray, R.E., & Doan, B.D. (1990). Heroic self-healing and cancer: Clinical issues for the health professions. *Journal of Palliative Care, 6*(1), 32–41.

Guralink, D.B. (Ed.). (1984). *Webster's new world dictionary of the American language* (2nd college ed.). New York: Prentice Hall.

Hill, H.L. (1991). Point and counterpoint: Relationships in oncology care. *Journal of Psychosocial Oncology, 9*(2), 97–112.

Koocher, G.P. (1980). Pediatric cancer: Psychosocial problems and the high costs of helping. *Journal of Clinical Child Psychology, 9*(1), 2–5.

Lerman, C., Croyle, R.T., Tercyak, K.P., & Hamann, H. (2002). Genetic testing: Psychosocial aspects and implications. *Journal of Consulting and Clinical Psychology, 70*, 784–797.

Lewis, C.E., O'Sullivan, C., & Barraclough, J. (Eds.). (1994). *The psychoimmunology of cancer: Mind and body in the fight for survival.* New York: Oxford University Press.

Malcarne, V.L., Compas, B.E., Epping-Jordan, J.E., & Howell, D.C. (1995). Cognitive factors in adjustment to cancer: Attributions of self-blame and perceptions of control. *Journal of Behavioral Medicine, 18*, 401–417.

Mate, G. (2003). *When the body says no: Understanding the stress-disease connection.* Hoboken, NJ: John Wiley.

Miller, H.H., Bauman, L.J., Friedman, D.R., & DeCosse, J.J. (1986). Psychosocial adjustment of familial polyposis patients and participation in a chemoprevention trial. *International Journal of Psychiatry in Medicine, 16*, 211–230.

NANDA International. (2005). *Nursing diagnoses: Definitions and classification, 2005–2006.* Philadelphia: Author.

Remen, R. (1996). *Kitchen table wisdom.* New York: Riverhead Books.

Saunders, E.J. (1988). Physical and psychological problems associated with exposure to diethylstilbestrol (DES). *Hospital and Community Psychiatry, 39*, 73–77.

Shanfield, S.B. (1980). On surviving cancer: Psychological considerations. *Comprehensive Psychiatry, 21*, 128–134.

Siegel, B. (1986). *Love, medicine, and miracles: Lessons learned about self-healing from a surgeon's experience with exceptional patients.* New York: Harper & Row.

Silberfarb, P.M., & Greer, S. (1982). Psychological concomitants of cancer: Clinical aspects. *American Journal of Psychotherapy, 36*, 470–478.

Simonton, C.O., Matthews-Simonton, S., & Creighton, J. (1978). *Getting well again: A step-by-step, self-help guide to overcoming cancer for patients and their families.* New York: St. Martin's Press.

Spiegel, D., Bloom, J., Kraemer, H., & Gottheil, E. (1989). Effect of psychosocial treatment on survival of patients with metastatic breast cancer. *Lancet, 2*, 888–891.

Vess, J.D., Moreland, J.R., Schwebel, A.I., & Kraut, E. (1988). Psychosocial needs of cancer patients: Learning from patients and their spouses. *Journal of Psychosocial Oncology, 6*(1/2), 31–51.

Welch-McCaffrey, D. (1988). Family issues in cancer care: Current dilemmas and future directions. *Journal of Psychosocial Oncology, 6*(1/2), 199–211.

CHAPTER 20

Altered Sexuality

PAULA J. ANASTASIA, RN, MN, AOCN®, OCN®

One day my lover is playful,
fondles the breast
beneath my shirt.
I wait a bit, then say,
You've got the wrong one.
We both laugh and are warm
in the knowledge that
it doesn't matter any more.

—Jean Bateman

Cancer affects an individual's total being, including the physical, emotional, spiritual, and sexual aspects of oneself. Sexuality in relation to cancer often is overlooked as a priority when treatment needs are assessed because of both practitioners' and patients' reluctance to address the subject. Although all types of cancer can interfere with sexual health, the sexuality literature identifies gynecologic and breast cancers for women and genitourinary cancer for men as the most disruptive to sexual function (Shell, 2002). Sexuality has no age restriction and therefore can be maintained until the end of life. Sexuality not only refers to sexual intercourse but also to intimacy such as body language, hugging, kissing, and touching. Self-esteem and body image are integral aspects of being sexual. Although cancer can alter a person's sexuality, it cannot take away his or her sexual self.

Important Principles About Sexuality

Many external and internal variables can affect sexual functioning, including disease processes, health status, pain, emotions, stress, interpersonal relationships, and religious and cultural norms. An individual's background, culture, value system, past experiences, and current relationship will influence how he or she views sex (e.g., dirty, shameful). What is normal for one person may be viewed as abnormal to another (e.g., vaginal-penile intercourse, oral stimulation, anal penetration) and, therefore, the definition of sexual dysfunction can be interpreted individually. Shell (2002) reported the prevalence of sexual dysfunction as ranging from 20%–100%. Ongoing evidence has shown that the change in sexual desire and function that results from cancer treatment often is experienced for prolonged periods of time (Thaler-DeMers, 2002; Wenzel et al., 2002). Therefore, communicating with patients and partners about possible sexual changes related to cancer treatment should be an ongoing part of the nursing assessment at each patient visit.

Altered Sexuality and Cancer

Table 20-1 lists various cancers and types of sexual dysfunction according to the three most common types of treatment. Psychological responses and behaviors that

Table 20-1. Type of Treatment and Its Effects on Sexuality

Malignancy	Medical Intervention	Adverse Effects
Head and neck	Surgical resection Laryngectomy Tracheostomy Radiotherapy Chemotherapy	Altered body image Facial disfigurement Difficulty kissing Mucositis, xerostomia Fatigue Nausea Pain Alopecia Weight loss Skin color/texture changes
Breast	Mastectomy Lumpectomy Radiotherapy Chemotherapy Hormone therapy Biotherapy	Altered body image Pain Fatigue Feelings of loss of femininity Breast edema Skin irritation Loss of nipple sensation Nausea Alopecia Neuropathy Decreased libido Fluid retention Hot flashes Postmenopausal bleeding

(Continued on next page)

Table 20-1. Type of Treatment and Its Effects on Sexuality *(Continued)*

Malignancy	Medical Intervention	Adverse Effects
Lung	Pneumonectomy Lobectomy Radiotherapy Chemotherapy Biotherapy	Dyspnea Altered body image Fatigue Pain Neuropathy Skin irritation Nausea Alopecia
Colorectal	Colectomy Colostomy Radiotherapy Chemotherapy Biotherapy	Altered body image Feelings of embarrassment Pain Fatigue Diarrhea Nausea Mucositis
Bladder	Radical cystectomy Ileal conduit Radiotherapy Chemotherapy	Altered body image Erectile dysfunction Vaginal atrophy/shortening Fatigue Pain Urinary frequency Diarrhea Nausea Alopecia
Gynecologic	Hysterectomy Oophorectomy Vaginectomy Vulvectomy Colostomy Ileal conduit Radiotherapy Chemotherapy Hormone therapy	Decreased libido Hot flashes Alopecia Nausea/vomiting Neuropathy Fatigue Pain Altered body image Vaginal atrophy Vaginal stenosis
Prostate	Prostatectomy Hormonal therapy Radiotherapy Chemotherapy	Erectile dysfunction Pain Urinary incontinence Fatigue Hot flashes Altered body image

Note. Based on information from Bruner & Berk, 2004; McKenzie & Carson, 2003; Schover, 2001a, 2001b; Shell, 2002; Sprunk & Alteneder, 2000; Young & Markman, 2000.

alter sexuality can be a result of treatment side effects (e.g., nausea, pain) or related to the emotional response to cancer (e.g., anxiety, depression, fatigue). These reactions can negatively affect desire or libido and sexual functioning (Schover, 2001a, 2001b).

The Impact of Surgery on Sexuality

Although sexual functioning and performance may not be directly affected, surgery can alter body image and self-esteem. For instance, head and neck cancer surgery may cause scarring and disfigurement. Radiation and chemotherapy after head and neck surgery may increase the risk for mucositis and xerostomia, causing difficulty with intimacy and kissing (Peterman, Cella, Glandon, Dobrez, & Yount, 2001). Another example of altered body image related to surgery is breast cancer, which may interfere with feelings of femininity. Because a mastectomy affects a woman's body image and feelings of attractiveness, more conservative types of surgery, such as lumpectomy, are offered for breast cancer management. Reconstruction can assist in maintaining body image but still may result in scarring and decreased nipple sensation (Yurek, Farrer, & Anderson, 2000). Recent studies comparing radical mastectomy to lumpectomy and radiation therapy revealed that women who underwent lumpectomy had fewer issues related to altered body image and therefore reported fewer changes in frequency of intercourse and less sexual dysfunction (Ganz et al., 2002; Nissen, Swenson, & Kind, 2002). However, in a study of 1,957 women with breast cancer, more women in the mastectomy with reconstruction group reported that breast cancer had a negative impact on their sex lives than those who underwent lumpectomy or mastectomy alone (Rowland et al., 2000).

Surgical impact related to prostate cancer: Prostate cancer is the most commonly occuring cancer in men and the second leading cause of death after lung cancer (Jemal et al., 2005). Regardless of treatment, varying reports exist on the sexual function and performance of male cancer survivors. Sexual dysfunction still may occur for men with prostate cancer, and potency may take up to a year to return, despite improvement in outcomes with the nerve-sparing prostatectomy for localized prostate cancer (Clark et al., 2003; Talcott et al., 1998, 2003). Men who have their prostate removed still may experience orgasmic pleasure, but they experience a "dry ejaculation" and therefore are infertile. Urinary incontinence is a side effect from surgery that does not interrupt sexual function, but it may alter patients' self-esteem and cause feelings of shame or embarrassment. The adverse effect of sexual dysfunction is one of the factors in the treatment decision-making process for men. Some men would rather choose a less aggressive treatment if it meant less sexual dysfunction (Holmberg, Bill-Axelson, & Helgesen, 2002).

Men who undergo abdominoperineal surgery may have erectile dysfunction (ED) because of nerve injury, regardless of whether a colostomy is performed (Shell, 2002). Little is known about how a stoma affects arousal and orgasm in women, although body image is the most common reason for sexual dysfunction in patients with an ostomy. The potential for interference with sexual organ function exists depending on the location of the colostomy. When nerve preservation is performed, there is a high probability that orgasmic function will be maintained. However, concerns about ostomy appearance, odors, and sounds can affect the individual's sense of attractiveness and self-esteem (Bruner & Berk, 2004). Partners may be apprehensive about becoming intimate for fear of causing damage to the colostomy. Single individuals may refrain from initiating a relationship for fear of rejection or negative reactions from new partners (Lee, 2000).

Surgical impact related to gynecologic cancer: The three most common gynecologic cancers, in order of incidence, are endometrial, ovarian, and cervical (Jemal et al., 2005).

Most sexual disruption from these types of cancer is caused by surgical interventions, including hysterectomy, bilateral salpingo-oophorectomy (BSO), and vaginal resection. Changes in sexual function can be acute or chronic and may present as dyspareunia and vaginal dryness. The psychosexual adjustment for women with a gynecologic malignancy is complex. Psychologically, the removal of the reproductive organs can have devastating effects for all women; however, if a BSO is performed on a premenopausal woman, the potential vasomotor symptoms can interfere with sexual relationships because of hot flashes, mood changes, and insomnia resulting in fatigue. The function of the cervix with regard to sexual arousal has been disputed based on a widely reported Finnish study of 212 women. Half of the women underwent a total hysterectomy, and the other half underwent a supracervical hysterectomy. The only statistically significant finding was a reported decrease in orgasmic frequency in the women who underwent the total hysterectomy (Kilkku, Gronroos, Hirvonen, & Rauramo, 1983). However, in a recent randomized study of 279 women with benign disease undergoing total abdominal hysterectomy or subtotal hysterectomy, no difference occurred in bladder, bowel, or sexual function at 12 months postoperative (Thakar, Ayers, Clarkson, Stanton, & Manyonda, 2002). Accounting for individual differences, some women have reported a decrease in intensity during sexual climax because of the absence of uterine contraction following hysterectomy, whereas others felt a loss of femininity after reproductive organs were removed (Bruner & Berk, 2004). A prospective study of 1,101 women 24 months posthysterectomy for benign gynecologic conditions showed an overall improvement in sexual functioning, including frequency of sexual activity and a decrease in dyspareunia (Rhodes, Kjerulff, Langenberg, & Guzinski, 1999).

Pelvic exenteration, a radical surgery that is performed for curative treatment of recurrent cervical cancer, involves removal of the uterus, ovaries, vagina, bladder, and rectum. Although an uncommon procedure, the surgical outcome causes severe alterations in psychosexual functioning because of changes in body appearance (Andersen, 2000). A neovagina is constructed so that women can maintain vaginal intercourse, but women continue to experience a lack of desire for sexual relations. In a study of 40 women who underwent pelvic exenteration, more than half reported that they had not resumed sexual activity because of body-image concerns (Hatch, 2000). Vulvar cancer requires a vulvectomy, which may involve minimal removal of the surrounding tissue or possibly an extensive disfiguring removal of the labia, clitoris, and lymph nodes. Although less radical surgery is now the standard, disruption of sexual arousal still occurs (Andersen, 2000).

The Impact of Radiation Therapy on Sexuality

The local effects from radiation therapy can have short-term and long-term effects, with fatigue as a common side effect. Women undergoing radiation to the pelvis involving the rectum, bladder, uterus, or cervix may develop interruption of hormonal function resulting in premature menopause. Menopausal effects can lead to hot flashes and vaginal dryness that may indirectly interfere with sexual function and desire. Vaginal narrowing is possible after pelvic radiation, especially if the cervix is involved. In a study of 118 women with cervical cancer who underwent radiation, 85% reported decreased or no sexual interest up to two years later, and 45% reported never or only occasionally being able to complete sexual intercourse (Jensen et al., 2003).

Lymphedema may occur after removal of or radiation to the lymph nodes. This commonly occurs following breast cancer treatment or groin dissection for gyne-cologic cancers. Lymphedema can affect appearance and self-esteem and decrease intimacy (Velanovich & Szymanski, 1999). In addition to altered body image, lower leg edema can interfere with mobility, activities, and even style of dress to conceal the enlarged limb (Ryan et al., 2003). Lymphedema of the lower limb can impair positioning the legs comfortably for sex. The affected limb may become heavy and large, requiring the support of pillows for comfort. In many cases, lymphedema also can cause the skin to be taut and fragile. Edema may contribute to pain and decreased sensation.

Men treated with radiotherapy for prostate cancer have reported a cluster of side effects that affect sexuality, including urinary and bowel changes and ED (Shrader-Bogen, Kjellberg, McPherson, & Murray, 1997). Lymphedema also may develop secondary to fibrosis. In a pilot study of men undergoing surgery and radiotherapy for bladder cancer, 71% reported a reduction in their sex life following radiation therapy, and 50% reported a decline in the quality of their erection (Little & Howard, 1998).

The Impact of Chemotherapy on Sexuality

High-dose chemotherapy, such as regimens used for bone marrow transplant (BMT), caused sexual difficulties in an estimated 20% of men and 67% of women three years after BMT, although the areas of sexual dysfunction were not identi-fied (Syrjala et al., 1998). Specific chemotherapeutic agents may cause infertility, azoospermia, or ovarian failure. Chemical menopause resulting from chemotherapy is the cessation of ovarian function and menstruation, which can occur over a few weeks or a few months (Moore, 2004). Many agents can affect sexual functioning and libido by interfering with the production of sex hormones (Kaplan, 1992; Young & Markman, 2000). These changes may be temporary or permanent and will depend on the cytotoxic agent, dosage, duration of chemotherapy, and patient's age. Alkylating agents (e.g., cyclophosphamide) are the class of drugs most known to cause ovarian failure (Bruner & Berk, 2004).

Chemotherapy's side effects (e.g., nausea, stomatitis, diarrhea, fatigue, depression) can inhibit sexual desire. Chemo-induced peripheral neuropathy can impair the sense of touch, thereby negatively affecting intimacy. Alopecia, from scalp only to total body hair loss, alters patients' self-image and self-esteem (Schwartz & Plawecki, 2002), decreasing feelings of sexual attractiveness. Bone marrow suppression from chemotherapy also may cause side effects that affect sexual activity. For example, neutropenia increases the risk for vaginal infection and sexually transmitted diseases. Fatigue may necessitate planning sexual activities to conserve energy, thereby reducing spontaneity. Lastly, thrombocytopenia must be taken into account if the patients are at risk for bleeding from oral stimulation and related activities.

Studies of long-term follow-up in women with breast cancer reported that women who received adjuvant chemotherapy had more sexual dysfunction as a result of vaginal dryness, dyspareunia, and decreased libido than those who did not receive chemotherapy (Broeckel, Thors, Jacobsen, Small, & Cox, 2002; Ganz et al., 2002). Chemo-induced menopause also can have a negative impact on the sexuality and quality of life of young women who have not yet entered natural menopause.

The Impact of Hormonal Therapy

A category of antiestrogen hormonal therapies for malignancies needs to be acknowledged because of the side effects that interfere with sexuality, desire, and function. The selective estrogen receptor modulators, such as tamoxifen (Nolvadex®, AstraZeneca Pharmaceuticals, Wilmington, DE), can cause hot flashes, loss of libido, and impotence in men. Tamoxifen is a standard treatment for breast cancer and also is used for treatment of malignant melanoma. Common side effects such as nausea, hot flashes, and fatigue have been reported with selective aromatase inhibitors, such as anastrozole (Arimidex®, AstraZeneca Pharmaceuticals) (Baum et al., 2002; Versea & Rosenzweig, 2003). Another category for hormonal therapy is the selective estrogen receptor downregulators, such as fulvestrant (Faslodex®, AstraZeneca Pharmaceuticals), which include side effects of vaginal dryness, urinary tract infections, and gastrointestinal upset (Carlson, 2002; Versea & Rosenzweig).

Men may receive luteinizing hormone-releasing hormone (LHRH) analogs, causing medical castration by preventing testosterone production in the testes. Medications include leuprolide acetate for depot suspension (Lupron Depot®, TAP Pharmaceuticals, Lake Forest, IL) and goserelin acetate implant (Zoladex®, AstraZeneca Pharmaceuticals). These treatments alter sexual function and self-esteem with side effects that include hot flashes, gynecomastia, and decreased desire and erection function (Bruner & Berk, 2004). Nonsteroidal antiandrogen therapy, such as flutamide (Eulexin®, Schering-Plough, Kenilworth, NJ) and bicalutamide (Casodex®, AstraZeneca Pharmaceuticals), blocks testosterone at the prostate and may cause fewer alterations in libido and arousal than LHRHs. Combination therapy of LHRH and antiandrogen therapy may improve survival (Prostate Cancer Trialists' Collaborative Group, 2000). Ongoing nursing assessment of a patient's medication list is important because hormonal therapies may be given as primary therapy or as adjuvant treatment for five years or more following standard treatment.

Long-Term Treatment Effects on Sexuality

Menopause: Menopause is the cessation of ovarian function resulting in the permanent absence of menses. Although the average age of menopause is 52 years, premature menopause may result secondary to surgery (hysterectomy/BSO), chemotherapy, or radiation therapy to the ovaries. It is estimated that women who undergo BSO experience up to 50% reduction in testosterone from presurgical levels, and up to half of these women report a decrease in libido (Buster et al., 2005). In premenopausal females, ovarian failure can have a tremendous impact on quality of life. Symptoms resulting from decreased estrogen production, such as hot flashes, mood changes (e.g., depression, irritability, fatigue, insomnia, memory loss), and loss of libido resulting from decreased androgen production, may further affect the sexual self already threatened by the cancer diagnosis. The use of hormone replacement has effectively managed vasomotor symptoms; however, long-term use is not without risk.

The Women's Health Initiative (Rossouw et al., 2002) studied the risks and benefits to women who took hormone replacement to determine whether it would potentially decrease heart disease, fractures, and breast and colorectal cancers. From 1993–1998, the study accrued 161,809 postmenopausal women who were assigned randomly to estrogen alone (for women without a uterus), a combination of estrogen and progestin (for women with a uterus), or a control arm (observation). The study was to continue until 2006 but was prematurely halted in 2002 when the results showed an increase in invasive breast cancers, heart disease, strokes, and thrombotic events in some study participants. The study concluded after a mean of 5.2 years of follow-up. Of the 8,506 women who were assigned to estrogen and progestin, an absolute excess risk of 8 cases per 10,000 women was found, or an estimated increase of 26%, in invasive breast cancer. This further calculated to 4 women out of 1,000 after five years (Love, 2003). However, women who had been on estrogen therapy prior to going on study had the highest rate of breast cancer. If women who had previously used hormone replacement had been excluded, no significant difference would exist between the two groups. Healthcare practitioners should review each patient's medical history to determine whether short-term use of low-dose hormone therapy would be indicated. Of note, the estrogen-only arm, for women without a uterus, still was continuing at the time of this writing (Rossouw et al.).

Infertility: For women with an intact uterus and at least one ovary, in vitro fertilization (IVF) may be a consideration. Alternatively, for women with an intact uterus and absence of both ovaries, IVF with donor oocytes is a possibility. The success of donor-recipient cycles depends upon the quality of the oocyte. Cryopreservation involves frozen embryos that can be thawed and transferred into the uterus. Semen can be cryopreserved for men who are not able to produce a sample on the day of embryo transfer. Men with male factor infertility may inquire about intracytoplasmic sperm injection, in which a single sperm is injected into the cytoplasm of an egg (Richlin, Shanti, & Murphy, 2003). These techniques provide no guarantee of success and are expensive. However, they offer alternatives to infertility for patients with cancer. The pregnancy success rates of assisted reproductive technology are dependent on many factors, and each clinic will have its own statistics. Since 1992, The Fertility Clinic Success and Certification Act (Richlin et al.) requires clinics to report their success rates to the Centers for Disease Control and Prevention (CDC, 2005). These data can be found on the CDC Web site (www.cdc.gov/reproductivehealth/art.htm).

The nurse's role for patients with infertility issues involves making a referral to a fertility specialist. The legal and ethical issues may challenge both nurses' and patients' cultural and religious values and beliefs. Adoption is a viable alternative that often is overlooked but should be discussed as a possible option for future parenting. Healthcare professionals should inform patients of the risks of infertility related to cancer treatments as part of the informed consent process. Nurses play a vital role in referring patients to social workers, therapists, and the appropriate technologic services for infertility support, sperm banking, and adoption.

Intimacy: Intimacy refers to the physical or emotional closeness shared with another individual. Individuals dealing with a cancer diagnosis may experience several psychological responses, such as anxiety, depression, and anger, which may alter their feelings about intimacy and sexual activity. For instance, patients who have ostomies or alterations in elimination patterns may worry about the loss of control of bodily functions and therefore refrain from intimate situations (Sprunk & Alteneder, 2000).

Cancer survivors who are not in a permanent sexual relationship may face unique challenges with treatment sequelae. Patients with cancer who are coping with meeting potential dating partners are at greater risk for sexual dysfunction than their married counterparts (Love, 2003; Schover, 2001a, 2001b). Uneasy feelings about when to tell the potential partner and doubts about attractiveness and acceptance are concerns that can make patients fearful of or resistant to starting a new relationship. Support groups for single patients with cancer can be a therapeutic way to facilitate sharing of similar anxieties and issues (Caldwell et al., 2003; Schover, 2001a, 2001b).

Intimacy in older adults often is ignored because of society's perception that older people are not sexual or intimate. Physiologically, older patients may experience changes with sexuality caused by comorbid disease, menopause in women, or erectile and ejaculatory changes in men. These changes may result in the couple needing to find ways to maintain intimacy without sexual intercourse, but, overall, many older individuals remain sexually active in their later years. Older patients whose spouse has died have greater difficulty meeting new partners. In addition to their loss, grief, and sense of isolation, a cancer diagnosis may threaten their independence and self-esteem, especially if their spouse was a significant source of support (Shell & Smith, 1994). As the population of older adults increases, these problems will become more apparent.

Healthcare Professionals' Responses to Altered Sexuality

Sexuality is a topic that is difficult for most healthcare professionals to initiate with patients. Professionals must understand their own sexuality and preconceived notions about what constitutes acceptable or expected sexual behavior before attempting to assess and intervene with patients (Bruner & Berk, 2004). Research has revealed that nurses and physicians are comfortable discussing sexuality only if patients initiate the topic (McKenzie & Carson, 2003). Patients may be hesitant and embarrassed to broach the topic of sexuality with their healthcare team. Using principles of patient education, identifying patient readiness will assist nurses in recognizing the patients' needs and willingness to discuss sexuality.

If patients are in pain or experiencing other side effects from treatment, discussing sexuality is not appropriate. Confidentiality and privacy are important to patients and are not always available in a clinical setting (Shell, 2002). Barriers to discussion may include patients' culture and values, age, gender, and sexual orientation. Information should be presented in a relaxed and nonjudgmental fashion so that the lines of communication remain open between the patient and nurse. However, this is a difficult and challenging aspect of care, and expertise comes only with personal insight, scientific understanding, and practice. Nurses do not need to be sex therapists to assist their patients who are experiencing sexual dysfunction. However, nurses need to be knowledgeable about the etiology and management of sexual dysfunction and how to make appropriate referrals.

Nursing Care of Patients Experiencing Altered Sexuality

Assessment

Identifying patients at risk for sexual dysfunction can assist the oncology team in facilitating counseling interventions in a timely manner. The literature has suggested that patients who have had sexual dysfunction or relationship discord prior to the cancer diagnosis will be at greater risk for sexual difficulties (Northouse, Caraway, & Appel, 1991). However, identifying these patients may not be easy unless thorough assessment skills and questioning are employed. This begins with nurses understanding basic principles about sexuality and the psychological and physiologic factors that affect sexual functioning.

Nurses should be familiar with the four phases of the sexual response cycle: desire, excitement, orgasm, and resolution (see Figure 20-1). Reproductive hormones and neurotransmitters affect the phases of the sexual response cycle. Sexual desire, for instance, is driven by estrogen, testosterone, and progesterone. The neurotransmitter dopamine promotes desire and arousal, and norepinephrine affects arousal (Clayton, 2003). Patients most often will identify concerns with the phases of desire (decreased libido) and excitement (performance issues related to dyspareunia or ED). Patient education primarily will focus on these two areas. Andersen (1990) developed the ALARM model as a framework to assess sexual behaviors and the sexual response cycle (see Figure 20-2). Primary causes of sexual dysfunction can result from hypoactive sexual desire or secondary causes such as emotional disorders (depression), situational and psychosocial stressors (illness, relationship stress, or job conflict), or endocrine (diabetes) and other physical factors (high blood pressure). Medications and substance abuse, including alcohol, also can interfere with sexual response.

Figure 20-1. Four Phases of a Sexual Response

1. **Desire:** Having an interest in sexual activity
2. **Excitement:** State of being aroused
3. **Orgasm:** Sexual climax
4. **Resolution:** Return to prearoused state

Note. Based on information from Schover, 2001a, 2001b.

Figure 20-2. ALARM Model for Sexual Functioning Assessment

A = Activity: Frequency and type of sexual practice
L = Libido/desire: Interest in sex
A = Arousal and orgasm: Ability to achieve orgasm
R = Resolution: Satisfaction with sexual activity
M = Medical history relevant to sexuality: Precipitating events

Note. Based on information from Andersen, 1990.

Sexual history: Obtaining a successful sexual health history includes providing privacy and confidentiality for patients and significant others. Nurses must remember that some patients will react with embarrassment or resistance when they try to discuss sexual issues. Establishing a trusting and professional relationship will facilitate open communication. When taking the health history, it may be helpful to inform patients that although the questions appear personal, they are necessary to assess total well-being, which includes sexual health. Another recommendation is moving from less sensitive questions to more personal ones, such as first asking if they are in a sexual relationship and then inquiring about sexual difficulties. Another nonthreatening approach may be to ask, "How do you think that your cancer and treatment will affect your sexual function and relationship?" Measurement tools are available for longitudinal assessment and research, including the Derogatis Interview for Sexual Functioning (DISF) (Derogatis, 1997) and the Sexual Adjustment Questionnaire (SAQ) (Shell, 2002). The DISF measures five domains of sexual functioning: sexual fantasy, arousal, experience, drive, and orgasm. The SAQ is a self-administered survey assessing desire, activity level, relationship, arousal, sexual techniques, and orgasm (Shell). In the clinical setting, identifying patients at risk for sexual dysfunction can be simplified by asking simple, straightforward questions such as, "Has your cancer or its treatment caused any changes in your sex life?" (Shell).

Differential Diagnosis

For some individuals, sexual expression is a release, a coping mechanism that validates closeness, reassurance, and love. For others, it is an extra stressor, an added responsibility or pressure to "perform" in addition to the demands of the cancer treatment. Sexual dysfunction may manifest from physical behaviors or from an emotional response, such as depression, anxiety, or fear (see Table 20-2). Patients who are depressed may experience decreased desire or motivation to engage in a relationship. Side effects from treatment (e.g., fatigue, pain, nausea) may compound an already depressed mood, further affecting desire, arousal, and orgasm. Treatment of underlying symptoms is the first step to removing the barrier that is masking patients' desires to respond sexually.

Attention to the types of medications patients are receiving for medical reasons other than cancer must be an ongoing part of the nursing assessment for sexual dysfunction. Certain classifications of antidepressants (e.g., selective serotonin reuptake inhibitors [SSRIs]) suppress libido and the sexual response. Different brands of antihypertensives cause ED, and other drugs that affect arousal and performance include antiadrenergics, anticholinergics, hormonal therapies, and recreational drugs.

Lastly, patients may present with a prior sexual dysfunction because of a history of emotional or psychiatric illness and psychotropic medication use or a history of substance abuse. Low self-esteem, feelings of hopelessness, and body dysmorphic syndrome can interfere with interpersonal relationships and sexual interest. Often, more than one variable is responsible for sexual dysfunction, and, therefore, psychosocial assessment and intervention are appropriate. An ongoing appraisal of individuals' physical and emotional health can assist in identifying secondary causes of sexual dysfunction (Andersen, 2000; Bruner & Berk, 2004).

Interventions

One of the most common models for sexual counseling is the PLISSIT model, a four-step process used to guide nurses through information seeking and counseling for the patient (Annon, 1976) (see Figure 20-3). The first three phases of the model, permission, limited information, and specific suggestions, are interventions commonly used by nurses. Once the nurse has identified a patient as being at risk for sexual dysfunction, education can begin on several levels. A proactive approach is discussing the potential impact of sexual dysfunction at the time of informed consent and treatment decision making (Bruner & Berk, 2004). Resources that can assist patients include books, videos, teaching pamphlets, and support groups. The American Cancer Society offers free booklets for men and women on sexuality and cancer (Schover, 2001a, 2001b). Support groups can be beneficial to patients, especially if they are

Table 20-2. Psychological and Behavioral Responses That Affect Sexuality

Response	Interventions
Anxiety	Assess anxiety and underlying fear. Provide information and correct misconceptions about resuming or initiating sexual activity, including the following suggestions. • Mood setting: Warm bath with dim lights, candles, and music • Relaxation tapes • Massage Suggest use of antianxiety medications or a glass of wine prior to activity if not contraindicated. (Note. May cause erectile dysfunction)
Depression	Assess cause (e.g., situational depression as a result of cancer, preexisting chronic depression). Encourage verbalization of feelings with a focus on short-term positive outcomes. Recommend involvement in a support group or referral to a therapist. Recommend couples therapy as needed (e.g., partner is having difficulty coping with mastectomy, patient feels rejected). Encourage discussion with patient and partner. Consider antidepressants if necessary. (Note. May cause erectile dysfunction)
Fatigue	Recommend scheduling time for sexual activity. Suggest planning naps or conserving energy prior to sexual activity. Provide illustrations of alternate, energy-conserving positions.
Pain	Schedule pain medication and monitor level of drowsiness prior to sexual activity. Recommend use of vaginal lubricants and changing of position to reduce discomfort. Recommend manual or oral stimulation.
Nausea	Time antiemetic dose according to expectation of nausea. Monitor for drowsiness. Provide a small snack, and encourage relaxation activities (e.g., dim lights, music, massage). Suggest passive sexual position if active movement causes nausea.
Decreased desire	Suggest initial use of intimacy without intercourse. Recommend patient and partner use touch and stimulation to achieve arousal or increase desire (e.g., massage, hugging, kissing). Remind patient to use strategies that have worked in the past to stimulate desire. Recommend mood setting with lights and candles. If not otherwise constrained, use a small amount of alcohol to increase desire. Consider referral to a sex therapist for treatment of chronic problems or for testosterone injections.

Note. Based on information from Bruner & Berk, 2004; Gossfeld & Cullen, 1996; Kaplan, 1992; Krebs, 1997; Moore, 2004; Schover, 2001a, 2001b.

cancer-specific groups (e.g., breast or prostate cancer) that allow patients to share similar areas of concern related to their disease and treatment.

In a pilot study of 19 women with gynecologic cancers who participated in a 12-week group intervention for psychosexual problems, results showed that the group

---

Figure 20-3. The PLISSIT Model

P = Permission: The nurse provides an open and trusting environment for the patient that gives permission to discuss sexual feelings and behaviors. This is the initial assessment phase when the nurse identifies any potential for sexual dysfunction.

LI = Limited Information: The nurse provides factual information regarding treatment and its effect on sexuality. The nurse should identify and clarify fears and misconceptions that the patient may be expressing (e.g., cancer is not contagious, intercourse will not cause the cancer to spread, fatigue from treatment may interfere with the desire for sexual activity).

SS = Specific Suggestions: These are provided after a thorough sexual health history that includes baseline sexual functioning, attitudes, and beliefs. Comfort and knowledge in discussing strategies and options for improving sexual expression are important for this phase.

IT = Intensive Therapy: This is recommended when the patient has prolonged or severe sexual dysfunction requiring referral to a sex therapist. Sexual dysfunction may be a preexisting condition or a result of the cancer treatment.

Note. Based on information from Annon, 1976; Bruner & Berk, 2004; Gossfeld & Cullen, 1996.

---

intervention improved overall sexual functioning and decreased mood disturbances (Caldwell et al., 2003). However, on the three-month follow-up assessment, the improvements dissipated over time, suggesting that ongoing intervention may be indicated. Oncology nurses should regularly reassess patients' responses to suggestions and interventions based upon their needs at each stage of the illness continuum. For example, at each follow-up appointment, nurses can intervene by again using the first three stages of the PLISSIT model, assisting patients to reevaluate their sexual needs and goals. Prior to surgery, the goal may be to help patients to establish open communication with their partner and find alternative ways of expressing sexuality during recovery. At postoperative follow-up appointments, nurses can intervene by giving patients permission and a safe environment to discuss any alterations in sexual functioning related to the surgery. Nurses can play a vital role in the ongoing assessment of patients' sexual health, making specific suggestions when appropriate and referring patients to a sex therapist if warranted by prolonged sexual dysfunction, the last phase of the PLISSIT model.

Female-Specific Considerations

Desire, or lack of, is one of the most common complaints from women going through or recovering from cancer treatment. Decreased libido can be a result of many variables. The most familiar is fatigue resulting from life's pressures and responsibilities along with the additional effects from cancer treatment. Validating how common the loss of libido is for women is the beginning phase in communicating with patients. Talking with patients about their ability to be aroused, whether it is with a current partner or by fantasizing, can offer patients hope in recapturing their libido.

Medications to stimulate libido have achieved limited success. The use of dehydroepiandrosterone, a hormone made by the adrenal glands and converted into testosterone, may increase libido in both men and women, but its safety in women with breast cancer remains unknown (Love, 2003). Testosterone may increase libido for some women, but the doses of injections, pills, patches, and gels are not standardized.

A recent study (Buster et al., 2005) of 533 women with hypoactive sexual desire who have undergone hysterectomy and BSO were randomized in a double-blind, placebo-controlled trial using 300 mcg/d testosterone patches twice weekly for 24 weeks. The group receiving the testosterone patches had an improvement in satisfying sexual activity and desire compared to the placebo group. The testosterone group also was receiving concomitant oral or transdermal estrogen therapy. Because the study was limited to 24 weeks, safety and long-term effects cannot be addressed (Buster et al.). Compounding pharmacies can make testosterone creams, such as 2% testosterone propionate, which are more natural. The side effects and long-term risks remain unknown but may include hepatocellular damage, lipid alterations, acne, hirsutism, clitoromegaly, and voice deepening (McKenzie & Carson, 2003). The use of sildenafil (Viagra®, Pfizer, New York, NY) currently is being studied in women with hypoactive sexual desire (Nurnberg, Hensley, Croft, et al., 2003).

The side effects from menopause, whether naturally occurring or treatment related, can interfere with sexual pleasure on many levels. Vaginal atrophy or thinning of the vaginal lining can cause dryness, irritation, burning, and dyspareunia, which make vaginal penetration uncomfortable. Without intervention, a woman may resist sexual relations for fear of pain, causing her partner to feel rejected. Several options are available for treating vaginal dryness, including estrogen and non–estrogen-based preparations. Water-soluble vaginal lubricants, such as Astroglide® (BioFilm, Vista, CA), and vaginal estrogen creams intended to increase epithelialization for severe vaginal thinning can ease problems resulting from vaginal atrophy or dryness. Vaginal estrogen creams such as Premarin® (Wyeth Pharmaceuticals, Philadelphia, PA) or Estrace® (Warner Chilcott, Rockaway, NJ) can be used daily for two to three weeks, then twice weekly after vaginal vascularization has increased (Schenken, 2003). Other estrogen preparations are the sustained-release formulations such as Vagifem® suppository(Novo Nordisk, Princeton, NJ) or the low-dose Estring® (Pfizer), which is inserted similar to a diaphragm every three months. The Estring is believed to have minimal systemic absorption and therefore is recommended for women with a history of breast cancer with whom the use of systemic estrogen often is contraindicated (Love, 2003).

Nonhormonal vaginal moisturizers, such as the nonprescription brand Replens® (Lil' Drug Store Products, Cedar Rapids, IA), will effectively treat vaginal dryness but will not reverse vaginal atrophy. Vaginal moisturizers can be used as often as once a day or as little as once a week. A randomized controlled study of 15 women comparing Replens with vaginal estrogen found that they were equal in treating vaginal dryness (Nachtigall, 1994). A study of 45 breast cancer survivors randomized to Replens and a placebo lubricating product showed that both appeared to relieve vaginal dryness and dyspareunia (Loprinzi et al., 1997).

Vasomotor symptoms, such as hot flashes, do not directly affect sexual function. However, intimacy and sexual stimulation may bring on a hot flash. Estrogen commonly had been the treatment of choice for treating menopause-induced hot flashes until the Women's Health Initiative study was published (Rossouw et al., 2002). Yet, estrogen often is not used in women with a history of breast cancer, so alternative remedies have been prescribed. Pharmacologic interventions that have been used with limited success for hot flashes include Bellergal® (Novartis, East Hanover, NJ), clonidine, and megestrol acetate. Clonidine has almost similar results as vitamin E and placebo but has unpleasant side effects such as dry mouth, dizziness, and drowsiness (Barton et al., 1998).

The class of antidepressants known as SSRIs, such as fluoxetine (Prozac®, Eli Lilly, Indianapolis, IN) and venlafaxine (Effexor®, Wyeth Pharmaceuticals), has been studied in women with breast cancer. In two randomized studies (Loprinzi et al., 2000, 2002), the use of an antidepressant compared to placebo showed a significant decrease in hot flashes. Each patient must be evaluated individually because the use of antidepressants causes side effects of nausea, dry mouth, and constipation.

Soy has been studied in various forms to ascertain whether the use of soy, or isoflavone in pill form, can decrease hot flashes. In one randomized study comparing soy to placebo, a statistically significant decrease occurred in hot flashes with the soy group, but after 12 weeks, the soy group was no longer statistically significant (Upmalis et al., 2000). Quella et al. (2000) reported no statistical benefit of soy tablets compared to placebo in 177 women. Herbal preparations that have shown success in reducing hot flashes are black cohosh and dong quai. Although many women have tried these and other products (such as red clover) to reduce menopausal symptoms, research does not support their effectiveness, and concerns include their cancer-promoting abilities (Love, 2003).

Lastly, treatment for cervical cancer may result in vaginal stenosis, which causes dyspareunia. Women may be instructed to use vaginal dilators in the form of a cylinder or to practice penile intercourse to keep the vagina from further narrowing (Andersen, 2000). After a hysterectomy, some women may notice that the effects of vaginal shortening result in discomfort during sexual intercourse. Instruct patients to experiment with changes in sexual positioning, such as side-to-side or the woman on top, to control the amount of penetration from her partner (Schover, 2001b). The vagina will expand with use, so patients can be reassured that the discomfort is reversible.

Male-Specific Considerations

ED affects up to 30 million American men and their partners and is not limited to those with a cancer diagnosis. According to the Health Consensus Development Conference (Laumann, Paik, & Rosen, 1999), the term "erectile dysfunction" has replaced what was previously termed "impotence" because of its less negative connotation. Many therapeutic options are available for ED, including pharmaceutical agents known as phosphodiesterase-5 (PDE) inhibitors. The first of its kind, sildenafil, also known as Viagra, revolutionized awareness of and open communication about ED. In 2003, two new products were approved for ED, vardenafil (Levitra®, Bayer Pharmaceuticals, West Haven, CT) and tadalafil (Cialis®, Eli Lilly), with the latter demonstrating effectiveness for up to 36 hours (Gaines, 2004). Although ED is not specific to patients with prostate cancer, the use of sildenafil has shown beneficial effects in men who have undergone nerve-sparing prostatectomy (Zippe et al., 2000). Predictors of patient success include patients younger than 55 and preservation of cavernosal nerves, as well as those who are having partial erections postprostatectomy. Patients should be counseled that it commonly takes 12–18 months postsurgery for recovery of nerve function, even with the use of sildenafil (Hong, Lepor, & McCullough, 1999; Martinez-Jabalovas et al., 2001). Patients should be assessed on an individual basis regarding their health history and medication history for possible drug interactions. The concomitant administration of PDE inhibitors with nitrates can cause a significant drop in blood pressure. Other agents that have been used for

ED include yohimbine (*Rauwolfia serpentina [L.] Benth*) and intracavernosal alprostadil (Caverject®, Pfizer), which is self-injected into the corpus cavernosum (Kunelius, Hakkinen, & Lukkarinen, 1997; Padma-Nathan et al., 1997). Nonpharmacologic treatments include vacuum erection devices, penile prostheses, and penile revascularization (Bosshardt, Farwerk, Sikora, Sohn, & Jakse, 1995).

Premature ejaculation is the most common male sexual dysfunction, and the use of SSRIs has been the standard of care (McMahon & Samali, 1999). Two Italian studies reported that the use of sildenafil combined with an SSRI had a more beneficial effect with improved ejaculatory latency periods and better erections (Chen, Greenstein, Mabjeesh, & Matzkin, 2002; Montorsi et al., 2002). Interesting to note is that sexual dysfunction is a common side effect of SSRIs. A retrospective subanalysis of 10 phase II/III double-blind, placebo-controlled, fixed and flexible dose trials (12–26 weeks) identified a group of ED patients taking SSRIs concomitantly with sildenafil (Nurnberg et al., 2001). The patients showed significantly greater improvement in their ability to achieve and maintain an erection, frequency of ejaculation, and frequency of orgasm with the use of sildenafil. The only exception for success was that little difference occurred between the placebo group and the sildenafil group on frequency of sexual desire. In a randomized study of 90 men with SSRI-induced sexual dysfunction, patients given sildenafil in addition to the SSRI showed significantly greater improvements in sexual functioning compared to patients taking placebo with an SSRI over a six-week period (Nurnberg, Hensley, Gelenberg, et al., 2003). Future research is needed to focus on male libido and sexual desire in addition to functional performance.

Young men treated for testicular cancer with an orchiectomy may request a testicular prosthesis, a silicone-filled sac inserted into the scrotal sac to retain presurgical appearance. Following unilateral orchiectomy, patients will remain fertile and sexually functional, provided this was their presurgical state. For men who experience decreased libido following treatment, testosterone levels should be evaluated to determine whether medication is necessary (Krebs, 1997). Men undergoing hematopoietic cell transplantation experience gonad failure largely because of the chemotherapy and radiation administered prior to the transplant. Evaluation of functional capacity of the penis can be achieved through imaging, biopsy, cavernosal electrical activity, penile tumescence monitoring, and neurologic testing of somatic and automatic innervation. Testosterone replacement via oral medications, a transdermal patch, or an intramuscular injection may be indicated for men with low hormone levels (Tierney, 2004).

Hormone therapy is prescribed for advanced-stage prostate cancer to decrease the circulating plasma testosterone levels to that of castration levels. Side effects from hormone therapy include decreased libido, impotence, gynecomastia, and nausea. If gynecomastia is severe, low-dose radiation may be administered to reduce the size of the breast tissue. Liposuction also has been used. An alternative to hormone treatment is bilateral orchiectomy, which some men may find psychologically unacceptable (Bruner & Berk, 2004). A steroidal antiandrogen, nilutamide (Nilandron®, Aventis Pharmaceuticals, Bridgewater, NJ) is used in combination with orchiectomy in the treatment of metastatic prostate cancer and has the additional side effect of hot flashes and nausea (Aventis Pharmaceuticals, 2004). Patients should receive information about the treatment options for advanced-stage prostate cancer combined with a referral to a physician who specializes in urologic surgery (see Figure 20-4).

Figure 20-4. Plan of Care

Assessment
- Sexual history
- Developmental age
- Learning needs regarding sexuality
- Nature of the sexual problem and its importance to the patient
- Partners' perceptions of the problem
- Extent of treatment- or cancer-related interference with normal sexual functioning
- Levels of anxiety and depression related to cancer or sexual alteration
- Patients' attitudes and beliefs regarding sexuality
- Additional life stressors that can impede sexual functioning

Nursing Diagnoses (NANDA International, 2005)
- Ineffective sexuality pattern
- Sexual dysfunction

***DSM-IV-TR* Diagnoses** (American Psychiatric Association, 2000)
- Sexual dysfunction due to (indicate the general medical condition)
- Female/male hypoactive sexual desire disorder due to (indicate the general medical condition)
- Male erectile disorder due to (indicate the general medical condition)
- Male/female dyspareunia due to (indicate the general medical condition)

Expected Outcomes
- Patients will verbalize perceptions of sexual concerns.
- Patients will identify ways to alter sexual functioning to adapt to physical changes.
- Patients will express satisfaction with sexual functioning.
- Patients will express satisfaction with ability to communicate sexual concerns with partners.

Interventions
- Be aware of own difficulties with discussion of sexual issues.
- Approach patients/partners with a nonjudgmental/accepting attitude.
- Encourage ongoing expression of sexual concerns, including the personal meaning of changes to the patients.
- Provide information about the reasons for the sexual alteration; correct misconceptions regarding cancer or its treatment or any long-standing notions in general.
- Instruct patients/partners regarding contraindications to sexual activity (e.g., myelosuppression, thrombocytopenia).
- Address stress-related, depression-related, anxiety-related or body-image and self-esteem issues as necessary.
- Provide specific suggestions for overcoming treatment-related impediments to sexual functioning.
  - Fatigue: Take a nap prior to sexual activity; plan activity according to fatigue patterns.
  - Dyspareunia: Use water-soluble lubricants, increase time of foreplay, and change positions. Use vaginal dilators for vaginal stenosis.
  - Decreased libido: Fantasize. Discuss with physician the use of estrogen or testosterone. Discover each other's erogenous areas with playful teasing techniques. Recommend mood setting with lights and candles, adult movies, sex toys, and magazines.
  - Erectile difficulty: Discuss probable etiology, including psychological and physical factors. Discuss available treatment options such as prescription medications, vacuum devices, and penile prostheses. Discuss other forms of self- and/or partner pleasure.
- Discuss ways to experience intimacy or alternate forms of sexual gratification. Suggest initial use of intimacy without intercourse (e.g., kissing, cuddling, manual/oral gratification). Recommend patients and partners use touch stimulation to achieve arousal or increase desire. Make touch playful, and communicate what part of the body is aroused when touched or teased. Remind patients to use strategies that have worked in the past to stimulate desire.
- Encourage frank and open discussions with partners, provide support to initiate discussions, and ensure that partners have necessary knowledge regarding cancer- or treatment-related sexual effects.
- Consider referral to a sex counselor if correctable problems persist.

Case Study

Cindy is a 45-year-old married Caucasian woman with grown children. She was diagnosed with stage IIIc ovarian cancer and underwent an exploratory laparotomy, total abdominal hysterectomy, and bilateral salpingo-oophorectomy. Cindy was started on chemotherapy consisting of carboplatin and paclitaxel. Menopause began soon after surgery and chemotherapy. She refused estrogen replacement. Upon initial assessment, Cindy stated that she had approximately eight hot flashes per day and night sweats that awaken her. She complained of being tired before starting her day. Cindy is a grade-school teacher but currently is not working. Her husband accompanies her to chemotherapy treatments and physician appointments. They drive an hour one way to their medical appointments. Cindy also takes care of her parents, although they do not live with her.

Cindy returned to the office for her routine assessment prior to her third cycle of chemotherapy. She met with the clinical nurse specialist (CNS), who carried out a review of systems and a physical exam. Cindy was asked if she and her husband had resumed their sexual relationship. Her husband was present in the office. She looked at her husband and responded that they had not. She said, "I'm too tired, and I'm afraid." She then began to cry. Her husband voiced irritation and said, "She is always tired."

The CNS validated Cindy's experience of fatigue and reminded both her and her husband that fatigue is one of the most common side effects after surgery and chemotherapy. The nurse explained that many women and their partners verbalize a change in lifestyle caused by the fatigue. Cindy smiled and agreed that was what she was experiencing. Her husband also agreed but stated, "Cindy seems to want to do less of everything since her treatments."

The CNS identified several issues after her brief assessment of Cindy's status. The CNS evaluated the possibility of depression as a primary symptom and diagnosis or as a secondary result from chemotherapy treatments. Obviously, Cindy's fatigue resulted from her recent surgery, current chemotherapy, and insomnia. Cindy's motivation and activity level decreased because of the fatigue, contributing to feelings of depression. She also was questioning her sexuality, and her relationship with her husband was strained.

The CNS further questioned Cindy about her level of fatigue (0–10 scale), her activities, and her stressors. Cindy reported that she was so tired from the hot flashes keeping her awake that she felt irritable and depressed (level 8). Also, her parents needed frequent assistance with transportation and errands, and she was feeling pressured to meet their needs. Cindy confided to the CNS that she had not told her parents of her diagnosis. Upon questioning Cindy's husband, he stated that his wife seemed to have less motivation to fight, and she was not as loving toward him as she used to be. "She feels like her body is ugly with her painful abdominal scar and because she lost all her hair from chemotherapy." After a heavy sigh, he said, "I still think that she is beautiful."

Cindy told the CNS that what her husband said was true. She did feel ugly and worn out, and although she felt guilty about not meeting his sexual needs, it was one more pressure she could not deal with right now.

(Continued on next page)

Case Study *(Continued)*

The CNS reassured Cindy that her feelings were normal, often temporary, and shared by many women in her situation. The CNS discussed with Cindy ways to prioritize her activities and ways to counteract the fatigue, such as taking rest periods when needed. A complete blood count was ordered to rule out anemia. Recommendations for treating hot flashes, especially night sweats, were discussed, and Cindy agreed to try over-the-counter black cohosh twice daily for three weeks. If Cindy found no relief after three weeks, she was willing to try a low-dose antidepressant. Cindy also decided to meet with the social worker to discuss getting assistance with the care of her parents and to attend a support group for patients with ovarian cancer.

The CNS included Cindy's husband in the education and care planning to make him aware of the reasons behind Cindy's feelings and behaviors. The CNS pointed out the relationship between Cindy's apprehension to resume sexual relations and her husband's feelings of neglect and isolation. Using the PLISSIT model, discussion focused on behaviors to renew the intimacy in their relationship without intercourse by holding hands, cuddling, and massage. Cindy and her husband agreed that they wanted to try these behaviors, and both expressed relief that communication between them had been reopened.

Cindy and her husband returned three weeks later. Cindy reported that she was sleeping better through the night, waking up only once, and she felt more rested each morning. The talking and closeness with her husband was helping her to feel more positive, and she had begun a light walking exercise routine to relieve stress. Cindy said she noticed increasing stamina throughout the day. The social worker had been helping Cindy to seek out community resources to assist her parents, and members of her new support group had helped her problem solve ways to tell her parents about her diagnosis and her own needs. Slowly, Cindy felt that she was feeling more like herself—happy, energetic, and lovable.

Cindy still expressed apprehension with resuming intercourse, but she and her husband were feeling more secure and intimate in their quiet discussions and cuddling. At this assessment, the CNS began anticipatory guidance to educate Cindy on interventions that would assist sexual intercourse when she felt psychologically ready. This included the use of lubricants for vaginal dryness along with a longer duration of foreplay or manual stimulation prior to penetration. She suggested that Cindy assume a side-lying position to aid in conserving energy and controlling the depth of penetration. The nurse asked the couple if they had experimented with other means of sexual pleasure besides intercourse. They stated that they often used manual and oral stimulation. The nurse recommended that they use these other forms of sexual expression if intercourse still remained too painful.

The important message the CNS gave to Cindy and her husband was validation of the emotional reactions to the cancer and treatment, including acknowledgment that neither partner was right or wrong in expressing sexual desire. The CNS suggested that Cindy let her husband know when she needed rest periods and time alone, recognizing that these behaviors did not mean that she did not love or appreciate him. In return, her husband was instructed to set aside a few

(Continued on next page)

Case Study *(Continued)*

minutes or hours a day when he could do whatever he wanted without feeling guilty for taking time away from Cindy. Both partners were encouraged to verbalize their feelings and needs without feeling insecure. When the nurse reevaluated the situation three weeks later, Cindy felt that her relationship with her husband had improved, and, as a result, she was coping better with her illness.

Discussion

This case illustrates some common themes that arise when helping patients to deal with some of the indirect effects of a cancer diagnosis and its treatment. A young wife who is both a mother and a daughter must not only struggle for her life but also shoulder guilt feelings when the illness interferes with her sexual relationship with a loving husband.

The nurse demonstrated expertise at assessing and identifying the underlying physical and emotional difficulties affecting Cindy's sexual concerns, including fatigue, depression, body-image changes, and fear. The nurse also modeled professional behavior by confronting the issues directly with the husband and facilitating their open communication. In addition, the nurse identified learning needs, supplied helpful and supportive teaching, and assisted the patient and her husband to identify personal resources and, at least partially, the difficulties they must overcome. Helping Cindy and her husband to understand the impact of the illness on their daily lives and marriage enabled them to begin communicating their needs to each other, helped them to provide support for each other, and finally, helped them to reestablish intimacy in their relationship. Lastly, encouraging Cindy to reach out to other resources such as the social worker and the support group provided more encouragement, understanding, and physical help, improving Cindy's ability to cope with rigorous but potentially successful therapy.

Conclusion

Research supporting evidence-based interventions for sexual dysfunction is limited in the nursing and health-related literature. A review by Shell (2002) reported that published literature from 1980–2000 found only eight intervention studies for sexual dysfunction. Thus, more randomized, controlled clinical trials is needed to test and support interventions to treat sexual dysfunction in patients with cancer. Additional research on disease-specific cancers and disease-specific interventions is needed to evaluate outcomes and improve sexual functioning for men and women with cancer. Prospective studies also are necessary to identify the relationship between symptom management and sexual functioning and to identify effective education and counseling techniques for nurses and other healthcare professionals.

Finally, nurses and physicians need to be aware of their own limitations in treating and counseling individuals with sexual dysfunction. A referral to a professional sex therapist is an appropriate plan after all other interventions have been initiated and the patient is still in crisis. The American Association of Sex Educators, Counselors, and Therapists can provide referrals (Schover, 2001a). The nurse is the liaison between patients and the resources that help to guide patients back to sexual wellness. Through trust, skilled assessment techniques, and education, nurses can assist patients by providing information in the areas of sexuality and sexual rehabilitation, supporting their quality of life.

References

American Psychiatric Association. (2000). *Diagnostic and statistical manual of mental disorders* (4th ed., text rev.). Washington, DC: Author.

Andersen, B.L. (1990). How cancer affects sexual functioning. *Oncology, 4*(6), 81–88.

Andersen, B.L. (2000). Psychological issues. In J.S. Berek & N.F. Hacker (Eds.), *Practical gynecologic oncology* (3rd ed., pp. 887–913). Philadelphia: Lippincott Williams and Wilkins.

Annon, J. (1976). The PLISSIT model: A proposed conceptual scheme for the behavioral treatment of sexual problems. *Journal of Sex Education and Therapy, 2,* 1–15.

Aventis Pharmaceuticals. (2004). Nilandron [Package insert]. Bridgewater, NJ: Author.

Barton, D.L., Loprinzi, C.L., Quella, S.K., Sloan, J.A., Veeder, M.H., & Egner, J.R. (1998). Prospective evaluation of vitamin E for hot flashes in breast cancer survivors. *Journal of Clinical Oncology, 16,* 495–500.

Baum, M., Budzar, A.U., Cuzick, J., Forbes, J., Houghton, J.H., Klijn, J.G., et al. (2002). Anastrozole alone or in combination with tamoxifen versus tamoxifen alone for adjuvant treatment of postmenopausal women with early breast cancer: First results of the ATAC randomised trial. *Lancet, 359,* 2131–2139.

Bosshardt, R.J., Farwerk, R., Sikora, R., Sohn, M., & Jakse, G. (1995). Objective measurement of the effectiveness, therapeutic success, and dynamic mechanisms of the vacuum device. *British Journal of Urology, 75,* 786–791.

Broeckel, J.A., Thors, C.L., Jacobsen, P.B., Small, M., & Cox, C.E. (2002). Sexual functioning in long-term breast cancer survivors treated with adjuvant chemotherapy. *Breast Cancer Research and Treatment, 75,* 241–248.

Bruner, D.W., & Berk, L. (2004). Altered body image and sexual health. In C.H. Yarbro, M.H. Frogge, & M. Goodman (Eds.), *Cancer symptom management* (3rd ed., pp. 596–634). Sudbury, MA: Jones and Bartlett.

Buster, J.E., Kingsberg, S.A., Aguirre, O., Brown, C., Breaux, J.G., Buch, A., et al. (2005). Testosterone patch for low sexual desire in surgically menopausal women: A randomized trial. *Obstetrics and Gynecology, 105*(5 Pt. 1), 944–952.

Caldwell, R., Classen, C., Lagana, L., McGarvey, E., Baum, L., Duenke, S.D., et al. (2003). Changes in sexual functioning and mood among women treated for gynecological cancer who receive group therapy: A pilot study. *Journal of Clinical Psychology in Medical Settings, 10,* 149–156.

Carlson, R. (2002). Fulvestrant: An estrogen receptor downregulator for postmenopausal breast cancer. *Cancer Investigation, 20*(Suppl. 1), 83–84.

Centers for Disease Control and Prevention. (2005, April). *Assisted reproductive technology: Home.* Retrieved April 8, 2005, from http://www.cdc.gov/reproductivehealth/art.htm

Chen, J., Greenstein, A., Mabjeesh, N.J., & Matzkin, H. (2002, May). *Role of sildenafil in the treatment of premature ejaculation (PE)* [Abstract 1104]. Program and abstracts of the 97th Annual Meeting of the American Urological Association, Orlando, FL.

Clark, J.A., Inui, T.S., Sillima, R., Bokhour, B.G., Krasnow, S.H., Robinson, R.A., et al. (2003). Patients' perceptions of quality of life after treatment for early prostate cancer. *Journal of Clinical Oncology, 21,* 3777–3784.

Clayton, A.H. (2003, May). *Sexual dysfunction in depression. Tricks of the trade in the long-term treatment of depression* [Abstract IS 17B]. Program and abstracts of the 156th annual meeting of the American Psychiatric Association, San Francisco, CA.

Derogatis, L.R. (1997). The Derogatis Interview for Sexual Functioning (DISF/DISF-SR): An introductory report. *Journal of Sex and Marital Therapy, 23,* 291–304.

Gaines, K.K. (2004). Tadalafil (Cialis) and vardenafil (Levitra) recently approved drugs for erectile dysfunction. *Urologic Nursing, 24,* 46–48.

Ganz, P.A., Desmond, K., Leedham, A., Rowland, J.H., Meyerowitz, B.E., & Beli, T.R. (2002). Quality of life in long-term, disease-free survivors of breast cancer: A follow-up study. *Journal of the National Cancer Institute, 94,* 39–49.

Gossfeld, L., & Cullen, M. (1996). Sexuality and fertility issues. In G. Moore (Ed.), *Women and cancer* (pp. 540–578). Sudbury, MA: Jones and Bartlett.

Hatch, K. (2000). Pelvic exenteration. In J.S. Berek & N.F. Hacker (Eds.), *Practical gynecologic oncology* (3rd ed., pp. 829–845). Philadelphia: Lippincott Williams and Wilkins.

Holmberg, L., Bill-Axelson, A., & Helgesen, F. (2002). Prostate cancer treatment: To wait or not. *New England Journal of Medicine, 347,* 781–789.

Hong, E.K., Lepor, H., & McCullough, A.R. (1999). Time dependent patient satisfaction with sildenafil for erectile dysfunction (ED) after nerve-sparing radical retropubic prostatectomy (RRP). *International Journal of Impotence Research, 11*(Suppl. 1), S15–S22.

Jemal, A., Murray, T., Ward, E., Samuels, A., Tiwari, R., Ghafoor, A., et al. (2005). Cancer statistics, 2005. *CA: A Cancer Journal for Clinicians, 55,* 10–30.

Jensen, P.T., Groenvold, M., Klee, M.C., Thranov, I., Petersen, M.A., & Machin, D. (2003). Longitudinal study of sexual function and vaginal changes after radiotherapy for cervical cancer. *International Journal of Radiation Oncology, Biology, Physics, 56,* 937–949.

Kaplan, H.S. (1992). A neglected issue: The sexual side effects of current treatments for breast cancer. *Journal of Sex and Marital Therapy, 18,* 3–19.

Kilkku, P., Gronroos, M., Hirvonen, T., & Rauramo, L. (1983). Supravaginal uterine amputation vs. hysterectomy. Effects on libido and orgasm. *Acta Obstetricia et Gynecologica Scandinavica, 62,* 147–152.

Krebs, L. (1997). Sexual and reproductive dysfunction. In S.L. Groenwald, M.H. Frogge, M. Goodman, & C.H. Yarbro (Eds.), *Cancer nursing: Principles and practice* (4th ed., pp. 742–767). Sudbury, MA: Jones and Bartlett.

Kunelius, P., Hakkinen, J., & Lukkarinen, O. (1997). Is high-dose yohimbine hydrochloride effective in the treatment of mixed-type impotence? *Urology, 49,* 441–444.

Laumann, E.O., Paik, A., & Rosen, R.C. (1999). The epidemiology of erectile dysfunction: Results from the National Health and Social Life Survey. *International Journal of Impotence Research, 11*(Suppl. 1), S60–S64.

Lee, C. (2000). Gynecologic cancers: Part II—risk assessment and screening. *Clinical Journal of Oncology Nursing, 4,* 73–88.

Little, F.A., & Howard, G.C.W. (1998). Sexual function following radical radiotherapy for bladder cancer. *Radiotherapy and Oncology, 40,* 157–161.

Loprinzi, C.L., Abu-Ghazaleh, S., Sloan, J.A., van Haelst-Pisani, C., Hammer, A.M., Rowland, K.M., Jr., et al. (1997). Phase III randomized double-blind study to evaluate the efficacy of a polycarbophil-based vaginal moisturizer in women with breast cancer. *Journal of Clinical Oncology, 15,* 969–973.

Loprinzi, C.L., Kugler, J.W., Sloan, J.A., Mailliard, J.A., LaVasseur, B.L., Barton, D.L., et al. (2000). Venlafaxine in management of hot flashes in survivors of breast cancer: A randomized controlled trial. *Lancet, 356,* 2059–2063.

Loprinzi, C.L., Sloan, J.A., Perez, E.A., Quella, S.K., Stella, P.J., Mailliard, J.A., et al. (2002). Phase III evaluation of fluoxetine for treatment of hot flashes. *Journal of Clinical Oncology, 20,* 1578–1583.

Love, S.M. (2003). *Dr. Susan Love's menopause and hormone book: Making informed choices* (Rev. ed.). New York: Three Rivers Press.

Martinez-Jabalovas, J.M., Gil-Salom, M., Villam-Fort, R., Pastor-Hernandez, F., Martinez-Garcia, R., & Garcia-Sisamon, F. (2001). Prognostic factors for response to sildenafil in patients with erectile dysfunction. *European Urology, 40,* 641–646.

McKenzie, L.J., & Carson, S.A. (2003). Human sexuality and female sexual dysfunction. In J.R. Scott, R.S. Gibbs, B.Y. Karlan, & A.F. Haney (Eds.), *Danforth's obstetrics and gynecology* (9th ed., pp. 739–755). Philadelphia: Lippincott Williams & Wilkins.

McMahon, C.G., & Samali, R. (1999). Pharmacological treatment of premature ejaculation. *Current Opinion in Urology, 9,* 553–561.

Montorsi, F., Salonia, A., Zanoni, M., Colombo, R., Pompa, P., & Rigatti, P. (2002). Counseling the patient with prostate cancer about treatment-related erectile dysfunction. *Current Opinion in Urology, 11,* 611–617.

Moore, S. (2004). Menopausal symptoms. In C.H. Yarbro, M.H. Frogge, & M. Goodman (Eds.), *Cancer symptom management* (3rd ed., pp. 571–595). Sudbury, MA: Jones and Bartlett.

Nachtigall, L.E. (1994). Comparative study: Replens versus local estrogen in menopausal women. *Fertility and Sterility, 61,* 178–180.

NANDA International. (2005). *Nursing diagnoses: Definitions and classification, 2005–2006.* Philadelphia: Author.

Nissen, M., Swenson, K.K., & Kind, E. (2002). Quality of life after postmastectomy breast reconstruction. *Oncology Nursing Forum, 29,* 547–553.

Northouse, L., Caraway, A., & Appel, C. (1991). Psychological consequences of breast cancer on partner and family. *Seminars in Oncology Nursing, 7,* 216–223.

Nurnberg, H.G., Gelenberg, A.J., Hargreave, T.B., Harrison, W.M., Siegel, R.L., & Smith, M.D. (2001). Efficacy of sildenafil citrate for the treatment of erectile dysfunction in men taking serotonin reuptake inhibitors. *American Journal of Psychiatry, 158,* 1926–1928.

Nurnberg, H.G., Hensley, P.L., Croft, H.A., Fava, M., Warnock, J.K., & Paine, S. (2003, May). *Sildenafil citrate treatment for SSRI-associated female sexual dysfunction.* Program and abstracts of the 156th annual meeting of the American Psychiatric Association, San Francisco, CA.

Nurnberg, H.G., Hensley, P.L., Gelenberg, A.J., Fava, M., Lauriello, J., & Paine, S. (2003). Treatment of antidepressant-associated sexual dysfunction with sildenafil: A randomized controlled study. *JAMA, 289,* 56–64.

Padma-Nathan, H., Hellstrom, W.J., Kaiser, F.E., Labasky, R.F., Lue, T.F., Nolten, W.E., et al. (1997). Treatment of men with erectile dysfunction with transurethral alprostadil. Medicated Urethral System for Erection (MUSE) Study Group. *New England Journal of Medicine, 336,* 1–7.

Peterman, A., Cella, D., Glandon, G., Dobrez, D., & Yount, S. (2001). Mucositis in head and neck cancer: Economic and quality of life outcomes. *Journal of the National Cancer Institute Monographs, 29,* 45–51.

Prostate Cancer Trialists' Collaborative Group. (2000). Maximum androgen blockade in advanced prostate cancer: An overview of the randomised trials. *Lancet, 355,* 1491–1498.

Quella, S.K., Loprinzi, C.L., Barton, D.L., Knost, J.A., Sloan, J.A., La Vasseur, B.I., et al. (2000). Evaluation of soy phytoestrogens for the treatment of hot flashes in breast cancer survivors: A North Central Cancer Treatment Group Trial. *Journal of Clinical Oncology, 18,* 1068–1074.

Rhodes, J.C., Kjerulff, K.H., Langenberg, P.W., & Guzinski, G.M. (1999). Hysterectomy and sexual functioning. *JAMA, 282,* 1934–1941.

Richlin, S.S., Shanti, A., & Murphy, A.A. (2003) Assisted reproductive technology. In J.R. Scott, R.S. Gibbs, B.Y. Karlan, & A.F. Haney (Eds.), *Danforth's obstetrics and gynecology* (9th ed., pp. 697–712). Philadelphia: Lippincott Williams & Wilkins.

Rossouw, J.E., Anderson, G.L., Prentice, R.L., La Croix, A.Z., Kooperberg, C., Stefanick, M.L., et al. (2002). Risks and benefits of estrogen plus progestin in healthy postmenopausal women: Principal results from the Women's Health Initiative randomized controlled trial. *JAMA, 288,* 321–333.

Rowland, J.H., Desmond, K.A., Meyerowitz, B.E., Belin, T.R., Wyatt, G.E., & Ganz, P.A. (2000). Role of breast reconstructive surgery in physical and emotional outcomes among breast cancer survivors. *Journal of the National Cancer Institute, 92,* 1422–1429.

Ryan, M., Stainton, C.M., Jaconelli, C., Watts, S., MacKenzie, P., & Mansberg, T. (2003). The experience of lower limb lymphedema for women after treatment for gynecologic cancer. *Oncology Nursing Forum, 30,* 417–423.

Schenken, R.S. (2003). Endometriosis. In J.R. Scott, R.S. Gibbs, B.Y. Karlan, & A.F. Haney (Eds.), *Danforth's obstetrics and gynecology* (9th ed., pp. 713–738). Philadelphia: Lippincott Williams & Wilkins.

Schover, L. (2001a). *Sexuality and cancer: For the man who has cancer, and his partner.* Atlanta, GA: American Cancer Society.

Schover, L. (2001b). *Sexuality and cancer: For the woman who has cancer, and her partner.* Atlanta, GA: American Cancer Society.

Schwartz, S., & Plawecki, H.M. (2002). Consequences of chemotherapy on the sexuality of patients with lung cancer. *Clinical Journal of Oncology Nursing, 6,* 212–216.

Shell, J.A. (2002). Evidence-based practice for symptom management in adults with cancer: Sexual dysfunction. *Oncology Nursing Forum, 29,* 53–66.

Shell, J.A., & Smith, C. (1994). Sexuality and the older person with cancer. *Oncology Nursing Forum, 21,* 553–558.

Shrader-Bogen, C.L., Kjellberg, J.L., McPherson, C.P., & Murray, C.L. (1997). Quality of life and treatment outcomes. *Cancer, 79,* 1977–1986.

Sprunk, E., & Alteneder, R.R. (2000). The impact of an ostomy on sexuality. *Clinical Journal of Oncology Nursing, 4,* 85–90.

Syrjala, K.L., Roth-Roemer, S.L., Abrams, J.R., Scanlan, J.M., Chapko, M.K., Visser, S., et al. (1998). Prevalence and predictors of sexual dysfunction in long-term survivors of marrow transplantation. *Journal of Clinical Oncology, 16,* 3148–3157.

Talcott, J.A., Manola, J., Clark, J.A., Kaplan, I., Beard, C.J., Mitchell, S.P., et al. (2003). Time course and predictors of symptoms after primary prostate cancer therapy. *Journal of Clinical Oncology, 21,* 3979–3986.

Talcott, J.A., Rieker, P., Clark, J.A., Propert, K.J., Weeks, J.C., Beard, C.J., et al. (1998). Patient-reported symptoms after primary therapy for early prostate cancer: Results of a prospective cohort study. *Journal of Clinical Oncology, 16,* 275–283.

Thakar, R., Ayers, S., Clarkson, P., Stanton, S., & Manyonda, I. (2002). Outcomes after total versus subtotal abdominal hysterectomy. *New England Journal of Medicine, 347,* 1318–1325.

Thaler-DeMers, D. (2002). Sexuality, fertility issues, and cancer. *Illness, Crisis, and Loss, 10,* 27–41.

Tierney, D.K. (2004). Sexuality following hematopoietic cell transplantation. *Clinical Journal of Oncology Nursing, 8,* 43–47.

Upmalis, D.H., Lobo, R., Bradley, L., Warren, M., Cone, F.L., & Lamia, C.A. (2000). Vasomotor symptom relief by soy isoflavone extract tablets in postmenopausal women: A multicenter, double-blind, randomized, placebo-controlled study. *Menopause, 7,* 236–242.

Velanovich, V., & Szymanski, W. (1999). Quality of life of breast cancer patients with lymphedema. *American Journal of Surgery, 177,* 184–187.

Versea, L., & Rosenzweig, M. (2003). Hormonal therapy for breast cancer: Focus on fulvestrant. *Clinical Journal of Oncology Nursing, 7,* 307–311.

Wenzel, L.B., Donnelly, J.P., Fowler, J.M., Habbal, R., Taylor, T.H., Azziz, N., et al. (2002). Resilience, reflection, and residual stress in ovarian cancer survivorship: A Gynecologic Oncology Group study. *Psycho-Oncology, 11,* 142–153.

Young, R.C., & Markman, M. (2000). Chemotherapy. In J.S. Berek & N.F. Hacker (Eds.), *Practical gynecologic oncology* (3rd ed., pp. 83–115). Philadelphia: Lippincott Williams & Wilkins.

Yurek, D., Farrer, W., & Anderson, B.L. (2000). Breast cancer surgery: Comparing surgical groups and determining individual differences in postoperative sexuality and body change stress. *Journal of Consulting and Clinical Psychology, 68,* 697–709.

Zippe, C.D., Jhaveri, F.M., Klein, E.A., Kedia, S., Pasqualotto, F.F., Kedia, A.W., et al. (2000). Role of Viagra after radical prostatectomy. *Urology, 55,* 241–245.

CHAPTER 21

Delirium and Dementia

Esther Muscari, RN, MSN, APRN, BC

Cogito ergo sum. I think, therefore I am.

—Descartes

Cognitive mental disorders, including delirium and dementia, in patients with cancer can be unrelated to the cancer or caused by it. Whatever the etiology, these disorders represent a disturbing but often overlooked aspect of dealing with this disease. The impact of these disorders on patients, families, and healthcare professionals adds to the stress of coping with the cancer. Cognitive and behavioral changes can increase patients' and families' emotional distress, thereby affecting the quality of the time they spend together.

Delirium

In the acute-care setting, a patient's affect, behavior, and cognition may change suddenly and unpredictably. A patient who was coherent, sociable, and cooperative in the morning may become restless, confused, and unable to remember simple instructions that evening. This phenomenon is known by many names, including acute psychosis, toxic psychosis, acute organic brain syndrome, delirium, and dementia. The diversity of names in the literature and among clinicians reflects imprecise and inconsistent identification and diagnosis of the problem. In the face of such confusing terminology, nurses must be aware of the many labels that are used to describe this situation (Trzepacz, 1994).

Signs and Symptoms

Delirium is a common, morbid condition in which the patient is in a confusional state that is acute in onset but can last as long as 12 months (Kiely et al., 2004; Mc-

Cusker, Cole, Dendukuri, Han, & Belzile, 2003). The mental status changes of delirium range from full consciousness to deep coma (Morrison, 2003). Delirium is a medical diagnosis made when the following symptoms are present: (a) clouding of consciousness and attention, (b) global disturbance of cognition with perceptual distortions, illusions, and hallucinations, (c) psychomotor disturbances that are reflected in either hypo- or hyperactive reaction times and flow of speech, (d) disturbance of the sleep/wake cycle, and (e) depression, anxiety, fear, irritability, euphoria, apathy, or wandering (Burns, Gallagley, & Byrne, 2004).

Delirium is characterized by a fluctuation in the intensity of the symptoms, often with the symptoms worsening over the course of the day and into the evening (Caeiro, Ferro, Albuquerque, & Figueira, 2004). The patient can be hyperactive or hypoactive or may fluctuate between the two within a few hours or a day. Activity is disorganized and without purpose. Hyperactivity combined with confusion can lead to self-injury. If patients are fearful or hallucinating, they may strike out at others. In patients who are critically ill, hypoactive behavior is difficult to differentiate from the illness or medication effects.

Despite its obvious nature, delirium often is unrecognized by healthcare providers and is undetected in approximately half of all cases (Morrison, 2003). The symptoms of these disorders (e.g., apathy, agitation, withdrawal) can be mistaken for depression or other emotional responses to the cancer. It is a common disorder of the older population, affecting up to 80% of hospitalized older adults (people older than 65 years) (Miller, 2004). Although age is a risk factor for the development of delirium, how much the association is independent from physical frailty is unclear. Medications in lower doses can precipitate delirium in older adults because of the altered metabolism and susceptibility of the aging brain to altered neurochemical activity (Burns et al., 2004; Miller).

Etiologies

Although the etiology of delirium usually is multifactorial in older adults, a single cause often is identifiable. Factors that predispose or contribute to older adults experiencing delirium include visual impairment, mood disorders, immobility/functional dependency, dehydration, alcoholism, hip fracture, fecal impaction, urinary retention, and stroke, but usually these are not independent causes (Burns et al., 2004; Lyketsos, Sheppard, & Rabins, 2000). Factors that can independently precipitate delirium include narcotic use, severe acute illness, stroke, metabolic abnormalities, shock, anemia, pain, physical restraints, indwelling urethral catheter, surgery, prolonged time on cardiac bypass, multiple invasive/noninvasive hospital procedures, and intensive care unit admission (Burns et al.; Caeiro et al., 2004; McNicoll et al., 2003; Miller, 2004). See Figure 21-1 for a more comprehensive list of causes of delirium. Other physical causes of delirium include new or worsening medical illnesses, drug abuse, poisons, drug withdrawal syndromes, mental illness, severe pain, immobilization, or sleep deprivation (Torpy, Lynm, & Glass, 2004).

Pathophysiology

The pathophysiology of delirium lies in widespread disruption of the higher cortical functioning of the brain. Dysfunction is evident in diffuse areas such as subcortical

---

Figure 21-1. Factors Associated With Delirium

Predisposing and Contributing Factors	Precipitating Factors and Causes
• Older age	• Hepatic failure
• Prior cognitive impairment	• Renal failure
• Severe/highly acute illness	• Hyperosmolality
• Multitude of comorbidities	• Hypernatremia
• Depression	• Hyponatremia
• Vision/hearing impairment	• Hypercalcemia
• Pain	• Hypoxia
• Emotional stress	• Hypercapnia
• Unfamiliar environment	• Anemia
• Presence of dementia	• Hyperglycemia
• Immobility	• Hypoglycemia
• Hip fracture	• Infection/sepsis
• Dehydration	• Brain metastasis
• Alcoholism	• Disseminated intravascular coagulation
• Metabolic abnormality	• Opioids
• Surgery	• Corticosteroids
• Chemotherapy (e.g., vincristine, vinblastine, L-asparaginase, intrathecal methotrexate, interferon, interleukin, amphotericin)	• Metoclopramide
	• Benzodiazepines
• Brain radiotherapy	• Tricyclic antidepressants
	• Scopolamine
	• Severe acute illness
	• H2 blockers
	• Intensive care unit admission
	• High number of hospital procedures
	• Physical restraint
	• Bladder catheter use
	• Iatrogenic event
	• Pain

Note. Based on information from Burns et al., 2004; Casarett & Inouye, 2001; Morita et al., 2001; Roth & Breitbart, 1996; Tuma & DeAngelis, 2000.

---

structures, the brain stem, the thalamus, the nondominant parietal lobe, the fusiform and prefrontal cortices, as well as focal areas of the frontal and parietal cortex in the right hemisphere (Burns et al., 2004).

Delirium is the result of multiple complex and interactive biologic, psychological, and social factors (e.g., infectious processes, electrolyte imbalances, hematologic abnormalities, nutritional deficiencies, metabolic encephalopathy, sensory deprivation, sleep deprivation, anxiety, fear, inadequate social supports, body-image changes, exotic environments found in the hospital) that interfere with normal neural transmissions in critical brain pathways. The delirium is attributable to temporary and often reversible neuronal tissue damage related to impaired cerebral oxygenation and neurochemical transmission.

The onset of acute confusion frequently signals a worsening of the primary illness or a complication of treatment. Patients who develop acute confusional states have higher morbidity and mortality during hospitalization and after discharge (Neelon, Champagne, Carlson, & Funk, 1996).

The clinical course of delirium in hospitalized adults is associated with adverse effects that often lead to loss of independence (Kiely et al., 2004). It has been associated with impairments in motivation and compliance, urinary incontinence, and falls (Franco, Litaker, Locala, & Bronson, 2001; Saravay et al., 2004). Delirium contributing to prolonged hospitalizations first manifests itself before the seventh day of hospitalization with mental signs of disorientation, memory loss, and impaired consciousness followed by behavioral manifestations of falls, need for restraints, incontinence, and pulled IV lines occurring 24 hours later (Saravay et al.). Delirium can persist into the postacute setting, particularly if the patient is cognitively impaired or an older adult (older than 85) and experiences any of the following while hospitalized: severe delirium, disorientation, sleep disturbance, perceptual disturbance, attention disturbance, consciousness disturbance, incoherent speech, abnormal psychomotor activity, and fluctuating behavior (Kiely et al.).

Delirium in People With Cancer

The prevalence of delirium in people with cancer has been reported to be as low as 18% to as high as 66% (Ljubisavljevic & Kelly, 2003; Tuma & DeAngelis, 2000). Typically, the delirium occurred by the third day of admission and lasted an average of 2.1 days. Consistent with other disease populations, the occurrence of delirium resulted in longer hospital stays. Factors that researchers noted as being associated with the development of the delirium were advanced age (older than 65), preexisting cognitive impairment, low albumin level, bone metastases, and the presence of a hematologic malignancy, with lymphoma being the most common diagnosis (Ljubisavljevic et al.). The association with the bone metastases was independent of elevated serum calcium levels.

Delirium can occur as a direct result of cancer. Primary brain tumors or metastatic spread of disease to the brain by hematogenous or lymphatic routes may result in either delirium or dementia. But, by far, the most frequent sources of delirium in patients with cancer are the indirect effects of organ dysfunction, electrolyte imbalances, and nutritional deficiencies, as well as medication- and treatment-related side effects.

Hospitalized patients with cancer are most at risk for developing a narcotic- or steroid-induced confusional state, a metabolic encephalopathy related to the consequences of disease- or treatment-related side effects, infection, or recent surgery (Tuma & DeAngelis, 2000). Respiratory compromise causes cerebral hypoxia and confusion. Hepatic encephalopathy produces a neuropsychiatric disorder that may vary from mild alterations in mental status to coma. Uremia, as well as thyroid and adrenal dysfunction, also can produce mental status changes. Similar to the general medical population, patients with cancer have multiple causes of delirium, but they differ in that a preexisting dementia as a contributory cause is considerably less likely (Tuma & DeAngelis). Resolution of delirium in patients with cancer can be expected in people with a new onset and an identifiable cause. Mortality associated with delirium in patients with cancer is related to the severity of the metabolic and structural abnormalities, hypoxia, critical organ failure (hepatic and renal), infection, and coagulopathies (Tuma & DeAngelis).

Chemotherapy usually is not associated with episodes of delirium. Although anecdotal reports exist, this is considered a rare adverse effect (Morrison, 2003).

The corticosteroids sometimes given with chemotherapy administration are associated more with the risk of a "steroid psychosis" than are the chemotherapy agents themselves.

Delirium in Patients With Terminal Cancer

Delirium is a frequent neuropsychiatric complication in the terminally ill oncology population, occurring in 28%–83% of the population (Casarett & Inouye, 2001; Lawlor & Bruera, 2002; Minagawa, Uchitomi, Yamawaki, & Ishitani, 1996; Morita, Tei, Tsunoda, Inoue, & Chihara, 2001). Lawlor et al. (2000) reported the occurrence of delirium in patients with advanced cancer to be 42% on admission, 45% for first onset after admission, and 88% in patients who died with advanced cancer. Delirium is a distressing experience for patients and families and may be a predictor of impending death for some patients (Breitbart, Gibson, & Tremblay, 2002; Casarett & Inouye).

Factors that contribute to mental status changes and delirium during the terminal stage are the same as those in nonterminal patients with cancer, but because of progressive disease, organ death, worsening hypoxemia, and increasing psychosocial stressors, terminally ill patients are at greater risk; therefore, the prevalence is greater than in the general oncology population. The main underlying pathologies of delirium in terminally ill patients with cancer include hepatic failure, medications, prerenal azotemia, hyperosmolality, hypoxia, disseminated intravascular coagulation, central nervous system damage, infection, and hypercalcemia (Morita et al., 2001).

The delirium seen in terminally ill patients can present as either hyperactive ("agitated"), hypoactive ("quiet, sedated"), or mixed behaviors. Underlying pathologies most often associated with hyperactive psychomotor activity are hepatic failure, opioids, and steroids. In patients with these presentations, symptomatic sedation usually is required (Morita et al., 2001). Hypoactive delirium often is correlated with dehydration pathologies and hypercalcemia (Morita et al.).

Because medication effects are the most common causes of delirium in both the general and terminally ill oncology population, patients' drug profiles require consideration (Casarett & Inouye, 2001). Numerous medications, including gastrointestinal drugs such as cimetidine, ranitidine, and metoclopramide, can contribute to delirium and may need to be tapered or stopped. When considering treatment options for pain, meperidine is the only opioid that is associated with a higher incidence of delirium than others and should be switched with another agent (Casarett & Inouye). Additional management of delirium in the terminal setting may be different than in the general oncology population because families may choose sedation over alertness, thereby narrowing the treatment choices. Additionally, metabolic causes of the delirium may not be easily treatable or possible at all in the hospice setting; therefore, diagnostic and therapeutic decision making requires careful consideration and discussion with the family of what treatment could entail. Delirium in combination with dementia is seen in 30%–60% of older hospitalized patients (Saravay et al., 2004). Duration of delirium in older adults with dementia tends to last longer than in those without dementia (McCusker et al., 2003).

Dementia

Dementia, a disorder mostly of older adults, also is an important risk factor for delirium (Burns et al., 2004). Dementia is a behavioral syndrome of persistent, acquired intellectual impairment caused by brain dysfunction (Mendez & Cummings, 2003). Deterioration of intellectual functioning is gradual over time, with cognition and behavior changes resulting in grave disability. Patients with dementia can be expected to have a continuing deteriorating course with progressive declines in cognition and function.

A determination that the mental impairment is acquired and permanent will depend on whether the patient previously was able to intellectually grasp the forgotten content. This characteristic excludes patients who are mentally impaired and simultaneously helps to distinguish dementia from delirium.

Etiologies

Dementia is considered a syndrome resulting from structural and metabolic changes. Alzheimer disease is the leading cause of the dementia syndrome. Other causes include vascular dementia, infectious disease dementias (e.g., AIDS, syphilis, Lyme disease), psychiatric diseases, toxic metabolic processes, and frontotemporal lobar degenerations (Mendez & Cummings, 2003). Eight to ten percent of older adults in the United States have dementia, with more than half of those affected by pure Alzheimer or a mixture of Alzheimer and cerebrovascular disease. It is important not to assume Alzheimer disease or label the dementia as Alzheimer but rather consider the possibility within the framework of other dementias. The pathology of Alzheimer disease can, and often does, overlap with other pathologies that result in dementia. Figure 21-2 provides other distinguishing facts and clarifications about dementia.

Causes of dementia that are purely oncologic in nature usually result from brain and spinal column involvement. Long-term effects of radiotherapy can include structural brain destruction. These effects can range from a short-lived period of somnolence to dementia. DeAngelis, Delattre, and Posner (1989) found that 3% of patients receiving radiation therapy to treat brain metastases exhibited signs of dementia within 5–36 months of treatment.

Care of Patients With Delirium and Dementia

Assessment

Increases in the prevalence of psychiatric complications have serious implications for inpatient cancer care. Because delirium has precipitating factors, it is a medical emergency, with time being of the essence. Interventions should focus on resolving precipitating factors that can result in decreased morbidity. Nurses and other healthcare professionals need to be educated regarding psychiatric assessment, differentiation of reversible and irreversible conditions, and specific interventions. The biggest problem to overcome is delayed detection of mild, but very important, signs

---

Figure 21-2. Characteristics of Dementia

- Is not a global impairment of mental function.
  Some cognitive areas are spared with deterioration of other areas.

- Does not always impair memory.
  Memory may be spared early in the dementia course, with other spheres of mental functioning affected.

- Does not always impair patients' insight into their condition.
  Despite insight being impaired early in the Alzheimer disease course, some patients with other types of dementia may be aware of their intellectual deterioration.

- Is not only a disorder of cognition but also is a behavioral disorder.
  Some dementias manifest predominantly as changes in behavior and personality (such as frontotemporal lobar degenerations).

- Does not always occur in older adults.
  Dementia is not an inevitable occurrence for people older than 65 years. The cognitive changes that occur because of aging are distinctly different than those associated with the pathology of the dementias.

- Is not synonymous with senility.

- Is not a predictable, constant progressive disorder.
  Dementia can plateau or be static at any point in the course of the syndrome and does not necessarily progress on any given schedule or course.

- Does not always have a delayed or gradual onset.
  Head trauma or hydrocephalus may result in acute dementia.

- Is treatable.
  Many dementias, including Alzheimer disease, are treatable or manageable. A few dementias are reversible, such as those caused by structural alterations from trauma or hydrocephalus.

Note. Based on information from Mendez & Cummings, 2003.

---

and symptoms of impending delirium before a crisis occurs. Frequent and systematic assessment of patients, including cognition, orientation, attention, wakefulness, mood, and psychomotor behavior, is key. Mental status assessment with objective evaluations using bedside testing, clinical rating scales, or neuropsychological testing documents mental function compromise.

Assessment of patients with altered mental status is best done at the bedside with careful attention to deficits in attention and cognition. Patients with dementia have alertness and attention that are relatively unaffected, whereas people with delirium have reduced alertness and lack direction and selectivity with fluctuation throughout the course of the day.

Because thinking becomes acutely disorganized and fragmented as manifested in changed speech patterns and an inability to make decisions (e.g., what to eat, where to sit) or complete tasks, self-care deficits may be an early indication of delirium, whereas thinking processes in patients with dementia are impoverished with decreases noted over time. Family members, possibly the patients themselves, and primary care providers most likely will have noted behavioral and cognitive changes and will recall those early observations during worsening episodes. The objective changes of dementia characteristically are an inability to learn and retain new information, short-term memory loss, and an inability to recall a list of items.

Patients with memory problems cannot easily take in new information, and what is taken in cannot be recalled. The initial signs of memory deficits may be repeated use of the call bell or forgetting the location of personal items (e.g., glasses, toothbrush). Short-term memory loss is seen early with delirium and dementia. Long-term memory loss is affected more often in patients with severe delirium. For patients with dementia, the memory loss is from the current point in time backward; therefore, they hold onto their long-term memory until the terminal stages. Patients can remain alert and conversant in the presence of serious memory impairment. Delirious patients may be either overattentive (i.e., hypervigilant) or inattentive. If patients cannot attend appropriately to what is occurring, decreased memory and disorganized thinking may result. Patients' conversations may wander randomly, and they may not respond to others' attempts to refocus or redirect their attention. Patients with dementia tend not to exhibit extremes in behavior or speech, such as being hyper- or hypoalert, unless experiencing a compounding delirium. Deterioration in the speech of people with a dementing disease is more empty or sparse, with aphasia notable in many cases. Patients with dementia often have difficulty finding words.

Orientation is dependent on healthy cognitive functioning. Patients may be oriented to person, place, and day (global orientation) but may confuse the time of day, the length of hospitalization, or where familiar, simple things in their room are located. Although global orientation usually is not impaired until delirium is severe, immediate orientation to the surrounding environment may decrease significantly before it is noticed. Mild symptoms of disorientation may be overlooked as staff members attribute the behavior to the strange environment, anxiety, or sleepiness. Orientation of delirious patients usually is impaired at times, with the tendency to mistake unfamiliar for familiar places and people (Jacobson & Schreibman, 1997).

Sleep-wake cycles are more disturbed in patients with delirium than in those suffering from dementia. Because a disturbance in the sleep-wake cycle can be characteristic of delirium, restlessness, agitation and disorientation, and "sundowning" all may be signs of decreasing mental status. The sleep-wake cycle always is disrupted in people with delirium, and patients with dementia experience more fragmented sleep. Sundowning is a transient worsening of delirium that occurs in the evening hours (Jacobson & Schreibman, 1997). In patients with Alzheimer dementia, sundowning may be exhibited in behavioral problems, such as becoming demanding, suspicious, upset, disoriented, or hallucinatory and believing things that are not true. Unless the patient is disruptive, these behaviors usually are interpreted as anxiety or insomnia, and staff members do not see them as early signs of delirium.

Standardized, objective measurement and reporting of delirium allow for quantification, evaluation of success of interventions, and communication to other clinicians. Objective tools assist in differentiating delirium and dementia from other causes of altered mental status. Once the correct diagnosis is made, potential treatable causes can be considered. Standard mental status screening instruments have emerged for use at the bedside. Those most frequently described in the literature are the Mini-Mental State Examination (MMSE) (Folstein, Folstein, & McHugh, 1975), the Delirium Rating Scale (DRS), the Confusion Assessment Method (CAM), and the Bedside Confusion Scale (BSCS) (Sarhill, Walsh, Nelson, LeGrand, & Davis, 2001). Because routine use of standardized assessment tools adds to the workload and has not been proved to affect outcome, their use should be considered on an individual basis as needed (Tanios, Epstein, & Teres, 2004).

The MMSE has the greatest advantage for early "flagging" of an abnormality because it is most familiar to clinicians and easy to conduct. The DRS uses a 10-point observational scale that rates temporal onset of symptoms (Caeiro et al., 2004). The CAM was designed to assist nonpsychiatric clinicians in their assessment of confusion, but it lacks a cognitive assessment component (Morrison, 2003). The BSCS is a validated two-item instrument tested in patients with cancer that assesses level of alertness and attention with totaled scores identifying borderline or confused mental states (Sarhill et al., 2001). These assessment tools assist clinicians in distinguishing the intellectual changes of dementia from those associated with delirium, normal aging effects, and other conditions.

Once staff members have observed changes in affect, behavior, and cognition, laboratory evaluation should be conducted to determine the specific etiology. An accurate assessment may include a psychiatric consultation, especially if no history of altered cognitive functioning exists. Evaluation should include electrolytes, kidney function, liver function, blood glucose, and oxygen levels. Drug screening, as appropriate, also may be needed. Other tests may include lumbar puncture, blood cultures, electroencephalogram, and computed axial tomography scans (Lesko & Fleishman, 1991).

Differential Diagnosis

Tuma and DeAngelis (2000) reported that the most common cause for a neurologic consultation at their institution was delirium, with lethargy and poor attention being the characteristics that precipitated the referral. Differentiating between delirium and dementia can be difficult, especially early in the course of dementia. Dementia, a condition seen more in older adults, is characterized by a less acute onset with progressive deterioration. Dementia appears in a relatively alert individual and is associated with impaired short-term memory, judgment, and abstract thinking. Delirium, on the other hand, occurs in all ages and is characterized by fluctuating levels of consciousness (attention) and disordered orientation, with symptoms usually worsening at night with hyperactivity.

In older individuals who are physically ill, delirium and dementia both may be present and manifest clinically as delirium superimposed on dementia. A further consideration in the differential diagnosis of cognitive mental disorders is the presence of a masked depression that presents as pseudodementia (Andersen, Vestergaard, Riis, & Ingeman-Nielsen, 1996; Baile, 1996). Depression and dementia present a major diagnostic dilemma, as misdiagnosis is common in older adults (Maynard, 2003).

Nurses obtain a great deal of useful information about their patients during normal nursing interactions and may be the first to detect cognitive changes in patients. These observations and impressions, along with the data collected by using a formal assessment tool, provide the information needed to make an accurate diagnosis and facilitate medical or psychiatric treatment.

Management

Delirium, if untreated, can severely complicate the course of patients who are critically ill. Because most cases of delirium are the result of physiologic, psychological, or environmental factors that are treatable with medical and nursing actions, the importance of early detection and accurate diagnosis cannot be overemphasized. Prompt assessment and management of the symptoms, even when they are only mild, are crucial to the patient's optimal outcome.

Nursing interventions for supportive management during the assessment process are important. Because delirium and dementia are associated with untoward and potentially deleterious events, such as self-extubation, IV line removal, lengthened hospital stay, and increased costs, nurses must respond to acute changes in patients' mental status as an emergency situation (Bowton, 2004; Dubois, Bergeron, Dumont, Dial, & Skrobik, 2001; Roth & Breitbart, 1996; Saravay et al., 2004; Skrobik, Bergeron, Dumont, & Gottfried, 2004).

Four major areas for interventions include environmental safety, interpersonal support, educational information, and biochemical manipulation. Because patients with delirium are especially sensitive to their surroundings, particular attention should be paid to lighting, noise, and activity. Rooms should be quiet and well lighted. A night-light will decrease disorientation when visual stimuli are decreased. Minimize sensory input by limiting the number of staff members entering patients' rooms and performing only required procedures.

Frequent, short contacts with a supportive family member who understands how to interact with the patient can be very helpful. Speaking in a calm reassuring voice can set a quiet and orderly tone. The addition of a clock, a calendar, and a few small, familiar items from home can help to reorient the patient. Encouraging the patient to walk, read, or participate in personal care can promote orientation and awareness of reality. The most effective interpersonal intervention is the presence of a familiar companion or nurse who monitors the patient's behavior, provides a stable schedule, and explains noises, procedures, and equipment.

A careful review of the patient's medication profile, noting the risks and benefits of drug treatment, should be considered before instituting new medications so that "deliriogenic" drugs can be avoided and the reduced use of medicines results (Burns et al., 2004). Close monitoring of all the medications the patient is taking also is important to determine whether they contribute to delirium. Neuroleptics/antipsychotics often result in patient improvement before the underlying causes are elucidated (Burns et al.). Benzodiazepines usually are instituted in cases of drug withdrawal syndromes or are added to the regimen, but alone they have limited benefit. Also, benzodiazepines are sedatives and will not improve sensorium or cognition (Morrison, 2003). Antipsychotics (e.g., haloperidol 0.5–10 mg/day, risperidone 0.75 mg/day) are the mainstay of treatment and are effective with all types of delirium. The low incidence of cardiovascular and sedative side effects is another reason for choosing haloperidol. Haloperidol produces less orthostatic hypotension and fewer anticholinergic side effects while providing the greatest degree of antipsychotic action. Risperidone and olanzapine are newer antipsychotic agents that have fewer neurologic side effects and can improve cognitive and behavioral symptoms in low doses (Mittal et al., 2004).

Other antipsychotics include chlorpromazine and thioridazine. A possible side effect of antipsychotics is extrapyramidal symptoms, including pseudoparkinsonism (shuffling gait, muscle twitching) and akathisia (the need to be in constant motion). Pretreating patients with diphenhydramine can prevent these conditions (Fleishman & Lesko, 1990).

When all other methods of intervention fail, patient safety may include physical restraints if the patients are a danger to themselves or others. Many institutions are a completely restraint-free environment; therefore, every other alternative should be considered. The Clinical Practice Committee of the American Geriatrics Society (2002) provided guidelines for restraint use, if needed in the uncommon instance, which can be found on its Web site (www.americangeriatrics.org). If restraints are used, frequent personal contact with the patients for support, reassurance, and orientation is essential. Special considerations are required if patients are dehydrated, have thrombocytopenia or a fever, or are septic. Patients never should be threatened with restraints; but, when deemed necessary, they should be applied immediately and carefully according to institutional policies. Contrary to most nurses' concerns, restraints usually do not interfere with a good nurse/patient relationship when the reason for their use is explained appropriately to the patients and family members.

Psychosocial Response to Delirium

The emotional response to delirium is different from patient to patient. The most frequent reactions are depression, anxiety, anger, or, possibly, mixed moods with fluctuating intensity. Family and friends usually are the first to notice changes in the patient's emotional state or behavior. If the patient is aware of the changes in mental functioning, the emotional response may be more intense.

Patients may recall more of the delirium experience than has been previously thought. Anecdotal reports have documented patients' awareness of profound disturbances in their consciousness and awareness (Burns et al., 2004). Schofield (1997) reported that 80% of patients queried about their experience with delirium were able to recall their experience, many with great clarity. For patients who are aware of losing their faculties, the fear of loss of control can be overwhelming. This loss may represent the patients' greatest fear. Loss of dignity as the patients say or do uncharacteristic things (e.g., foul language, incontinence) can be devastating to the patients and families. Patients who are aware of mental changes are prone to anxiety, depression, and suicide attempts.

The impact of delirium or dementia on family members can be profound. The rapid onset of symptoms associated with delirium adds to the fear and anxiety of those caring for the patients. Family members may be at a loss to understand what is happening. Their initial response may be that the patients are reacting to the stress of the diagnosis or treatment. This, of course, can delay determining the etiology of the mental changes. Others may fear that the symptoms represent brain metastases and become depressed or anxious at this prospect. Not realizing that the symptoms may be treated readily, family members may assume that the patients now have advanced or terminal disease. Concerns about how to care for the patients, as well as the need for restraints or tranquilizers, add additional stress to an already difficult situation.

Caring for a loved one with dementia can take a considerable physical and emotional toll on an individual or family because the problems are ongoing and become more complex as the deteriorations progress. In addition, it is depressing for loved ones to anticipate the changes ahead because of the progressive and downward nature of dementia. Therefore, families require assistance and support with the acute needs of their loved one while also planning for future needs. A multidisciplinary approach consisting of nursing, social work, spiritual direction, and ongoing medical intervention assists in meeting the complex needs of patients and families. Palliative care standards and hospice care assist in meeting patients' needs during the terminal phase regardless of patients' cognition and are a necessary comfort and support for families. Respite care, either in the home or at a facility, should be encouraged for the family who needs a break. Often, they need to be encouraged to trust in respite care and reminded that they are not abandoning their loved one but tending to the needs of their own bodies and minds (see Figure 21-3).

Figure 21-3. Plan of Care

Assessment
- Assess for physiologic and psychological factors that could contribute to cognitive impairment.
- Ensure that appropriate testing is completed.
- Monitor for signs of change in affect, behavior, and cognition. Consider performing systematic mental status exam. Assess orientation on a regular basis.
- Determine patients' baseline personality and behavior.
- Identify current medication regimen, including dosages.
- Monitor sleep schedule.

Nursing Diagnoses (NANDA International, 2005)
- Disturbed sensory perception
- Disturbed thought processes
- Disturbed sleep pattern
- Risk for injury
- Risk for violence, self-directed or other-directed
- Acute or chronic confusion

DSM-IV-TR Diagnoses (American Psychiatric Association, 2000)
- Delirium because of medical condition
- Delirium because of multiple etiologies
- Dementia
- Dementia with delirium
- Opioid intoxication delirium
- Sedative-, hypnotic-, or anxiolytic-induced psychotic disorder

Expected Outcomes
- Patients will demonstrate improved orientation and awareness of environment.
- Patients will experience an increase in frequency and length of sleep periods and increased periods of restful sleep.
- Patients will remain injury-free.
- Patients will experience a decrease in frequency and severity of misperceptions, delusions, and hallucinations.

Interventions: Patients
- Use side rails appropriately, provide adequate lighting, and keep bed in lowest position.
- Orient patients to immediate environment at least every two hours; give cues such as name, time, and activities about to occur.

(Continued on next page)

Figure 21-3. Plan of Care *(Continued)*

- Provide clock, calendar, and schedule of patients' daily routines.
- Provide simple, concise information related to patients' concerns.
- Reassure patients of the staff's attention to physical status and safety.
- Assess patients' feelings about hospitalization and treatment.
- Clarify and discuss worries and fears; provide reassurance when possible.
- Limit extraneous stimuli (e.g., intercom communications) as much as possible.
- Administer antipsychotic medication regimen as prescribed.
- Explain the purpose of psychotropic medication.
- Assess the effectiveness of psychotropic medication, and monitor for adverse side effects.
- Discuss with patients and families the rationale for physical restraints and the nursing care regimen.
- Assess patients' response to restraints to determine the continued need.

Interventions: Family Members
- Instruct family members about how to orient patients to time, place, and purpose of hospitalization as necessary; have them bring in photos or other personal items.
- Educate families regarding patterns of interactions with patients (e.g., simple, short explanations or directions, focus on one activity or problem at a time).
- Encourage families to reinforce information and communication from staff.
- Encourage family members to participate in patients' care according to their ability.
- Educate family members about the physical causes of an impaired mental state.
- Inform families about the purpose and expected outcomes of medications or restraints.
- Reassure families of the staff's concern for patients' safety.

Healthcare Professionals' Responses to Delirium

Because behavior, cognition, and mood can be unpredictable when patients are experiencing delirium, staff members may feel frustrated and angry about the situation. Most staff members have a more positive attitude and will take more active measures in caring for these patients if they believe the confusion and disorientation are reversible. Patients with more serious delirium or dementia may need constant repetition of instructions, tasks broken down into very small steps, or more time to accomplish activities of daily living. The staff may feel helpless to improve the patient's condition. Feeling as if their interventions do not make much difference in patients' outcomes may lead to low morale and decreased job satisfaction if staff members are responsible for a number of these patients. Staff members may detach emotionally and avoid those patients to decrease their own feelings of inadequacy. They may tend to give only impersonal care and stop trying to communicate with confused or hostile patients. Staff members may be concerned about a confused patient's possible violence. They mistakenly may believe that patients have control over their own behavior and become frustrated with negative, hostile, or impulsive patients who are slow to respond. Sometimes, staff members may feel repulsed by poor hygiene, messy eating habits, incontinence, lack of ability to communicate, and other difficult behaviors (Gorman, Raines, & Sultan, 2002). The challenge of caring for these patients on top of the demands of providing the cancer treatment can be very difficult for healthcare professionals.

Healthcare staff should be encouraged to acknowledge the stress of caring for patients experiencing dementia or delirium and simultaneously reminded that their response is normal and does not reflect negatively on them. Rotating care providers to these patients instead of a few primary care nurses repeatedly caring for the same patients injects forced breaks from constant care. Educating the staff about the causes, compounding factors, and management strategies can empower them so that they feel the support of working as a group for complex patients. Suggesting self-care activities such as exercise, time away, support groups, and sharing of feelings, frustrations, and concerns with a trusted colleague are ideas for relieving the constant stress.

Case Study

Mr. R, a 75-year-old Hispanic male with lung cancer, was hospitalized for evaluation of pneumonia and dehydration related to chemotherapy and radiation therapy. He completed his chemotherapy a few weeks ago and had just started the daily outpatient radiation therapy. He has required large doses of pain medication. He has been unable to eat or drink much because of severe nausea and anorexia related to the chemotherapy. His normal weight of 150 pounds dropped to 122 pounds. Because of the radiation therapy schedule and severe fatigue, Mr. R had been sleeping before and after his radiation treatments; however, he is up most of the night going to the bathroom or vomiting. His 74-year-old wife, no longer able to care for him at home and concerned about his rapid weight loss and daily increase of pain medication, called his oncologist, who admitted him to the hospital.

Shortly after admission, the patient became increasingly incoherent and lapsed in and out of deep sleep. When aroused, he became agitated and restless; he had visual hallucinations and alternated between being withdrawn and anxious. He was not oriented to date, time, or place and did not remember when his wife or other family members came to visit. He could not concentrate on eating or bathing or recall any information given by the nurses.

He was treated with IVs for dehydration and antibiotics for a lung infection. Because the doctor believed many of Mr. R's symptoms were the result of his increasing doses of liquid morphine before admission, Mr. R also was weaned off the short-duration narcotics and closely observed for any mental status changes. The staff discussed the patient's behavioral and cognitive changes with his wife and family so that they could better understand his behavior and support his needs rather than be frightened by his behavior and avoid visiting.

Within two days of admission to the hospital, Mr. R began to stay awake for longer periods of time and his orientation improved. He stopped hallucinating and was able to recognize visitors and participate more actively in bathing and eating routines. He started to stay awake during the day and to sleep more at night. He began to remember what he was told and started asking questions about his condition and discharge. Within another five days, virtually all the symptoms of delirium had cleared, his lung infection was resolved, and he had begun to gain some weight. Mr. R was discharged with a prescription for the analgesic that had controlled his pain in the hospital. A referral for follow-up visits by the home-health nurse was initiated. According to his wife, Mr. R had difficulty sleeping at home, but he did not suffer any recurrence of delirium after discharge and was able to tolerate the completion of his radiation therapy.

(Continued on next page)

Case Study (Continued)

Discussion

This case demonstrates the complex, multiple causes of delirium in a patient with cancer. The cumulative effects of chemotherapy and radiation, along with nutritional deficits and increased use of narcotics for prolonged pain in an older patient, progressed to severe delirium. Observation of the cognitive and behavioral changes led to timely identification and correction of the underlying causes. The patient's treatment regimen, although interrupted to treat complications of pneumonia and narcotic toxicity, was completed successfully with appropriate posthospital care.

Family members were adequately informed about the cause and management of the patient's delirium, and, as a result, they continued to be supportive and participate fully in the patient's care in the hospital and at home.

Conclusion

Delirium and dementia are significant clinical problems because of their prevalence, the increasing age of society, and the subsequent likelihood that the problem will grow and continue to affect healthcare costs and care requirements. As a complication of cancer, delirium compromises treatment and causes significant distress for patients and families. Nurses are able to assess and intervene with the physiologic, psychological, and environmental causes of delirium and its cognitive, behavioral, and affective sequelae because of their frequent and close contact with patients and families. The staff of an oncology unit must be able to recognize and treat this complication. Early diagnosis and management of these serious clinical problems will enhance the quality of life for patients and family members as fewer days will be lost to the disorientation, fear, disabilities, and confusion involved in the delirium and dementia experience.

Special thanks to Marcia L. Raines, RN, PhD, MN, CS, who served as the author of this chapter in the first edition.

References

American Geriatrics Society. (2002). *AGS position statement: Restraint use.* New York: Author. Retrieved April 12, 2005, from http://www.americangeriatrics.org/staging/products/positionpapers/restraintsupdate.shtml

American Psychiatric Association. (2000). *Diagnostic and statistical manual of mental disorders* (4th ed., text rev.). Washington, DC: Author.

Andersen, G., Vestergaard, K., Riis, J.O., & Ingeman-Nielsen, M. (1996). Dementia of depression or depression of dementia in stroke? *Acta Psychiatrica Scandinavica, 94,* 272–278.

Baile, W.F. (1996). Neuropsychiatric disorders in cancer patients. *Current Opinion in Oncology, 8,* 182–187.

Bowton, D.L. (2004). Delirium—The cost of inattention. *Critical Care Medicine, 32,* 1080–1081.

Breitbart, W., Gibson, C., & Tremblay, A. (2002). The delirium experience: Delirium recall and delirium-related distress in hospitalized patients with cancer, their spouses/caregivers, and their nurses. *Psychosomatics, 43,* 183–194.

Burns, A., Gallagley, A., & Byrne, J. (2004). Delirium. *Journal of Neurology, Neurosurgery, and Psychiatry, 75,* 362–367.

Caeiro, L., Ferro, J.M., Albuquerque, R., & Figueira, M.L. (2004). Delirium in the first days of acute stroke. *Journal of Neurology, 251,* 171–178.

Casarett, D.J., & Inouye, S.K. (2001). Diagnosis and management of delirium near the end of life. *Annals of Internal Medicine, 135,* 32–40.

DeAngelis, L.M., Delattre, J., & Posner, J.B. (1989). Radiation-induced dementia in patients cured of brain metastases. *Neurology, 39,* 789–796.

Dubois, M.J., Bergeron, N., Dumont, M., Dial, S., & Skrobik, Y. (2001). Delirium in an intensive care unit: A study of risk factors. *Intensive Care Medicine, 27,* 1297–1304.

Folstein, M.F., Folstein, S.E., & McHugh, P.R. (1975). Mini-mental state: A practical method for grading the cognitive state of patients for the clinician. *Journal of Psychiatric Research, 12,* 189–198.

Franco, K., Litaker, D., Locala, J., & Bronson, D. (2001). The cost of delirium in the surgical patient. *Psychosomatics, 42,* 68–73.

Gorman, L.M., Raines, M.L., & Sultan, D.F. (2002). *Psychosocial nursing for general patient care* (2nd ed.). Philadelphia: F.A. Davis.

Jacobson, S., & Schreibman, B. (1997). Behavioral and pharmacologic treatment of delirium. *American Family Physician, 56,* 2005–2012.

Kiely, D.K., Bergmann, M.A., Jones, R.N., Murphy, K.M., Orav, E.J., & Marcantonio, E.R. (2004). Characteristics associated with delirium persistence among newly admitted post-acute facility patients. *Journals of Gerontology Series A: Biological Sciences and Medical Sciences, 59A,* M344–M349.

Lawlor, P.G., & Bruera, E.D. (2002). Delirium in patients with advanced cancer. *Hematology/Oncology Clinics of North America, 16,* 701–714.

Lawlor, P.G., Gagnon, B., Mancini, I.L., Pereira, J.L., Hanson, J., Suarez-Almazor, M.E., et al. (2000). Occurrence, causes and outcome of delirium in patients with advanced cancer: A prospective study. *Archives of Internal Medicine, 160,* 786–794.

Lesko, L.M., & Fleishman, S. (1991). Treatment and support in confusional states. *Recent Results in Cancer Research, 121,* 378–392.

Ljubisavljevic, V., & Kelly, B. (2003). Risk factors for development of delirium among oncology patients. *General Hospital Psychiatry, 25,* 345–352.

Lyketsos, C.G., Sheppard, J.M., & Rabins, P.V. (2000). Dementia in elderly persons in a general hospital. *American Journal of Psychiatry, 157,* 704–707.

Maynard, C.K. (2003). Differentiate depression from dementia. *Nurse Practitioner, 28*(3), 18–19, 23–27.

McCusker, J., Cole, M., Dendukuri, N., Han, L., & Belzile, E. (2003). The course of delirium in older medical inpatients: A prospective study. *Journal of General Internal Medicine, 18,* 696–704.

McNicoll, L., Pisani, M.A., Zhang, Y., Ely, E.W., Siegel, M.D., & Inouye, S.K. (2003). Delirium in the intensive care unit: Occurrence and clinical course in older patients. *Journal of the American Geriatrics Society, 51,* 591–598.

Mendez, M.F., & Cummings, J.L. (2003). *Dementia: A clinical approach* (3rd ed.). Philadelphia: Butterworth-Heinemann.

Miller, C.A. (2004). What nurses need to know about drugs as a cause of delirium. *Geriatric Nursing, 25,* 124–125.

Minagawa, H., Uchitomi, Y., Yamawaki, S., & Ishitani, K. (1996). Psychiatric morbidity in terminally ill cancer patients. *Cancer, 78,* 1131–1136.

Mittal, D., Jimerson, N.A., Neely, E.P., Johnson, W.D., Kennedy, R.E., Torres, R.A., et al. (2004). Risperidone in the treatment of delirium: Results from a prospective open-label trial. *Journal of Clinical Psychiatry, 65,* 662–667.

Morita, T., Tei, Y., Tsunoda, J., Inoue, S., & Chihara, S. (2001). Underlying pathologies and their associations with clinical features in terminal delirium of cancer patients. *Journal of Pain and Symptom Management, 22,* 997–1005.

Morrison, C. (2003). Identification and management of delirium in the critically ill patient with cancer. *AACN Clinical Issues, 14,* 92–111.

NANDA International. (2005). *Nursing diagnoses: Definitions and classification, 2005–2006.* Philadelphia: Author.

Neelon, V.J., Champagne, M.T., Carlson, J.R., & Funk, S.G. (1996). The NEECHAM Confusion Scale: Construction, validation, and clinical testing. *Nursing Research, 45,* 324–330.

Roth, A.J., & Breitbart, W. (1996). Psychiatric emergencies in terminally ill cancer patients. *Hematology/Oncology Clinics of North America, 10,* 235–259.

Saravay, S.M., Kaplowitz, M., Kurek, J., Zeman, D., Pollack, S., Novik, S., et al. (2004). How do delirium and dementia increase length of stay of elderly general medical inpatients? *Psychosomatics, 45,* 235–242.

Sarhill, N., Walsh, D., Nelson, K.A., LeGrand, S., & Davis, M.P. (2001). Assessment of delirium in advanced cancer. The use of the bedside confusion scale. *American Journal of Hospice and Palliative Care, 18,* 335–341.

Schofield, I. (1997). A small exploratory study of the reaction of older people to an episode of delirium. *Journal of Advanced Nursing, 25,* 942–952.

Skrobik, Y.K., Bergeron, N., Dumont, M., & Gottfried, S.B. (2004). Olanzapine vs haloperidol: Treating delirium in a critical care setting. *Intensive Care Medicine, 30,* 444–449.

Tanios, M.A., Epstein, S.K., & Teres, D. (2004). Are we ready to monitor for delirium in the intensive care unit? *Critical Care Medicine, 32,* 295–296.

Torpy, J.M., Lynm, C., & Glass, R.M. (2004). JAMA patient page: Delirium. *JAMA, 291,* 1794.

Trzepacz, P.T. (1994). The neuropathogenesis of delirium. *Psychosomatics, 35,* 374–391.

Tuma, R., & DeAngelis, L.M. (2000). Altered mental status in patients with cancer. *Archives of Neurology, 57,* 1727–1731.

CHAPTER 22

Powerlessness

LINDA M. GORMAN, RN, MN, APRN, BC, OCN®, CHPN

God, grant me the serenity to
Accept the things I cannot change,
Courage to change the things I can,
And the wisdom to know the difference.

—Reinhold Niebuhr

Despite dramatic progress in screening, early diagnosis, improved treatment outcomes, and survivor rates, cancer continues to be one of the most feared diseases (Holland, 2002). Many people still associate cancer with inevitable death, terrible suffering, disfigurement, and intractable pain. Although individuals may have coped well with many other serious problems or losses, when they learn that they have a new or recurrent diagnosis of cancer, many feel overwhelmed and unable to cope. These patients and their families often describe feeling helpless, hopeless, and powerless to deal with the cancer, the stress, and the decision making associated with coping with the disease.

Important Principles About Powerlessness

An important part of the human experience is the extent to which people feel able to obtain good outcomes and avoid undesirable situations as a result of their own efforts. A sense of personal control is associated with a variety of positive outcomes for those living with a serious illness, such as better emotional well-being and health outcomes, enhanced ability to cope with stress, and improved motor and intellectual tasks. These effects emphasize the usefulness of perceived control and its opposite, lack of control or powerlessness, in understanding reactions to a traumatic situation, such as receiving a cancer diagnosis. Research studies on perceptions of control are based on social learning theory and learned helplessness. Rotter (1966) developed the notion of internal-external locus of control to measure how much an individual believes that outcomes depend on his or her own actions or on circumstances outside the individual's control. Powerlessness is not exactly synonymous with locus of control. Locus of control is a stable personality trait, whereas powerlessness generally is situationally determined (Carpenito, 2002). However, understanding this concept can assist nurses in understanding why some patients actively participate in their cancer care, yet others are passive or seem apathetic. For example, according to locus of control theory, a patient with internal locus of control believes that a treatment outcome can be affected by active involvement, such as regular exercise, reading literature about the diagnosis, and learning assertiveness skills. A person with external locus of control believes that treatment outcomes are outside of personal control and attributes outcomes to others' actions or to fate. Internally controlled people usually are more self-motivated, whereas externally controlled people usually need others to motivate them (see Figure 22-1).

Figure 22-1. Assessment of External and Internal Locus of Control

External	**Internal**
• Talks of fate or luck being needed to control illness	• Expresses belief that one can actively control the course of the illness
• Has less interest in educational materials and self-monitoring programs	• Actively seeks information about the illness
• Looks to family or healthcare professionals to make decisions and plan treatment	• Participates in self-care strategies such as exercise programs and self-help groups
• Looks to others for motivation and encouragement	• Does not need prodding or reminding to follow through with self-monitoring
• Needs to be repeatedly prodded to follow through on making appointments or to complete self-monitoring	• Looks at how one's behavior can affect treatment
• May respond to rewards	

Seligman (1975) further explained that people feel helpless and become depressed when there seems to be no connection between what they do and the outcomes they experience. Conversely, people will feel that what they do can make a difference if they can see a connection between their behavior or choices and later results or outcomes. Learned helplessness is reflected in victims of abuse who become unable to act on their own to escape the victimizer (Townsend, 2000). Bandura (1977) found that people will change their behavior if they believe they can perform the desired action and that it will result in the desired outcome (e.g., "I can stop smoking, and when I stop smoking, my chances of avoiding lung cancer will improve").

The final connection among perceptions of control, good coping, and mental health is the notion that cognitive adaptation strategies that can be learned and used by those dealing with traumatic life experiences can enhance adjustment to traumatic events (Taylor, Helgeson, Reed, & Skokan, 1991). These strategies include assessing how threatening the situation is, assessing what resources are available for dealing with the situation, and deciding what other options or outcomes would be satisfactory if the ideal cannot be achieved. Stuart (2001) pointed out that individuals who are more resistant to depression and learned helplessness have a greater sense of mastery of life.

In a similar vein, Averill (1973) described three types of control (behavioral, cognitive, and decisional) that individuals can use when a threatening or unpredictable situation has decreased their perceived sense of control. Any action that allows people to participate in their own care will enhance behavioral control. Providing information, asking for feelings about an event, and giving feedback about a situation are examples of supporting patients' cognitive control. Allowing patients to make choices and give input into planning for treatments and evaluating outcomes are ways to increase their decisional control.

Powerlessness and Age-Specific Considerations

Young children usually are externally controlled; that is, they see their parents and teachers as responsible for determining outcomes. However, they can be taught internal control as they learn more independence and coping skills. Hospitalized children often experience powerlessness. Interventions can be directed at manipulating the environment to provide opportunities for children to make choices and gain mastery over their illness experience through play activities.

Older adults are at high risk for powerlessness because as they age, they experience many more changes (e.g., loss of role responsibilities, independence, income, health, friends) that are out of their control (Garrison, 2000). Normal changes from aging can result in feelings of powerlessness. Patients with a more external locus of control may accept those changes more easily. Increased dependence on caregivers can lead to an increase in perceived loss of control. Also, feelings of alienation and boredom, especially in institutionalized older adults, have a high correlation with powerlessness (Mor, Allen, & Malin, 1994).

Powerlessness and Illness

Any disease process, whether acute or chronic, can cause or contribute to perceived loss of control. Inability to perform usual activities, dietary restrictions, progressive immobility, or mental deterioration resulting from advancing disease or side effects of treatments may lead to feelings of powerlessness and vulnerability. In turn, individuals can begin to believe in the inevitability of a chronic condition or death. Powerlessness is a feeling that all people will experience to varying degrees when dealing with illness. Realizing that a disease, such as arthritis or diabetes, will never be cured and will always be a part of their lifestyle can cause some to feel helpless. For many, some aspect of the disease process (e.g., the psychological effects of hospitalization, fear of disapproval or isolation by family or friends, increased financial burden related to the illness) contributes to their increased perception of loss of control.

An individual's response to loss of control depends on the meaning of the loss, usual coping patterns, personal characteristics (e.g., age, culture, occupation, spirituality), and the response of others. Every individual, whether healthy or ill, wants to have control. Feeling powerless in some situations is expected and appropriate. When people do not expect to have much control in a situation, they will reduce their attention to that situation as they focus on other outcomes that can be controlled. Increased support or control in other related areas may counterbalance a loss or decrease of perceived control in one area. The healthcare system itself can induce a sense of powerlessness and frustration (Sundeen, 2001). Some healthcare settings, especially critical care units, are associated with increased risk for patients to experience loss of control (Ursano, Epstein, & Lazar, 2002). Patients with mental illness particularly are vulnerable to a sense of powerlessness (Fitzsimmons & Fuller, 2002).

Powerlessness and Cancer

A diagnosis of cancer brings an individual's normal life to a halt. After receiving a cancer diagnosis, an individual's focus is on the illness, which pervades all thoughts and paralyzes the individual, demands attention, and creates anxiety, pain, and uncertainty. According to patients, time drags on—seconds seem like hours, and hours seem like days. As one patient explained, "I just couldn't do anything. I couldn't think. I couldn't read. I couldn't work. And it went on for weeks" (quoted in Hagopian, 1993, p. 759).

People who are diagnosed with cancer go through an existential crisis (Halldorsdottir & Hamrin, 1996). During the first 100 days following the diagnosis, the individual attempts to address some of the issues raised by the diagnosis of cancer: the future, the meaning life has had, and the possibility of dying (Weisman & Worden, 1976–1977). The significance of this existential plight should not be underestimated. Nothing is "normal" about receiving a cancer diagnosis, nor is there a "right" way to react to a life-threatening disease. Healthcare professionals must refrain from labeling patients' or families' responses as maladaptive or abnormal. Patients and families exhibit a wide range of responses as they struggle to adapt to an overwhelming situation.

The number of cancer survivors has increased steadily over the past several years (Jemal et al., 2005). Patients who are newly diagnosed can expect to survive their treatments and live longer, on average, than ever before. Having cancer today is similar to being diagnosed with a chronic illness. Pollin (1994), who described commonly experienced fears related to long-term illness, cited the fear of losing control as the most common fear that patients experience. Patients with long-term illnesses must make decisions and navigate a course through an experience they did not choose, and over which they have no control, toward an uncertain future that defies prediction.

Massey (1989) found that hopelessness was significantly related to powerlessness in a sample of patients with cancer. Thompson and Collins (1995) found that a sense of personal control (i.e., the absence of perceived powerlessness) was associated with positive outcomes for those living with a chronic illness. Having a sense of control is a determinant of hopefulness; therefore, interventions that decrease patients' powerlessness will promote hope and coping. Hope, in turn, helps patients to maintain a sense of control (Bunston, Mings, Mackie, & Jones, 1995).

The Influence of Culture on Powerlessness

Oncology nurses have known for a long time that culture is an important factor to consider when caring for patients with cancer (Sugarek, Deyo, & Holmes, 1988).

Differences in cancer screening rates and mortality rates, as well as variances in types of cancer by ethnicity, are evidence of the role of culture in the development, detection, and treatment of cancer.

Many researchers believe that a severe form of powerlessness, called cancer fatalism, is a barrier to participation by African Americans and Hispanics in cancer screening and other health-promoting behaviors. Powe (1996) described cancer fatalism as the perception of hopelessness, helplessness, powerlessness, and social isolation related to the cycle of cancer and death within families and communities resulting from segregation, substandard health care, and poverty. Within this context, many African Americans, especially older women, believe that cancer is inevitable regardless of the person's actions. As a result of these beliefs, many do not seek cancer care until their cases are advanced, and their chances of cure or even survival are greatly reduced.

Preferred coping strategies also vary in different cultural groups. Potts (1996) found that African Americans with cancer frequently "turned it over to the Lord." That is, they realized the limits of human knowledge and personal control and put their trust in God.

The implications of these findings for psychosocial oncology are significant. Understanding how patients' culture shapes beliefs about the meaning of illness and modes of responding to illness will lead to more culturally sensitive and effective interventions (Jecker, Carrese, & Pearlman, 1995). Chadiha, Adams, Biegel, Auslander, and Gutierrez (2004) reported that older African American women who are caregivers particularly are vulnerable to powerlessness, which intensifies the stress of their roles (see Chapter 6).

Healthcare Professionals' Responses to Powerlessness

To render quality psychosocial care to patients with cancer and their families, nurses must consider their perception of the impact of the disease. The meaning a cancer diagnosis holds for a particular nurse is framed within the nurse's own life experience and the many patients he or she has seen. With each patient who has a new or recurrent cancer, the nurse may be reminded of his or her own or a family member's existential plight. Such thoughts may be positive or negative and accumulate over time (McCray, 1994).

Nurses must be aware of their personal feelings of powerlessness. Nurses who feel powerless often develop ineffective, dictatorial, and regimented management styles to deal with their sense of loss of control. This coping style makes it difficult for these nurses to implement nursing interventions that will prevent or minimize perceived loss of control in their patients as well as in themselves (Gorman, Raines, & Sultan, 2002).

The challenge for nurses is to find the balance between feeling powerless to help patients and a sense that it is possible to make a difference. The strain of facing a stream of neverending physical and psychosocial needs of large numbers of patients can lead to physical and emotional exhaustion for nurses. Experimental-protocol clinics and bone marrow transplant units are two of the most difficult places in which to work because of the high number of recurrent diagnoses and patients who are dying.

Oncology nurses need to pause occasionally to reflect on the essence of oncology nursing and the impact of their presence on patient care (Cohen, Haberman, Steeves, & Deatrick, 1994). Henderson (2003) studied the power balance between patients and nurses. She found that nurses often were unwilling to share their decision-making powers, which created a power imbalance. This author felt that nurses need to make efforts to equalize this imbalance to promote more open communication.

Evidence-Based Practice

Limited research exists in the area of powerlessness as it relates to illness, but some small studies give a perspective on its impact. Braga and Cruz (2003) interviewed postoperative cardiac surgery patients about their experience of powerlessness. They found that powerlessness most frequently was associated with verbal expression of having no control or influence over a situation, doubts about planning future objectives, and expression of doubts about role performance. Ryan, Hassell, Dawes, and Kendall (2003) identified factors that influence whether patients felt they had control over their rheumatoid arthritis. Factors that contributed to a greater sense of control included reduction of physical symptoms, matching of social support with perceived need, the provision of information, and the nature of the clinical consultations. These studies give support to the importance of many nursing interventions to enhance patients' sense of control over their illness.

Nursing Care of Patients Experiencing Powerlessness

Assessment

Because powerlessness is a subjective state, nurses must validate any inferences about patients' feelings of this experience. Nurses must assess each individual to determine his or her usual level of control and decision making and past experiences with powerlessness (Carpenito, 2002). Whether the patient has an internal or external locus of control also contributes to his or her choices and reactions.

The major characteristics of powerlessness are overt or covert expressions of dissatisfaction, such as anger or apathy, over the inability to control a situation (e.g., diagnosis of cancer, poor prognosis, treatment complications, loss of one's job because of the illness) that is negatively affecting the patient's goals, future, and lifestyle. Other characteristics of powerlessness include depression, acting-out or violent behaviors, apathy and resignation, passivity, dissatisfaction with dependence on others, and inability to problem solve, make decisions, or seek information.

Once nurses determine that a patient is feeling powerless, they should try to identify factors that may be contributing to the perception of loss of control. Asking questions about usual patterns of coping with uncontrollable events and previous experiences with illness will provide that information. In addition, asking how the patient makes decisions and what his or her roles and responsibilities are will help nurses to assess potential problems the patient may be having with adjusting to the diagnosis or future treatment plans. Nurses need to pay special attention to the patient's information-seeking behaviors and motivation for involvement in treatment decision making. Emotional reactions to new information are important to note and discuss with the patient and family.

Differential Diagnosis

Powerlessness is part of a triad of often concurrent feelings that includes hope-lessness and helplessness. Powerlessness also may be related to denial. The use of denial temporarily may produce a sense of control, enabling the patient to be more functional. When this individual begins to think about the causes or consequences of the illness (i.e., when denial begins to break down or decrease), feelings of pow-erlessness may emerge or increase. It may be difficult to differentiate hopelessness and denial from powerlessness in some patients.

Stephenson (1979) described two types of powerlessness: situational powerless-ness, which occurs in reaction to a specific event and usually is short-lived, and trait powerlessness, which is more pervasive and permanent in nature, affecting the individual's general outlook, goals, relationships, and lifestyle. Nurses should assess which type of powerlessness the patient is experiencing before selecting a nursing diagnosis and interventions. For example, a patient may feel anxiety and fear as well as some powerlessness related to a first hospitalization for a biopsy or reactions to chemotherapy. If the hospitalization is expected to be short, it would be most ap-propriate to focus on the patient's anxiety related to the unfamiliar environment, loss of usual routines, and invasion of privacy as an example of situational powerlessness. If, however, the hospitalization is a readmission for a recurrence, and the illness has had ongoing effects on the patient's career, marriage, or financial status, then the use of a diagnosis of powerlessness may be more appropriate.

Interventions

Depending on the stage of the patient's illness, he or she may demonstrate varying amounts of symptom distress, perceived self-care burden, and different mood states (Andrykowski & Brady, 1994; Gorman et al., 2002; Munkres, Oberst, & Hughes, 1992). Patients' perceptions of their condition as improving or deteriorating will influence the level of powerlessness and associated behaviors and feelings. Although patients' anger, and possibly violence, over a recurrence may be harder for nurses to tolerate, it shows that the patients are verbalizing their feelings; nurses then can intervene with emotional support, more information, or active listening skills. Conversely, apathetic and passive patients are much harder to assess and motivate, although this behavior usually is easier for a busy oncology unit's staff to tolerate.

When initially intervening with patients who are feeling powerless, nurses should use a supportive, accepting approach to interviewing the patients and family members about past crises and illness experiences. If patients are demonstrating pain or anxiety, these problems should be further assessed and reduced before expecting patients to pay attention to new information or try new coping skills. Providing information about the illness also can give patients a sense of control and power. Controllability of a given illness is a crucial variable in coping behavior (Ursano et al., 2002) (see Figure 22-2).

Figure 22-2. Plan of Care

Assessment
- Recognize the types of powerlessness and differences in individual locus of control.
- Reassess patients' levels of powerlessness at different stages of the illness continuum (e.g., at diagnosis, during different treatments or hospitalizations, at time of recurrence).
- Consider patients' past coping behaviors related to uncontrollable events, especially illness.
- Differentiate among denial, hopelessness, and powerlessness.
- Determine patients' ability to use new information and motivation to change sense of control.
- Identify other people or events that can assist in reducing patients' feeling of powerlessness.

Nursing Diagnoses (NANDA International, 2005)
- Powerlessness
- Deficient knowledge
- Hopelessness
- Ineffective coping

***DSM-IV-TR* Diagnoses** (American Psychiatric Association, 2000)
- Adjustment disorder with anxiety or depression
- Major depression

Expected Outcomes
- Patients will identify factors that they can control or influence.
- Patients will make decisions regarding care, treatment, and future.
- Patients will verbalize a realistic ability to control/influence situations and outcomes.
- Patients will select and use alternative methods for increasing sense of control in illness-related situations.

Interventions
- Provide effective communication regarding all procedures, rules, and options relevant to patients and families.
- Provide an opportunity for patients to express feelings.
- Allow time to answer questions; encourage patients and families to write down questions. If possible, plan specific meeting times with patients and family members.
- Keep patients and families informed about the schedule, changes, treatments, and results; anticipate questions/interests, and offer information.
- If pain or anxiety is a contributing factor, provide assessment and appropriate interventions (e.g., relaxation, deep breathing, prescribed medication).
- Provide consistent staffing and opportunities for family members to identify with selected nurses; keep promises, and follow through on agreed-upon care.
- While being realistic, identify positive changes in patients' conditions.
- Acknowledge patients' usual response style (e.g., internal or external locus of control); be sensitive to cultural differences.
- Provide as many opportunities as possible for patients to control decisions; assist patients to identify controllable factors and to accept what cannot be changed.
- Allow patients and families to participate in care; keep needed items within reach.
- Increase decision-making opportunities for patients as their condition progresses.
- Emphasize what patients can do; set short-term, achievable goals.
- Use encouragement, and reward small gains/achievements (e.g., walked five more feet, ate two more bites).
- Provide information about the illness and treatment plan.

(Continued on next page)

Figure 22-2. Plan of Care *(Continued)*

- Assist patients in identifying power from other sources (e.g., support groups, chaplain, prayer, food, pets, special rituals).
- When feelings of powerlessness decrease, evaluate with patients and family members what strategies have been effective, and discuss how they will manage feelings of powerlessness in the future.

Case Study

Tommy, a 16-year-old boy who was diagnosed with bone cancer in his left humerus three months ago, was rehospitalized for evaluation of increased pain and swelling in the upper left arm. He had been receiving pain medication and diagnostic tests for the past 36 hours, and he had just been told that the limb salvage procedure was not successful. Although Tommy had cooperated over the past several months with all the diagnostic tests and chemotherapy and the experimental procedure to replace his own diseased bone with a bone graft, now the doctors tell him he will need to have the arm amputated at the shoulder to prevent the spread of the cancer and to ultimately save his life. As the doctors started to tell him about other young patients with the same kind of cancer who have undergone arm or leg amputation and how they adjusted to a prosthetic limb and went on to play sports or pursue a desired career, Tommy started crying and said he does not want to hear about other people. His parents, who were present, tried to console him. As soon as the doctors walked out of his room, he got out of bed and threw his IV pole and dinner tray to the floor. He refused to speak to his parents and wanted to be discharged immediately. He called his girlfriend to pick him up.

Until this morning, the staff felt that, for his age, Tommy had coped very well with his cancer and the difficult treatments. Although Tommy had some short periods of mild depression and withdrawal from his family and friends during the chemotherapy and right after the surgery, he "bounced back to normal" after regaining his physical strength. Both the staff and Tommy's family had treated him as an adult throughout this illness, discussing all the options and letting him make the final decisions about his treatment. His angry reactions were more difficult to deal with, and the nurses felt uncertain about what to do.

The nursing staff tried to give Tommy some quiet time; nurses also tried to sit and talk with him. These interventions had worked before, but this time Tommy seemed inconsolable and would not let anyone stay in his room. He repeatedly said, "I just want to leave the hospital." The parents reacted with disbelief and disappointment that the limb salvage procedure had been unsuccessful. They were very worried about Tommy's threat to leave the hospital. Tommy yelled at his parents, "There is nothing more to do. The doctors can't do any more, and I can't do any more. I don't want to die, but I can't do anything without my arm, so what's the use?"

(Continued on next page)

Case Study *(Continued)*

Discussion

The staff in this case observed the young patient's feelings of powerlessness displayed mostly as anger. Over the previous several months, they had seen this mature adolescent cope well with the first three stages of his illness: diagnosis, treatment, and recovery. He coped with the support of family and friends and the belief that his arm could not only be saved but also that he would be able to use it normally. He had hoped to play baseball during his junior and senior years of high school. In facing recurrence of the bone cancer and loss of the arm, he felt helpless to control or change the situation.

Everyone was surprised by the intensity of Tommy's anger and his refusal to accept help. He always had been able to "talk out" his feelings, let others help him to gather information, and discuss his decisions about what to do throughout his illness. The staff realized that Tommy is experiencing situational powerlessness related specifically to the loss of his arm and his dream of playing baseball next year. His usual coping style of asking questions and getting information before making decisions had been effective up to this point. Tommy was not denying the reality of his illness, nor did he seem hopeless about his overall chances to survive. Staff members had observed that Tommy tended to use internal locus of control; that is, he generally made decisions based on the belief that what he does will make a difference in the final outcome. For instance, he had learned that the more he practices, the better his batting average becomes.

Having made these assessments of Tommy's current behavior and his past coping skills, staff members wanted to find out more about what he is thinking and feeling about this new development in his illness. In addition, they wanted to ascertain what he needs to know or do to be able to cope with the feelings of powerlessness resulting from the recurrence of his cancer.

The nurses requested that an interdisciplinary family conference be arranged as soon as possible. Tommy would be informed about the meeting and asked to attend. The goals of the meeting were to (a) discuss the doctor's recommendations, (b) discuss any possible alternatives and their advantages and disadvantages, (c) determine time frames for making decisions, and (d) determine potential outcomes for all possible choices. Any questions and concerns would be addressed. All staff members involved with Tommy's care were asked to contribute to the conference.

At the conference, Tommy heard that he does not have to make a decision about the amputation immediately. He requested to be discharged so he can go home and think everything over for a while. Once out of the hospital, he asked to speak to other patients, especially young athletes, who have had the same experience. He asked questions about prosthetics and rehabilitation and was amazed at what some of the amputees he met can do. After a week or two, he was ready to proceed with the surgery.

This case demonstrates the effectiveness of good nursing assessment in selecting the most appropriate interventions for each patient. The staff's prior knowledge of Tommy's coping skills and preferred locus of control were helpful

(Continued on next page)

Case Study *(Continued)*

in determining that providing more information and time to make a decision were appropriate actions with this adolescent. Accepting his angry behaviors as normal reactions to expected feelings of powerlessness, rather than diagnosing his responses as abnormal and maladaptive, allowed Tommy to feel increased control in his difficult situation. By supporting the need for decisional and cognitive control in this stage of his illness, Tommy's family and the nursing staff supported his efforts to accept what he could not control (i.e., the recurrence of his cancer). This reduced the potential long-term negative consequences of powerlessness during the recovery stage of his amputation.

Nurses should allow as much time as possible to listen and, depending on the patients' locus of control, provide information about scheduled or changed procedures, treatments, and results. Allow patients to ask questions, and point out realistic, positive changes in their condition. Encourage patients and family members to write down their questions. Setting a specific time of the day for patients and families to ask questions and get new information can help them to feel as though they have some control.

Provide as many opportunities as possible for patients to make or participate in decisions (e.g., having access to personal possessions, choosing clothing, determining when visitors can come). Emphasize what patients can do rather than what they cannot do. Only offer options that are relevant and possible for them. Reinforce participation in self-care and decision making. Be sensitive to patients' culturally determined and usual ways of coping with uncontrollable events. If a patient has a strong external locus of control and a high level of powerlessness, work with a family member or friend who may be more able to assist the patient in making the decision or learning the necessary information about chemotherapy or radiation treatments.

Arrange for patients to meet other patients with a similar diagnosis and visit a hospital- or clinic-based support group early in the cancer experience. Encourage and allow patients and families to use other control strategies (e.g., prayer, meditation, special foods) and their own stress-reduction techniques (e.g., pet visitation). Finally, provide discharge teaching and follow-up care instructions to both patients and family members. As feelings of powerlessness decrease, patients and families will be able to learn and retain this information more effectively.

Conclusion

Similar to denial and hopelessness, feelings of powerlessness and behaviors and thoughts indicative of perceived loss of control in the face of life-threatening illness tend to surface at the most stressful points in the cancer experience: when first diagnosed, at the time of metastases or recurrence, and when facing end-stage disease. Having moderate to strong feelings of powerlessness at these times is appropriate and should not be considered abnormal. However, if patients or family members continue to experience such a level of loss of control that adaptive behaviors such as information seeking or decision making are impeded, then healthcare professionals must assess the factors contributing to the ongoing perception of loss of control. Prolonged powerlessness may lead to hopelessness and depression that may, in turn, negatively affect cancer treatment and outcomes.

Staff can use three types of control to assist patients dealing with feelings of powerlessness: behavioral, cognitive, and decisional. Regardless of patients' preferred locus of control, interventions supporting small gains or achievements in dealing with their illness or small efforts to accept what is not controllable may ameliorate the negative effects of powerlessness in the cancer experience.

Special thanks to Marcia L. Raines, RN, PhD, MN, CS, who served as the author of this chapter in the first edition.

References

American Psychiatric Association. (2000). *Diagnostic and statistical manual of mental disorders* (4th ed., text rev.). Washington, DC: Author.

Andrykowski, M.A., & Brady, M.J. (1994). Health locus of control and psychological distress in cancer patients: Interactive effects of context. *Journal of Behavioral Medicine, 17,* 439–458.

Averill, J. (1973). Personal control over aversive stimuli and its relationship to stress. *Psychological Bulletin, 80,* 286–290.

Bandura, A. (1977). Self-efficacy: Toward a unifying theory of behavioral change. *Psychological Review, 84,* 191–215.

Braga, C.G., & Cruz, D.A.L. (2003). [The powerlessness psycho-social response in the postoperative period in cardiac surgery patients]. *Revista da Escola de Enfermagem da USP, 37*(1), 26–35.

Bunston, T., Mings, D., Mackie, A., & Jones, D. (1995). Facilitating hopefulness: The determinants of hope. *Journal of Psychosocial Oncology, 13*(4), 79–103.

Carpenito, L. (Ed.). (2002). *Nursing diagnosis: Application to clinical practice* (9th ed.). Philadelphia: Lippincott.

Chadiha, L.A., Adams, P., Biegel, D.E., Auslander, W., & Gutierrez, L. (2004). Empowering African American women informal caregivers: A literature synthesis and practice strategies. *Social Work, 49,* 97–108.

Cohen, M.Z., Haberman, M.R., Steeves, R., & Deatrick, J.A. (1994). Rewards and difficulties of oncology nursing. *Oncology Nursing Forum, 21*(Suppl. 8), 9–17.

Fitzsimmons, S., & Fuller, R. (2002). Empowerment and its implications for clinical practice in mental health: A review. *Journal of Mental Health, 11,* 481–499.

Garrison, T.M. (2000). Chronic illness and rehabilitation. In A.G. Lueckenotte (Ed.), *Gerontologic nursing* (2nd ed., pp. 348–369). St. Louis, MO: Mosby.

Gorman, L.M., Raines, M.L., & Sultan, D.F. (2002). *Psychosocial nursing for general patient care.* Philadelphia: F.A. Davis.

Hagopian, G.A. (1993). Cognitive strategies used in adapting to a cancer diagnosis. *Oncology Nursing Forum, 20,* 759–763.

Halldorsdottir, S., & Hamrin, E. (1996). Experiencing existential changes: The lived experience of having cancer. *Cancer Nursing, 19,* 29–36.

Henderson, S. (2003). Power imbalance between nurses and patients: A potential inhibitor of partnership in care. *Journal of Clinical Nursing, 12,* 501–508.

Holland, J.C. (2002). The history of psychooncology: Overcoming attitudinal and conceptual barriers. *Psychosomatic Medicine, 64,* 206–221.

Jecker, N.S., Carrese, J.A., & Pearlman, R.A. (1995). Caring for patients in cross-cultural settings. *Hastings Center Report, 25*(1), 6–14.

Jemal, A., Murray, T., Ward, E., Samuels, A., Tiwari, R., Ghafoor, A., et al. (2005). Cancer statistics, 2005. *CA: A Cancer Journal for Clinicians, 55,* 10–30.

Massey, V.H. (1989). Relationships between powerlessness, hardiness, diagnosis, and hopelessness in persons hospitalized for cholecystectomy or metastatic carcinoma. *Dissertation Abstracts International, 50,* 2339B. (UMI No. 8920776)

McCray, N.D. (1994). Psychosocial issues. In S.E. Otto (Ed.), *Oncology nursing* (2nd ed., pp. 720–736). St. Louis, MO: Mosby.

Mor, V., Allen, S., & Malin, M. (1994). The psychosocial impact of cancer on older versus younger patients and their families. *Cancer, 74*(Suppl. 7), 2118–2127.

Munkres, A., Oberst, M.T., & Hughes, S.H. (1992). Appraisal of illness, symptom distress, self-care burden, and mood states in patients receiving chemotherapy for initial and recurrent cancer. *Oncology Nursing Forum, 19,* 1201–1209.

NANDA International. (2005). *Nursing diagnoses: Definitions and classification, 2005–2006.* Philadelphia: Author.

Pollin, I. (with Golant, S.). (1994). *Taking charge: Overcoming the challenges of long-term illness.* New York: Times Books.

Potts, R.G. (1996). Spirituality and the experience of cancer in an African-American community: Implications for psychosocial oncology. *Journal of Psychosocial Oncology, 14*(1), 1–19.

Powe, B.D. (1996). Cancer fatalism among African-Americans: A review of the literature. *Nursing Outlook, 44,* 18–21.

Rotter, J.B. (1966). Generalized expectations for internal versus external control of reinforcement. *Psychological Monographs, 80*(1), 1–28.

Ryan, S., Hassell, A., Dawes, P., & Kendall, S. (2003). Perceptions of control in patients with rheumatoid arthritis. *Nursing Times, 99*(13), 36–38.

Seligman, M.E. (1975). *Helplessness: On depression, development, and death.* San Francisco: W.H. Freeman.

Stephenson, C.A. (1979). Powerlessness and chronic illness: Implications for nursing. *Baylor Nursing Educator, 1*(1), 17–28.

Stuart, G.W. (2001). Emotional responses and mood disorders. In G.W. Stuart & M.T. Laraia (Eds.), *Principles and practice of psychiatric nursing* (7th ed., pp. 345–380). St. Louis, MO: Mosby.

Sugarek, N., Deyo, R., & Holmes, B. (1988). Locus of control and beliefs about cancer in a multi-ethnic clinic population. *Oncology Nursing Forum, 15,* 481–486.

Sundeen, S.J. (2001). Psychiatric rehabilitation. In G.W. Stuart & M.T. Laraia (Eds.), *Principles and practice of psychiatric nursing* (7th ed., pp. 246–264). St. Louis, MO: Mosby.

Taylor, S.E., Helgeson, V.S., Reed, G.M., & Skokan, L.A. (1991). Self-generated feelings of control and adjustment to physical illness. *Journal of Social Issues, 47,* 91–109.

Thompson, S.C., & Collins, M.A. (1995). Applications of perceived control to cancer: An overview of theory and measurement. *Journal of Psychosocial Oncology, 13*(1/2), 11–26.

Townsend, M.C. (2000). *Psychiatric mental health nursing. Concepts of care* (3rd ed.). Philadelphia: F.A. Davis.

Ursano, R.J., Epstein, R.S., & Lazar, S.G. (2002). Behavioral responses to illness: Personality and personality disorders. In M.G. Wise & J.R. Rundell (Eds.), *American Psychiatric Publishing textbook of consultation-liaison psychiatry: Psychiatry in the medically ill* (2nd ed., pp. 107–126). Washington, DC: American Psychiatric Publishing.

Weisman, A.D., & Worden, J.W. (1976–1977). The existential plight in cancer: Significance of the first 100 days. *International Journal of Psychiatry in Medicine, 7,* 1–15.

SECTION IV

Psychosocial Interventions

CHAPTER 23

Interpersonal and Therapeutic Skills Inherent in Oncology Nursing

KATHRYN E. PEARSON, RN, CNS, MN, AOCN®

I did not hear the words you said. Instead I heard the love.
–Joan Walsh Anglund

As patients and families experience the myriad of emotional challenges along the continuum of cancer care, nurses frequently face feelings of being inadequately prepared to respond in a supportive manner. Nurses also may become overwhelmed by the anxiety, fears, uncertainties, grief, anger, and depression that patients and families experience. Nurses who are uncomfortable responding to patients' and families' emotional behavior are at risk for causing more harm by escalating the intensity of the situation or by avoiding and withdrawing from needed interventions. The inadvertent outcome may contribute to patients' and families' feelings of dissatisfaction, abandonment, and isolation (Bailey & Wilkinson, 1998). In contrast, psychosocially skilled oncology nurses are instrumental in assisting patients and families to achieve a sense of control and well-being during times of stress.

When educated in appropriate interpersonal and social skills, nurses will be prepared to provide the needed emotional support for patients and families. These communication skills include attentive listening, reflection, and supportive problem solving. The goal of professional communication is to facilitate a trusting relationship. First, oncology nurses must take into account the social, cultural, and ethnic background of the patients and families and be aware of how these belief systems influence the response to health and illness. Second, caring for patients and family members when they are confronting life-changing and life-threatening illness also will challenge nurses' own belief systems and emotions. This especially is true in circumstances when cultural, language, or healthcare settings contribute to patients and families feeling threatened and compounding their fears and anxiety. To establish a trusting relationship, nurses must carry out interventions that are evidence-based to promote comfort and provide psychosocial care in a safe environment and therapeutic manner. Figure 23-1 outlines personal beliefs, attitudes, and behaviors that can interfere with therapeutic communication and support.

Social Skills

Initiating professional interactions requires the use of basic social skills that are considered "good manners." This begins as the nurse offers a professional introduction and shows respect by explaining to the patient the nurse's role and purpose. Simply approaching a patient and family in a nonthreatening manner increases their comfort in the nurse's presence (Berk, 1997; Ross & Johansen, 2002). Nonverbal behaviors such as a handshake, smile, and eye contact reinforce spoken words. The physical environment should be adjusted to allow for privacy and comfort (Arnold, 2003c), and nurses should avoid separating themselves from patients by standing behind physical barriers such as tables and desks. Skilled nurses adjust their verbal

---

Figure 23-1. Beliefs, Attitudes, and Behaviors That Interfere With Therapeutic Communication

- Discounting or devaluing emotional symptoms
- Believing that talking about sensitive issues with patients takes too much time
- Believing that talking about emotions (or becoming tearful) is detrimental for patients
- Believing that talking about death is taboo
- Believing that there is no hope
- Believing that anger is an unwarranted emotion that interferes with patient care
- Labeling (stereotyping) patients as
  - Noncompliant
  - Lazy
  - Manipulative
  - Attention seeking
- Personalizing patients' anger by becoming defensive or feeling out of control
- Overcompensating to be the "nice nurse"
- Giving false reassurance (e.g., saying "Don't worry" when you do not know what the patient is worried about)
- Changing the topic, ignoring cues, or making jokes (putting off patients' true concerns)
- Being judgmental
- Giving trite advice
- Lecturing
- Excessive questioning
- Ill-timed use of emotionally charged words and phrases
- Self-focusing behaviors
- Using double-bind messages (conflicting verbal and nonverbal messages)

Note. Based on information from Frost et al., 1997; Heaven & Maguire, 1996; Lovejoy & Matteis, 1997; Maguire, 1985; Parle et al., 1997; Peterson, 1988; Smith & Hart, 1994; Wilkinson, 1991; with additional information from Haber, 1997.

Note. From "Coping With Cancer: Patient Issues" (p. 9), by D.M. Sivesind and J.A. Rohaly-Davis in C.C. Burke (Ed.), *Psychosocial Dimensions of Oncology Nursing Care,* 1998, Pittsburgh, PA: Oncology Nursing Society. Copyright 1998 by the Oncology Nursing Society. Adapted with permission.

tone and behavior to suit each patient's and family's situation. For example, if the nurse is aware that the patient has just received bad news, he or she may adjust a normally cheery introduction to one conveying respect and empathy.

One's interpersonal skills (i.e., verbal and nonverbal communication) and attitudes can positively or negatively influence how an individual treats others while performing professional roles (Berk, 1997). Ross and Johansen (2002) found, in their qualitative study of psychosocial home visits to patients with colon cancer, that nurses' attitudes toward patients are crucial to the outcome of interactions. Effective nurse-patient and nurse-family interactions resulted when patients and families were authentically viewed as fellow human beings and not merely as people experiencing a cancer diagnosis (Ross & Johansen). Being authentic requires nurses to recognize personal vulnerabilities, strengths, and limitations and to be able to engage with patients on a human level (Arnold, 2003c). Oncology nurses who are able to behave in a trustworthy, dependable manner are secure enough within themselves to establish professional boundaries and yet feel warmth, caring, fondness, interest, and respect toward patients. The result is a rewarding professional relationship that is healing to patients and families (Arnold, 2003c).

Interacting with patients in a sensitive, caring, and helpful manner may be challenging to nurses if personal emotional responses are triggered by patients' or families' behavior or by other environmental or personal factors. By gaining insight into their own feelings, nurses are better equipped to choose the behavior appropriate to the situation and therefore act and respond professionally although they may feel differently. Nurses must be aware of nonverbal language, which may lead to what Berk (1997) referred to as "emotional leakage." Emotional leakage occurs when one really thinks or feels leaks out in nonverbal behaviors, conflicting with what is communicated verbally. For example, a family member may be convinced that the patient's confused behavior is related to chemotherapy and be unable to accept that the patient is experiencing functional decline. The nurse may feel frustrated by the family member's denial but may attempt to explore the family's understanding in greater depth. The nurse may ask, "How do you think the confusion is caused by the chemotherapy?" but at the same time, the nurse's deep sigh or perturbed expression creates emotional leakage by communicating frustration nonverbally.

Communication Skills

Communication skills that elicit information from patients and families are required to establish the psychosocial data upon which to base nursing diagnoses and interventions. Allowing patients and families to "story" the illness experience is an effective therapeutic tool that provides an opportunity to problem solve and find meaning in what is happening. Stories tell "who people are, where they've been, and where they are going" (Smith & Liehr, 2003, p. 167). People will tell their story when they believe the nurse is listening (Liehr, 2005). Skilled nurses employ a *facilitating* communication style using open-ended questions, reflection, clarification, and empathy. In contrast, a *blocking* style of communication is superficial and ignores the verbal and behavioral cues that may indicate areas of psychosocial distress that patients and family members are feeling. Behaviors that characterize a blocking style of communication include using closed-ended or leading questions, changing the focus of conversation prematurely, giving inappropriate advice, or using stereotypical comments. A study aimed at investigating how nurses communicate with patients with cancer found that nurses who used blocking techniques tended to have less self-awareness, poor communication techniques, and poor relationships with colleagues (Wilkinson, 1991). Blocking communication techniques most often were used by nurses when patients disclosed feelings and interpreted that the nurses were uncomfortable with emotional distress. Conversely, nurses who were more comfortable confronting patient distress tended to employ a facilitative style of communication (Wilkinson).

A variety of questioning techniques can facilitate the telling of the patient's story. Open-ended questions are intended to let the patient and family members answer in their own words without being influenced or "led" by the interviewer (Arnold, 2003b; Paice, 2002). Open-ended questions usually begin with "how," "why," "what," "where," "can you tell me about," and "in what way" (Arnold, 2003b; Haber, 1997). An example of an open-ended question is "Tell me how you felt after your last chemotherapy administration." In contrast to general open-ended questions that allow for a variety of answers, open-ended but focused questions are more directed, such as "Tell me more about the fatigue you experienced after your last chemotherapy administration." Closed-ended questions are those that elicit a yes/no response or a definitive answer (Arnold, 2003b), such as "What was your level of fatigue after your last chemotherapy administration on the 0–10 scale?"

Circular questions focus on the interpersonal context in which the illness occurs (Arnold, 2003b) and are useful in therapeutic communication designed to help to solve problems. Categories of circular questions include difference, behavioral, hypothetical, triadic, and future oriented (Arnold, 2003b; Leboeuf, 2000). One might use a difference question, such as "What is the best and worst advice that you have received from family and friends after your diagnosis?" An example of a behavioral question is "In your opinion, which member of your family is the most affected by your cancer? In what way has this person been affected?" Hypothetical and future-oriented questions pose a "what-if" scenario that can be useful in problem solving (e.g., "If you were to tell your wife about your concerns regarding your cancer, what would she say and do?"). Triadic questions bring in the behaviors of a third party, such as "How do your wife's coworkers help to support her after her chemotherapy treatments?"

Listening Skills

Active listening is an interactive process in which the listener not only hears the words being said but also interprets and finds meaning within the attached attitudes and feelings (Arnold, 2003b; Stanley, 2002). Active listeners observe the tone of voice and nonverbal expressions in posture, gestures, and affect. Listening or "attending" behaviors communicate one's interest and respect. Attending behaviors include making eye contact, nodding, and making listening responses such as "yes," "OK," and "um-hum." Active listeners clarify meaning by asking questions such as "Are you saying that . . . ?" or ensure understanding by paraphrasing or summarizing what has been said (e.g., "Do you mean . . . ?"). Interpretation of nonverbal behaviors also should be acknowledged during communication, for instance, "You are clenching your fist. How are you feeling right now?"

If patients or family members are rambling or giving too much information in an anxious or insistent manner, nurses can intervene by writing down major points to help them to focus and become more specific. With this technique, nurses confirm the points for accuracy by repeating, rephrasing, or summarizing the information. Another way to focus the communication is to ask for more information, examples, or details at key junctures (Berk, 1997), such as asking specifically how many episodes of vomiting the patient experienced after chemotherapy.

Touch is another response that active listeners can use. Touch has been identified as an important aspect of supportive communication that can convey concern and empathy. However, patients' attitudes toward touch vary according to personal belief systems. Some patients see supportive touch as being comforting and empathetic, whereas others may find it unnecessary and intrusive (Sapir et al., 2000). Strategies to assess whether patients would welcome touch include asking their permission, taking cues from their body language, and being aware of the meaning of touch in diverse cultures.

Silence is a useful tool in giving patients time to gather thoughts to make a significant point. During quiet pauses, nurses remain silent but maintain attentive behaviors to preserve the interpersonal connection (Arnold, 2003c). Comfortable silences also convey concern, acceptance, and presence and support (Stanley, 2002). Mark Twain best described the valuable use of silence: "The right word may be effective, but no word was ever as effective as a rightly timed pause" (Andrews, Biggs, & Seidel, 1996).

Language Skills

Effective communication requires nurses to be aware of the language and communication styles that patients and families use. Words and phrases commonly used in medical terminology frequently have different meanings in lay language. Mark Twain stated that "the difference between the right word and the almost right word is the difference between lightning and a lightning bug" (Andrews et al., 1996). Words such as "progressing" and "positive nodes" may hold different, the same, or opposite meanings to patients and family members (Fallowfield, Jenkins, & Beveridge, 2002). The word "tumor" may imply a benign process that is not cancer. Patients and families may interpret an "incurable" condition as one that is imminently life threatening. Staging classifications can be perceived as a step process in which an unspoken "stage V" is interpreted as a death sentence. Therefore, patients diagnosed with stage III or IV cancers often inaccurately interpret that death is imminent. The use of "complete response" or "partial response" to treatment may imply cure to lay individuals unfamiliar with the terminology. Active listening and directed questioning will help nurses to verify how the patients and families interpret medical information to avoid misunderstanding and unnecessary fears.

The cultural and ethnic interpretation of words, phrases, and communication styles also will influence how patients and families understand information regarding diagnosis, treatment, and prognosis. Present education regarding the disease and treatment in a clear, concise, and understandable manner. Medical terminology "must make sense to the patient and family in terms of their lay view of ill health, and should acknowledge and respect the patients' experience and interpretation of their own condition" (Helman, 2001, p. 106). Helman identified a major criterion for successful communication as "reflexivity," a heightened sense of self-awareness. Health professionals communicate from their own perspective on health and illness, and these perspectives are personal and cultural as well as professional. Therefore, unless one is aware of one's own beliefs, it will be difficult to understand and communicate with other people's beliefs and perspectives (Helman).

Many of the words and phrases used in oncology have multiple metaphors and myths attached (Sontag, 1978). To a layperson, the word "cancer" may imply a painful death sentence. The word "hospice" frequently is emotionally charged and may be perceived as "giving up" or "abandonment." However, one should not avoid using correct words such as "cancer" but instead should explore the meaning of the word with patients and families to dispel myths and misconceptions. In describing the psychological responses of patients receiving a cancer diagnosis, Schofield et al. (2003) exemplified this point by concluding that higher patient satisfaction occurred among those patients when the word "cancer" was directly used to inform them of their diagnosis.

Words can positively or negatively influence how patients and families cope along the different phases of the cancer journey. An example is the word "victim." The patient who is perceived or labeled as being a victim is one who feels powerless in the face of the illness. To combat "victimization," the National Coalition for Cancer Survivorship (NCCS) describes all people experiencing cancer as cancer "survivors" (Donaldson, 2004). In using the word "survivor," the perception is reframed to represent a person who is empowered and one who can successfully cope with the challenges of cancer. The word "survivor" also implies patient-active decision making and reflects hopefulness, not powerlessness (Mullan, 1996).

A point on the cancer continuum that demands expert counseling and communication skills is the emotional time of transition from active treatment to palliative care or hospice. To identify patients' interpretations of communication regarding ending active treatment, Friedrichsen, Strang, and Carlsson (2002) identified words and phrases that proved confusing for patients and families. Indirect warning words were evasive words from which patients had to decipher an implied message. Words such as "unfortunately" or other words of forewarning caused patients and family members to anticipate something unpleasant. Evasive, vague phrases, such as "You may have three months to five years" leave patients and families confused and anxious as to the actual meaning of the message (Friedrichsen et al.). Bad news often is couched in vague phrases in an effort to provide hope or to protect the messenger, but doing so robs patients and family members of the information needed to understand the situation and interferes with decision making and problem solving. Using medical terminology also can be evasive if patients and families do not have a reference point by which to interpret its meaning. For example, a statement such as "The tumor marker is going up" delivered in an ominous verbal tone and without accompanying explanation leaves patients and families without the information needed to process the meaning or its implications accurately. Researchers also have found that when benefits from treatment are discussed primarily in terms of statistics and probabilities, patients' and families' feelings of uncertainty increase (Mishel et al., 2002). Finally, emotionally charged words and phrases elicit an emotional response above and beyond the original message. Phrases such as "There is nothing more to do" bring forth feelings of abandonment and fear (Friedrichsen et al.), and patients may believe that even comfort measures such as pain medicine will be withdrawn.

In contrast, fortifying and supportive words communicate strength and confirmation. Examples include "We are going to help you with this" and "There are things that can be done to . . . " The goal of supportive language is to communicate and present information in a positive manner that gives patients and families a measure of control and assures them that they will not be abandoned. Verbal confirmation of patients' and families' feelings, thoughts, and decisions through statements such as "This must be a difficult time for you" is supportive and helpful (Friedrichsen et al., 2002).

Humor as Communication

When used appropriately, humor can lighten many situations and break down communication barriers. Using humor can "test the waters" to see how the listener will receive sensitive topics or concerns. It also may be used to break away from a line of thought that is too painful to explore in the moment. Humor and laughter also have been found to be therapeutic in relieving stress. Humor can help to reframe perception. In spite of the benefits, nurses must be sensitive to patients' and families' interpretations of humor and be cautioned that humor is used to laugh with and not at others (MacDonald, 2004).

Communicating Bad News

In recent years, focus has increased on the most effective and least harmful way to deliver bad news in healthcare settings. Robert Buckman's (1992) book *How to Break Bad News: A Guide for Health Care Professionals* outlined interventions appropriate for supporting both professionals and patients when they must discuss bad news. Later termed the SPIKES model (Baile et al., 2000), these practical, step-by-step directions were designed to improve the outcomes of these sensitive encounters so that the communication itself does not increase the distress of those patients and family members on the receiving end of the bad news (Fallowfield et al., 2002; Ptacek, Fries, Eberhardt, & Ptacek, 1999) (see Figure 23-2).

When the doctor leaves the room after disclosing bad news to a patient, the role of the oncology nurse often involves "picking up the pieces." The most supportive technique for nurses at this point is to stand by quietly while patients and family members absorb the information (Higgins, 2002) and give support by answering questions, providing safety and privacy to handle emotions, and staying present. Ptacek et al. (1999) found that oncologists may follow many of the "bad news telling" guidelines of the SPIKES model but often did not identify members of the patients' support network to be present and did not make a plan of action prior to meeting with the patients. Depending on the ability of patients and family members to absorb the information or which family members were present, it frequently fell to nurses to repeat the SPIKES process (Higgins).

Figure 23-2. SPIKES Model of Communication

Step 1: Setting up the interview
- Mental rehearsal
- Arrange for privacy
- Involve significant others
- Sit down
- Make connection with the patient (eye contact)
- Manage time constraints and interruptions

Step 2: Assessing the patient's **P**erception
- What have you been told . . . ?

Step 3: Obtaining the patient's **I**nvitation
- How much information does the patient want?

Step 4: Giving **K**nowledge and information to the patient

Step 5: Addressing the patient's **E**motions

Step 6: **S**trategy and **S**ummary
- What will we do now?

Note. From "SPIKES—A Six-Step Protocol for Delivering Bad News: Application to the Patient With Cancer," by W.F. Baile, R. Buckman, R. Lenzi, G. Glober, E.A. Beale, and A.P. Kudelka, 2000, *Oncologist, 5,* pp. 305–308. Copyright 2000 by AlphaMed Press. Adapted with permission.

Communication to Support Decision Making

Nurses are in a pivotal position to be a resource for patients and families as they search for solutions at stressful transition points, especially at the time of diagnosis, throughout treatment, and during end-of-life decision making. Keys to effective communication include mutual respect between the patient and nurse, the sharing of intimate feelings in confidence, and reflection. As patients and families grapple with issues of quality of life, treatment options, and mortality, nurses should encourage them to consider available choices within the framework of their own beliefs, values, and life circumstances (MacDonald, 2002; Shannon-Dorcy & Wolf, 2003). During the decision-making process, questions such as "Did you think about . . . " or "How did you reach that decision?" help and support patients and families to explore the issues (Shannon-Dorcy & Wolf). Additionally, nurses must be knowledgeable to respond to questions to ensure that patients have adequate, accurate, and thorough information to guide their decisions (Chelf et al., 2001; MacDonald, 2002; Shannon-Dorcy & Wolf). The more active patients are in their own decision making, the more information they require. Therefore, nurses must be able to recognize priority educational needs and provide information in a concise and clear manner. Chelf et al. identified the primary information areas that influence patients' decisions: the recommendations of healthcare providers, the potential for cure and recurrence, and information regarding symptoms and side effects.

Hope is essential throughout the cancer care continuum (Nail, 2001), but during decision-making processes, it is essential that it not be used in a coercive manner, nor should it be taken away. In situations where hope for a good long-term prognosis is unrealistic, nurses can help to refocus hope in terms of incremental steps in daily life (Shannon-Dorcy & Wolf, 2003) and quality of life as defined by patients and families.

Nurses' mediation and conflict-management skills become critical when families and patients disagree about decisions (Zhang & Siminoff, 2003). Although patients and families may not bring up their distress over disagreements in decision making, sensitively asked questions such as "How do you each feel about this decision?" will give permission for patients and family members to acknowledge disagreement. This technique will allow for open discussions that can elucidate the concerns of each individual, clarify assumptions, identify problems, and work to find resolution to conflicts or disagreements (Arnold, 2003a). Acknowledging family roles in providing support and care to patients can decrease the risk of family members feeling helpless and out of control of the circumstances. Including families in the decision-making process opens channels of communication within the family, solidifying their support and understanding of the patients' experiences.

Behavioral Therapeutic Techniques

Nurses can use several cognitive restructuring and behavioral techniques described in psychiatric nursing literature (Barry, 2002; Haber, 1997; Stuart, 1998) in daily interactions with patients to strengthen their coping and decision-making skills. The goals of these techniques are to increase patients' self-esteem, increase their sense of control, and modify thoughts that negatively affect them (Haber).

Problem-Solving Skills

Problem solving occurs within the context of cognitive restructuring. As patients confront the stressors of the cancer experience, the mind appraises the internal feelings of threat and modifies internal and external choices to cope effectively (Barry, 2002). If patients are able to successfully solve problems and confront challenges associated with cancer and cancer treatment, then these events become less threatening. Problem-solving steps include defining the problem, generating alternatives, choosing among the alternatives, and implementing possible solutions (Mishel et al., 2002). The nurse's role as educator, providing patients with information, resources, and alternatives, enhances problem-solving and communication skills. Cognitive reframing allows patients to interpret events as manageable, thereby reducing uncertainties as they encounter new stresses and challenges at different stages of the cancer continuum. For example, if a nurse explains to a patient the rationale behind taking pain medication around the clock, the fear commonly associated with the pain experience can be reframed by assisting the patient to be in control. Therefore, the nurse's role as competent clinician, educator, and counselor can help the patient to reframe the cancer experience as a challenging rather than a threatening event if mastery results in positive outcomes (Barry).

Emotional Support

In addition to strengthening problem-solving skills, cognitive reframing can be used to strengthen and support coping mechanisms. Patients experiencing cancer will react and cope according to their previous life experiences. Their perceptions or internal viewpoints will influence how they experience the situation (Haber, 1997).

Nurses can assist patients and families in reframing their perceptions by offering insight into why they may be experiencing feelings such as fear, anxiety, and anger. Nurses also can help patients to apply another meaning to the event. For example, patients and families often interpret "Keep a good attitude" to mean "Do not feel sad or depressed." This creates an unrealistic emotional expectation, blocks communication, and creates a sense of failure for patients. Reframing the perception of keeping a good attitude to mean that patients try to maintain a positive, problem-solving approach to coping with the cancer separates the perception from the feelings being experienced. Then nurses can normalize feelings to the cancer experience (e.g., grief, loss) that are to be expected.

Reframing gives patients permission to share and address these feelings and explore effective ways in which to cope with them. This may include both problem-solving coping and emotion-focused coping (Barry, 2002), a balanced approach to adapting to the challenges confronting the patients (see Chapter 4). Maliski, Heilemann, and McCorkle (2002) found that providing specific information to newly diagnosed patients with prostate cancer and their spouses enabled them to reframe the appraisal of their cancer from a "death sentence" to a "good cancer" and increased their ability to problem solve, make decisions, and cope with the diagnosis.

Thought-Stopping Techniques

Patients confronting cancer may find that they have ruminating thought processes grounded in uncertainty and fear. Unlike reviewing alternative solutions in the problem-solving process, these ruminations are circular and serve only to reinforce feelings of helplessness and fear. This may be especially true for patients who have a history of generalized anxiety disorder (see Chapter 13). Typically, the individual is unable to sleep or concentrate and constantly may worry about real or perceived threats. A thought-stopping technique may be useful to stop these repeated, unproductive thoughts. In thought stopping, individuals are taught to put up a mental stop sign to interrupt the thought cycles. For example, a patient is unable to sleep because of continued ruminations of self-blame related to having delayed seeking medical care. Teaching the patient to self-talk and carry out a mental "stop" to the repeated thought processes can provide distraction and help to interrupt the course.

Other interventions such as guided imagery and relaxation techniques also can be used to help patients to relax. Finally, nurses can help patients to learn to redirect their thoughts toward a more positive perspective. Nurses can encourage patients to stop negative self-talk and replace it with positive self-talk with simple communication techniques (e.g., "I understand that you are upset with yourself because you are so tired from chemotherapy, but tell yourself how well you are doing to be setting your priorities and reaching out to your family for help"). If patients continue to experience overwhelming feelings that interfere with their ability to function, then nurses should refer them to a mental health professional for support.

Journaling

Journaling is a therapeutic tool that enables patients to externalize their internal experiences and emotions, taking a positive step toward active problem solving. Journaling techniques can vary between structured journaling (i.e., writing about reactions to certain feelings or events) and free-thought, free-floating journaling. Ullrich and Lutgendorf (2002) asserted that journaling to address both cognitive (factual) and emotional expression provides more personal growth and healing after traumatic events than a purely expressive style of journaling. For example, the patient writes about an actual experience and its meaning (e.g., finding a breast lump and the possibility that it is cancer) and then writes about her emotional reaction to the event (e.g., fear).

Although journaling can be a sophisticated technique used by psychologists and counselors, it also can be a valuable technique for nurses to teach patients. Rancour and Brauer (2003) described the use of letter writing as a healing method to address altered body image in a patient with breast cancer. A method of journaling that frequently is used in outpatient clinics is journals that serve as day planners, side effect monitoring tools, and self-care journals (e.g., *The Write Track: Personal Health Tracker* [Bristol Myers Squibb, Princeton, NJ, 2001]). In line with cognitive reframing, patients should include positive aspects of their experience as well as the negative to gain beneficial insight from their journaling experience (Ullrich & Lutgendorf, 2002).

Role-Play Techniques

Role-play techniques are another constructive tool that can help patients to build confidence in a desired behavior and help them to explore useful alternatives of action. For example, a patient who is having difficulty asking the physician questions can safely role play strategies of asking the questions in different ways until a level of comfort is felt. The nurse can participate by providing feedback and by role playing different responses. The nurse can suggest that the patient play out different scenarios mentally (e.g., "What would happen if . . . ?"). In psychoeducational groups, role play has been used successfully to promote learner interaction and to improve interest (Collins, 1988). Participants can act out scenarios without restriction on how roles are to be played or interpreted. Through supporting or defending a behavior in role play, participants can become aware of other behaviors and their personal bias (Collins), experiencing a broader perspective on an issue or situation.

Nurses' Responses to Patient and Family Emotions

The acting out of strong emotions by patients and families frequently elicits strong feelings in nurses. A sobbing or angry patient may trigger the desire to protect oneself by withdrawing from the patient or, conversely, prompt the nurse to become overinvolved in the moment. Instead of withdrawing or participating in displays of emotion, nurses can maintain a professional stature by being calm and present. Helpful nurse responses include role modeling positive behaviors, using helpful communication skills, and actively listening (Stanley, 2002).

The ultimate challenge occurs when patients' or family members' anger is projected directly at the nurse. Frequently, the nurse's initial reaction is to feel personally attacked and withdraw or disengage from the situation in self-defense. Unfortunately, defensive behavior is more likely to increase the anger (Thomas, 2003). Figure 23-3 outlines interventions that can help to defuse anger. The emotional reactions of patients and families can be very intense at transitional points in the cancer journey

---

Figure 23-3. Nursing Interventions to Defuse Anger in Patients

- Remain calm, maintain calm body postures, and speak softly (e.g., "Ride out the storm").
- Implement communication and listening skills to identify why patients are angry. Do not say "Calm down."
- Maintain respectful body language and eye contact. Do not stand or sit too close. Position one-self at an angle (nonconfrontive).
- Validate the complaint (e.g., "I can understand why you are upset").
- Set limits on inappropriate anger expression, such as punching the wall.
- Avoid doing anything that can be perceived as controlling or dismissive.
- As the anger expression settles, utilize open-ended questions and problem-solving techniques to work toward resolution.
- Reassure patients that you are concerned and want to understand.
- Maintain one-on-one dialogue. Avoid temptation to involve two to three people in the immediate situation to avoid confusion.
- Teach patients how to communicate concerns in more effective manner.

Note. Based on information from Garnham, 2001; Sachs, 1999; Thomas, 2003.

---

when apprehension and fear of the unknown are heightened (e.g., diagnosis, beginning and cessation of active treatment, recurrence, end of life). Many interventions are available to support nurses to deal effectively with patient and family emotions. How nurses respond will influence positively or negatively how the patients and families respond. First, nurses must be aware of their own feelings regarding what is happening to patients (e.g., is the nurse also grieving the impending death of the patient?). Second, nurses must be knowledgeable regarding the normal, expected emotional reactions to the cancer experience and be able to identify and differentiate these emotions from abnormal emotions that interfere with patients' ability to cope. Lastly, nurses must carry out self-care strategies to remain emotionally healthy and nourished to deal with the challenges of oncology nursing. Stress management and interventions for nurses' self-care can be found in Chapter 35.

Nurses' Role in Support Groups

Patients and families often seek out support groups and self-help groups (see Appendix) to find a place to share experiences and to obtain new knowledge from patients in similar situations. This, in turn, helps to normalize and destigmatize individual emotions and counteracts feelings of isolation. Most group participants verbalize that involvement in a group gives them a community feeling and a safe place to expose feelings and affirm each other (Adamsen & Rasmussen, 2003). For many, groups offer inspiration by experiencing the courage of others, witnessing the motivation to fight, and being exposed to the role modeling of other patients with cancer. Johnson (2000) encouraged the use of supportive groups to help patients and families to feel control over specific aspects of the survival experience.

In addition to referring patients and families to support groups, nurses are qualified to participate directly in support groups as therapeutic leaders who create the group framework and identify the ground rules (e.g., confidentiality). In support groups, the nurse's role is that of an initiator, social networker, consultant, resource person, and catalyst (Adamsen & Rasmussen, 2003). Nurses promote the exchange of experience and offer guidance. Nurses as group leaders can make major contributions to psychoeducational groups by providing expert knowledge of treatment, side effects, nutrition, and disease processes. Whether the group is a psychoeducational group, a closed-focus group, a self-help group, or an open-continuing group, participation calls for emotional and intimate contact by the nurse therapist. Nurse facilitators and group members together establish a culture or social network that fosters closeness and reduces social isolation (Adamsen & Rasmussen; Johnson, 2000). Additional responsibilities are to provide safety and support for participants to share their stories and articulate their feelings and provide validation for both (see Figure 23-4). A major goal of group therapy is to promote and strengthen the coping skills of participants; the focus of therapeutic groups is not about the leader. However, nurses will gain a great deal of wisdom and insight from the intimate connection with group members. These valuable life lessons are gifts that most often are incorporated into nurses' personal attitudes and belief systems, further contributing to their expertise and knowledge as caring and compassionate professionals.

Figure 23-4. Practical Tips for Group Facilitation

- *Nurses' role is to facilitate*—Do not monopolize the discussion. Nurses do not have to have all the answers.
- *Respond to all input in a positive manner*—Find something positive to say about all participant contributions, no matter how off target they may be.
- *Reaffirm individual input by referring back to what the person may have said or discussed earlier*—Use reflective listening and feedback.
- *Give participants full credit for ideas*—Promote active problem solving.
- *Use a conversational approach*—Address participants by names.
- *Reinforce participant contributions*—Use validating statements, such as "Good point" or "I'm glad you raised that issue."
- *Summarize or rephrase for emphasis*—"Did I hear you say . . . ?"
- *Use statements as a "bridge" to move the discussion*—"Let's move on to . . . "
- *Keep discussions from being monopolized by one or two people*—Prepare for members who inadvertently monopolize or disrupt group dynamics (e.g., "Thank you for your input, but . . . ").
- *Elicit responses from all participants by asking for their ideas/feelings*—"Mr. X, how do you feel about that?"
- *Corroborate group response*—"Is this consistent with how all of you are feeling?"
- *Observe nonverbal behaviors within the group*—facial expressions, body movements.
- *Confirm information if a point is being made in a convoluted manner*—Clarify by saying "Let's see if I understand" or "Are you saying . . . ?"

Note. Based on information from Berk, 1997; McMahon & Presswalla, 1997.

The Role of Oncology Nurses in Interdisciplinary Cancer Care

Nurses are strategic members of the oncology interdisciplinary team throughout the cancer care continuum (Rieger, 2002). The interdisciplinary team approach to cancer care provides patients with access to comprehensive specialty care. Team members working together elevate the quality of care given. Interdisciplinary pathways such as the National Comprehensive Cancer Network (NCCN, 2005) distress management guidelines have been developed to help to define the different roles of team members to optimize psychosocial outcomes. The use of standardized psychosocial assessments has yet to be consistently implemented or validated outside of clinical trials (McLachlan et al., 2001), but the standard set for oncology professionals is to identify psychosocial problems and refer to appropriate interdisciplinary team members when necessary (NCCN).

As a valuable team member, the nurse's role is to participate and support interdisciplinary care and carry out interdisciplinary referrals when needed. Nurses have a responsibility, along with team members, to monitor patient outcomes in psychosocial care, to create evidence-based practice, to evaluate cost-effective pathways that promote psychosocial interventions, and to help to coordinate interdisciplinary team communication (Rieger, 2002).

The interdisciplinary team not only serves to bring rich resources to the complex problems presented by patients with cancer and their families but also serves to bring those same resources to support the team members themselves. Medland, Howard-Ruben, and Whitaker (2004) described using the resources of the interdisciplinary team to develop a "Circle of Care" retreat. The goal of this retreat was to create a community among nurses and team members to examine work stress, promote effective coping mechanisms, and reduce burnout among interdisciplinary team members. Massachusetts General Hospital holds noon-time "Schwartz Center Rounds," which are multidisciplinary forums that explore the patient-caregiver relationship (Lynch, 2002). As a result of these rounds, healthcare professionals involved have expressed an enhanced sense of team building and community (Lynch). The interdisciplinary team approach also decreases the risks of professional isolation and feelings of professional inadequacy by supporting and validating the challenges that each member faces when involved in meeting the complex needs of patients experiencing cancer. Team members can find comfort and safety to express their feelings in a supportive atmosphere. Oncology nurses must recognize that they are an integral part of the patient's team, which is made up of all the professionals who are involved in the care of the patients and families. This includes members in settings from the hospital to outpatient and home care, including nurses and physicians, social workers, chaplains, and mental health professionals. Nurses must recognize all members who contribute to the psychosocial care of patients and family members as valuable resources to consult. This may include hospital volunteers or nurse aides who take part in patients' experience of care.

Conclusion

Patients with cancer and their families respond emotionally to the experience of cancer in many different ways, based upon their own life experiences, belief systems, coping mechanisms, culture and ethnicity, and communication styles. Therefore, oncology nurses must be prepared for a myriad of emotional responses, of which many are not always evident and easy to assess (e.g., in patients who display outwardly stoic behavior). The emotional pain of these patients may go unaddressed and unattended in contrast to the patients who demonstrate visible emotions and behaviors such as tearfulness or anger. Through mastering professional communication skills and active listening techniques, oncology nurses can recognize cues to enhance patient and family communication, problem solving, and coping. Oncology nurses who are competent in interpersonal and therapeutic skills and who are skilled members of an interdisciplinary team are better equipped to provide holistic psychosocial care to patients and families.

References

Adamsen, L., & Rasmussen, J.M. (2003). Exploring and encouraging through social interaction. *Cancer Nursing, 26,* 28–36.

Andrews, R., Biggs, M , & Seidel, M. (1996). *The Columbia world of quotations.* New York: Columbia University Press. Retrieved August 13, 2004, from http://www.bartleby.com/66

Arnold, E. (2003a). Communicating with families. In E. Arnold & K.U. Boggs (Eds.), *Interpersonal relationships: Professional communication skills for nurses* (4th ed., pp. 332–364). St. Louis, MO: Saunders.

Arnold, E. (2003b). Developing therapeutic communication skills in the nurse-client relationship. In E. Arnold & K.U. Boggs (Eds.), *Interpersonal relationships: Professional communication skills for nurses* (4th ed., pp. 232–265). St. Louis, MO: Saunders.

Arnold, E. (2003c). Structuring the relationship. In E. Arnold & K.U. Boggs (Eds.), *Interpersonal relationships: Professional communication skills for nurses* (4th ed., pp. 113–142). St. Louis, MO: Saunders.

Baile, W.F., Buckman, R., Lenzi, R., Glober, G., Beale, E.A., & Kudelka, A.P. (2000). SPIKES—A six-step protocol for delivering bad news: Application to the patient with cancer. *Oncologist, 5,* 302–311.

Bailey, K., & Wilkinson, S. (1998). Patients' views on nurses' communication skills: A pilot study. *International Journal of Palliative Nursing, 4,* 300–305.

Barry, P.D. (2002). *Mental health and mental illness* (7th ed.). Philadelphia: Lippincott Williams & Wilkins.

Berk, S. (1997). *Spirit in action: Reviewing our commitment to excel in service.* Fullerton, CA: St. Jude Medical Center.

Buckman, R. (1992). *How to break bad news: A guide for health care professionals.* Baltimore: Johns Hopkins University Press.

Chelf, J.H , Agre, P., Axelrod, A., Cheny, L., Cole, D.D., Conrad, K., et al. (2001). Cancer-related patient education: An overview of the last decade of evaluation and research. *Oncology Nursing Forum, 28,* 1139–1147.

Collins, J.A. (1988). The effectiveness of role playing in cardiac care rehabilitation education. *Military Medicine, 153,* 464–468.

Donaldson, S. (2004). Introduction. In B. Hoffman (Ed.), *A cancer survivor's almanac: Charting your journey* (3rd ed., pp. 1–2). Minneapolis, MN: Chronimed.

Fallowfield, L.J., Jenkins, V.A., & Beveridge, H.A. (2002). Truth may hurt but deceit hurts more: Communication in palliative care. *Palliative Medicine, 16,* 297–303.

Friedrichsen, M.J., Strang, P.M., & Carlsson, M.E. (2002). Cancer patients' interpretations of verbal expressions when given information about ending cancer treatment. *Palliative Medicine, 16,* 323–330.

Frost, M.H., Brueggen, C., & Mangan, M. (1997). Intervening with the psychosocial needs of patients and families: Perceived importance and skill level. *Cancer Nursing, 20,* 350–358.

Garnham, P. (2001). Understanding and dealing with anger, aggression and violence. *Nursing Standard, 16*(6), 37–42.

Haber, J. (1997). Therapeutic communication. In J. Haber, B. Krainovich-Miller, A.L. McMahon, & P. Price-Hoskins (Eds.), *Comprehensive psychiatric nursing* (5th ed., pp. 136–140). St. Louis, MO: Mosby.

Heaven, C., & Maguire, P. (1996). Training hospice nurses to elicit patient concerns. *Journal of Advanced Nursing, 23,* 280–286.

Helman, C.G. (2001). *Culture, health and illness* (4th ed.). London: Arnold.

Higgins, D. (2002). Breaking bad news in cancer care part 2: Practical skills. *Professional Nurse, 17,* 670–671.

Johnson, J. (2000). An overview of psychosocial support services. *Cancer Nursing, 23,* 310–313.

Leboeuf, I. (2000). Impact of a family-centered approach on a couple living with a brain tumour: A case study. *Axon, 22*(1), 24–31.

Liehr, P. (2005, April). Story theory for practice and research. In L. Williams (Coordinator), *Stories of oncology family caregiving.* Instructional session presented at the 30th Annual Congress of the Oncology Nursing Society, Orlando, FL.

Lovejoy, N., & Matteis, M. (1997). Cognitive-behavioral interventions to manage depression in patients with cancer: Research and theoretical initiatives. *Cancer Nursing, 20,* 155–167.

Lynch, T. (2002). Introduction. *Oncologist, 7*(Suppl. 2), 3–4.

MacDonald, C.M. (2004). A chuckle a day keeps the doctor away: Therapeutic humor and laughter. *Journal of Psychosocial Nursing, 42*(3), 18–25.

MacDonald, D.J. (2002). Women's decisions regarding management of breast cancer risk. *MEDSURG Nursing, 11,* 183–186.

Maguire, P. (1985). For debate: Barriers to psychological care of the dying. *BMJ, 29,* 1711–1713.

Maliski, S.L., Heilemann, M.V., & McCorkle, R. (2002). From "death sentence" to "good cancer": Couples' transformation of a prostate cancer diagnosis. *Nursing Research, 51,* 391–397.

McLachlan, S., Allenby, A., Matthews, J., Wirth, A., Kissane, D., Bishop, M., et al. (2001). Randomized trial of coordinated psychosocial interventions based on patient self-assessments versus standard care to improve the psychosocial functioning of patients with cancer. *Journal of Clinical Oncology, 19,* 4117–4125.

McMahon, A.L., & Presswalla, J.L. (1997). Working with groups. In J. Haber, B. Krainovich-Miller, A.L. McMahon, & P. Price-Hoskins (Eds.), *Comprehensive psychiatric nursing* (5th ed., pp. 178–198). St. Louis, MO: Mosby.

Medland, J., Howard-Ruben, J., & Whitaker, E. (2004). Fostering psychosocial wellness in oncology nurses: Addressing burnout and social support in the workplace. *Oncology Nursing Forum, 31,* 47–54.

Mishel, M.H., Beylyea, M., Germino, B.B., Stewart, J.L., Bailey, D.E., Robertson, C., et al. (2002). Helping patients with localized prostate carcinoma manage uncertainty and treatment side effects. *Cancer, 94,* 1854–1866.

Mullan, F. (1996). Survivorship: A powerful place. In B. Hoffman (Ed.), *A cancer survivor's almanac: Charting your journey* (pp. xvii–xix). Minneapolis, MN: Chronimed.

Nail, L.M. (2001). I'm coping as fast as I can: Psychosocial adjustment to cancer and cancer treatment. *Oncology Nursing Forum, 28,* 967–970.

National Comprehensive Cancer Network. (2005). Distress management. *Clinical practice guidelines in oncology v.1.2005.* Jenkintown, PA: Author. Retrieved April 14, 2005, from http://www.nccn.org/professionals/physician_gls/default.asp

Paice, J.A. (2002). Managing psychological conditions in palliative care. *American Journal of Nursing, 102*(11), 36–43.

Parle, M., Maguire, P., & Heaven, C. (1997). The development of a training model to improve health professionals' skills, self-efficacy and outcome expectancies when communicating with cancer patients. *Social Science and Medicine, 44,* 231–240.

Peterson, M. (1988). The norms and values held by three groups of nurses concerning psychosocial nursing practice. *International Journal of Nursing Studies, 25,* 85–103.

Ptacek, J.T., Fries, E.A., Eberhardt, T.L., & Ptacek, J.J. (1999). Breaking bad news to patients: Physicians' perceptions of the process. *Supportive Care in Cancer, 7,* 113–120.

Rancour, P., & Brauer, K. (2003). Use of letter writing as a means of integrating an altered body image: A case study. *Oncology Nursing Forum, 30,* 841–846.

Rieger, P. (2002). Collegiality. *Oncologist, 7*(Suppl. 2), 7.

Ross, L., & Johansen, C. (2002). Psychosocial home visits in cancer treatment. *Cancer Nursing, 25,* 350–357.

Sachs, P.R. (1999). Deflecting harsh words when tempers flare. *Nursing, 29*(3), 62–64.

Sapir, R., Catane, R., Kaufman, B., Isacson, R., Seagal, A., Wein, S., et al. (2000). Cancer patient expectations of and communication with oncologists and oncology nurses: The experience of an integrated oncology and palliative care service. *Supportive Care in Cancer, 8,* 458–463.

Schofield, P.E., Butow, P.N., Thompson, J.F., Tatersall, M.H.N., Beeney, L.J., & Dunn S.M. (2003). Psychological responses of patients receiving a diagnosis of cancer. *Annals of Oncology, 14,* 48–56.

Shannon-Dorcy, K., & Wolf, V. (2003). Decision making in the diagnosis and treatment of leukemia. *Seminars in Oncology Nursing, 19,* 142–149.

Smith, M., & Hart, G. (1994). Nurses' response to patient anger: From disconnecting to connecting. *Journal of Advanced Nursing, 20,* 643–651.

Smith, M.J., & Liehr, P. (2003). The theory of attentively embracing story. In M.J. Smith & P.R. Liehr (Eds.), *Middle range theory for nursing* (pp. 167–187). New York: Springer.

Sontag, S. (1978). *Illness as metaphor.* New York: Farrar, Straus and Giroux.

Stanley, K. (2002). The healing power of presence: Respite from the fear of abandonment. *Oncology Nursing Forum, 29,* 935–940.

Stuart, G.W. (1998). Cognitive behavioral therapy. In G.W. Stuart & M.T. Laraia (Eds.), *Principles and practice of psychiatric nursing* (6th ed., pp. 641–653). St. Louis, MO: Mosby.

Thomas, S.P. (2003). Anger: The mismanaged emotion. *MEDSURG Nursing, 12,* 103–110.

Ullrich, P.M., & Lutgendorf, S.K. (2002). Journaling about stressful events: Effects of cognitive processing and emotional expression. *Annals of Behavioral Medicine, 24,* 244–250.

Wilkinson, S. (1991). Factors which influence how nurses communicate with cancer patients. *Journal of Advanced Nursing, 16,* 677–688.

Zhang, A.Y., & Siminoff, L.A. (2003). The role of the family in treatment decision making by patients with cancer. *Oncology Nursing Forum, 30,* 1022–1028.

CHAPTER 24

Crisis Intervention

SHARON VAN FLEET, MS, APRN, BC

Man is not imprisoned by habit. Great changes in him can be wrought by crisis—once the crisis can be recognized and understood.
—Norman Cousins

A crisis is an event that threatens one's equilibrium, challenging usual coping mechanisms (Aguilera, 1998). Aguilera specified three balancing factors that determine whether a crisis has occurred: the individual's perception of the event, the situational supports available to the individual, and the individual's coping mechanisms. When one has a realistic perception of the event, has adequate supports available, and uses effective coping mechanisms, equilibrium is maintained, and a crisis is less likely to occur. When one or more of these factors are absent, a crisis occurs. Figure 24-1 illustrates the development of a crisis. A crisis represents a turning point with potential for growth, but it also poses a risk of regression through the development or perpetuation of maladaptive behaviors. Intervention, with the goal of expanding available coping strategies, increases the likelihood of returning to a healthy equilibrium after a crisis, as well as being able to withstand future stressors (Roberts, 2000). Caring for people in crisis is part of the daily practice for many oncology nurses. Developing skills to identify and assist people at these difficult times is an important role for nurses.

Crisis Assessment

The Patient

During a crisis or a potential crisis, nurses must assess and then intervene quickly. Early intervention can eliminate the need for later assistance (Roberts, 2000). The person in a crisis related to cancer is unable to effectively reduce his or her distress

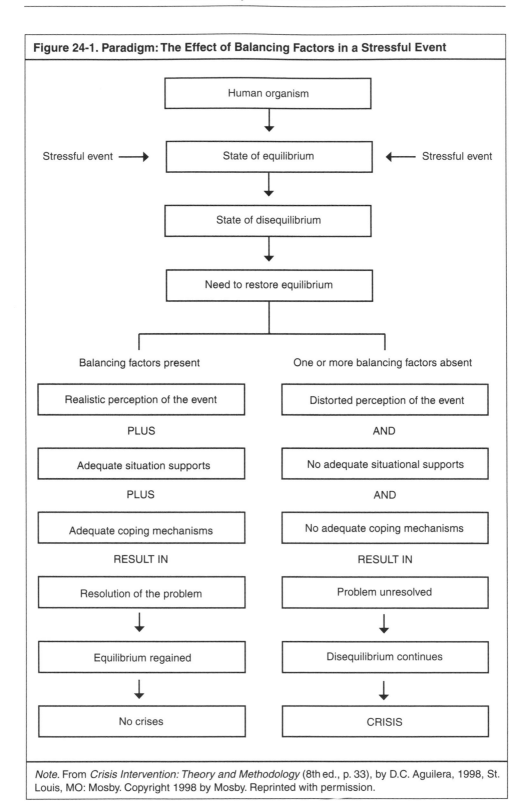

Figure 24-1. Paradigm: The Effect of Balancing Factors in a Stressful Event

Human organism

Stressful event → State of equilibrium ← Stressful event

State of disequilibrium

Need to restore equilibrium

Balancing factors present

Realistic perception of the event

PLUS

Adequate situation supports

PLUS

Adequate coping mechanisms

RESULT IN

Resolution of the problem

Equilibrium regained

No crises

One or more balancing factors absent

Distorted perception of the event

AND

No adequate situational supports

AND

No adequate coping mechanisms

RESULT IN

Problem unresolved

Disequilibrium continues

CRISIS

Note. From *Crisis Intervention: Theory and Methodology* (8th ed., p. 33), by D.C. Aguilera, 1998, St. Louis, MO: Mosby. Copyright 1998 by Mosby. Reprinted with permission.

with characteristic coping strategies when the development of an illness necessitates significant and destabilizing changes in lifestyle (Shulman & Shewbert, 2000). Slaikeu (1990a) offered a framework to structure assessment and intervention termed "BASIC." The acronym BASIC represents five areas of function: Behavioral, Affective/mood, Somatic, Interpersonal, and Cognitive.

Crisis behavior shows several characteristic patterns: fight-flight, which is demonstrated by blaming others or avoiding responsibility; conflicted behavior, which entails partially completed tasks and indecisive or inconsistent behavior; helpless, incompetent, immature behavior with responsibility placed on others; and hopeless, apathetic, passive behavior (Janosik & Davies, 1996). Nurses should watch for signs of increased disorganization, including changes in self-care and habits, and assess coping strategies that have been used as well as the potential for violence against self or others.

Assessment of affect/mood is the second BASIC component. Is the individual withdrawn, numbed, depressed, angry, or sad? Does the person express feelings? Does he or she appear out of control? Is the response typical of an individual in this situation? The presenting affective state may provide clues regarding the degree to which the crisis has been worked through and which stage(s) of the grieving process the person is experiencing (Slaikeu, 1990b).

Somatic complaints related to anxiety and depression are numerous and need to be evaluated (van Servellen, 1997).

Assessment of interpersonal functioning, the fourth system, involves examining the relationships within the patient's interpersonal sphere; the patient's interpersonal style, skill, and difficulties in relating to others; and the level of support that the patient receives (Slaikeu, 1990b).

The final system, cognitive functioning, incorporates the individual's self-image, perceptions of the past and future, and beliefs and values. Nurses should determine whether the patient possesses a realistic understanding of the crisis or is minimizing or exaggerating the severity of the situation, keeping in mind that if the patient believes a situation is a crisis, that perception must be the starting point, with the nurse being able to view the crisis as the patient sees it (James & Gilliand, 2004). In some situations, a patient's contact with reality may be impaired, and at times, this may be evident in hallucinations or delusions. Several other factors influence how a person perceives and adjusts to his or her situation, including age, developmental level, impact of the illness, prior experiences with loss, as well as history of depression or substance abuse, socioeconomic factors and level of social support (Ferszt, 1995, Roberts, 2000; Zabora, 1998). Van Servellen (1997) advised nurses to assess other factors, including the patient's current medical status, awareness of such, and knowledge regarding the illness. Denial (whether of specific facts, the implications of such facts, or the actual illness) should be assessed as well. Figure 24-2 lists questions for assessing individual coping mechanisms and perceptions. The National Comprehensive Cancer Network (2005) has developed a patient-rated distress measurement scale intended to assist with screening. In addition to the distress measure, the tool also provides a checklist for the patient to identify specific potential sources of distress under several categories.

The Family

Family assessment is essential because a crisis involves and affects the family, whose response, in turn, affects the patient (Blanchard, Albrecht, & Ruckdeschel, 1997).

Figure 24-2. Questions for Assessing Individuals in Crisis

1. When did the crisis begin? Why did the crisis occur when it did? When did family members begin to feel anxious? What happened at that time? What was the problem or event that pushed them to their limit? What is their knowledge regarding the illness?
2. What does the illness mean to the patient? How has it affected his or her life? What are the greatest stressors secondary to the illness? How does the patient think it will affect the future? What is the greatest concern now? How strong is his or her sense of control and self-confidence? What stressors in addition to the illness are present?
3. What is it about the situation that makes it different from events in the past? What happened today (or this week or month) to make it different? Why now?
4. Have other family or friends experienced cancer? How did cancer affect them? How did it affect the other family members?
5. How does the patient usually relieve tension and anxiety and solve problems? Has he or she tried this method this time? If not, why? What does patient think would reduce the stress?
6. How well is he or she able to cope with and manage symptoms related to the illness? What strategies are not helping him or her to cope? How does the patient's current health limit him or her from doing what he or she wants to do?
7. What does patient wish the nurse or other healthcare providers would do? What is needed? What is expected from treatment?
8. What kinds of losses (physical, social, emotional, or psychological) did the patient experience previously? What was the response? What helped him or her to deal with the crisis?
9. Does the patient have a support system? Does he or she feel it is adequate?

Note. Based on information from Baird, 1987; Barry, 1996; James & Gilliland, 2004; van Servellen, 1997.

Figure 24-3 outlines questions that nurses can use to help to guide family assessment. The BASIC framework can be used to assess the functioning of individual family members (Slaikeu, 1990b). Nurses must approach the family as a system. Slaikeu (1990b) described four tasks of crisis resolution with families. One task is for the family to physically survive the crisis, managing financially and without developing additional illness. The second task is to manage feelings and the resultant effects on individual members, family life, other generations of family members, and social networks. The third task is cognitive mastery of the crisis. The nurse assesses family norms and values and how the family manages boundaries, power, and alignments. The final task is making the necessary interpersonal and behavioral adjustments precipitated by the crisis. Determining how family roles and relationships have changed since the crisis can provide important information regarding potential problems, including financial matters, role conflicts, and family needs that are unmet (Blanchard et al.; Lederberg, 1998). The nurse helps to determine what additional changes will be needed in roles, division of responsibility, communication, and decision making.

Other Assessment Factors

Cultural influences significantly affect families' behaviors, attitudes, and beliefs and are an important part of the assessment (Bernal, 1996). Although conventional crisis intervention theory has been promoted throughout the world, differences exist in the use of crisis services as well as the degree and type of symptoms that prompt different ethnic groups to obtain assistance (Congress, 2000). Congress suggested that emphasizing strengths and positive coping skills rather than deficits is especially important in working with diverse cultures. Factors to consider in such situations include health beliefs, value systems, legal status, duration of time living in the community, and contact with cultural institutions (see Chapter 6).

Healthcare professionals must assess possible risk factors that may contribute to the development of a crisis. Kornblith (1998) listed several factors deemed important in affecting vulnerability to stressors related to cancer: (a) medical problems involving comorbid states as well as cancer- and treatment-related conditions, (b) social support, (c) economic factors, (d) intrapsychic factors, and (e) length of time since treatment completion. Given the complexity of many crises, nurses may have difficulty determining when a situation exceeds their abilities. Nursing intervention may be appropriate for those circumstances involving minimal to moderate levels of anxiety or depression (Barry, 1996).

If a problem is moderate to severe or if the nurse has questions, he or she should consider a consultation with a psychiatry clinical nurse specialist (Van Fleet & Hughes, 1996), social worker, or other mental health professional (Barry, 1996). Barry listed instances when nursing intervention would likely be insufficient: situations involving mental disorders resulting from medical causes (e.g., anxiety or depression directly caused by medical factors, delirium, dementia), noncompliance, or the presence of multiple complicated factors. Significant history involving severe or chronic depression, suicidal behavior, addiction, severe anxiety, potential for violence, psychosis, or antisocial behavior should generate a referral as well because individuals with these problems require more long-term intervention (Janosik & Davies, 1996). Other warning signs include complete withdrawal, denial

---

Figure 24-3. Questions for Assessing Families in Crisis

1. Who does the family consider to be its leader? Who is the decision maker? Which family members need to be consulted when decisions need to be made? How often are issues discussed? How are problems solved? Which members are included, and which members are excluded? How do they handle conflict? Are there topics that are not discussed?
2. What are the family's religious beliefs? If there is a religious preference, what role does it play? What is its ethnic orientation? How important are these factors to family members?
3. What expectations do the patient and family members have?
4. What is the developmental level of the family? What are the developmental levels of individual members?
5. How does the family perceive the problem?
6. What does the illness mean to the family members? How has it changed their lives? How do they think it will affect their future? Is there hopelessness or powerlessness? Are there concerns about which family members have hope? Is the illness viewed as a challenge or a threat?
7. Has the family experienced a similar event in the past? What did the family members do to cope? What was most helpful to the family?
8. What are the educational levels of the family members? Are family members employed?
9. What emotional assistance do the family members require? Whom do they ask for help when they have questions or needs? On whom do they rely? Do the people they live with help? Are they involved with other healthcare professionals?
10. How do family members express their needs to one another?
11. What information do they need to or want to know?

Note. Based on information from Baird, 1987; Caine, 1989; Gray-Price & Szczesny, 1985; Hendricks-Ferguson, 2000; Shaw & Halliday, 1992.

of illness severity, blaming self or others, or inability to express feelings or thoughts (Hendricks-Ferguson, 2000).

Interventions

Roberts (2000) developed a seven-stage model for crisis intervention that is useful in acute situations and illnesses such as cancer (see Figure 24-4).

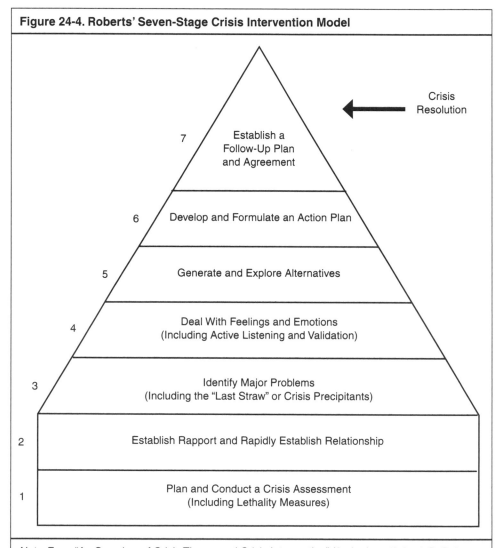

Figure 24-4. Roberts' Seven-Stage Crisis Intervention Model

Crisis Resolution

7 Establish a Follow-Up Plan and Agreement

6 Develop and Formulate an Action Plan

5 Generate and Explore Alternatives

4 Deal With Feelings and Emotions (Including Active Listening and Validation)

3 Identify Major Problems (Including the "Last Straw" or Crisis Precipitants)

2 Establish Rapport and Rapidly Establish Relationship

1 Plan and Conduct a Crisis Assessment (Including Lethality Measures)

Note. From "An Overview of Crisis Theory and Crisis Intervention" (2nd ed., p. 2), by A.R. Roberts in A. R. Roberts (Ed.), *Crisis Intervention Handbook: Assessment, Treatment, and Research,* 2000, New York: Oxford University Press. Copyright 2000 by Oxford University Press. Reprinted with permission.

Establishing Rapport and Developing the Relationship

Generally, given the anxiety inherent in crisis situations, nurses play a directive role, especially in situations involving serious risk to their physical or mental well-being (van Servellen, 1997). The primary initial goal is to stabilize the situation by listening and providing support (Loscalzo & BrintzenhofeSzoc, 1998). Establishing a calm, reassuring atmosphere conducive to the development of an empathic, supportive, and trusting relationship is essential for nurses who join patients and families in problem solving (Loscalzo & BrintzenhofeSzoc). Patients and families must have the opportunity to vent but also must be accepted, supported, and assisted in discovering the options available to resolve the crisis (Roberts, 2000). Remember that individuals in crisis often do not communicate clearly (van Servellen). Active listening skills are essential but not sufficient. Not only is the content of patients'/families' messages important but also the underlying affect (van Servellen). Patients and families need to feel heard and understood, and, therefore, nurses should validate the experiences expressed. Nurses should avoid making false promises or reassurances or insisting on a positive outlook, which patients may find burdensome (Wilkes, O'Baugh, Luke, & George, 2003), but rather they should help patients to maintain a focus on reality (Kruger, 1992). Healthcare professionals should gather information in a direct, straightforward manner while focusing on the current situation (van Servellen).

Dealing With Feelings and Emotions

The nurse's role involves controlling the intensity of interactions to prevent patients and family members from becoming overwhelmed. By emphasizing that crying does not signify loss of control but rather a normal reaction (Rando, 1984) and avoiding prematurely ending expression of intense feeling, nurses can promote beneficial expression (Loscalzo & BrintzenhofeSzoc, 1998). At the same time, nurses can educate patients and families about how working through emotional reactions can provide relief as well as improve energy and problem solving. Anxiety needs to be reduced before effective communication and problem solving can occur. Mild anxiety is essential for learning, but moderate anxiety can limit functioning. Anxiety at severe levels alters perception and attention. At this point, motor activity as well as cognitive and emotional expression may be helpful to reduce anxiety. When anxiety reaches panic levels, nurses need to be more directive. An active, commanding approach provides needed structure and creates a secure atmosphere while communicating an expectation that the crisis will be resolved. "Hope is a by-product of directed and meaningful action" (Loscalzo & BrintzenhofeSzoc, p. 672). However, nurses must avoid the urge to offer advice and solutions without actively assisting patients in finding solutions (Greene, Lee, Trask, & Rheinscheld, 2000). Figure 24-5 lists some general principles for intervening in a crisis.

Identifying Problems and Solutions, Formulating a Plan, and Performing Follow-Up

Once the initial phase of shock has subsided and patients are sufficiently calm to participate in a discussion, nurses can assist patients to review their thoughts and feelings, as well as fears (van Servellen, 1997). Nurses should help patients in review-

---

Figure 24-5. Principles of Crisis Intervention

1. The individual's perception of the event and the meaning attributed are the key factors in determining whether a crisis exists.
2. Each patient and crisis situation are unique.
3. The focus remains on the current problem.
4. The focus is on immediate intervention. Crises usually are not emergencies but require prompt action.
5. The nurse takes an active, directive, problem-solving stance, but the decision regarding the solution remains with the patient.
6. The nurse reinforces patient's and family's strengths and resources and facilitates the use of support systems.
7. The nurse communicates patience, hope, self-confidence, and knowledge and uses appropriate communication strategies.
8. The more severe the crisis, the more directive the nurse must be.
9. The nurse helps the patient to identify previous ways of coping and possible strategies to help to solve the current problem.
10. The nurse allows opportunities for identification and expression of feelings.
11. The nurse provides an opportunity for the patient and family to learn skills to help with future crises.
12. Crises usually are self-limiting, but intervention can prevent sequelae and increase the likelihood of optimal resolution.

Note. Based on information from Aguilera, 1998; Barry, 1996; Greene et al., 2000; Roberts, 2000.

---

ing the events related to the crisis and ask about strategies used to cope. The specific meaning of the illness for patients is explored, along with the effect the illness has had on their life goals, expectations, and assumptions (Roberts, 2000). Nurses need to listen for cues regarding concerns, seek specific concrete details, and help to break concerns into manageable components for discussion, ultimately assisting in prioritizing problems (Greene et al., 2000). Nurses can offer information and suggest alternatives to enable families to plan appropriate actions. The BASIC framework (Slaikeu, 1990b) is useful in terms of considering the areas in which interventions can be undertaken: behavioral (What can people do differently that will help?), affect/mood (How can depression, anger, and other negative effects be reduced?), somatic (How can individuals mitigate the amount of anxiety so that their physical distress can be lessened?), interpersonal (How can social support be optimized?), and cognitive (How can the crisis be looked at more adaptively?).

Of importance is accepting patients' and families' psychological status and responses when planning interventions (van Servellen, 1997). A strategy is adaptive if it helps one to function, effectively solve problems, and prevent significant emotional deterioration. A person's strengths should be sought actively and used to enhance coping (Greene et al., 2000). Nurses can offer empathy while communicating confidence that the distress will lessen (Loscalzo & BrintzenhofeSzoc, 1998). Because anxiety interferes with ordinary patterns of interactions, family members and friends may need assistance in maintaining interactions with the patient and each other that are as close to normal as possible.

Rickel (1987) offered a structured method for negotiating problem identification and addressing solutions (see Figure 24-6). The nurse, patient, and family list the problems as each sees them and place the problems into three categories. The patient and family separate them into things they can change soon, things they may be able to change in the future, and things they cannot change. The nurse separates problems into life threatening, those with which the nurse can assist, and those for which the nurse can get assistance. Rickel suggested visualizing a "mountain" of problems, with the most challenging problem at the base and the most solvable at the apex. The metaphor of a ladder then is employed. The ladder is constructed of four Hs: hope, helpfulness, harmony, and humor. The nurse assists by promoting hope, encouraging people to decrease helplessness using support systems, developing and promoting relationships based on trust and harmony, and using humor to reduce anxiety. The ladder is used to climb to the top of the mountain. With the tools of coping mechanisms, supports, and strengths, the mountain becomes more manageable.

Patients and families should be encouraged to discuss, and ultimately to understand, the crisis event's personal meaning and not only how it interferes with attaining their life goals but also how the event challenges cherished expectations and assumptions (Roberts, 2000). Nurses, while avoiding prematurely confronting irrational beliefs and errors or distortions in thinking, which are very common during

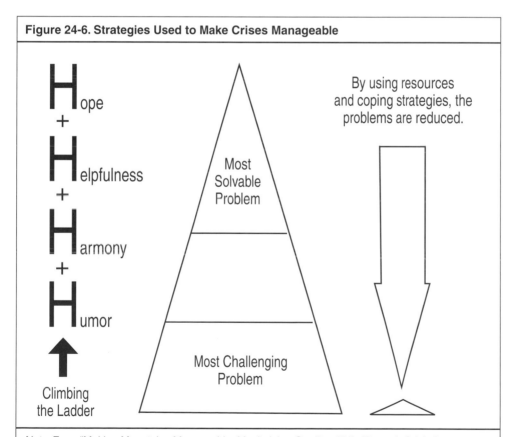

Figure 24-6. Strategies Used to Make Crises Manageable

Hope
+
Helpfulness
+
Harmony
+
Humor
↑
Climbing
the Ladder

Most Solvable Problem

Most Challenging Problem

By using resources and coping strategies, the problems are reduced.

Note. From "Making Mountains Manageable: Maximizing Quality of Life Through Crisis Intervention," by L.M. Rickel, 1987, *Oncology Nursing Forum, 14*(4), p. 32. Copyright 1987 by the Oncology Nursing Society. Adapted with permission.

a crisis, should attend to these sensitively and address them more indirectly through further questioning (Roberts).

Hendricks-Ferguson (2000) emphasized the role of nurses along the entire process in continuing to clarify issues, assessing the impact of stressors on coping, and assessing current coping strategies. Hendricks-Ferguson also specified the importance of nurses reviewing the adjustments and goals achieved and acknowledged that assistance may be needed at other points throughout the illness trajectory.

Cancer as a Crisis

The diagnosis and treatment of cancer, and increasingly the reality of survival (Loscalzo & BrintzenhofeSzoc, 1998), present challenges for patients and families. Whereas a crisis generally is thought to be short-term and self-limited, cancer potentially can precipitate intermittent crises throughout the illness trajectory. Not all individuals will experience a crisis at a particular phase of the illness. Loscalzo and BrintzenhofeSzoc referred to seven crisis events within the cancer experience: diagnosis, treatment, remission, recurrence/new primary, advanced disease, and terminal disease, with the final crisis event of bereavement for the family. Intervention is needed and can be most helpful at these points when new coping strategies may be required (Greene et al., 2000).

Diagnosis

Diagnosis engenders a variety of emotional responses, including disbelief, initial partial denial, anxiety, depressed mood, and anger (Loscalzo & BrintzenhofeSzoc, 1998). Several necessary tasks emerge during diagnosis: accepting dependency, establishing and understanding the treatment, accepting the diagnosis, making decisions, and establishing new routines. Nurses should be alert for certain maladaptive responses that may occur during this phase: denial, with refusal of treatment; refusal of treatment based on feelings of hopelessness; major depression; or seeking out unconventional, alternative therapies (Fawzy, Servis, & Greenberg, 2002). Patients require information to begin to make needed treatment decisions, and nurses serve as a resource, remembering that they may need to repeat information more than once. Education regarding typical emotional responses and validation of feelings can reduce anxiety. Referrals for other sources of information and assistance, such as a support group, may be appropriate.

Treatment

In planning for initial treatment, patients and families require information about expected length of hospitalization, type and length of treatment, anticipated side effects, expected limitations upon their activities, effects of the illness on significant others, and availability of support groups and other resources (Loscalzo & BrintzenhofeSzoc, 1998). Patients fear treatment side effects, pain, and death, as well as body-image changes. Some may fear abandonment by family and friends. Maladaptive responses include major depression; mental disorders related to the treatment, such as delirium; medication-induced psychoses; and mood, anxiety, or cognitive disorders related to the treatment. These responses should prompt referral for psychiatric consultation. Nurses may attempt to intervene in situations where, for example, a patient expresses an interest in postponing or avoiding surgery. In this case, the nurse could explore concerns and provide pertinent information.

Remission

During the adaptation phase, patients and families attempt to return to some level of their previous lifestyles and must balance the ill member's needs with the needs of other family members (Loscalzo & BrintzenhofeSzoc, 1998). Further, support from others may decline despite a possibly increased need for assistance. When treatment concludes, some mild anxiety and depressed mood commonly occur, along with fear of recurrence, which can precipitate a number of other difficulties (Lee-Jones, Humphris, Dixon, & Hatcher, 1997). Patients and families require information regarding follow-up and normalization of their emotional responses, as well as information regarding support groups and cancer education resources (Loscalzo & BrintzenhofeSzoc). If distress becomes moderate or severe, thus interfering with functioning, assessment by a psychiatric specialist is warranted (Pasacreta, n.d.).

Recurrence/New Primary

Recurrence often requires different strategies because physical problems often affect problem solving (van Servellen, 1997). Patients and families experience a wide variety of psychological responses, including initial denial, fear, anxiety, and depression (Loscalzo & BrintzenhofeSzoc, 1998). Patients may experience guilt, anger, and dissatisfaction with the initial treatment choice. They may have to face the possibility of death. Mahon (1991) suggested questions to ask upon recurrence.
- What difficulties are being caused by the recurrence or its treatment?
- How are the patient and family managing these problems?
- Do they have anyone they can ask for help?
- What does the recurrence mean?
- What worries them?
- How is life at work and at home?

Fears of more limitations, increased dependency, and uncontrollable pain often develop. The threat of death frequently is greater after recurrence, and acknowledging this can promote discussion. Nurses should provide information regarding planned treatment, anticipated side effects, common emotional responses, community resources, and strategies to maintain hope (Loscalzo & BrintzenhofeSzoc, 1998). Maladaptive reactions involving significant distress, behavior changes, or suicidal ideation necessitate a psychiatric referral (Pasacreta, n.d.).

Advanced and Terminal Illness

When palliative care becomes the focus, nurses can offer information that will help to make this transition as comfortable as possible. The increased awareness of death, anxiety, lack of control, the need for role changes, and limited time create challenges that can precipitate a crisis (Loscalzo & BrintzenhofeSzoc, 1998). One nursing role involves assessment of the patient's specific fears. Each fear is addressed separately. The family's primary interest and informational needs are concerned with the dying family member and his or her comfort. Reassurance that staff will continue to serve as resources for information and support is essential. Nurses prepare family members for the future at a pace they can tolerate. Family members need time to release outdated views of themselves and each other and to take on new definitions of themselves, the patient, and their relationships and interactions with each other (Reimer, Davies, & Martens, 1991). This process does not always correlate with factual information given to the family nor with observable physical changes in the patient. These shifts occur simultaneously in everyone involved and therefore can lead to conflict because changes that some family members make may be incompatible with those made by others.

Patients' independence should be fostered, and nurses can help families to understand patients' need for inclusion in family life (Rando, 1984). Discussing expectations that family members have regarding themselves and others helps to promote the sharing of tasks to avoid overloading particular individuals. Discussion also allows an opportunity to consider how members can relieve each other. Normalizing feelings such as anger and guilt and emphasizing that these feelings do not negate the positive feelings people have for each other is therapeutic. Nurses can encourage life review, acknowledging that it may include regret and pain. Fully eliminating a family's pain is not possible, and helping does not always involve a specific answer or solution. Instead, nurses can acknowledge the family's role in and commitment to providing comfort to their loved one (Ferrell, 1998). The nurse's role with a dying patient involves supporting family members by enabling them to be present with the dying person and emphasizing the importance of their presence (Rando). Nurses can further assist patients and families in enhancing communication, which often is the source of most difficulty in advanced illness (Ferrell). Family members should not be forced to talk about difficult topics, but nurses should determine whether any hesitation to talk about such topics comes from within themselves or the family (Rando). The family should be assisted to understand the normal withdrawal and detachment that the dying person shows and not to interpret this as abandonment. Family members will be fearful of the death and may feel an urge to initiate more aggressive treatment (Loscalzo & BrintzenhofeSzoc, 1998). Nurses can assist family members by encouraging them to view the situation according to the dying person's preferences. Family members need concrete information about what to expect in the final days, and nurses often must be prepared to repeat this information.

Interventions at Bereavement

After a patient's death, nurses must allow adequate time for loved ones who wish to be alone with the body. Nurses also must provide support and encourage expressions of sorrow (Rando, 1984). Focusing on concrete items, such as helping to make phone calls to other family members or ensuring that a family member is not left alone and will not have to drive home alone, can be important interventions at this time of crisis. Nurses must assess the family members' ability to adjust to the loss. Questions about how the loss is experienced, the adequacy of social support, coping behaviors, and history of loss can elicit useful information. Family members at greatest risk for complicated mourning include those who experience a death that is unexpected and sudden and/or involves the loss of a child (Sanders, 1999). These bereaved individuals may need more follow-up services, including phone calls to assess coping several days or weeks after the death and referrals to bereavement support programs or mental health counseling.

Evaluation of Interventions Across All Phases of Cancer

Generally, successful resolution of a crisis is apparent through reduced distress and improved coping (Hendricks-Ferguson, 2000). Rickel (1987) recommended a brief evaluation to review the experience with the patient or family to determine whether the crisis is resolved. Nurses may ask questions such as What was the problem? Is the problem solved or is it at least manageable? Are the usual coping mechanisms now effective? Are members functioning as they were before the crisis? What new strategies did they learn? When the usual coping mechanisms are working adequately again and the problem seems surmountable, the crisis can be considered to be over. If a decrease in symptoms is not seen fairly quickly, nurses should help to develop another plan. When the crisis has resolved, nurses can make referrals to address the remaining concerns.

Evidence-Based Practice

Newell, Sanson-Fisher, and Savolainen (2002) found more than 150 randomized controlled trials investigating the use of various forms of psychological therapies for patients with cancer, with measurement of outcomes on factors such as psychological adjustment, treatment side effects, quality of life, immune function, and survival. Most of the psychotherapeutic interventions employed in studies inherently apply at least some aspects of crisis intervention theory and techniques, such as information giving and cognitive reappraisal, as appropriate without necessarily being specifically defined as, or limited to, strict crisis intervention. In a meta-analysis of 37 controlled studies assessing the effectiveness of intervention on quality of life, Rehse and Pukrop (2003) commented on the heterogeneity of strategies used and called for more specific definitions of interventions to ascertain their effects. Other authors have lamented the state of psycho-oncology outcome research (Owen, Klapow, Hicken, & Tucker, 2001). Given the lack of consistency in defining and applying specific strategies, it is impossible to replicate studies and make conclusions regarding the effectiveness of crisis intervention in the oncology setting. Measured outcomes vary and currently make comparisons difficult.

As noted by Owen et al. (2001), likely differences occur in outcomes among various patient populations based on disease type (which often differ among demographic groups, with resultant differences in relevant psychosocial issues) and disease stage, as well as within specific homogeneous groups, as a result of individual differences. Most studies, other than those addressing outcomes in breast cancer, melanoma, and hematologic disorders, have not been disease-specific, and results may not be generalized to all patients with cancer.

Another issue is that of the applicability of research results to oncology nurses as providers without advanced preparation in mental health. Studies generally have involved mental health professionals with expertise in offering interventions such as various forms of psychotherapy or coping skills training to patients with cancer (Newell et al., 2002). Crisis intervention generally is considered to require at least basic counseling skills not necessarily possessed by all nurses (Kruger, 1992). Only a few authors have addressed the topic of crisis intervention for oncology nurses, and these usually have consisted of a limited review of theory along with discussion of case examples, such as Hendricks-Ferguson (2000) and Kruger. Studies have investigated the impact of nursing intervention on coping, mostly involving the provision of support and information, but the interventions were offered at treatment initiation rather than in response to identified crises (Rawl et al., 2002; Roberts et al., 2002; Wengström, Häggmark, & Forsberg, 2001).

Conclusion

Nurses in any oncology setting will encounter patients and families experiencing the crisis of cancer. Crises will occur across all phases of the cancer continuum. Nurses must recognize the various crises that patients and families face and how they can effectively intervene to assist them with a successful resolution and restoration of equilibrium.

References

Aguilera, D.C. (1998). *Crisis intervention: Theory and methodology* (8th ed.). St. Louis, MO: Mosby.

Baird, S.F. (1987). Helping the family through a crisis. *Nursing87, 17*(6), 66–67.

Barry, P.D. (1996). Crisis intervention with physically ill persons and their families. In P.D. Barry (Ed.), *Psychosocial nursing: Care of physically ill patients and their families* (3rd ed., pp. 284–300). Philadelphia: Lippincott.

Bernal, H. (1996). Delivering culturally competent care. In P.D. Barry (Ed.), *Psychosocial nursing: Care of physically ill patients and their families* (3rd ed., pp. 78–99). Philadelphia: Lippincott.

Blanchard, C.G., Albrecht, T.L., & Ruckdeschel, J.C. (1997). The crisis of cancer: Psychological impact on family caregivers. *Oncology, 11,* 189–194.

Caine, R.M. (1989). Families in crisis: Making the critical difference. *Focus on Critical Care, 16,* 184–189.

Congress, E.P. (2000). Crisis intervention with culturally diverse families. In A.R. Roberts (Ed.), *Crisis intervention handbook: Assessment, treatment, and research* (2nd ed., pp. 430–449). New York: Oxford University Press.

Fawzy, F.I., Servis, M.E., & Greenberg, D.B. (2002). Oncology and psychooncology. In M.G. Wise & J.R. Rundell (Eds.), *The American Psychiatric Publishing textbook of consultation-liaison psychiatry: Psychiatry in the medically ill* (2nd ed., pp. 657–678). Washington, DC: American Psychiatric Publishing.

Ferrell, B.R. (1998). The family. In D. Doyle, G.W.C. Hanks, & N. MacDonald (Eds.), *Oxford textbook of palliative medicine* (2nd ed., pp. 909–917). New York: Oxford University Press.

Ferszt, G.G. (1995). Performing a crisis assessment. *Nursing95, 25*(5), 88–89.

Gray-Price, H., & Szczesny, S. (1985). Crisis intervention with families of cancer patients: A developmental approach. *Topics in Clinical Nursing, 7*(1), 58–70.

Greene, G.J., Lee, M.Y., Trask, R., & Rheinscheld, J. (2000). How to work with clients' strengths in crisis intervention: A solution-focused approach. In A.R. Roberts (Ed.), *Crisis intervention handbook: Assessment, treatment, and research* (2nd ed., pp. 31–55). New York: Oxford University Press.

Hendricks-Ferguson, V.L. (2000). Crisis intervention strategies when caring for families of children. *Journal of Pediatric Oncology Nursing, 17,* 3–11.

James, R.K., & Gilliland, B.E. (2004). *Crisis intervention strategies* (5th ed.). Belmont, CA: Thomson Brooks/Cole.

Janosik, E.H., & Davies, J.L. (1996). *Mental health and psychiatric nursing* (2nd ed.). Boston: Little, Brown.

Kornblith, A.B. (1998). Psychosocial adaptation in cancer survivors. In J.C. Holland (Ed.), *Psycho-oncology* (pp. 223–254). New York: Oxford University Press.

Kruger, S. (1992). Parents in crisis: Helping them cope with a seriously ill child. *Journal of Pediatric Nursing, 7,* 133–140.

Lederberg, M.S. (1998). The family of the cancer patient. In J.C. Holland (Ed.), *Psycho-oncology* (pp. 981–993). New York: Oxford University Press.

Lee-Jones, C., Humphris, G., Dixon, R., & Hatcher, M.B. (1997). Fear of cancer recurrence—A literature review and proposed cognitive formulation to explain exacerbation of recurrence fears. *Psycho-Oncology, 6,* 95–105.

Loscalzo, M., & BrintzenhofeSzoc, K. (1998). Brief crisis counseling. In J.C. Holland (Ed.), *Psycho-oncology* (pp. 662–675). New York: Oxford University Press.

Mahon, S.M. (1991). Managing the psychosocial consequences of cancer recurrence: Implications for nurses. *Oncology Nursing Forum, 18,* 577–583.

National Comprehensive Cancer Network. (2005). Distress management. *Clinical practice guidelines in oncology v.1.2005.* Jenkintown, PA: Author. Retrieved April 26, 2005, from http://www.nccn. org/professionals/physician_gls/f_guidelines.asp#care

Newell, A.A., Sanson-Fisher, R.W., & Savolainen, N.J. (2002). Systematic review of psychological therapies for cancer patients: Overview and recommendations for future research. *Journal of the National Cancer Institute, 94,* 558–584.

Owen, J.E., Klapow, J.C., Hicken, B., & Tucker, D.C. (2001). Psychosocial interventions for cancer: Review and analysis using a three-tiered outcomes model. *Psycho-Oncology, 10,* 218–230.

Pasacreta, J.V. (n.d.). Distress management training for nurses. *Psychiatric complications associated with cancer: Principles and guidelines for psychotherapy and referral.* Retrieved May 23, 2005, from http://www.apos-society.org/professionals/meetings-ed/webcasts/webcasts-ican2.aspx

Rando, T.A. (1984). *Grief, dying and death: Clinical interventions for caregivers.* Champaign, IL: Research Press.

Rawl, S.M., Given, B.A., Given, C.W., Champion, V.L., Kozachik, S.L., Barton, D., et al. (2002). Intervention to improve psychological functioning for newly diagnosed patients with cancer. *Oncology Nursing Forum, 29,* 967–975.

Rehse, B., & Pukrop, R. (2003). Effects of psychosocial interventions on quality of life in adult cancer patients: Meta analysis of 37 published controlled outcome studies. *Patient Education and Counseling, 50,* 179–186.

Reimer, J.C., Davies, B., & Martens, N. (1991). Palliative care. The nurse's role in helping families through the transition of "fading away." *Cancer Nursing, 14,* 321–327.

Rickel, L.M. (1987). Making mountains manageable: Maximizing quality of life through crisis intervention. *Oncology Nursing Forum, 14*(4), 29–34.

Roberts, A.R. (2000). An overview of crisis theory and crisis intervention. In A.R. Roberts (Ed.), *Crisis intervention handbook: Assessment, treatment, and research* (2nd ed., pp. 3–30). New York: Oxford University Press.

Roberts, S., Schofield, P., Freeman, J., Hill, D., Akkerman, D., & Rodger, A. (2002). Bridging the information and support gap: Evaluation of a hospital-based cancer support nurse service. *Patient Education and Counseling, 47,* 47–55.

Sanders, C.M. (1999). *Grief: The mourning after: Dealing with adult bereavement.* New York: John Wiley.

Shaw, M.C., & Halliday, P.H. (1992). The family, crisis and chronic illness: An evolutionary model. *Journal of Advanced Nursing, 17,* 537–543.

Shulman, N.M., & Shewbert, A.L. (2000). A model of crisis intervention in critical and intensive care units of general hospitals. In A.R. Roberts (Ed.), *Crisis intervention handbook: Assessment, treatment, and research* (2nd ed., pp. 412–429). New York: Oxford University Press.

Slaikeu, K.A. (1990a). Crisis theory: A general framework. In K.A. Slaikeu (Ed.), *Crisis intervention: A handbook for practice and research* (2nd ed., pp. 14–41). Boston: Allyn and Bacon.

Slaikeu, K.A. (1990b). Second-order intervention: Multimodal crisis therapy. In K.A. Slaikeu (Ed.), *Crisis intervention: A handbook for practice and research* (2nd ed., pp. 142–182). Boston: Allyn and Bacon.

Van Fleet, S.K., & Hughes, M.K. (1996). Psychiatric clinical specialist consultation model in a medical setting. *Clinical Nurse Specialist, 10,* 204–211.

van Servellen, G.M. (1997). *Communication skills for the health care professional: Concepts and techniques.* Gaithersburg, MD: Aspen.

Wengström, Y., Häggmark, C., & Forsberg, C. (2001). Coping with radiation therapy: Effects of a nursing intervention on coping ability for women with breast cancer. *International Journal of Nursing Practice, 7,* 8–15.

Wilkes, L.M., O'Baugh, J., Luke, S., & George, A. (2003). Positive attitude in cancer: Patients' perspectives. *Oncology Nursing Forum, 30,* 412–416.

Zabora, J.R. (1998). Screening procedures for psychosocial distress. In J.C. Holland (Ed.), *Psychooncology* (pp. 653–661). New York: Oxford University Press.

CHAPTER 25

Programmatic Approaches to Psychosocial Support

MARGARET I. FITCH, RN, MScN, PhD

Separate reeds are weak and easily broken; but bound together they are strong and hard to tear apart.

—The Midrash

When cancer strikes, it has more than a physical impact. Cancer and its treatment also have emotional, psychological, social, and spiritual consequences that create myriad changes for an individual. For most, life is altered irrevocably when a definitive diagnosis of cancer is made. Dealing with the various changes can present many challenges and difficult issues for the person diagnosed with the disease and family members (Kristjanson & Ashcroft, 1994; Northouse, 1988). Whether individuals have timely access to appropriate assistance will influence their ability to cope effectively and their quality of life (Wyatt, Kurtz, & Liken, 1993).

Supportive care is the provision of the necessary services as defined by those living with or affected by cancer to meet their physical, informational, emotional, psychological, social, spiritual, and practical needs throughout the full spectrum of their experiences with cancer (Fitch, 2000). "Supportive care" is an overarching or umbrella term that encompasses a range of services and areas of expertise required for comprehensive, high-quality care of patients with cancer, including psychosocial oncology, rehabilitation oncology, and palliative care. Ultimately, supportive care services are designed to assist patients in meeting their needs, maintaining or improving quality of life, and optimizing their sense of well-being.

The specific focus of this chapter is on the psychosocial needs of patients with cancer and programs designed to help to meet those needs. The term "psychosocial" refers to the relationship between social conditions and mental health; it relates to how a person feels about the way the disease or its treatment has affected social functioning at work and home; relationships with partner/spouse, children, extended family, and friends; and one's self and one's body (Nicholas & Veach, 2000). Disturbances and changes in these areas can evoke intense feelings of distress.

The past decade has seen a remarkable increase in the attention paid to psychosocial needs of patients with cancer and understanding of the impact of psychosocial distress. Patients and survivors have shown a keen interest in finding ways to enhance coping and to reduce the psychosocial distress they experience. In turn, they have been instrumental in the development and growth of psychosocial programs. Unfortunately, systematic literature validating the use of specific interventions has not kept pace with the popular enthusiasm for them.

Background Context

Some individuals experience cancer as a single event with a defined beginning and ending. For others, the cancer experience takes on a chronic nature. Everyone undergoes a spectrum of experiences with a cancer care system that includes a peridiagnostic interval, diagnosis, treatment, and follow-up care. Depending upon the situation, follow-up care may encompass long-term survivorship with no further clinical evidence of disease or recurrent disease, metastatic spread, and death. Throughout this spectrum of experiences, patients diagnosed with cancer and their family members are likely to confront social, psychological, and spiritual issues and require access to supportive care services (see Figure 25-1).

Individuals may enter the cancer care delivery system at different points and move through the system along various pathways. Some will enter at the point of screening and may never proceed further. Others will enter at the point of diagnosis and move through phases of treatment, rehabilitation, and follow-up. Some of those in follow-up will live without further evidence of disease, whereas others will face the cycle of recurrence and treatment several times, depending on the type of cancer. Some may require palliative care services at diagnosis. Death as a result of cancer remains the final outcome for approximately half of those diagnosed with the disease, although the time between diagnosis and death can vary widely. Each person travels a unique and personal journey in living with cancer.

Regardless of the journey's pathway for any individual, that person carries physical, social, emotional, psychological, spiritual, informational, and practical needs. These needs will vary from person to person, as well as within the same person, as the course of the disease and treatment unfolds. No two individuals respond exactly the same way to the diagnosis of cancer and its impact on their lives or desire exactly the same assistance in dealing with their situation (see Figure 25-2).

The onset of an illness can influence a person's ability to meet his or her own needs. Physical discomfort, disability, emotional distress, and a sense of personal crisis may interfere with an individual's capacity to act, and the usual ways of meeting one's needs may be compromised. The patient may require new knowledge, new skills, or a different network of supports to manage the new demands of the illness situation, whether it is acute, chronic, or palliative. Having to learn new information and seek out resources in times of emotional vulnerability, especially when faced with a heightened sense of life threat, adds to the burden of suffering that patients feel (Taylor, 1983). Services to assist individuals in meeting this broad range of needs must be

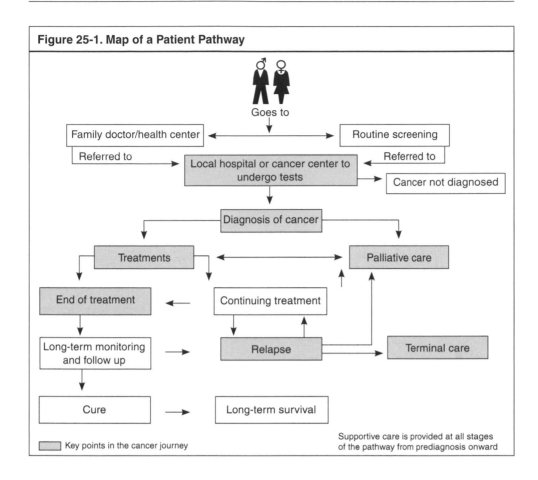

Figure 25-1. Map of a Patient Pathway

Goes to

Family doctor/health center ↔ Routine screening

Referred to → Local hospital or cancer center to undergo tests ← Referred to

→ Cancer not diagnosed

Diagnosis of cancer

Treatments ↔ Palliative care

End of treatment ← Continuing treatment

Long-term monitoring and follow up → Relapse → Terminal care

Cure → Long-term survival

▭ Key points in the cancer journey

Supportive care is provided at all stages of the pathway from prediagnosis onward

clearly visible and easily accessible to patients and their family members. Individuals may want to access these services at various points during their cancer journey.

One of the challenges in providing services to assist patients in meeting a broad range of needs is that needs are met in different ways from person to person. The intervention, or set of interventions, that may be helpful to one person will not necessarily be useful to another person. People have different styles of learning and ways of dealing with what happens to them. Ideally, they ought to be able to choose specific interventional approaches from a menu of options.

A person's perception of the situation will influence how he or she copes with life-threatening illness and adapts to its aftermath (Lazarus & Folkman, 1984), as well as a number of factors such as socioeconomic status, educational background, social support, culture, religion, and geographic location (Muzzin, Anderson, Figueredo, & Gudelis, 1994). The success of an intervention for an individual must be judged on the basis of whether it has been tailored sufficiently to attend to the person's unique situational factors. In the practice environment, this means the assessment process must identify the expectations and goals of the individual across all need areas within an existing situation and then tailor the intervention plan to those parameters in collaboration with the person. This process of assessment, mutual goal setting, and tailoring interventions is necessary throughout the course of a patient's cancer journey.

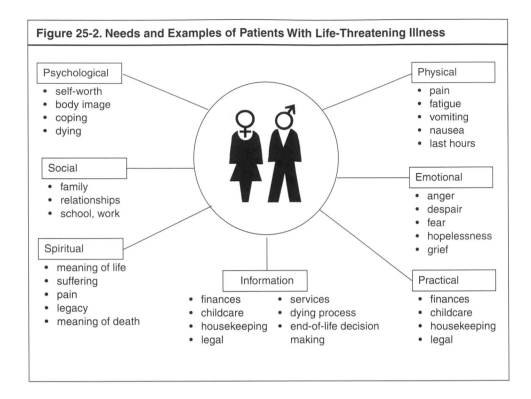

Figure 25-2. Needs and Examples of Patients With Life-Threatening Illness

Psychological
- self-worth
- body image
- coping
- dying

Social
- family
- relationships
- school, work

Spiritual
- meaning of life
- suffering
- pain
- legacy
- meaning of death

Information
- finances
- childcare
- housekeeping
- legal
- services
- dying process
- end-of-life decision making

Physical
- pain
- fatigue
- vomiting
- nausea
- last hours

Emotional
- anger
- despair
- fear
- hopelessness
- grief

Practical
- finances
- childcare
- housekeeping
- legal

Emotional or psychosocial distress is a natural response to life-threatening illness that all patients experience to some degree. Some patients with cancer, given relevant information, good symptom management, and good communication with their care providers, will mobilize their own supports or resources and cope effectively with their cancer situation (Bakker, Fitch, Gray, Reed, & Bennet, 2001). Others will require additional help to manage. Some, if needs remain unmet, will continue to experience ongoing distress and upheaval. This distress can escalate to significant levels, thus compromising compliance with tumor therapy, increasing utilization of other healthcare services, and elevating costs for care (Browne, Arpin, Corey, Fitch, & Gafni, 1990; Holland, 1999; Zabora, BrintzenhofeSzoc, Curbow, Hooker, & Piantadosi, 2001).

For mixed groups of outpatients with cancer, the prevalence of significant psychosocial distress (i.e., where intervention by professionals would be beneficial) has been reported as 20%–37% (Derogatis et al., 1983; Farber, Weinerman, & Kuypers, 1984; Fitch, Vachon, Greenberg, & Franssen, 1996; Holland & Rolland, 1989; Stam, Bultz, & Pittman, 1986; van't Spijker, Trijsburg, & Duivenvoorden, 1997; Zabora, BrintzenhofeSzoc, Curbow, et al., 2001). When patients were grouped on the basis of disease stage, the prevalence of significant psychosocial distress was 39% for those on active treatment, 79% for those receiving palliative care, and 17% for those who did not have any clinical evidence of disease (Fitch et al., 1996). However, the presence of psychosocial distress in itself does not reveal the reason for that distress or point to a specific course of intervention. Nurses must talk with patients to uncover the reason for the distress and their desire for assistance.

Individuals who receive appropriate emotional or psychosocial care experience less anxiety and depression and generally are able to return to a productive life. Both patients and families experience significant improvement in quality of life (Blake-Mortimer, Gore-Felton, Kimberling, Turner-Cobb, & Spiegel, 1999; Coates, 1997; Spiegel, Bloom, Kraemer, & Grottheil, 1989). Evidence also exists regarding the efficacy of interventions designed to augment coping skills, problem solving using behavioral training, stress management, cognitive therapy, and support of patients with cancer. Better outcomes have been reported in areas such as psychological state, coping response, quality of life, and compliance with therapy (Bucher, 1999; Fawzy, 1999; Greer, 1992; Moorey, Greer, Bliss, & Law, 1998; Richardson & Johnson, 1999). Evidence has shown that heightened psychosocial distress, if left unchecked, is associated with poor prognosis (Degner & Sloan, 1995; Kaasa, Mastekaasa, & Lund, 1989) and that psychosocial intervention potentially may extend survival (Carlson & Bultz, 2002; Cunningham et al., 2000).

Helping Patients to Meet Their Psychosocial Needs

Patients and their families require comprehensive, quality cancer care or an integrated approach that ensures that person-centered care is incorporated with tumor-centered care. Cancer programs must focus on biopsychosocial care and ensure that structures and processes are in place to allow (a) ongoing identification of needs in all domains, (b) a dialogue with patients and families about their desire for assistance, (c) provision of information about available resources, and (d) referral (if required). Cancer programs need to ensure psychosocial interventions/programs are available in addition to systemic, radiation, surgical, and symptom management interventions. This requires collaborative partnerships among a range of institutionally based and community-based providers, as well as among professional and volunteer initiatives. Currently, there remains wide variation among cancer programs in the availability of psychosocial programming by professionals and uneven access for patients who live in different regions. Additionally, volunteer-based community support agencies offer different programs from region to region. Patients and families often feel that they do not know where to turn for help with psychosocial concerns.

Helping patients to meet their psychosocial needs must begin with their entry into the cancer care system. Aspects of psychosocial care must be integral to the practice of all healthcare professionals and demonstrated in actions such as offering patients and families emotional support and information during the course of their interactions, communicating in a person-centered and sensitive manner, and referring them to psychosocial programs or experts as required. How sensitively that communication is handled is of importance to patients and can have a significant impact on their coping (Butow et al., 1996; Reynolds, Sanson-Fisher, Poole, Harker, & Byrne, 1981; Tattersall, Butow, & Clayton, 2002). In addition to the basic psychosocial interventions provided by nurses, oncologists, pharmacists, and radiation therapists, more focused and specialized therapeutic psychosocial interventions may be provided by social workers, psychologists, chaplains, advanced practice nurses, psychiatrists, and therapists in the fields of art, music, and touch. Peer support and volunteer-led initiatives also have an important role in helping patients to meet their psychosocial needs. Linking all of these providers in a way that allows patients with cancer and families easy access to the full range of services remains a challenge in many jurisdictions. Yet, this linkage is imperative if patients are to experience continuity and comprehensiveness in their care experience.

Programmatic Approaches to Psychosocial Care

Successful cancer programs have created programmatic mechanisms to (a) provide basic information and support to all patients with cancer and their families, (b) identify those who need additional assistance, and (c) link those who need additional assistance with appropriate services in a timely fashion. Figure 25-3 provides an illustration of various psychosocial services that may be involved in meeting the psychosocial needs of patients with cancer and their families at some point in the illness experience. At the very least, healthcare providers need to know about the services available in their local areas and be able to talk with patients about the benefits of the services (i.e., how that service might be able to help).

The following descriptions present information about programmatic approaches designed to help patients and their families to meet psychosocial needs during the cancer experience. These can be brought together in one facility or coordinated within a geographic area (see Table 25-1 and Appendix).

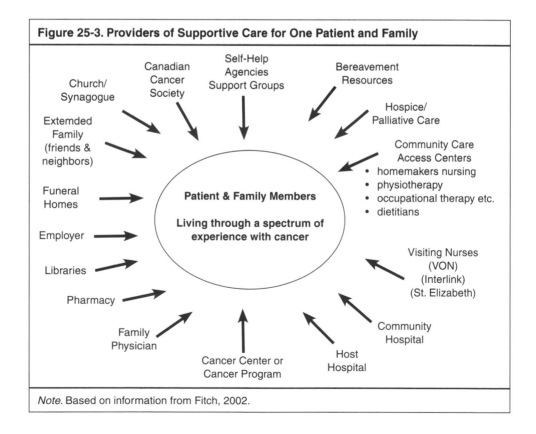

Figure 25-3. Providers of Supportive Care for One Patient and Family

Church/ Synagogue

Canadian Cancer Society

Self-Help Agencies Support Groups

Bereavement Resources

Extemded Family (friends & neighbors)

Hospice/ Palliative Care

Community Care Access Centers
• homemakers nursing
• physiotherapy
• occupational therapy etc.
• dietitians

Funeral Homes

Patient & Family Members

Living through a spectrum of experience with cancer

Employer

Libraries

Visiting Nurses (VON) (Interlink) (St. Elizabeth)

Pharmacy

Family Physician

Community Hospital

Cancer Center or Cancer Program

Host Hospital

Note. Based on information from Fitch, 2002.

Table 25-1. Supportive Care Program Model

Service or Activity	Target Group	Purpose	Leadership
Orientation	All new patients and family members	Introduces the cancer center and the cancer care system, offers information about resources, provides links to contacts to follow-up	Staff/patients Volunteers
Emotional support and peer information (e.g., Reach to Recovery, Cansurmount, self-help groups)	Individuals who wish to talk with another patient either in a group setting or on a one-to-one-basis	Provides an opportunity to talk with other patients with cancer about their experiences, feelings, concerns; allows sharing of experiences and information on a peer basis	Patients with cancer Volunteers
Psychoeducational (group or one-to-one)	Individuals who want to learn new coping skills and express difficulty coping with the cancer experience	Provides an opportunity to learn coping skills and problem-solving skills regarding issues confronting them	Professionally trained group leaders
Adjustment/supportive counseling (group or one-to-one)	Individuals who require help to adjust to their diagnosis and treatment	Provides regular assistance/support for individuals during their treatment	Professional
Crisis intervention (one-to-one)	Individuals requiring immediate intervention regarding emotional, spiritual, or psychosocial distress	Provides immediate intervention focused on managing or resolving emotional/psychosocial distress crises	Professional
Psychotherapy (group or one-to-one) Short-term Long-term	Individuals requiring ongoing intervention regarding emotional, spiritual, or psychosocial distress	Provides ongoing intervention focused on managing or resolving significant emotional/psychosocial distress	Professional
Nutritional intervention	Individuals who want advice regarding nutrition and who are experiencing difficulties regarding eating	Provides advice regarding nutrition/intervention for those with eating difficulties	Nutritionist
Pain and symptom management	Individuals experiencing difficulties with management of pain or other symptoms (e.g., lymphedema, fatigue)	Reduces or eliminates distress caused by symptoms	Healthcare professional
Practical assistance	Individuals who require help with activities of daily living, child care, financial assistance, transportation	Provides services designed to assist with practical matters	Staff/patients Volunteers

Note. Based on information from Fitch, 2002.

Patient Orientation, Information, and Education Approaches

Patients have cited timely access to relevant, understandable information as a key element in their capacity to cope with their cancer and gain a sense of control over what is happening to them (Adams, 1991; Ashbury, Findley, Reynolds, & McKerracher, 1998; Davison & Degner, 1997; Gray et al., 1998; Houts et al., 1988). However, the importance of providing information extends beyond this perceived need. Patients with cancer who receive information experience significant benefits, including increased participation in treatment decision making (Davison, Degner, & Morgan, 1995; Hinds, Streater, & Mood, 1995); increased satisfaction with treatment choices and interactions with healthcare professionals (Damian & Tattersall, 1991); increased control and coping with the stress of the diagnosis (Fisher & Britten, 1993); decreased levels of anxiety, mood disturbance, and affective distress (Rainey, 1985); increased ability to cope during and after treatment (Johnson, Nail, Lauver, King, & Keys, 1988); and assistance in communicating illness-related information to their families (Hogben & Fallowfield, 1989).

Patients have identified the importance of receiving information about cancer, treatment options, side effects, and available resources from their healthcare providers, especially at diagnosis (Fitch, Gray, & Franssen, 2000; Gray, Fitch, Phillips, Labrecque, & Fergus, 2000). Typically, satisfaction with the information provided about these topics is higher than for topics such as emotional issues, impact on personal and social relations, lifestyle and body-image changes, and emotional needs of family members (Canadian Cancer Society, 1992; Fitch et al., 2000). These latter topics tend to emerge with more intensity later in the course of the cancer experience (i.e., during or after treatment) (Gray et al., 1998; Hinds et al., 1995; Luker, Beaver, Lenster, & Owens, 1996). The majority of the work on reporting patient information needs focuses on newly diagnosed individuals, despite the recognition that information and education needs and topics of importance will change throughout the course of the cancer experience. Recommendations for program development emphasize the importance of targeting the information program to the stage of disease for maximum benefit (Ashbury, 1999; Houts, Rusenas, Simmonds, & Hufford, 1991).

Providing patient information and education programs has been identified as an important function of cancer programs for a number of years. As a result, healthcare professionals have organized initiatives in many forms, including written pamphlets, brochures, and books; patient/family libraries and resource centers; videos; teleconferences; audiotapes; Web-based programs; CD-ROMs; education lectures/discussion groups; orientation programs; posters/bulletin boards; newsletters; and teaching cards and demonstration models (Agre, Dougherty, & Pirone, 2002; Butow, Bundle, McConnell, Boakes, & Tattersall, 1998; Edgar, Greenberg, & Remmer, 2002; Hack et al., 1999; McQuellon et al., 1998; Shaw, McTavish, Hawkins, Gustafson, & Pingree, 2000; Till, 2003).

Although not always specified in the literature, providing information and offering education may be conceptualized as having different goals or intended outcomes. Goals for providing patient information include the communication of facts and practical guidance. Most frequently, information programs are designed with the intent of helping patients to navigate the cancer system, reducing anxiety, and encouraging patients' active participation in decision making about their treatment and rehabilitation. Educational programs aim to influence attitudes and behavior and maintain or improve health. It is an active process that assists people in changing behavior and improving decision-making and coping skills (Padilla & Bulcavage, 1991). Education programs can assist patients psychosocially by helping them to recognize their anxieties and develop strategies for dealing with them. Studies have demonstrated that anxiety decreases significantly when patients are informed and prepared emotionally for their treatment (Vahabi & Ferris, 1995).

The challenge for healthcare professionals is to be clear about the intended outcomes of the program of information provision or patient and family education. Each type of program requires appropriate methods of content delivery and outcome evaluation. These methods must be adjusted for the specific target audience. The notion of "one size fits all" is not useful. Programs need to be tailored to the specific patient population. Unfortunately, comparatively few rigorous evaluation studies have been undertaken to determine the most effective methods of designing and implementing patient education materials and the extent to which the materials influence patient outcomes (Ashbury, 1999; Kaegi, 1999). Consensus exists, however, regarding the principles of successful program development and delivery (see Figure 25-4).

Figure 25-4. Principles Associated With Successful Information and Education Program Development and Implementation

- Program development must include audience participation.
- Materials must be audience specific.
- Messages must be personalized.
- Materials must present information in plain language.
- Materials must be culturally sensitive.
- Active strategies to provide materials directly to patients are more successful.
- Materials should be introduced at key moments in the cancer trajectory.
- Materials should be relevant and comprehensive, present options, and facilitate communications with providers.
- Vehicles other than print can be beneficial.
- Dissemination of patient education materials must correspond to the needs of the patient audience.
- Multiple strategies are more effective than single strategies.

Note. Based on information from Ashbury, 1999.

This area of health care, providing information and education, remains challenging. The pace of knowledge development and availability of information is escalating exponentially. Healthcare professionals are no longer the sole provider of healthcare information and may have difficulty remaining up to date with all available information. They are struggling with ever-increasing caseloads. Patients are becoming educated consumers (Tyson, 2000). Approximately 100,000 Web sites provide information to 98 million individuals in the United States alone; up to 6 million Americans per day go online for medical advice—more than the number visiting healthcare professionals (Fox & Rainie, 2002). This makes the Internet an important tool for information dissemination. At the same time, patients can be overwhelmed with detailed information and experience difficulty knowing what truly applies to them. Finding local solutions to these challenges is important given that the provision of relevant, understandable information is a critical influence on coping with cancer.

Peer Information and Support Approaches

Although many patients with cancer want information from their healthcare providers, some also want information and support from fellow patients or peers. Many describe the information and support gathered from peers as different from that provided by healthcare professionals and as tremendously helpful in coping and in navigating the cancer system. This latter observation has been influential in the development and growth of self-help cancer organizations. These groups often have objectives related to support as well as providing information. In addition to their face-to-face group meetings, many of the groups have initiated other activities aimed at helping patients with cancer and their families. Examples of these activities include writing booklets, distributing newsletters, creating Web sites, providing one-on-one peer support, and delivering telephone-based peer support (long distance).

One-on-one peer support programs facilitate a patient's ability to interact with another patient who has undergone a similar experience. The matching of the patient and the peer may be made on the basis of cancer type (e.g., breast cancer), age, or life circumstance (e.g., rural dwelling, mother with children). Peer volunteers are trained for this role and in most instances focus on providing emotional support and practical information. Care is taken to not provide medical information. Evaluations of face-to-face peer support programs (Ashbury, 1999) and telephone peer support (Canadian Cancer Society, 1998) have cited benefits similar to those of self-help groups. The one-on-one approach works well for those who do not care for the group setting or who are unable to attend the group meetings. More recently, Internet-based peer support has been available (Till, 2003).

A solid body of evidence has accumulated regarding the positive relationship between social support and health (House, 1987). As well, solid documentation has shown the effect that social support has on helping individuals to adjust to and cope with cancer (Broadhead & Kaplan, 1991; Dunkel-Schetter, 1984; Nelles, McCaffrey, Blanchard, & Ruckdeschel, 1991). Various definitions of social support have been developed, but all share a common theme of being cared for by others and feeling emotionally connected. A social network can provide both tangible and intangible support. When coping with new situations, human beings often search out others who have similar experiences as an avenue to finding meaningful support. Individuals can feel an intense sense of isolation and loneliness, especially with diseases that carry an element of stigma.

Self-help groups are defined as "member-governed voluntary associations of persons who share a common problem, and who rely on experiential knowledge at least partly to mutually solve or cope with their common concerns" (Borkman, 1990, p. 321). Specifically excluded are support or psychoeducational groups run by healthcare professionals. From the self-help perspective, these are quite different models, with distinct philosophies and approaches (Riessman & Carroll, 1995).

During the past decade, a tremendous growth has occurred in the number of self-help groups for patients with cancer. These groups exist because of a belief in the value of peer information and support, as well as perceived gaps in the cancer system. In many instances, the groups are organized for individuals with a particular cancer (e.g., breast, prostate, colon). The groups range from those that are highly structured in terms of time and membership to groups that are drop-in and rather loosely structured. Usually, leaders have had some preparation for or orientation to leading a group and are survivors themselves. Several studies have described the benefits that patients and survivors feel from attending self-help groups (Ashbury, Cameron, Mercer, Fitch, & Nielsen, 1998; Gray, Fitch, Davis, & Phillips, 1996, 1997a, 1997b; Kurtz, 1990). These benefits include sharing common experiences/talking about difficulties, being accepted and affirmed, feeling supported, sharing information, reconstructing a positive identity, gaining a sense of affiliation and community, experiencing personal transformation, and finding opportunities for advocacy and empowerment. Attendees also have cited some drawbacks in attending a self-help group: dominance by some members, inability to help with complex or intimate issues, and lack of training of and poor facilitation by group leaders.

Many of the established self-help groups have an interest in linking with healthcare professionals to obtain endorsement or support for their groups. That support is evidenced through informing new patients about the group's existence and how the group may benefit them. In one study, encouragement by the cancer care team to attend self-help groups was an independent predictor of patient interest in the support group (Bui et al., 2002). In general, most healthcare professionals are positively predisposed to self-help groups but have relatively little awareness about the groups and how they operate (Gray et al., 1998). In one study of oncology nurses' perspectives about self-help groups for patients, only 20% mentioned the groups to their patients on a regular basis (Fitch et al., 2001).

Identifying Those Who Need Additional Assistance

In many cancer centers, screening programs for psychosocial distress have been implemented to help to routinely identify, monitor, and refer patients who are experiencing heightened levels of distress and could benefit from intervention by a psychosocial expert. Both the National Comprehensive Cancer Network (2005) and the National Cancer Institute (2002) have recommended a range of standardized screening tools for psychosocial distress and suggest that all patients with cancer should be screened at their initial visit, at appropriate intervals, and as clinically indicated. The actual tools being used differ among cancer centers, but the basic approach is the same: Individuals with high scores are seen immediately by a mental health professional, those with mid-range scores are called to schedule an appointment, and those with low scores are informed about available support and education programs. Table 25-2 provides examples of screening approaches in several institutions. The use of screening procedures has been reported as useful for identifying patients with greater psychological, social, and physical impairment (Carlson & Bultz, 2003; Patrick-Miller, Much, & Axelrod, 2002). Using standardized programmatic approaches to screening helps to overcome some of the stigma associated with emotional issues, identify distress before it erupts as a crisis, and reduce costs associated with health service utilization (Weisman, 1979; Zabora, BrintzenhofeSzoc, Jacobson, et al., 2001).

Table 25-2. Screening for Psychosocial Distress: Examples of Tools in Use

Institution	Instrument	Description
Northwestern Regional Cancer Center Thunder Bay, Ontario, Canada	Hospital Anxiety and Depression Score (HADS) (Zigmond & Snaith, 1983)	Patients complete the 14 forced-choice HADS on the second visit. Scores are generated for both anxiety and depression, and a follow-up discussion occurs with patients based on the scores and focuses on the source of distress and their desire for assistance (Sellick, 2001).
Memorial Sloan-Kettering Cancer Center New York, NY	Distress thermometer with a scale of 0–10 (0 = no distress) and a patient problem list (Roth et al., 1998)	Patients circle the number on the thermometer that best describes how much distress they have been feeling in the past, including today, and then indicate whether any of the items on the problem list has caused distress over the same period.
Johns Hopkins Oncology Center Baltimore, MD	18-item Brief Symptom Inventory (BSI-18) and a 16-item patient problem checklist (Zabora, BrintzenhofeSzoc, Jacobson, et al., 2001)	Patients complete the 18-item inventory in terms of how they have been feeling in the past week (rate each item on a 5-point scale from 0 (not at all) to 4 (always). The problem list has 16 common problems, with fatigue and pain included as visual analogs.
Dana-Farber Cancer Institute Boston, MA	Functional Assessment of Cancer Therapy—General (FACT-G) (Cella et al., 1993)	Patients use handheld computers to complete the form. Results are downloaded into a personal computer and given to the clinical team so they are available at the time of the patient visit.

Support, Education, and Therapy by Professionals

The past 15 years has witnessed a remarkable increase in the amount of literature describing psychosocial interventions for patients with cancer that are delivered by healthcare professionals or professionals and cancer survivors working in a collaborative model. Interventions are provided to promote coping and enhance quality of life. More specifically, they aim to reduce feelings of stigma, isolation, anxiety, helplessness, and hopelessness while promoting understanding about cancer and its treatment, awareness of self, and personal skill development. They may focus on reducing or resolving the individual's psychosocial distress immediately (crisis intervention), or on a short-term (adjustment counseling, brief psychotherapy) or long-term (psychotherapy) basis. Perhaps the most straightforward way of categorizing the interventions is by mode of delivery, whether group or individual.

Group programs for patients with cancer exist in many forms and have been designed to achieve various purposes. **Psychoeducational** groups usually are structured, time-limited education provided in a supportive environment. Participants learn about specific topics and often gather a sense of confidence or empowerment as they learn. Participants become informed consumers and feel more capable to take control in their care. **Psychotherapy** groups may offer cognitive restructuring, stress management training, and behavioral training (e.g., biofeedback, hypnosis, progressive relaxation). These groups must have a licensed professional with training in psychology, behavioral medicine, or psychiatry as a leader. **Support** groups tend to bring individuals together for mutual learning, sharing, and understanding. These groups tend to be more open-ended in terms of time frame and agenda and provide participants an opportunity to talk about their feelings and current concerns. Some operate on a "drop-in" format. **Expressive-supportive** groups use art, music, or other expressive forms as an avenue to express feelings and stimulate discussions. Additionally, group programs may be offered as a workshop or as a retreat, lasting various lengths of time (e.g., day, weekend, week). Some programs include only patients, whereas others also embrace family members.

Ideally, cancer centers should offer a structured psychosocial program that consists of health education, stress management, behavioral training, instruction in coping and problem-solving techniques, and support groups, especially for those newly diagnosed or in the early stages of treatment (Fawzy, Fawzy, Arndt, & Pasnau, 1995). Unfortunately, significant variation remains in the availability of these programs as standard offerings in cancer centers (Coluzzi et al., 1995). Lack of qualified staff and lack of funding are critical factors influencing this variation.

Individual therapy may be more appropriate for people with an aversion to group settings, those needing crisis intervention, or those with well-entrenched problems needing in-depth psychotherapy. Individual therapy is particularly helpful for patients who use inappropriate or ineffective methods of coping with stress and resolving their illness-related problems. The individual therapy format offers the best opportunity to tailor interventions to the specific person. The desired outcomes for individual intervention are similar to those of the psychotherapy group intervention and can be achieved through this modality (Smith & Glass, 1977).

Several challenges exist in trying to review the cancer literature on psychosocial interventions. Authors have reported on a wide range of techniques and have combined various interventions in their programs. Authors are inconsistent in their use of terminology, and various definitions exist for the same word. The combination of specific techniques within similarly labeled programs frequently differs, as do the desired outcomes of interest. Some programs focus on physical symptoms (e.g., pain, fatigue) as well as psychosocial issues (e.g., anxiety, worries, family concerns), whereas others focus only on psychosocial matters. Finally, similarly named outcomes (e.g., quality of life, emotional well-being) are defined somewhat differently and measured differently from study to study. This situation makes it difficult to compare across studies, and the variability has contributed to slow uptake and clinical utilization of the research in this field. Additionally, small sample sizes, the use of specific tumor types, and the application of less rigorous methodologies (e.g., quasi-experimental) to evaluate interventions have been cited as barriers. Evidence has shown, overall, that psychosocial interventions are beneficial for patients, but no clear evidence supports the use of one specific model of care or framework over another. For the most part, the expressed preference clinically is for an eclectic approach to available psychosocial interventions or models and choices made on the basis of specific patient need. This is supported by several meta-analyses and systematic reviews of psychosocial intervention studies (Devine & Westlake, 1995; Iacovino & Reesor, 1997; Meyer & Mark, 1995; Watson, 1991).

Meyer and Mark (1995) used meta-analytic methods to synthesize the results of published, randomized controlled outcome studies of psychosocial interventions with adult patients with cancer. The focus was on nonpharmacologic interventions intended to improve the quality of life of adults diagnosed with cancer. Outcomes of interest included measures of emotional adjustment, functional adjustment, treatment- or disease-related symptoms, medical status, or some combination of these categories. Forty-five studies reporting 62 treatment-controlled comparisons were identified. The samples predominately were white females living in the United States. The treatment type categories included cognitive-behavioral, informational/educational, nonbehavioral counseling/psychotherapy, supportive, and unusual/combination. The results clearly indicated that psychosocial interventions have positive effects on emotional adjustment (effect size d = 0.24), functional adjustment (effect size d = 0.19), and treatment- and disease-related symptoms (effect size d = 0.26). The authors recommended further investigations to isolate the effects of specific interventions, increase the impact of the interventions, and reduce the cost of delivering the interventions. This study was similar to Meyer's (1992) meta-analysis of 92 controlled studies of informational, counseling, hospice, and nonprofessional social support interventions used in the care of adults with cancer. Meyer reported modest beneficial effects on the outcomes of functional adjustment (d = 0.25, n = 36 studies), symptoms related to treatment and disease (d = 0.28, n = 41 studies), emotional adjustment (d = 0.31, n = 77 studies), and medical measures (d = 0.34, n = 6 studies).

Devine and Westlake (1995) explored the effects of psychoeducational care provided to adults with cancer in a meta-analysis of 116 studies. The outcomes of interest included anxiety, depression, mood, nausea, vomiting, pain, and knowledge. Across all types of psychoeducational care, statistically significant beneficial effects were found on all seven outcomes examined. The authors suggested that clinicians could use many types of psychoeducational care to reduce both anxiety and depression, but fewer research-based interventions were available for other outcomes. Behavioral strategies (e.g., relaxation, relaxation with guided imagery, systematic desensitization) have been well tested and are effective for nausea; relaxation strategies are effective for pain; and teaching interventions result in increased knowledge. These authors also indicated that little evidence supported the choice of one specific psychoeducational approach/technique over another.

A more recent review by Iacovino and Reesor (1997) described the practical benefits of 33 studies evaluating the effects of psychosocial interventions on patients' adjustment to cancer. The studies were classified according to methodology (i.e., descriptive, quasi-experimental, retrospective, and controlled clinical outcome trials) and included a range of interventional approaches (i.e., individual, group, behavioral, educational, multiple components). These authors concluded that a variety of interventions can be effective and enhance how patients cope with psychosocial issues. No one intervention appeared to be more effective than others in helping people to adapt to their situation. It is important to note, however, that the 33 studies included different interventions directed to different and specific issues, all of which contributed to overall adjustment. For example, educational approaches helped with lack of information, behavioral interventions helped to manage stress reactions to treatment, and support-oriented forms of intervention helped with interpersonal or existential concerns. Overall, these authors determined by their critical review that individual and group interventions did not differ in effectiveness, and higher levels of adjustment were attained more on the basis of preferences and personality than on therapeutic approaches or content.

Finally, Abbey, Stewart, and Katz (2002) assessed the level of evidence available for specific psychosocial interventions in breast cancer. The team focused on the interventions of education, integrated programs, stress management, cognitive-behavioral, behavioral, psychotherapy, social support, exercise, and nutrition. Level 1 evidence (D'Agostino & Kwan, 1995) exists only for specific interventions of education, cognitive-behavioral, and psychotherapy as single modalities with quality-of-life outcomes (Edmonds, Lockwood, & Cunningham, 1999; Fawzy & Fawzy, 1998; Helgeson, Cohen, Schulz, & Yasko, 1999; Spiegel, Bloom, & Yalom, 1981; Spiegel et al., 1989). These authors called for more research regarding individual modalities and use of psychosocial interventions in special populations of women (e.g., rural, lesbian, aboriginal, at risk for familial breast cancer). Part of the challenge in studying specific group therapies has been the lack of standardization. Recently, several authors have begun to try to standardize psychosocial group interventions and investigate their efficacy. Successes have been reported for supportive expressive therapy for metastatic (Classen et al., 2001) and early-stage (Spiegel et al., 1999) breast cancers; mindfulness meditation-based stress reduction for patients with many different types of cancer (Carlson, Ursuliak, Goodey, Angen, & Speca, 2001; Speca, Carlson, Goodey, & Angen, 2000); and standardized group psychoeducation for patients with any kind of cancer diagnosis (Cunningham, Edmonds, Jenkins, & Lockwood, 1995).

Conclusion

In summary, providing access to psychosocial interventions is an important part of supportive care for patients with cancer and their family members to achieve quality-of-life outcomes. Systematic approaches are needed to inform patients about what psychosocial services are available, to identify what type of assistance is both needed and desired, and to refer to the appropriate services (professional and peer) as required. A range of psychosocial programs ought to be available so that individuals may select the type of program that best matches their style of learning, personality, and way of coping.

Special thanks to Judi Johnson, RN, PhD, FAAN, and Mary B. Johnson, RN, PhD, OCN®, who served as the authors of this chapter in the first edition.

References

Abbey, S., Stewart, D., & Katz, M. (2002). *Literature review: Behavioural guidelines for adjusting to medical conditions.* Toronto, Ontario, Canada: Ontario Women's Health Council.

Adams, M. (1991). Information and education across the phases of cancer care. *Seminars in Oncology Nursing, 7,* 105–111.

Agre, P., Dougherty, J., & Pirone, J. (2002). Creating a CD-ROM program for cancer-related patient education. *Oncology Nursing Forum, 29,* 573–580.

Ashbury, F.D. (1999, March). *Literature review to determine the optimal means for design and disseminate clinical practice guidelines to persons who are "underserved."* Unpublished report submitted to Adult Health Division, Health Canada, Ottawa, Ontario.

Ashbury, F.D., Cameron, C., Mercer, S.L., Fitch, M., & Nielsen, E. (1998). One-on-one peer support and quality of life for breast cancer patients. *Patient Education and Counseling, 35,* 89–100.

Ashbury, F.D., Findley, H., Reynolds, B., & McKerracher, K. (1998). A Canadian survey of patients' experiences: Are their needs being met? *Journal of Pain and Symptom Management, 16,* 298–306.

Bakker, D.A., Fitch, M.I., Gray, R., Reed, E., & Bennet, J. (2001). Patient–health care provider communication during chemotherapy treatment: The perspectives of women with breast cancer. *Patient Education and Counseling, 43,* 61–71.

Blake-Mortimer, J., Gore-Felton, C., Kimberling, R., Turner-Cobb, J.M., & Spiegel, D. (1999). Improving the quality and quantity of life among patients with cancer: A review of the effectiveness of group psychotherapy. *European Journal of Cancer, 35,* 1581–1586.

Borkman, T. (1990). Self-help groups at the turning point: Emerging egalitarian alliances with the formal health care system? *American Journal of Psychology, 18,* 321–332.

Broadhead, W.E., & Kaplan, B.H. (1991). Social support and the cancer patient: Implications for future research and clinical care. *Cancer, 67*(Suppl. 3), 794–799.

Browne, G.B., Arpin, K., Corey, P., Fitch, M., & Gafni, A. (1990). Individual correlates of health service utilization and the cost of poor adjustment to chronic illness. *Medical Care, 18,* 43–58.

Bucher, J. (Ed.). (1999). *The application of problem-solving therapy to psychosocial oncology care.* New York: Haworth Medical Press.

Bui, L., Last, L., Bradley, H., Law, C., Maier, B., & Smith, A. (2002). Interest and participation in support group programs among patients with colorectal cancer. *Cancer Nursing, 24,* 150–157.

Butow, P., Bundle, E., McConnell, D., Boakes, R., & Tattersall, M.H.N. (1998). Information booklets about cancer factors influencing patient satisfaction and utilization. *Patient Education and Counseling, 33,* 129–141.

Butow, P.N., Kazemi, J.N., Beeney, L.J., Griffin, A., Dunn, S.M., & Tattersall, M.H. (1996). When the diagnosis is cancer. *Cancer, 77,* 2630–2637.

Canadian Cancer Society. (1992). *The final report of the needs of persons living with cancer across Canada.* Toronto, Ontario, Canada: Author.

Canadian Cancer Society. (1998). *Cancer Connection evaluation report.* Toronto, Ontario, Canada: Author.

Carlson, L.E., & Bultz, B.D. (2002). Efficacy vs. cost of psychosocial interventions. *Oncology Exchange, 1*(2), 34–39, 49–51.

Carlson, L.E., & Bultz, B.D. (2003). Cancer distress screening: Needs, models, and methods. *Journal of Psychosomatic Research, 55,* 403–409.

Carlson, L.E., Ursuliak, Z., Goodey, E., Angen, M., & Speca, M. (2001). The effects of a mindfulness meditation-based stress reduction program on mood and symptoms of stress in cancer outpatients: 6-month follow-up. *Supportive Care in Cancer, 9,* 112–123.

Cella, D.F., Tulsky, D.S., Gray, G., Sarafian, B., Linn, E., Bonomi, A., et al. (1993). The Functional Assessment of Cancer Therapy Scale: Development and validation of the general measure. *Journal of Clinical Oncology, 11,* 570–579.

Classen, C., Butler, L.D., Koopman, C., Miller, E., Dimiceli, S., Giese-Davis, J., et al. (2001). Supportive expressive group therapy and distress in patients with metastatic breast cancer: A randomized clinical intervention. *Archives of General Psychiatry, 58,* 494–501.

Coates, A. (1997). Quality of life and supportive care. *Supportive Care in Cancer, 5,* 435–438.

Coluzzi, P.H., Grant, M., Doroshow, J.H., Rhiner, M., Ferrell, B., & Rivera, L. (1995). Survey of the provision of supportive care services at National Cancer Institute-designated cancer centers. *Journal of Clinical Oncology, 13,* 756–764.

Cunningham, A.J., Edmonds, C.V., Jenkins, G., & Lockwood, G.A. (1995). A randomized comparison of two forms of a brief group. *International Journal of Psychiatric Medicine, 25,* 173–189.

Cunningham, A.J., Edmonds, C.V., Phillips, C., Soots, K.I., Hedley, D., & Lockwood, G.A. (2000). A prospective longitudinal study of the relationship of psychological work to duration of survival in patients with metastatic cancer. *Psycho-Oncology, 9,* 323–339.

D'Agostino, R.B., & Kwan, H. (1995). Measuring effectiveness: What to expect without a randomized control group. *Medical Care, 33*(Suppl. 4), AS95–AS105.

Damian, D., & Tattersall, M.H. (1991). Letters to patients: Improving communication in cancer care. *Lancet, 338,* 923–925.

Davison, B.J., & Degner, L.F. (1997). Empowerment of men newly diagnosed with prostate cancer. *Cancer Nursing, 20,* 187–196.

Davison, B.J., Degner, L.F., & Morgan, T.R. (1995). Information and decision-making preferences of men with prostate cancer. *Oncology Nursing Forum, 22,* 1401–1408.

Degner, L.F., & Sloan, J.A. (1995). Symptom distress in newly diagnosed ambulatory cancer patients as an indicator of survival in lung cancer. *Journal of Pain and Symptom Management, 10,* 423–431.

Derogatis, L.R., Morrow, G.R., Fetting, J., Penman, D., Piasetsky, S., Schmale, A.M., et al. (1983). The prevalence of psychiatric disorders among cancer patients. *JAMA, 11,* 751–757.

Devine, E.C., & Westlake, S.K. (1995). The effects of psychoeducational care provided to adults with cancer: Meta-analysis of 116 studies. *Oncology Nursing Forum, 22,* 1369–1381.

Dunkel-Schetter, C. (1984). Social support and cancer: Findings based on patient interviews and their implications. *Journal of Social Issues, 40*(4), 77–98.

Edgar, L., Greenberg, A., & Remmer, J. (2002). Providing Internet lessons to oncology patients and family members: A shared project. *Psycho-Oncology, 11,* 439–446.

Edmonds, C.V., Lockwood, G.A., & Cunningham, A.J. (1999). Psychological response to long-term group therapy: A randomized trial with metastatic breast cancer patients. *Psycho-Oncology, 8,* 74–91.

Farber, J.M., Weinerman, B.H., & Kuypers, J.A. (1984). Psychosocial distress in oncology outpatients. *Journal of Psychosocial Oncology, 2*(3/4), 109–118.

Fawzy, F.I. (1999). Psychosocial interventions for patients with cancer: What works and what doesn't. *European Journal of Cancer, 35,* 1559–1564.

Fawzy, F.I., Fawzy, N., Arndt, L., & Pasnau, R. (1995). Critical review of psychosocial interventions in cancer care. *Archives of General Psychiatry, 2,* 100–114.

Fawzy, F.I., & Fawzy, N.W. (1998). Psychoeducational interventions. In J.C. Holland (Ed.), *Psycho-oncology* (pp. 676–693). New York: Oxford University Press.

Fisher, B., & Britten, N. (1993). Patient access to records: Expectations of hospital doctors and experiences of cancer patients. *British Journal of General Practice, 43,* 52–56.

Fitch, M. (2000). Supportive care for cancer patients. *Hospital Quarterly, 3,* 39–46.

Fitch, M. (2002, April). *Providing supportive care to cancer patients.* Presentation report to the Cancer Quality Council, Cancer Care Ontario, Toronto, Canada.

Fitch, M., Gray, R.E., & Franssen, E. (2000). Women's perspectives regarding the impact of ovarian cancer. *Cancer Nursing, 23,* 359–366.

Fitch, M., Gray, R.E., Greenberg, M., Carroll, J., Chart, P., & Orr, V. (2001). Self-help groups: Oncology nurses' perspectives. *Canadian Oncology Nursing Journal, 11,* 76–81.

Fitch, M.I., Vachon, M., Greenberg, M., & Franssen, E. (1996, August). *Needs of cancer patients and their family members attending a comprehensive cancer centre.* Paper presented at the 9th International Conference on Cancer Nursing, Brighton, England.

Fox, S., & Rainie, L. (2002). *Vital decisions: How Internet users decide what information to trust when they or their loved ones are sick.* Washington, DC: Pew Internet and American Life Project.

Gray, R., Fitch, M., Davis, C., & Phillips, C. (1996). Breast cancer and prostate cancer self-help groups: Reflections on differences. *Psychosocial Oncology, 5,* 137–142.

Gray, R.E., Fitch, M., Davis, C., & Phillips, C. (1997a). Interviews with men with prostate cancer about their self-help group experience. *Journal of Palliative Care, 13*(1), 15–21.

Gray, R.E., Fitch, M., Davis, C., & Phillips, C. (1997b). A qualitative study of breast cancer self-help groups. *Psychosocial Oncology, 6,* 279–289.

Gray, R.E., Fitch, M., Phillips, C., Labrecque, M., & Fergus, K. (2000). Managing the impact of illness: The experiences of men with prostate cancer and their spouses. *Journal of Health Psychology, 5,* 525–542.

Gray, R.E., Greenberg, M., Fitch, M., Sawka, C., Hampson, A., Labrecque, M., et al. (1998). Information needs of women with metastatic breast cancer. *Cancer Prevention and Control, 2,* 57–62.

Greer, S. (1992). The management of denial in cancer patients. *Oncology, 6*(12), 39–40.

Hack, T.F., Pickles, T., Bultz, B., Degner, L., Katz, A., & Davison, B. (1999). Feasibility of an audiotaped intervention for patients with cancer: A multicenter, randomized, controlled pilot study. *Journal of Psychosocial Oncology, 17*(2), 1–15.

Helgeson, V.S., Cohen, S., Schulz, R., & Yasko, J. (1999). Education and peer discussion group interventions and adjustment to breast cancer. *Archives of General Psychiatry, 56,* 340–347.

Hinds, C., Streater, A., & Mood, D. (1995). Functions and preferred methods of receiving information related to radiotherapy. *Cancer Nursing, 18,* 374–384.

Hogben, B., & Fallowfield, L. (1989). Getting it taped: The "bad" news consultation with cancer patients. *British Journal of Hospital Medicine, 41,* 330–333.

Holland, J.C. (1999). NCCN practice guidelines for the management of psychosocial distress. *Oncology, 13*(5A), 113–147.

Holland, J.C., & Rolland, D. (Eds.). (1989). *Handbook of psychooncology: Psychological care of the patient with cancer.* New York: Oxford University Press.

House, J.S. (1987). Social support and social structure. *Social Forum, 2,* 135–146.

Houts, P.S., Rusenas, I., Simmonds, M.A., & Hufford, D.L. (1991). Information needs of families of cancer patients: A literature review and recommendations. *Journal of Cancer Education, 6,* 255–261.

Houts, P.S., Yasko, J.M., Harvey, H.A., Kahn, S.B., Hartz, A.J., Hermann, J.F., et al. (1988). Unmet needs of persons with cancer in Pennsylvania during the period of terminal care. *Cancer, 62,* 627–634.

Iacovino, V., & Reesor, K. (1997). Literature on interventions to address cancer patients' psychosocial needs: What does it tell us? *Journal of Psychosocial Oncology, 15*(2), 47–71.

Johnson, J.E., Nail, L.M., Lauver, D., King, K.B., & Keys, H. (1988). Reducing the negative impact of radiation therapy on functional status. *Cancer, 61,* 46–51.

Kaasa, S., Mastekaasa, A., & Lund, E. (1989). Prognostic factors for patients with inoperable non-small cell lung cancer, limited disease: The importance of patients' subjective experience of disease and psychosocial well-being. *Radiotherapy and Oncology, 15,* 235–242.

Kaegi, E. (1999, January). *Effective communication strategies to reach selected population groups with cancer-related educational materials.* Unpublished report submitted to Cancer Care Ontario, Toronto, Canada.

Kristjanson, L.J., & Ashcroft, T. (1994). The family's cancer journey: A literature review. *Cancer Nursing, 17,* 1–17.

Kurtz, L.F. (1990). The self-help movement: Review of the past decade of research. *Social Work Groups, 13,* 101–115.

Lazarus, R.S., & Folkman, S. (1984). *Stress, appraisal and coping.* New York: Springer.

Luker, K.A., Beaver, K., Lenster, S.J., & Owens, R.G. (1996). Information needs and sources of information for women with breast cancer: A follow-up study. *Journal of Advanced Nursing, 23,* 487–495.

McQuellon, R.P., Wells, M., Hoffman, S., Graven, B., Russell, G., Cruz, J., et al. (1998). Reducing distress in cancer patients with an orientation program. *Psycho-Oncology, 7,* 207–217.

Meyer, J.T. (1992). Meta-analysis of controlled studies of psychosocial interventions with adult cancer patients. *Dissertation Abstracts International, 52,* 4475B. (UMI No. 92 of 252)

Meyer, J.T., & Mark, M.M. (1995). Effects of psychosocial interventions with adult cancer patients: A meta-analysis of randomized experiments. *Health Psychology, 14,* 101–108.

Moorey, S., Greer, S., Bliss, J., & Law, M. (1998). A comparison of adjuvant psychological therapy and supportive counseling in patients with cancer. *Psycho-Oncology, 7,* 218–228.

Muzzin, L.J., Anderson, N.J., Figueredo, A.T., & Gudelis, S.O. (1994). The experience of cancer. *Social Science and Medicine, 38,* 1201–1208.

National Cancer Institute. (2002, November). *Normal adjustment, psychosocial distress, and the adjustment disorders (PDQ®).* Retrieved May 6, 2005, from http://cancer.gov/cancertopics/pdq/supportivecare/adjustment/patient

National Comprehensive Cancer Network. (2005, February). Distress management. *Clinical practice guidelines in oncology v.1.2005.* Jenkintown, PA: Author. Retrieved April 29, 2005, from http://www.nccn.org/physician_gls/index.html

Nelles, W.B., McCaffrey, R.J., Blanchard, C.G., & Ruckdeschel, J.C. (1991). Social supports and breast cancer: A review. *Journal of Psychosocial Oncology, 9*(2), 21–34.

Nicholas, D.R., & Veach, T.A. (2000). The psychosocial assessment of the adult cancer patient. *Professional Psychology: Research and Practice, 31,* 206–215.

Northouse, L.L. (1988). Family issues in cancer care. *Advanced Psychosomatic Medicine, 18,* 82–101.

Padilla, G.V., & Bulcavage, L.M. (1991). Theories used in patient health education. *Seminars in Oncology Nursing, 7,* 87–96.

Patrick-Miller, L., Much, J., & Axelrod, A. (2002). Psychosocial distress screening of ambulatory oncology patients [Abstract 1519]. *Proceedings of the American Society of Clinical Oncology, 21.*

Rainey, L.C. (1985). Effects of preparatory patient education for radiation oncology patients. *Cancer, 56,* 1056–1061.

Reynolds, P.M., Sanson-Fisher, R.W., Poole, A.D., Harker, J., & Byrne, M. (1981). Cancer and communication: Information-giving in an oncology clinic. *BMJ, 282,* 1449–1451.

Richardson, G.E., & Johnson, B.E. (1999). The biology of lung cancer. *Seminars in Oncology, 20,* 105–127.

Riessman, F., & Carroll, D. (1995). *Redefining self-help.* San Francisco: Jossey-Bass.

Roth, A.J., Kornblith, A.B., Batel-Copel, L., Peabody, E., Scher, H.I., & Holland, J.C. (1998). Rapid screening for psychologic distress in men with prostate carcinoma: A pilot study. *Cancer, 82,* 1904–1908.

Sellick, S.M. (2001, October). *Screening for psychosocial distress.* Presentation at Cancer Care Ontario Conference, "Working Together: Across the Cancer Continuum," Toronto, Ontario, Canada.

Shaw, B.R., McTavish, F., Hawkins, R., Gustafson, D.H., & Pingree, S. (2000). Experiences of women with breast cancer: Exchanging social support over the CHESS computer network. *Journal of Health Communication, 5,* 135–159.

Smith, M.L., & Glass, G.V. (1977). Meta-analysis of psychotherapy outcome studies. *American Psychologist, 32,* 752–760.

Speca, M., Carlson, L.E., Goodey, E., & Angen, M. (2000). A randomized wait-list controlled clinical trial: The effect of a mindfulness meditation stress reduction program on mood and symptoms of stress in cancer outpatients. *Psychosomatic Medicine, 62,* 613–622.

Spiegel, D., Bloom, J.R., Kraemer, H.C., & Grottheil, E. (1989). Effect of psychosocial treatment on survival of patients with metastatic breast cancer. *Lancet, 2,* 888–891.

Spiegel, D., Bloom, J.R., & Yalom, I. (1981). Group support for patients with metastatic cancer: A randomized outcome study. *Archives of General Psychiatry, 38,* 527–533.

Spiegel, D., Morrow, G.R., Classen, C., Raubertas, R., Stott, P.B., & Mudaliar, N. (1999). Group psychotherapy for recently diagnosed breast cancer patients: A multi-center feasibility study. *Psycho-Oncology, 8,* 482–493.

Stam, H.J., Bultz, B.D., & Pittman, C.A. (1986). Psychosocial problems and interventions in a referred sample of cancer patients. *Psychosomatic Medicine, 48,* 539–548.

Tattersall, M.H.N., Butow, P.N., & Clayton, J.M. (2002). Insights from cancer patient communication research. *Hematology/Oncology Clinics of North America, 16,* 731–743.

Taylor, S.E. (1983). Adjustment to threatening events: A theory of cognitive adaptation. *American Psychologist, 38,* 1161–1173.

Till, J.E. (2003). Evaluation of support groups for women with breast cancer: Importance of the navigator role. *Health and Quality of Life Outcomes, 1,* 16.

Tyson, T. (2000). The Internet: Tomorrow's portal to non-traditional health care services. *Journal of Ambulatory Care Management, 23*(2), 1–7.

Vahabi, M., & Ferris, L. (1995). Improving written patient education materials: A review of the evidence. *Health Education Journal, 54,* 99–106.

van't Spijker, A., Trijsburg, R.W., & Duivenvoorden, H.J. (1997). Psychological sequelae of cancer diagnosis: A meta-analytical review of 58 studies after 1980. *Psychosomatic Medicine, 59,* 280–293.

Watson, M. (1991). Breast cancer. In M. Watson (Ed.), *Cancer patient care: Psychosocial treatment methods* (pp. 222–237). Cambridge, England: British Psychological Society and Cambridge University Press.

Weisman, A.D. (1979). A model of psychosocial phasing in cancer. *General Hospital Psychiatry, 1,* 187–195.

Wyatt, G., Kurtz, M.E., & Liken, M. (1993). Breast cancer survivors: An exploration of quality of life issues. *Cancer Nursing, 16,* 440–448.

Zabora, J., BrintzenhofeSzoc, K., Curbow, B., Hooker, C., & Piantadosi, S. (2001). The prevalence of psychosocial distress by cancer site. *Psycho-Oncology, 10*(1), 19–28.

Zabora, J., BrintzenhofeSzoc, K., Jacobson, P., Curbow, B., Piantadosi, S., Hooker, C., et al. (2001). A new psychosocial screening instrument for use with cancer patients. *Psychosomatics, 42,* 241–246.

Zigmond, A.S., & Snaith, R.P. (1983). The hospital anxiety and depression scale. *Acta Psychiatrica Scandinavica, 67,* 361–370.

CHAPTER 26

Technologic Advances: Psychosocial Implications for Patient Care

PAULA KLEMM, DNSc, RN, OCN®

Although the world is full of suffering, it is also full of the overcoming of it.

—Helen Keller

The current revolution in computer technology has affected both the physical and psychosocial aspects of health care. However, "computers" are not new. People have used some device for counting and computing as far back as recorded history shows. The abacus was used for centuries in Egypt and appeared in the Near East and China about 2,000 years ago. In the 1600s, John Napier used numbered white rods that, when arranged side by side, were used to multiply numbers. Jacquard's Loom (1804) used paper cards that were prepunched with coded information to program and control the weaving process. In the 1800s, Charles Babbage proposed an analytical engine designed to carry out multiple mathematical calculations that integrated the basic components used in modern computers. "Babbage's folly" was never built, but he was years ahead of his time. It was not until the 1940s that a Harvard University engineer built the first large-scale, automatic, electric computer incorporating the ideas of Charles Babbage (Griffiths, 2002; Gromov, 2003; Richey, 1997).

In the early 1950s, the UNIVAC1 became the first commercially available electronic computer that used the binary system to process data. It was expensive, contained 5,000 vacuum tubes, and required an air conditioner to keep the components cool. Soon after this, President Eisenhower created the Advanced Research Projects Agency to fund high-powered space and scientific research. Computer technology advanced steadily from the use of vacuum tubes to transistors and then integrated circuits. In 1971, the introduction of the silicon chip allowed large amounts of data to be stored in much smaller computers. Today's descendents of these early computers are smaller, faster, and smarter and have led to the technologic revolution in health care (Gray, 1996; Griffiths, 2002).

Technology and Health Care

The psychosocial impact of a cancer diagnosis can be devastating for patients, families, and caregivers. Patients confronted with an uncertain future may experience a sense of helplessness, anxiety, depression, and a fear of death. In addition, patients facing a serious illness often experience existential and financial concerns (Manne, Glassman, & DuHamel, 2001; Zabora, BrintzenhofeSzoc, Curbow, Hooker, & Piantadosi, 2001). However, technologic advances have important psychological and social implications for patient care. For example, advances in computer capabilities have led to improvements in laparoscopic services, radiation therapy, and diagnostic procedures. Computer technology has furnished healthcare professionals with rapid access to the most up-to-date medical information in the world. Physicians are able to provide timely information to patients regarding diagnosis, treatment options, prognosis, and risk factors for cancer. As a result, the diagnosis of a malignancy may take a matter of hours rather than days or weeks, with treatment beginning earlier in the course of the disease. Technologic advances in molecular biology and gene therapy have led to a better understanding of the risk factors for some cancers and to new treatment options for others. Individuals with a familial history of malignancy (e.g., breast, thyroid, ovarian) may undergo genetic testing to help to determine their risk of developing cancer. The results of these tests may have profound positive (or negative) psychological effects.

Although not currently used in most hospitals, computerized physician order entry may help to prevent transcription errors, eliminate duplication of laboratory/diagnostic tests, shorten length of stay, and improve prescribing (Kuperman & Gibson, 2003; Teich et al., 2000). One report indicated that medication turnaround times, radiology procedure completion times, and laboratory result reporting times were significantly reduced as a result of computerized order entry and electronic medication administration record use (Mekhjian et al., 2002). In addition, the authors of these studies reported that all physician and nurse transcription errors were eliminated. The financial and psychological benefits of this technology to patients are self-evident.

Recently, the U.S. Food and Drug Administration approved a proposed regulation requiring the use of bar codes on single packages of prescription drugs, over-the-counter medications, and biologics (e.g., blood) (Becker, 2003). The Agency for Healthcare Research and Quality estimated that medication errors cost between $2,500 and $5,000 for each adverse drug event in 2001 (Haugh, 2003). Bar coding may cut medication errors by up to 80% and minimize associated financial and emotional consequences to patients as a result (Haugh).

Mobile computing devices are growing in popularity among healthcare workers, who use them to access, record, and transmit information (Waegemann & Tessier, 2002). Personal digital assistants (PDAs) can be used to review pharmaceutical information, chart patient care, or organize daily activities. Nurses are choosing PDAs because they can be used at patients' bedsides to document care, thus leaving more time for psychosocial and educational interventions (Lewis & Sommers, 2003; Stolworthy, 2003). Other devices known as mobile healthcare computing devices (MHCDs) combine several functions and can be used as a pager, cell phone, PDA, and port to the Internet. In addition, MHCDs can be used to prescribe medications, enter orders related to patient care, and keep track of health-related charges (Waegemann & Tessier). These examples illustrate how technologic advances can improve and augment comprehensive health care.

A recent report indicated that more than 60% of Americans currently have Internet access, with 40% having been online for three years or more (Horrigan & Rainie, 2002). Americans frequently access the Internet for healthcare information, with 67% stating that they can find reliable health-related information online (Horrigan & Rainie). Advantages associated with Internet use include access 24 hours a day, 7 days a week, availability to the disabled, lack of geographic boundaries, support for people with rare diseases, anonymity, and the greater likelihood that men may join an online support group (Fawcett & Buhle, 1995; Gustafson et al., 1993; Klemm, Reppert, & Visich, 1998). Another major psychosocial benefit of Internet access is that it may help to decrease the sense of isolation for individuals who are homebound as a result of disability or disease (Bradley & Poppen, 2003). Costs (e.g., computer, modem, Internet access), unreliable information, lack of physical contact, and large volumes of information are disadvantages associated with Internet use. In addition, disability, ethnic minority status, economic disadvantage, low literacy levels, visual impairments, and lack of culturally appropriate or age-specific information may impede Internet use (Fogel, 2003; Han & Belcher, 2001; Kaye, 2000; Larrison, Nackerud, Risler, & Sullivan, 2002; Sperazza, 2001).

Telemedicine

The ready availability of computer technology has led to the rise of telemedicine, a term that was first coined in the early 1970s. Although several definitions exist, "telemedicine" essentially refers to the practice of patients and healthcare workers exchanging medical information at a distance through the use of electronic communications. Information exchange may occur via audio, video, or computer networks and has been used for education, consultation, diagnosis, treatment, and transfer of information (ADV Communications, 2003). Healthcare professionals can earn continuing education credit or research specific diseases using Internet sources.

Online communication is a nontraditional means of offering informational and psychosocial support to people with cancer. E-mail offers quick and easy communication between patients and healthcare workers. Similar to other forms of communication, problems inherent to e-mail exist. Subtleties that are obvious in verbal or face-to-face communication may be missed in textual messages, or messages may become lost in "cyberspace." However, e-mail communication has evolved over the years, and a cyber-language has developed to help to overcome the textual limitations of messages posted online. For example, individuals may send "cyber hugs," use emoticons (e.g., a smiley face), or write abbreviations (e.g., LOL [laugh out loud]) to express emotions. Inserting appropriate Internet links, diagrams, photos, or videos may enhance the textual aspect of e-mail as well (Finichel et al., 2003).

People who are hearing impaired, those who travel extensively, or those suffering from the side effects of cancer therapy may prefer e-mail communications with healthcare professionals. The benefits associated with e-mail communications between healthcare providers and patients include simplicity and convenience. However, these are tempered by threats to patient privacy, potential security breaches, and legal liability issues (Baker, 2003; Mandl, Kohane, & Brandt, 1998) (see Figure 26-1). The American Medical Association has published guidelines for physician-patient electronic communications to help to diminish problems related to this form of communication (Robertson, 2003). Even so, one report indicated that physicians have yet to adopt e-mail communications on a wide scale with their patients (Eysenbach, 2003). Reasons attributed to this include fear of increased demands on practitioner time, insufficient time during office hours to respond to patients' e-mails, inability to provide responses in a timely manner, confidentiality issues, and lack of reimbursement (Moyer, Stern, Dobias, Cox, & Katz, 2002; Patt, Houston, Jenckes, Sands, & Ford, 2003).

Figure 26-1. Risks and Benefits of Provider-Patient E-Mail Communication

Benefits
- Convenient access to care
- 24-hour availability
- Creation of a written record of what information was covered
- Inexpensive
- Inclusion of educational material to reinforce teaching
- Asynchronous communication
- Improved compliance with care
- Use of graphics, videos, and photos to enhance information

Risks
- Threats to patient privacy and confidentiality
- Barriers to access (i.e., "digital divide")
- Delayed responses to urgent messages
- Large volume of e-mail to healthcare providers
- Inappropriate use of e-mail by providers/patients
- Legal liability issues
- Threats to security of information
- Messages lost in "cyberspace"

Online Support

Not surprisingly, the use of a telemedicine tool (e.g., the Internet) helps individuals to cope with the psychosocial issues related to a cancer diagnosis. For more than 30 years, people with cancer have turned to support groups to help them to cope with their disease (Fobair, 1997). More recently, individuals with cancer and their care-givers have turned to the Internet for online support. Traditionally, cancer support groups used a face-to-face format and met on a regular basis with a trained healthcare facilitator (Cella & Yellen, 1993; Colon, 1996; Pillon & Joannides, 1991). However, the majority of online (i.e., Internet, computer-mediated) support groups do not engage the services of a professional facilitator. In general, people with cancer join online support groups to find information about their disease, provide cancer-related information, offer encouragement to others who have cancer, and problem solve (Gustafson et al., 1993; Klemm, Hurst, Dearholt, & Trone, 1999; Klemm & Wheeler, 2005; McTavish et al., 1995; Sharf, 1997).

Online cancer support groups are offered in several formats. For example, a "chat room" offers real time (synchronous) interaction with other members. Listservs offer asynchronous interaction in which messages are posted online and members may respond to them whenever they choose (Madara & White, 1997). Essentially, people interested in online support "subscribe" or sign up and then are allowed to send and receive messages to a particular group. Most groups post simple rules called "netiquette" (net etiquette) to guide new subscribers ("newbies") when they interact with the online group. For example, users are instructed not to use all capital letters because it implies that they are shouting. Other rules may instruct users not to advertise, post chain letters, or speak harshly about group participants, a process known as "flaming."

Although the research base is limited, studies suggest that the Internet has changed the format but not the benefits of cancer support. Weinberg, Schmale, Uken, and Wessel (1996) reported that women with breast cancer were able to quickly master the skills needed for online participation and that messages generally focused on medical or personal concerns. Eight African American women with breast cancer were recruited to participate in a private online support group by McTavish et al. (1995). The researchers found that the women, all from impoverished neighborhoods, used the group most often for social support and information seeking. Sharf (1997) explored communication patterns in a private online group designed for women with breast cancer and identified three primary functions: information exchange, social support, and empowerment.

Two qualitative studies described categories of information exchanged on cancer support listservs (Klemm et al., 1999; Klemm & Nolan, 1998). Data analysis revealed that information exchange, encouragement/support, personal opinion, and personal experiences accounted for almost 80% of the messages posted. However, a difference existed between messages posted by men and those posted by women. Men who posted to a prostate cancer support group were more likely to give or seek information. Women who posted to a breast cancer support group were more likely to relate their personal experiences. As a group, men and women who posted to a colorectal support group were more likely to give or seek information, followed by offering encouragement/support (Klemm et al., 1999). Men may be more likely to subscribe to an online support group than join a face-to-face group. Although women outnumber men in face-to-face support groups (Cella & Yellen, 1993), one research study reported that men and women were represented equally on an online colorectal cancer support group (Klemm et al., 1998).

Internet use may have detrimental psychosocial effects under certain conditions. Kraut et al. (1998) reported that depression rates were higher the more time people spent on the Internet. Nie and Erbring (2000) studied Internet use in a representative sample of more than 4,000 individuals in the United States and reported that as Internet use increased, less time was spent with family and friends. A follow-up study indicated that depression rates decreased when the subjects were tested two years later (Kraut et al., 2002). Klemm and Hardie (2002) compared depression rates between face-to-face and online cancer support groups and found that 92% of the online group (as compared to 0% in the face-to-face group) had major depressive symptoms as measured by the Center for Epidemiologic Studies Depression Scale. Depression rates trended downward as the number of months on the online group increased. Additional research to explore the long-term effects of Internet use on depression needs to be conducted.

Contrasting results occurred in a study conducted in California that used professional therapists to facilitate online support groups for women with breast cancer. The researchers reported that depression rates decreased as a result of participation in the online groups (*Americans Use Net*, 2002). Winzelberg et al. (2003) explored the effects of participation in a 12-week, professionally facilitated online support group on depression, cancer-related trauma, and perceived stress in 72 women with breast cancer. Results indicated that the women had decreased scores on all three variables. Although a number of studies have focused attention on Internet support groups, most have focused on women with breast cancer. Outcome data on the psychological and psychosocial efficacy of these groups are limited (Bessell et al., 2002; Eysenbach, 2003; Klemm et al., 2003).

A problem that must be addressed before online social support can become universally available is that of the "digital divide." The digital divide has been described as a difference in computer ownership between the general population of the United States and the economically disadvantaged (Larrison et al., 2002). Kaye (2000) reported that Americans who were disabled were more than 50% less likely to own a computer than individuals without disabilities and were 75% less likely to use the Internet. In addition, older adults, people with low incomes, and minorities are less likely to have computer access (Davis & Lafrado, 2003; Larrison et al.; Opalinski, 2001). Usability issues should be considered as well. For example, although older adults may have access to the Internet, vision changes may impair their ability to read the print on a computer screen. People who speak English as a second language or who cannot read or write English may have difficulty using available Internet resources, although they may have computer access. A great deal of healthcare information is available via the Internet, yet Web sites in the United States that focus on specific ethnic groups and incorporate culturally sensitive information are limited (Fogel, 2003). Consideration should be given to creating age-appropriate healthcare information on the Internet, especially for children and adolescents.

Ethical Issues

According to Bishop and Scudder (1996), nurses have a moral obligation to become competent practitioners. Healthcare professionals cannot practice effectively without the use of advanced technology, including computers. This being said, nurses should become competent in using the newest technologic advances that are available to them. Nurses and other healthcare professionals should be knowledgeable and competent with regard to using computer technology because it can influence overall patient care. In addition, nurses should follow appropriate guidelines for evaluating health-related Internet sites and share this information with their patients. Tools designed to evaluate Internet sites for healthcare information and continuing education units abound. Formats vary, but Web sites that provide healthcare information to the lay public should be evaluated according to author, audience, information, reliability, links, and graphics (see Table 26-1). Nurses and other healthcare professionals may find it useful to create a list of appropriate Internet sites for patients who have informational needs or who wish to subscribe to an online support group (see Table 26-2). Information changes rapidly on the Internet, and

Table 26-1. Suggested Criteria for Evaluation of Healthcare-Related Web Sites Designed for the Lay Public

Criterion	Details
Author/sponsoring organization	• Author/sponsoring organization is clearly identified. • Qualified: Author/sponsoring organization is qualified to address this topic. • Credible: Author/sponsoring organization has appropriate credentials. • Contact information: Content includes a means to contact the author/sponsoring organization.
Audience	• Site identifies the intended audience (e.g., patients, caretakers, adults, healthcare professionals).
Information	• Accuracy: Information is accurate and not based on testimonials, secondhand information, or hearsay. • Timeliness: Site creator provides current date or recent revision date. • Clarity: Information is concise and easy to understand for lay readers. • Comprehensiveness: Site sufficiently covers the topic.
Reliability	• Content includes references/bibliography. • Complete: Site is not "under construction." • Grammar, spelling, and punctuation are correct. • Site is not trying to "sell" a product. • Information is evidence based.
Links	• Links are functional and clearly visible. • URL (i.e., Web address) is correct. • Links on secondary pages lead back to home page.
Graphics	• Images load quickly. • Graphics are appropriate to the topic.

reviewing health-related Web sites occasionally to ensure that they are still active and that information is up to date is a good practice.

Several ethical issues are relevant with regard to computerized medical records, research conducted online, and e-mail communication. The Health Insurance Portability and Accountability Act of 1996 set new security standards to protect health-related information (Office for Civil Rights, U.S. Department of Health and Human Services, 2005). Preserving patient privacy and confidentiality are critical components of the healthcare environment, especially when patient information is stored in computerized medical files. Although firewalls and encrypted records may prevent hackers from accessing patient information, maintaining these standards often rests in the hands of healthcare professionals. A recent report indicated that more than 80% of all security breaches in patient privacy are enacted by healthcare employees (Leestma, 2003). The balance between easy access to health information and maintaining patient privacy must be maintained (Eysenbach & Till, 2001; Meaney, 2003).

Researchers are required to conduct ethical cyberspace research. The Belmont Report, published in 1978, stated that the principles of respect for persons (autonomy and avoidance of harm), beneficence (acting for the good of the patient), and justice (equal distribution of the risks and benefits) should guide scientists in the conduct

Table 26-2. Selected Cancer Information Sites on the Internet

Organization	Web Address
Association of Cancer Online Resources	www.acor.org
American Cancer Society	www.cancer.org
Centers for Disease Control and Prevention	www.cdc.gov
National Cancer Institute	http://cancer.gov/cancerinformation
National Center for Complementary and Alternative Medicine	http://nccam.nih.gov
National Institutes of Health	www.nih.gov
OncoLink	www.oncolink.com
Oncology Nursing Society	www.ons.org

of research (Department of Health, Education, and Welfare, 1978). Healthcare professionals who use technology (e.g., the Internet) to conduct research must be cognizant of the social element that is involved and the inherent risks to participants (Boehlefeld, 1996; Klemm & Nolan, 1998). Researchers must take care to protect patient privacy and obtain informed consent, unless doing so would compromise the integrity of the study. Furthermore, proposed research should be approved by an ethics committee, human subjects review board, or other appropriate authority before data collection begins. Decisions with regard to protection (e.g., firewalls, passwords, encryption), access, and storage of electronic data should be made prior the beginning the study.

Conclusion

The use of technology in health care continues to grow. The competent use of telemedicine by healthcare professionals has far-reaching implications for patient care. Children who were born in the 1990s are growing up in a digital world, where instant messaging, e-mail, PDAs, and chat rooms are commonplace. The Internet is becoming the place where Americans of all ages, races, and incomes are turning for healthcare information. E-mail has become an acceptable communication device between patients and their care providers. Healthcare professionals must have a working knowledge of the latest communication technology to comprehensively care for the medical, informational, and psychosocial needs of people with cancer.

References

ADV Communications. (2003). *Telemedicine.* Retrieved November 28, 2003, from http://www.advcomms.co.uk/telemedicine/definition.htm

Americans use Net to look after themselves. (2002, May). Retrieved September 21, 2003, from http://www.nua.ie/surveys/index.cgi?f=VS&art_id=905357995&rel=true

Baker, D.B. (2003). Provider-patient e-mail: With benefits come risks. *American Health Information Management Association, 74*(8), 22–29.

Becker, C. (2003, June 16). Scanning for higher profits: The FDA's plan to require bar codes on commonly used medical products will do more than improve patient safety. *Modern Healthcare, 33*(24), 6–7, 16.

Bessell, T.L., McDonald, S., Silagy, C., Anderson, J.N., Hiller, J.E., & Sansom, L.N. (2002). Do Internet interventions for consumers cause more harm than good? A systematic review. *Health Expectations, 5*, 28–37.

Bishop, A.H., & Scudder, J.R. (1996). *Nursing ethics: Therapeutic caring presence.* Sudbury, MA: Jones and Bartlett.

Boehlefeld, S. (1996). Doing the right thing: Ethical cyberspace research. *Information Society, 12*, 141–152.

Bradley, N., & Poppen, W. (2003). Assistive technology, computers, and Internet may decrease sense of isolation for homebound elderly and disabled persons. *Technology and Disability, 15*(1), 19–25.

Cella, D.F., & Yellen, S.B. (1993). Cancer support groups: The state of the art. *Cancer Practice, 1*, 56–61.

Colon, Y. (1996). Telephone support groups: A nontraditional approach to reaching underserved cancer patients. *Cancer Practice, 4*, 156–159.

Davis, L.M., & Lafrado, L.J. (2003). Addressing senior needs in the accessibility of Internet health-related information. *Journal of Hospital Librarianship, 3*(1), 7–14.

Department of Health, Education, and Welfare. (1978). *The Belmont Report: Ethical principles and guidelines for the protection of human subjects of biomedical and behavioral research.* Washington, DC: Author.

Eysenbach, G. (2003). The impact of the Internet on cancer outcomes. *CA: A Cancer Journal for Clinicians, 53*, 356–371.

Eysenbach, G., & Till, J.E. (2001). Ethical issues in qualitative research on Internet communities. *BMJ, 323*, 1103–1105.

Fawcett, J., & Buhle, E. (1995). Using the Internet for data collection: An innovative electronic strategy. *Computers in Nursing, 13*, 273–279.

Finichel, M., Suler, J., Barak, A., Zelvin, E., Jones, G., Munro, K., et al. (2003). *Observations on the phenomena of online behavior, experience and therapeutic relationships.* Retrieved December 5, 2003, from http://ismho.org/casestudy/myths.htm

Fobair, P. (1997). Cancer support groups and group therapies: Part I. Historical and theoretical background and research on effectiveness. *Journal of Psychosocial Oncology, 15*(1), 63–81.

Fogel, J. (2003). Internet use for cancer information among racial/ethnic populations and low literacy groups. *Cancer Control, 10*(Suppl. 5), 45–51.

Gray, J. (1996). *Data management: Past, present, and future.* Retrieved February 10, 2004, from http://cne.gmu.edu/pjd/cs491/RES/gray.pdf

Griffiths, R. (2002, October). *History of the Internet, Internet for historians (and just about everyone else).* Retrieved May 2, 2005, from http://www.let.leidenuniv.nl/history/ivh/frame_theorie.html

Gromov, G. (2003). Internet pre-history: Ancient roads of telecommunications and computers. Retrieved December 6, 2003, from http://www.netvalley.com/intval_intr.html

Gustafson, D., Wise, M., McTavish, F., Taylor, J.O., Wolberg, W., Stewart, J., et al. (1993). Development and pilot evaluation of a computer-based support system for women with breast cancer. *Journal of Psychosocial Oncology, 11*(4), 69–93.

Han, H., & Belcher, A.E. (2001). Computer-mediated support group use among parents of children with cancer: An exploratory study. *Computers in Nursing, 19*, 27–33.

Haugh, R. (2003, May). Bar code bandwagon. *Hospitals and Health Networks, 77*(5), 54–56. Retrieved November 28, 2003, from http://www.hospitalconnect.com/hhnmag/jsp/articledisplay.jsp?dcrpath=AHA/PubsNewsArticle/data/0305HHN_FEA_BarCode&domain=HHNMAG

Horrigan, J., & Rainie, L. (2002, December). *Counting on the Internet.* Washington, DC: Pew Internet and American Life Project. Retrieved December 1, 2003, from http://www.pewinternet.org/reports/toc.asp?Report=80

Kaye, H. (2000). *Disability and the digital divide* [Abstract 22]. Washington, DC: U.S. Department of Education, National Institute on Disability and Rehabilitation Research.

Klemm, P., Bunnell, D., Cullen, M., Soneji, R., Gibbons, P., & Holecek, A. (2003). Online cancer support groups: A review of the research literature. *Computers in Nursing, 21*, 136–142.

Klemm, P., & Hardie, T. (2002). Depression in Internet and face-to-face cancer support groups: A pilot study [Online exclusive]. *Oncology Nursing Forum, 29,* E45–E51. Retrieved May 3, 2005, from http://www.ons.org/publications/journals/ONF/Volume29/Issue4/290445.asp

Klemm, P., Hurst, M., Dearholt, S.L., & Trone, S. (1999). Cyber solace: Gender differences on Internet cancer support groups. *Computers in Nursing, 17,* 65–72.

Klemm, P., & Nolan, M. (1998). Internet cancer support groups: Legal and ethical issues for nurse researchers. *Oncology Nursing Forum, 25,* 673–676.

Klemm, P., Reppert, K., & Visich, L. (1998). A nontraditional support group: The Internet. *Computers in Nursing, 16,* 31–36.

Klemm, P., & Wheeler, E. (2005). Cancer caregivers online: Hope, emotional roller coaster, and physical/emotional/psychological responses. *Computers, Informatics, Nursing, 23,* 38–45.

Kraut, R., Kiesler, S., Boneva, B., Cummings, J., Helgeson, V., & Crawford, A. (2002). Internet paradox revisited. *Journal of Social Issues, 58*(1), 49–74.

Kraut, R., Patterson, M., Lundmark, V., Kiesler, S., Mukophadhyay, T., & Scherlis, W. (1998). Internet paradox: A social technology that reduces social involvement and psychological well-being? *American Psychologist, 53,* 1017–1031.

Kuperman, G., & Gibson, R. (2003). Improving patient care. Computer physician order entry: Benefits, costs, and issues. *Annals of Internal Medicine, 139,* 31–39.

Larrison, C.R., Nackerud, L., Risler, E., & Sullivan, M. (2002). Welfare recipients and the digital divide: Left out of the new economy? *Journal of Technology in Human Services, 19*(4), 1–12.

Leestma, R. (2003). Implementing technological safeguards to ensure patient privacy. *Caring, 22*(2), 16–18.

Lewis, J., & Sommers, C. (2003). Personal data assistants: Using new technology to enhance nursing practice. *American Journal of Maternal Child Nursing, 28,* 66–73.

Madara, E., & White, B. (1997). On-line mutual support: The experience of a self-help clearinghouse. *Information and Referral: The Journal of the Alliance of Information and Referral Systems, 19,* 91–107.

Mandl, K., Kohane, I., & Brandt, A. (1998). Electronic patient-physician communication. *Annals of Internal Medicine, 129,* 495–500.

Manne, S., Glassman, M., & DuHamel, K. (2001). Intrusion, avoidance, and psychological distress among individuals with cancer. *Psychosomatic Medicine, 63,* 658–667.

McTavish, F.M., Gustafson, D.H., Owens, B.H., Hawkins, R.P., Pingree, S., Wise, M., et al. (1995). CHESS: An interactive computer system for women with breast cancer piloted with an underserved population. *Journal of Ambulatory Care Management, 18*(3), 35–41.

Meaney, B. (2003). Ethics, security, and quality on the Net: Online resources can help healthcare organizations establish and comply with high standards. *Medicine on the Net, 9*(4), 1–3, 5–9.

Mekhjian, H., Kumar, R., Kuehn, L., Bentley, T., Teater, P., Thomas, A., et al. (2002). Immediate benefits realized following implementation of physician order entry at an academic medical center. *Journal of the American Medical Informatics Association, 9,* 529–539.

Moyer, C.A., Stern, D.T., Dobias, K.S., Cox, D.T., & Katz, S.J. (2002). Bridging the electronic divide: Patient and provider perspectives on e-mail communication in primary care. *American Journal of Managed Care, 8,* 427–433.

Nie, N., & Erbring, L. (2000, February). *Internet and society: A preliminary report.* Retrieved May 3, 2005, from http://news-service.stanford.edu/news/2000/february16/internetsurvey-216.html

Office for Civil Rights, U.S. Department of Health and Human Services. (2005, April). *Medical privacy—National standards to protect the privacy of personal health information.* Washington, DC: Author. Retrieved May 5, 2005, from http://www.hhs.gov/ocr/hipaa

Opalinski, L. (2001). Older adults and the digital divide: Assessing results of a Web-based survey. *Journal of Technology in Human Services, 18,* 203–221.

Patt, M.R., Houston, T.K., Jenckes, M.W., Sands, D.Z., & Ford, D.E. (2003). Doctors who are using e-mail with their patients: A qualitative exploration. *Journal of Medical Internet Research, 5,* Article e9. Retrieved May 3, 2005, from http://www.jmir.org/2003/2/e9

Pillon, L., & Joannides, G. (1991). An 11-year evaluation of a Living With Cancer program. *Oncology Nursing Forum, 18,* 707–711.

Richey, K.W. (1997, February). *The ENIAC.* Retrieved May 2, 2005, from http://qubit.plh.af.mil/RelatedArticles/related/TheEniac-Richey97.pdf

Robertson, J. (2003). *Guidelines for physician-patient electronic communications.* Retrieved February 4, 2004, from http://www.ama-assn.org/ama/pub/category/2386.html

Sharf, B.F. (1997). Communicating breast cancer on-line: Support and empowerment on the Internet. *Women and Health, 26*(1), 65–84.

Sperazza, L.C. (2001). Rehabilitation options for patients with low vision. *Rehabilitation Nursing, 26,* 148–151, 163.

Stolworthy, Y. (2003, October). *RNs are mobilizing.* Retrieved December 1, 2003, from http://www.pdacortex.com/RNs_are_Mobilizing.htm

Teich, J.M., Merchia, P.R., Schmiz, J.L., Kuperman, G.J., Spurr, C.D., & Bates, D.W. (2000). Effects of computerized physician order entry on prescribing practices. *Archives of Internal Medicine, 160,* 2741–2747.

Waegemann, C., & Tessier, C. (2002). Documentation goes wireless: A look at mobile healthcare computing devices. *Journal of the American Health Information Management Association, 73*(8), 36–39.

Weinberg, N., Schmale, J., Uken, J., & Wessel, K. (1996). Online help: Cancer patients participate in a computer-mediated support group. *Health and Social Work, 21*(1), 24–29.

Winzelberg, A., Classen, C., Alpers, G., Roberts, H., Koopman, C., Adams, R., et al. (2003). Evaluation of an Internet support group for women with primary breast cancer. *Cancer, 97,* 1164–1173.

Zabora, J., BrintzenhofeSzoc, K., Curbow, B., Hooker, C., & Piantadosi, S. (2001). The prevalence of psychological distress by cancer site. *Psycho-Oncology, 10,* 19–28.

CHAPTER 27

The Close of Life

LINDA M. GORMAN, RN, MN, APRN, BC, OCN®, CHPN

A good death does honor to a whole life.
—Francesco Petrarch

When patients and their families face the news that the cancer cannot be cured and is, in fact, advancing, end-of-life care needs to be addressed. In recent years, much has been published about the importance of good end-of-life care, yet it continues to elude some patients (Institute of Medicine [IOM], 2003; SUPPORT Principal Investigators, 1995). Transitioning from a "cure" mode to a "care" mode often is frightening. Patients and their loved ones may feel abandoned, helpless, and frustrated. As improved efforts are under way to provide oncology professionals with training in this area, more inroads will be made to improve access to high-quality end-of-life care. See Table 27-1 for a list of some current programs. The recent proliferation of palliative care programs should also help to promote better access to improved end-of-life care. The National Cancer Institute in 2001 emphasized access to palliative care and provided guidelines to integrate palliative care into cancer care (Foley & Gelband, 2001).

Where People Die

In 2003, approximately 50% of deaths in the United States occurred in hospitals, 25% in nursing homes, and 25% in homes (National Hospice and Palliative Care Organization [NHPCO], n.d.-a). As recently as 1994, 73% of deaths occurred in hospitals (NHPCO, n.d.-a). The number of home and nursing home deaths has increased significantly over the past decade. This may be the result of the growing access to hospice and palliative care.

Table 27-1. End-of-Life Training Programs

Program	Contact Information
American Medical Association End-of-Life Care	www.ama-assn.org/ama/pub/category/14730.htm
DELEtCC—Disseminating End-of-Life Education to Cancer Centers	http://deletcc.coh.org
ELNEC—End-of-Life Nursing Education Consortium	www.aacn.nche.edu/ELNEC
EPEC—Education in Palliative and End-of-Life Care	http://epec.net/EPEC/webpages/index.cfm
EPERC—End-of-Life/Palliative Education Resource Center	www.eperc.mcw.edu
IPPC—Initiative for Pediatric Palliative Care	www.ippcweb.org

The hospital as the place of death is a relatively new phenomenon. Historically, family members cared for the sick in their own homes throughout the dying process. After World War II, as advances in healthcare technology grew, the hospital became the most frequent location of death. Today, nearly all Medicare beneficiaries spend at least some time in a hospital during their last year of life (Center to Advance Palliative Care [CAPC], 2005). Although the number of home deaths has increased in recent years, the hospital remains the focus for many people. Teno et al. (2004) identified that family members expressed a higher rate of concerns when patients died in the hospital or nursing home. Common concerns found in this large national study included unmet needs for symptom management, lack of emotional support, belief that their dying family member was not always treated with respect, and poor communication with the physician. Being in the hospital increases access to technologic advances and, therefore, increases the likelihood that they will be used to treat problems when a patient is close to death. Use of the intensive care unit at the end of life is increasing. A large epidemiologic study found that 22% of hospital deaths in the United States in 1999 occurred in the intensive care unit (Angus et al., 2004).

Dying in one's home remains the wish of most people (IOM, 2003; NHPCO, n.d.-a). Fifty percent of patients who died under hospice care died at home in 2003 (NHPCO, n.d.-a). Home hospice care resulted in significantly higher satisfaction for family members compared to the hospital setting (Teno et al., 2004).

As the U.S. population ages, dying in a nursing home is expected to become increasingly more common (Zerzan, Stearns, & Hanson, 2000). As a result of shorter lengths of stay in the acute hospital setting and the lack of availability of home caregivers, for many people, the delivery of end-of-life care in the nursing home setting will be increasingly more common. Hospice care can be provided in a nursing home under some circumstances, but it often is underutilized (Casarett et al., 2005). Underutilization, in part, may be caused by reimbursement policies that encourage nursing homes to focus on restorative care (Zerzan et al.). Nursing home residents under hospice care are less likely to be hospitalized in their final days than similar patients who are not receiving hospice care (Miller, Gozalo, & Mor, 2001). In 2003, 23% of hospice patients died in nursing facilities (NHPCO, n.d.-a). Miller, Mor, and Teno (2003) found that hospice patients in nursing homes had improved pain management compared to nonhospice patients. Providing palliative care in the nursing home is a concept that is just beginning to generate more interest. The nursing home environment presents many challenges, including staff with many different knowledge and education levels as well as a high turnover rate. Regulations and reimbursement can impede quality end-of-life care in nursing homes (Wilson, 2001). For example, giving sedatives or analgesics may require additional documentation to justify their administration. In addition, infrequent physician visits also may contribute to poor symptom management (Wilson). The environment may not be set up for family involvement or unrestricted visitors, which can contribute to family anxiety. IOM recommended that future study should focus on the following areas of research for end-of-life care in nursing homes: how well-informed residents and families are about who is responsible for care and what they can expect, how residents' and families' preferences are assessed, what practice guidelines and protocols are in place to guide care of the dying, what palliative care expertise is available, and whether dying residents are segregated from other residents (Wunderlich, Sloan, & Davis, 1996). Studies indicate that pain management continues to be a concern in many facilities (Ferrell, 2000; Hall, Schroder, & Weaver, 2002). Because of the expected increase in the number of deaths occurring in nursing homes, these problems must be addressed.

Components of High-Quality End-of-Life Care

Singer, Martin, and Kelner (1999) reported on the wishes of 126 people with advanced illnesses. Their wishes included (a) management of pain and other distressing symptoms of the illness, (b) a sense of control, (c) not wanting to be a burden, (d) avoidance of inappropriate prolongation of dying, and (e) strengthened relationships with loved ones. Steinhauser et al. (2000) studied a group of patients who expressed additional wishes, including having the opportunity to gain a sense of completion in their lives, wanting support from healthcare professionals beyond disease management, and wishing to be mentally aware. These points provide a rallying call to all oncology professionals to examine how they can address these quality-of-life issues for their patients. Few of these wishes can be achieved if advancing illness is not acknowledged and the opportunity to plan is not provided.

Adequate symptom control is an essential component of end-of-life care. Only when pain and symptoms are controlled can patients focus on their emotional, spiritual, and social needs (Hermann & Looney, 2001).

End-of-Life Programs

Palliative Care

In recent years, the proliferation of palliative care programs has played a role in transitioning patients from cure-oriented treatment to supportive care. Palliative care has been a tradition in Canada and throughout Europe, whereas it just now is spreading throughout the United States. Although palliative care can be appropriate throughout the course of illness (see Figure 27-1), it often is thought of as an approach to care when the focus is no longer on cure. The World Health Organization (2005) has defined palliative care as an approach that improves the quality of life of patients facing life-threatening illness and their families, through the prevention, assessment, and treatment of pain and other physical, psychosocial, and spiritual problems. CAPC (2005) described a palliative care program as one that uses an interdisciplinary model to relieve suffering and improve the quality of life for patients with advanced illness. Palliative care is more likely to be a hospital-based program, although some palliative care is provided in home health care, clinics, and nursing facilities. Working in an acute hospital setting provides the opportunity to promote education, appropriate policy development, research, and services to these patients. This can be provided in a consultative model or in a specialized palliative care unit (CAPC; Whedon, 2001). Cancer centers are in key roles to improve access to palliative care to patients throughout their disease course (Whedon, 2002). Hospitals now are learning that high-quality palliative care not only contributes to high-quality patient care but also may contribute to lower costs (CAPC; Smith et al., 2003).

Palliative care can provide access to expert symptom management as patients are pursuing curative therapy. If the focus changes to supportive care, then the palliative care team can take a larger role in providing support, managing symptoms, addressing goals, and assisting with plans for the future. Potentially, referral to palliative care will increase access to hospice care earlier in the course of the illness.

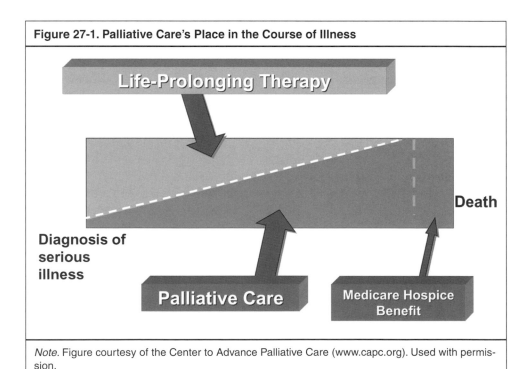

Figure 27-1. Palliative Care's Place in the Course of Illness

Life-Prolonging Therapy

Death

Diagnosis of serious illness

Palliative Care

Medicare Hospice Benefit

Note. Figure courtesy of the Center to Advance Palliative Care (www.capc.org). Used with permission.

Hospice

Hospice is a philosophy of care for terminally ill people and their families that focuses on palliating symptoms and enhancing the quality of life during however much time patients have remaining. Based on the Medicare model, hospice care has been limited to patients with a life expectancy of six months or less if the disease takes its expected course. Hospice affirms life and neither hastens nor postpones death.

The modern hospice movement began in London, England, in 1967 when Dame Cecily Saunders started St. Christopher's Hospice. The first U.S. hospice was started in 1974 in New Haven, CT. Hospice care in the United States usually is a home-based program. "Home" can be a nursing home or an assisted-living setting. NHPCO (n.d.-a) reported that more than 3,200 hospice programs exist in the United States.

Many of the early U.S. hospices were small agencies with largely volunteer staffs that provided services in the home. Dedicated people who believed in the hospice concept were the backbone of this grassroots movement. In 1981, the National Hospice Study attempted to validate the impact of hospice care (Mor & Kidder, 1985). The study compared the care and costs involved in meeting the needs of the dying in traditional oncology units and hospices. The study revealed that hospice care, particularly home hospice care, was significantly less costly than conventional care in the final two months of life. It also revealed that improved symptom control and increased caregiver satisfaction existed in the hospice program. This study led to Congress passing the Medicare Hospice Benefit in 1983.

Medicare's coverage of hospice has played a major role in shaping hospice care as it exists today. At least 80% of hospice patients are Medicare beneficiaries (NHPCO, 2003). Medicare beneficiaries who are certified by a physician to have less than six months to live and who are receiving no curative treatment for the illness can select the benefit. Hospice patients are able to receive noncurative medical and support services, many of which would not otherwise be covered in regular home care. Hospice care allows for ongoing visits by a hospice nurse without the need to identify a skilled need for care (as is required in home health care). Signing up for the hospice benefit means the beneficiary waives all rights to Medicare payment for curative treatment of the terminal condition. The individual can revoke the benefit at any time to pursue aggressive treatment or because of a change in condition. The patient or surrogate usually signs a "do not resuscitate" form and is advised to call the hospice agency rather than emergency medical services in case of an emergency. However, it is not mandated that patients on hospice have a "do not resuscitate" order. Hospice care cannot be denied to someone who meets the qualifications but continues to wish an attempt at resuscitation (National Hospice Organization, 1992).

Hospices are paid on a daily basis per patient rather than per visit, and Congress determines the amount that Medicare pays. The daily rate paid to hospices covers all services, including nursing, equipment, symptom management medications, home health aides, social work, and clergy visits (NHPCO, n.d.-b). Since the inception of the Medicare Hospice Benefit, many private insurers, as well as Medicaid in many states, also have a hospice benefit. The Medicare benefit will continue to pay for hospice care beyond the six-month life expectancy if patients continue to meet the qualifications.

The benefit provides for different levels of care depending on the variations in care intensity needed by the patient and family (Egan & Labyak, 2001). **Routine**

home care is the most common level of care provided by the interdisciplinary team in the patient's residence. **Continuous care** covers patients in brief periods of crisis by providing a minimum of eight hours per day of care in the home, at least 50% of which must be provided by a licensed nurse. **Inpatient respite care** covers patients who need a short stay in an inpatient facility to relieve their caregivers. Respite care can be provided for up to five days. **General inpatient care** is appropriate when patients need symptom management that requires an inpatient setting, and the hospice can arrange admission to a contracted nursing home, hospice facility, or acute hospital. This is particularly useful if the patient's symptoms become too complex to manage in the home.

Hospice programs must provide care using an interdisciplinary team. This team provides a variety of services, including pain and symptom management, psychosocial and spiritual support, and bereavement services (see Figure 27-2). All members of the team should participate in providing these services. All of these components contribute to meeting the goal of administering comfort care to patients and support to family members. Symptom management is key to providing good end-of-life care. McMillan and Small (2002) found that dry mouth, pain, lack of energy, and shortness of breath are the most frequently reported symptoms that affect the quality of life of hospice patients.

Figure 27-2. Components of Hospice Care

- Patient and family as unit of care
- Focus on symptom management, addressing physical, psychosocial, and spiritual distress
- Interdisciplinary team
- Service available 24 hours a day, seven days a week
- Physician-directed, nurse-coordinated care
- Volunteers, family, and friends active in providing care and support
- Bereavement services for survivors
- Coordinated homecare services with inpatient care available

Note. Based on information from McNally et al., 1996.

Barriers to Effective End-of-Life Care

The SUPPORT Study (SUPPORT Principal Investigators, 1995), which is the largest study of end-of-life care in U.S. hospitals to date, demonstrated that even when physicians had clear information on patient prognosis, they consistently overestimated patients' life expectancies. Tang and McCorkle (2003) found that two-thirds of a group of patients with cancer wanted to die at home, yet less than one-third of this group actually did. These two studies provide some evidence of the continuing problem that end-of-life care often is not addressed until very late in the disease course and, thus, becomes a barrier to access to palliative care and hospice. Research has documented the declining median length of stay in hospice programs, despite widespread information available to patients and their families about hospice (Christakis & Escarce, 1996; NHPCO, n.d.-a). NHPCO (n.d.-a) reported that in 2003, the median length of stay in hospice programs nationally was 22 days. This was down from 29 days in 1995. More than 30% of patients admitted to hospice programs were on service seven days or less in 2003 (NHPCO, n.d.-a). Barriers to good end-of-life care continue to affect access to these services (Egan & Labyak, 2001; Ellershaw & Ward, 2003; Jennings, Ryndes, D'Onofrio, & Baily, 2003; Last Acts, 2002).

A lack of acknowledgment of the limited life expectancy of some patients is an important factor contributing to hospice referrals being made in the last days of life instead of the last months. Also, the increasing number of therapeutic agents being developed for patients with cancer may lead to delays in hospice referrals. Oncologists may continue to promote aggressive treatment in the face of far-advanced disease because of the new therapies that continue to become available (Earle et al., 2004; Weissman & von Gunten, 2004). It has become more difficult to determine the right time to stop aggressive treatments. In addition, the U.S. healthcare system tends to focus on the search for more treatment rather than on looking realistically at patients' quality of life.

Physicians need to promote communication early in the treatment process to address patients' wishes, goals, and values. Paice (interviewed by Fromer, 2003) pointed out that patients usually will not be comfortable addressing end-of-life care, so it is the physician's responsibility to initiate the conversation. As a patient's disease progresses, his or her wishes in the face of advancing disease need to be reassessed (Quill, 2000). Oncology nurses play an important role in initiating conversations with patients about their wishes. End-of-life discussions should begin long before the patient is imminently terminal.

Denial of terminal illness remains a frequent barrier that may be fostered by patients, families, and physicians who are unable to acknowledge the poor prognosis. This may be coupled with the fear that hospice may represent giving up hope or even accelerating death. Oncology nurses can assist patients in considering hospice care by exploring fears about what hospice represents and refocusing hope on pain relief and resolving family conflicts. A decision to end curative treatment is not the same as ending life (Gurafino & Dumas, 1994). Emphasizing quality of life and palliative care will enhance the patient's life for whatever time is left.

A lack of knowledge on the part of physicians about hospice also exists. Physicians sometimes inaccurately believe that they will lose control over their patient's care once a patient starts a hospice program. In reality, the attending physician remains responsible for and is expected to be a key participant in establishing the treatment plan. The attending physician can continue to bill for seeing patients who are receiving the Medicare hospice benefit. Palliative care teams need to communicate to physicians that their role as consultants will not interfere with the doctor-patient relationship.

Another frequent barrier is the desire of patients, families, or physicians to continue treatments such as blood transfusions, chemotherapy, total parenteral nutrition, and IV fluids because of the belief that these interventions will enhance the patient's quality of life. Individual hospices may allow some of these interventions if they seem to help the patient without creating added burdens. If patients cannot begin hospice care because of the aggressive treatments they are still receiving, efforts to engage a palliative care approach in the home and nursing home settings need to be pursued. In addition, patients often can continue to pursue phase I clinical trials while on a hospice program (Byock, 2003; Goodman, 2003; Meyers & Linder, 2003).

Families and friends often are overwhelmed with the idea of taking a loved one home to die, which creates another potential barrier to choosing home hospice care. Supporting potential caregivers and educating them about how to prepare and what to expect can help to eliminate this barrier. Berry and Ward (1995) noted that a common fear of caregivers is their belief that they will be unable to control the pain and will be required to give the patient injections for analgesia. Teaching caregivers that most pain can be controlled with oral, sublingual, transdermal, and rectal preparations will address these fears.

Patients may not access hospice or palliative care because it never has been explained to them. Many programs conduct community and physician education programs to increase community awareness of the service.

In addition, some cultural and ethnic groups may be uncomfortable with accepting hospice professionals in their homes. Hospice programs need to identify populations in their community that are underserved, undertake programs to educate staff on the needs of these groups, and hire staff from these groups to make patients and families more comfortable (Gaffin, Hill, & Penso, 1996).

Coping With a Death at Home

Anticipating a home death can provide the patient and family with an intimate, personal experience that brings them closer together during a time of tremendous stress. The close presence of the family may allow time for working through conflicts and obtaining forgiveness for past hurts. Being in one's home surrounded by family, friends, pets, and cherished possessions can provide a sense of peace and control for the patient. Loss of control can be one of the most distressing feelings for dying patients (Schachter & Coyle, 1998). Families can gain a sense of accomplishment by knowing that they helped to meet the patient's wish to die at home. Even young children can gain from this experience by being active participants with the family during this crisis (Sankar, 1991).

A major disadvantage to the patient dying at home is that caregivers can become overwhelmed by the patient's care needs and may not have the energy or time to actually grieve, which can negatively affect caregivers' quality of life (Meyers & Gray, 2001). Family members lacking in social support and social outlets are most likely to feel unable to handle the stress of the death (Martinez & Wagner, 1993). Steele and Fitch (1996b) reported that families identify the need for rest, time to themselves, access to a 24-hour hot line, and education as important needs. Wilbert, Beckwith, Holm, and Beckwith (1995) reported that encouraging increased socialization for family caregivers can reduce anxiety. Redinbaugh, Baum, Tarbell, and Arnold (2003) found that family caregivers who accepted their loved one's illness, redefined illness-related problems in a more manageable way, and felt capable of solving illness-related problems had less caregiver strain.

Poorly managed physical symptoms are among the most stressful aspects of caring for a dying person at home (Rabow, Hauser, & Adams, 2004). Close supervision by a hospice or palliative care team generally can ensure that most symptoms will be managed (Egan & Labyak, 2001). Hospice team members also work with the family regarding what to do at the time of death. Many times, family members have little experience with the actual dying process. It is common for people to rely on myths and stories they hear from others, which can increase the fear of what will occur during the dying process. Oncology nurses play a key role in assessing the family's readiness to care for their loved one at home, identifying fears, and providing much-needed education about the dying process. More research on how best to provide support to caregivers needs to be done.

Pediatric End-of-Life Care

Much has been written about the end-of-life care for adults, but the needs of dying infants and children have long been underemphasized and understudied (Sumner, 2001). Yet, cancer is the leading cause of nonaccidental death in childhood (Jemal et al., 2005). Facing the loss of a child may be the most traumatic event in a person's life (Ashton & Ashton, 2000). Parents face multiple losses—not only losing the relationship with the child but also all that the child represented for the family's hopes and dreams. Pediatric oncology professionals must develop special skills to address the needs of the children, parents, and siblings. Traditionally, children receive aggressive treatment until the very end. Accepting when it is time to stop aggressive treatment may be unthinkable for parents (Wolfe et al., 2000). Wolfe et al.'s study of parents of children with advanced cancers found that only 13% of parents reported lessening suffering as a primary goal of therapy. The majority remained focused on extending life. However, the child often understands what is happening (Ashton & Ashton). Parents may resist facing the reality of the poor prognosis. At times, communication within a family can be difficult if the child wants to address his or her fears and concerns and the parents are unable to bear this. Other families may feel abandoned by their healthcare team if the team is unable to address the needs of the patient and family when the end is near. Special training in providing pediatric end-of-life care is essential. Several initiatives now are under way to increase the training and support for healthcare professionals in this area, including the Initiative for Pediatric Palliative Care (Solomon et al., 2002). More children's hospitals are adding palliative care teams that can promote education and services to these patients and their families and also help the pediatric staffs to address the many issues.

Whereas more than 80% of hospice patients are older than age 65, less than 1% are younger than age 18 (NHPCO, 2003). Children's Hospice International (2005) found that less than 1% of children needing hospice care receive it. Hospice care for children has been underutilized by parents and healthcare professionals because life expectancy often is more difficult to estimate in children, aggressive treatment is more likely to be continued because of the patient's age or denial of the prognosis, and parents often do not have experience with death, resulting in fear of hospice care (Martinson, 1993; Sumner, 2001). Not all communities will have access to a hospice program that specializes in care of infants and children, so efforts should be made to work with local hospice programs to determine how to provide quality end-of-life care.

Pediatric hospice care provides the same services for patients and families as hospice programs for adults. Specialized services include preparing parents for the dying process in regard to children, addressing the emotional needs of siblings, and coordinating specialized bereavement services (Martinson, 1995).

End-of-Life Nursing

Along with the increase in research and education on the end of life, the specialty of hospice and palliative nursing has grown and developed. Hospice nurses generally function as case managers and coordinators of the interdisciplinary treatment plan with the goal of maintaining patient comfort. Often asked to make treatment decisions, hospice nurses need to have a wide range of skills in areas such as home health, oncology, pain management, and skin care, in addition to excellent psychosocial skills (Brett, 1996). The Hospice and Palliative Nurses Association (HPNA) has developed *Scope and Standards of Hospice and Palliative Nursing Practice* (2002). HPNA (2003) also has developed a position statement titled *Value of Professional Nurse in End-of-Life Care*. Certification exams also exist for all levels of nursing from advanced practice nurses, RNs, licensed vocational/practical nurses, and nurse's aides. The ability to handle a caseload of terminal patients and their distressed families requires an individual to be mature, flexible, and creative. For example, a hospice nurse may enter a home and find a patient who is suddenly close to death, no longer able to swallow, and in pain with only morphine tablets in the house. The nurse must find a way to relieve the pain immediately and address the fears of the caregivers.

Zervekh (1994) described hospice nurses as "truth-tellers" because they find themselves having to ask difficult questions and speak the truth with people facing the greatest crisis of their lives. Working with dying patients forces nurses to address the truth when others may be trying to avoid it (e.g., preparing families when the patient has only days to live). Wright (2002) studied groups of hospice nurses and found that the most prominent trait was attending, or being humanly present. Other traits included independence, the ability to work with a team, a sense of calling, spirituality, confidence, intuitiveness, and a sense of humor. Gaydos (2004) found that hospice nurses in her study had a sense of endurance and resilience.

The specialty of palliative nursing is newer than other specialties. Nurses working in palliative care are in a variety of settings, including hospitals, radiation therapy, clinics, nursing homes, and home health. In reality, many nurses who work in palliative care are not in an identified palliative care program. Critical care nurses and oncology nurses, among others, may consider themselves to be palliative care specialists. Working closely within the interdisciplinary team model and championing good symptom management are hallmarks of a palliative care nurse (Coyle, 2001). The advanced practice role in palliative care attained certification status in 2003. It is a specialty recognized as contributing to improved quality and access to care (Kuebler, 2003).

Conclusion

The importance of addressing the care needs of patients at the end of life is beginning to attain more attention and research. Hospice and palliative nursing can provide care and services to patients and their families to help them to achieve their goals of comfort and enhanced quality of life throughout the disease progression. Oncology professionals are in key positions to promote improved end-of-life care. In cancer centers, clinics, hospitals, nursing facilities, and homes, patients with cancer can receive high-quality care throughout the progression of the disease.

References

Angus, D.C., Barnato, A.E., Linde-Zwirble, W.T., Weissfeld, L.A., Watson, R.S., Rickert, T., et al. (2004). Use of intensive care at the end of life in the United States: An epidemiologic study. *Critical Care Medicine, 32,* 638–643.

Ashton, J., & Ashton, D. (2000). Dealing with chronic/terminal illness or disability of a child: Anticipatory mourning. In T.A. Rando (Ed.), *Clinical dimensions of anticipatory mourning* (pp. 415–454). Champaign, IL: Research Press.

Berry, P., & Ward, S. (1995). Barriers to pain management in hospice: A study of family caregivers. *American Journal of Hospice and Palliative Care, 10*(4), 19–33.

Brett, R. (1996). A tribute to hospice nurses. *American Journal of Hospice and Palliative Care, 12*(1), 3–10.

Byock, I. (2003). Palliative care and the ethics of research: Medicare, hospice and phase I trials. *Journal of Supportive Oncology, 1,* 130–141.

Casarett, D., Karlawish, J., Knashawn, M., Crowley, R., Mirsch, T., & Asch, D.A. (2005). Improving the use of hospice services in nursing homes. *JAMA, 294,* 211–217.

Center to Advance Palliative Care. (2005). *Building a hospital-based palliative care program.* New York: Author. Retrieved May 4, 2005, from http://www.capc.org/building-a-hospital-based-palliative-care-program

Children's Hospice International. (2005). *About children's hospice, palliative and end-of-life care.* Retrieved May 9, 2005, from http://www.chionline.org/resources/about.phtml

Christakis, N.A., & Escarce, J.J. (1996). Survival of Medicare patients after enrollment in hospice programs. *JAMA, 335,* 172–178.

Coyle, N. (2001). Introduction to palliative care. In B.R. Ferrell & N. Coyle (Eds.), *Textbook of palliative nursing* (pp. 3–6). New York: Oxford University Press.

Earle, C.C., Neville, B.A., Landrum, M.B., Ayanian, J.Z., Block, S.D., & Weeks, J.C. (2004). Trends in the aggressiveness of cancer care near the end of life. *Journal of Clinical Oncology, 22,* 315–321.

Egan, K.A., & Labyak, M.J. (2001). Hospice care: A model for quality end-of-life care. In B.R. Ferrell & N. Coyle (Eds.), *Textbook of palliative nursing* (pp. 7–26). New York: Oxford University Press.

Ellershaw, J., & Ward, C. (2003). Care of the dying patient: The last hours or days of life. *BMJ, 326,* 30–34.

Ferrell, B.A. (2000). Pain management. *Clinics of Geriatric Medicine, 16,* 853–874.

Foley, K.M., & Gelband, H. (Eds.). (2001). *Improving palliative care for cancer: Summary and recommendations.* Washington, DC: National Academies Press.

Fromer, M.J. (2003, December 25). Innovations in end of life care. *Oncology Times,* pp. 15–17.

Gaffin, J., Hill, D., & Penso, D. (1996). Opening doors: Improving access to hospice and specialist palliative care services by members of the black and minority ethnic communities. *British Journal of Cancer, 74*(Suppl.), S51–S53.

Gaydos, H.L. (2004). The living end: Life journeys of hospice nurses. *Journal of Hospice and Palliative Nursing, 6,* 17–26.

Goodman, A. (2003, May 10). A largely unnoticed problem: Medicare won't pay for both hospice and phase I trials. *Oncology Times,* pp. 35–36.

Gurafino, V., & Dumas, L. (1994). Hospice nursing: The concept of palliative care. *Nursing Clinics of North America, 29,* 533–546.

Hall, P., Schroder, C., & Weaver, L. (2002). The last 48 hours of life in long-term care: A focused chart audit. *Journal of the American Geriatrics Society, 50,* 501–506.

Hermann, C., & Looney, S. (2001). The effectiveness of symptom management in hospice patients during the last 7 days of life. *Journal of Hospice and Palliative Nursing, 3*(3), 88–96.

Hospice and Palliative Nurses Association. (2002). *Scope and standards of hospice and palliative nursing practice.* Dubuque, IA: Kendall/Hunt.

Hospice and Palliative Nurses Association. (2003, October). *HPNA position statement. Value of professional nurse in end-of-life care.* Retrieved May 9, 2005, from http://www.hpna.org/pdf/Value_of_professional_nurse_Position_Statement_PDF.pdf

Institute of Medicine. (2003). *Describing death in America.* Washington, DC: National Academies Press.

Jemal, A., Murray, T., Ward, E., Samuels, A., Tiwari, R., Ghafoor, A., et al. (2005). Cancer statistics, 2005. *CA: A Cancer Journal for Clinicians, 55,* 10–30.

Jennings, B., Ryndes, T., D'Onofrio, C., & Baily, M.A. (2003). Access to hospice care: Expanding boundaries, overcoming barriers. *Hastings Center Report, 33*(Suppl.), S3–S7, S9–S13, S15–S21.

Kuebler, K. (2003). The palliative care advanced practice nurse. *Journal of Palliative Medicine, 6,* 707–714.

Last Acts. (2002). *Means to a better end: A report on dying in America today.* Retrieved May 25, 2005, from http://www.rwjf.org/files/publications/other/meansbetterend.pdf

Martinez, J., & Wagner, S. (1993). Hospice care. In S.L. Groenwald, M. Goodman, M.H. Frogge, & C.H. Yarbro (Eds.), *Cancer nursing: Principles and practice* (3rd ed., pp. 1432–1450). Sudbury, MA: Jones and Bartlett.

Martinson, I.M. (1993). Hospice care for children: Past, present, and future. *Journal of Pediatric Oncology Nursing, 10,* 93–98.

Martinson, I.M. (1995). Improving care for dying children. *Western Journal of Medicine, 163,* 258–262.

McMillan, S.C., & Small, B.J. (2002). Symptom distress and quality of life in patients with cancer newly admitted to hospice home care. *Oncology Nursing Forum, 29,* 1421–1428.

McNally, J.C., Bohnet, N.L., & Lindquist, M.E. (1996). Hospice nursing. *Seminars in Oncology Nursing, 12,* 238–243.

Meyers, F.J., & Linder, J. (2003). Simultaneous care: Disease treatment and palliative care throughout illness. *Journal of Clinical Oncology, 21,* 1412–1415.

Meyers, J.L., & Gray, L.N. (2001). The relationship between family primary caregiver characteristics and satisfaction with hospice care, quality of life, and burden. *Oncology Nursing Forum, 28,* 73–82.

Miller, S.C., Gozalo, P., & Mor, V. (2001). Hospice enrollment and hospitalization of dying nursing home patients. *American Journal of Medicine, 111,* 38–44.

Miller, S.C., Mor, V., & Teno, J.M. (2003). Hospice enrollment and pain assessment and management in nursing homes. *Journal of Pain and Symptom Management, 26,* 791–799.

Mor, V., & Kidder, D. (1985). Cost savings in hospice: Final results of the National Hospice Study. *Health Services Research, 20,* 407–422.

National Hospice and Palliative Care Organization. (2003). *National trend summary—2000–2002.* Alexandria, VA: Author. Retrieved June 23, 2005, from http://www.nhpco.org/files/members/2002Nationaldataset.pdf

National Hospice and Palliative Care Organization. (n.d.-a). *Hospice facts and figures.* Alexandria, VA: Author. Retrieved May 4, 2005, from http://www.nhpco.org/files/public/Hospice_Facts_110104.pdf

National Hospice and Palliative Care Organization. (n.d.-b). *Medicare Hospice Benefit.* Retrieved May 5, 2005, from http://www.nhpco.org/i4a/pages/index.cfm?pageid=3283

National Hospice Organization. (1992). *Do-not-resuscitate decisions in the context of hospice care.* Arlington, VA: Author.

Quill, T.E. (2000). Perspectives on care at the close of life. Initiating end-of-life discussions with seriously ill patients: Addressing the "elephant in the room." *JAMA, 284,* 2502–2507.

Rabow, M.W., Hauser, J.M., & Adams, J. (2004). Supporting family caregivers at the end of life. *JAMA, 291,* 483–491.

Redinbaugh, E.M., Baum, A., Tarbell, S., & Arnold, R. (2003). End of life caregiving: What helps family caregivers cope? *Journal of Palliative Medicine, 6,* 901–909.

Sankar, A. (1991). *Dying at home.* Baltimore: Johns Hopkins Publishers.

Schachter, S.R., & Coyle, N. (1998). Palliative home care—Impact on families. In J.C. Holland (Ed.), *Psycho-oncology* (pp. 1004–1015). New York: Oxford University Press.

Singer, P.A., Martin, D.K., & Kelner, M. (1999). Quality end-of-life care: Patients' perspectives. *JAMA, 281,* 163–168.

Smith, T.J., Coyne, P., Cassel, B., Penberthy, L., Hopson, A., & Hager, M.A. (2003). A high-volume specialist palliative care unit and team may reduce in-hospital end-of-life care costs. *Journal of Palliative Medicine, 6,* 699–705.

Solomon, M.Z., Dokken, D.L., Fleischman, A.R., Heller, K.S., Levetown, M., Rushton, C.H., et al. (2002). *IPCC background and goals.* Newton, MA: Education Development Center, Inc. Retrieved May 9, 2005, from http://www.ippcweb.org/initiative.pdf

Steele, R.G., & Fitch, M.I. (1996b). Needs of family caregivers of patients receiving home hospice care for cancer. *Oncology Nursing Forum, 23,* 823–828.

Steinhauser, K.E., Christakis, N.A., Clipp, E.C., McNeilly, M., McIntyre, L., & Tulsky, J.A. (2000). Factors considered important at the end of life by patients, family, physicians, and other care providers. *JAMA, 284,* 2476–2482.

Sumner, L.H. (2001). Pediatric care: The hospice perspective. In B.R. Ferrell & N. Coyle (Eds.), *Textbook of palliative nursing* (pp. 556–569). New York: Oxford University Press.

SUPPORT Principal Investigators. (1995). A controlled trial to improve care for seriously ill hospitalized patients. The Study to Understand Prognoses and Preferences for Outcomes and Risks of Treatments (SUPPORT). *JAMA, 274,* 1591–1598.

Tang, S.T., & McCorkle, R. (2003). Determinants of congruence between the preferred and actual place of death for terminally ill cancer patients. *Journal of Palliative Care, 19,* 230–237.

Teno, J.M., Clarridge, B.R., Casey, V., Welch, L.C., Wetle, T., Shield, R., et al. (2004). Family perspectives on end-of-life care at the last place of care. *JAMA, 291,* 88–93.

Weissman, D.E., & von Gunten, C.F. (2004). Oncology and hospice. *Community Oncology, 1,* 85–91.

Whedon, M.B. (2001). Hospital care. In B.R. Ferrell & N. Coyle (Eds.), *Textbook of palliative nursing* (pp. 584–608). New York: Oxford University Press.

Whedon, M.B. (2002). Revisiting the road not taken: Integrating palliative care in oncology nursing. *Oncology Nursing Forum, 6,* 27–33.

Wilbert, M.G., Beckwith, B., Holm, J., & Beckwith, S. (1995). A preliminary study of the impact of terminal illness on spouses: Social support and coping strategies. *Hospice Journal, 10*(4), 35–48.

Wilson, S.A. (2001). Long-term care. In B.R. Ferrell & N. Coyle (Eds.), *Textbook of palliative nursing* (pp. 531–542). New York: Oxford University Press.

Wolfe, J., Klar, N., Grier, H.E., Duncan, J., Salem-Schatz, S., Emanuel, E.J., et al. (2000). Understanding of prognosis among parents of children who died of cancer. *JAMA, 284,* 2469–2475.

World Health Organization. (2005). *WHO definition of palliative care.* Retrieved May 5, 2005, from http://www.who.int/cancer/palliative/definition/en

Wright, D.J. (2002). Researching the qualities of hospice nurses. *Journal of Hospice and Palliative Nursing, 4,* 210–216.

Wunderlich, G.S., Sloan, F.A., & Davis, C.K. (Eds.). (1996). *Nursing staff in hospitals and nursing homes: Is it adequate?* Washington, DC: National Academies Press.

Zervekh, J. (1994). The truth-tellers: How hospice nurses help patients confront death. *American Journal of Nursing, 94*(2), 31–34.

Zerzan, J., Stearns, S., & Hanson, L. (2000). Access to palliative care and hospice in nursing homes. *JAMA, 284,* 2489–2494.

CHAPTER 28

Psychoneuroimmunology: The Mind-Body Connection

JANICE E. POST-WHITE, PHD, RN, FAAN,
AND SUSAN BAUER-WU, DNSC, RN

Serenity is not freedom from the storm, but peace within the storm.
—Author Unknown

Psychoneuroimmunology (PNI) is the study of interactions among behavior, neural and endocrine function, and immune processes of adaptation (Ader, 1996). The field of PNI examines and tests for evidence of mind-body interactions. In 1981, Ader published the first comprehensive overview of PNI. This text examined the evidence that related psychosocial factors to disease, explained the effects of stress and neuroendocrine influences on immune function, and extensively reviewed the research validating conditioned immune suppression in rats. The second edition of *Psychoneuroimmunology* (Ader, Felten, & Cohen, 1991) reflected the burgeoning growth of the field with very detailed investigations of specific neurochemical links, the role of psychoneuroimmune responses in autoimmune and inflammatory diseases, and preliminary evidence for the effects of exercise, imagery, and relaxation on PNI outcomes. The 2001 edition encompasses two volumes, emphasizes an interdisciplinary team approach, and acknowledges the role of psychosocial responses and behavioral effects on immunity (Ader, Felten, & Cohen, 2001). As further evidence of research progress in PNI, the Basic and Biobehavioral Research Branch of the Division of Cancer Control and Population Sciences at the National Cancer Institute sponsored a multidisciplinary scientific meeting in 2002 to review current knowledge related to the biologic mechanism of psychosocial effects on disease and the specific effects on cancer control. This meeting went beyond investigations of the role of PNI on disease and addressed quality-of-life concerns, such as the role of sleep in host defense and the relationship of loneliness, mood, and fatigue to immunity.

Although PNI involves the testing of interventions, it does not refer to the use of the interventions themselves. PNI provides the framework, or model, in which interventions are selected, carried out, and evaluated. Determining the mechanism of action of mind-body interventions is the next step in validating their efficacy. The study of PNI has implications along the cancer continuum, from cancer prevention to survivorship, and increasingly is viewed as a multidisciplinary field relevant to oncology nurses.

Evidence for Mind-Body Interaction

The discovery of Pavlovian conditioning in the 1920s first shed light on communication between the brain and the immune system. In 1975, Ader and Cohen demonstrated conditioned vomiting and immune suppression in rats exposed to immunosuppressive cyclophosphamide. More recently, immune enhancement has been demonstrated in response to conditioned stimuli. The ability to positively influence physiologic and immune responses in humans has important implications in cancer. Other evidence early on in the field of PNI linked the sympathetic nervous system (SNS) to the immune system, leading the way to the discovery of the effects of stress on immune function and the hypothesized effects of stress on cancer, mediated by immune responses. Studies continue to demonstrate interactions among the nervous, endocrine, and immune systems, with increasingly complex interactions and recognition of multiple triggers and mediators affecting immune and disease outcomes (Ader et al., 2001; Rabin, 1999).

Conditioned Immune Suppression and Immune Enhancement

Classical conditioning is a form of learning that Ader and Cohen (1975) discovered unexpectedly when rats' immune systems were suppressed following one episode in which they drank saccharin water paired with cyclophosphamide. On the second exposure, the rats' immune systems responded as though the water contained the powerful immunosuppressant drug, when, in fact, it did not. A series of studies in rats followed, verifying that conditioning occurs when an event is paired with a stimulus that subsequently is withdrawn. These early studies provided evidence that the brain could signal the immune system to respond in an anticipated way.

Conditioning involves training a particular response to a specific stimulus. Anticipatory nausea and vomiting is a conditioned response. The initial experience of nausea and vomiting associated with the first course of emetogenic chemotherapy can precipitate nausea and vomiting prior to receiving the same chemotherapy a second time. Merely anticipating further chemotherapy (i.e., the specific stimulus) can result in the conditioned response of nausea and vomiting. Conditioned nausea or anxiety may last for years when patients return to the oncology clinic for follow-up visits (Bovbjerg, 2003). However, not all patients experience conditioned nausea and vomiting, even if they have symptoms with their first course of chemotherapy. Several factors are thought to influence conditioned responses, including the type, duration, and frequency of the stimuli, as well as individual responses such as age, gender, anxiety, and underlying immune and genetic factors (Ader et al., 2001).

In conditioned responses, the body reacts to the mind's perception of the expected response. Placebo effects and stress responses also are conditioned responses. Placebo responses occur when the individual has specific expectations (perceived by the cortex) and emotional responses (triggering the limbic system) that determine the desired and expected outcomes. Conditioned stress responses occur when a stimulus, initially associated with a negative response, activates the sympathetic nervous and endocrine systems on subsequent exposures. Perception of the stimulus is important to the individual response.

Conditioning has been a consistent and reproducible phenomenon. However, the mechanism remains unclear, in part because different stimuli can elicit different autonomic, neuroendocrine, and immune responses, and the effects on the immune system are a function of the immune status of the host. Several neuroendocrine mechanisms appear to explain these immune responses, including the mediating effects of adrenocortical steroids, opioids, and catecholamines.

The biologic significance and clinical implications of conditioning increasingly are becoming evident, with several studies confirming that immune responses can be conditioned in humans (Longo et al., 1999). Conditioning can enhance immune responses and improve clinical outcomes in lupus-prone mice (Ader, 2003) and in children with asthma receiving a placebo (Castes, Palenque, Canelones, Hagel, & Lynch, 1998). Future research is needed to determine whether conditioning can influence the development of and recovery from autoimmune, infectious, and neoplastic diseases.

Central Nervous System and Immune System Interactions

The nervous and immune systems communicate through recognition and binding of hormones and neurotransmitters to lymphocytes and macrophages, which have receptors for cortisol and catecholamines (Rabin, 1999). Once activated, these immune cells produce and secrete an array of neuropeptides and cytokines (e.g., interferons, interleukins, growth factors) that influence central nervous system (CNS) responses, including increased firing of neurons (Maier & Watkins, 2003), thus resulting in changes in mood states, energy, and behavior. For example, when interferon alpha or interleukin 2 (IL-2) is given systemically as cancer treatment to trigger a cell-mediated immune response to a tumor, the result is fever, anorexia, fatigue, and profound emotional and cognitive changes.

Targeted immunotherapy once was considered the goal of cancer therapy. However, it now is recognized that multiple processes play a role in immune regulation of cancer, and targeting a single immune response is unlikely to be effective (Moynihan, 2003). The complexity of immune interactions is a protective process in which compensatory mechanisms restore homeostasis. It now is known that interactions between the SNS and the immune system always occur in the context of other potent immune modulators, some of which activate and some which suppress immune responses (Madden, 2001). Figure 28-1 presents evidence for bidirectional effects among the CNS, neuroendocrine responses, and the immune system.

Specific evidence for the effects of CNS and neuroendocrine influences on immunity predominantly has been derived from rat models demonstrating that damage to or interference with the neurons in central brain regions (e.g., locus coeruleus, hippocampus, hypothalamus) affects the secretion of neurohormones and cytokines and alters the function and trafficking of lymphocytes and other immune cells. The immune system also responds to more subtle neurohormone changes, such as

---

Figure 28-1. Evidence for Central Nervous and Immune System Interactions

Central Nervous System (CNS) and Neuroendocrine Effects on Immunity
- Lymphocytes have receptors for hormones, neurotransmitters, and opioids.
- Catecholamines, opioids, growth hormones, and adrenocortical steroids alter immune responses.
- Biologic and circadian rhythms alter immune responses.
- Changes in hormone or neurotransmitter levels alter immune responses.
- Sympathetic nervous system activation innervates lymphoid tissue.
- Acute stress can increase or decrease immune response.
- Chronic stress decreases immune cell–mediated and humoral immune responses.
- Sensory stimulation, cognitive thought, and emotion affect immune response.
- Classic (Pavlovian) conditioning can modify immune responses.
- Pain suppresses cellular and humoral immune responses.
- Psychosocial factors influence autoimmune disorders, infections, and cancer.
- Psychosocial and behavioral interventions can alter immune response.

Immune Effects on Behavioral and CNS Responses
- Cytokines and neuropeptides secreted from activated lymphocytes influence behavior and CNS responses.
- Firing of neurons increases in response to immunization and infection.
- Select cytokines cross the blood-brain barrier via several mechanisms.
- The CNS has receptors for cytokines.
- Glial cells in the brain produce and secrete identical cytokines.
- Immune changes signal hypothalamic-pituitary-adrenal responses and release of catecholamines.
- Proinflammatory cytokines cause predictable "sickness behavior."
- Cytokines contribute to depression, memory loss, and hyperresponsiveness to pain.

---

dysregulation of the autonomic nervous system, alterations in sex hormones (e.g., menopause, pregnancy), and inefficient binding of neurotransmitters (e.g., depression). Immune and inflammatory processes can be influenced by physical stressors, behavioral conditioning, unconditioned stimuli (antigens), and opioids, which trigger SNS responses and release of catecholamines. Catecholamines and neuropeptides modulate leukocyte migration and adhesion to endothelial cells, resulting in an inflammatory response. Lymph tissue is richly innervated by sympathetic fibers and nerve fibers containing numerous neuropeptides that affect immune and inflammatory responses (e.g., substance P, somatostatin, cell adhesion molecules, vasoactive intestinal peptide, neuropeptide Y) (Carlson, 2001). The behavioral science approach to PNI centers on the role of stress and psychosocial factors modulating immune function and how changes in immune status influence behavior. Greater evidence supports the direct role of cytokines as mediators of central and peripheral immune and neuroendocrine responses.

Cytokines as Mediators of PNI Responses

Cytokines are considered to be any protein released by an immune cell that can, in turn, affect itself or other immune cells. Whereas hormones, neurotransmitters, and neuropeptides are the mediators of the nervous and endocrine systems, cytokines appear to be the main messengers from the immune system to the brain (Besedovsky & Del Rey, 2001). Peripheral and central cytokines influence brain–immune system

---

communication, with neurotransmitters assisting in cytokine transfer. Cytokines are thought to follow humoral and neural routes to influence brain functions, with some crossing the blood-brain barrier (Banks, 2001; Besedovsky & Del Rey). The presence of receptors for cytokines in the nervous system and the production of cytokines by glial cells and certain neurons provide evidence for their central effect. However, the actual physiologic effect of central cytokines has yet to be determined.

Immune cells produce cytokines in response to antigen or cell signaling. Monocytes secrete IL-1. Type 1 helper (Th1) T-cell subsets regulate cellular immunity and express interferon gamma and tumor necrosis factor-alpha (TNF-α), and type 2 helper (Th2) T-cell subsets regulate humoral immunity and express cytokines IL-4, 6, and 10 (Mosmann & Sad, 1996). IL-1 is one of the most studied cytokines because of its powerful stimulation of the hypothalamus to release cortisol and its ability to cross the blood-brain barrier through a saturable transport system and exert specific neurologic effects (Besedovsky & Del Rey, 2001). Known as an endogenous pyrogen that causes fever, IL-1 has been shown to reduce dopamine and serotonin by stimulating metabolism, inducing slow-wave sleep, triggering release of prostaglandins that increase pain and inflammation, and exerting profound effects on learning, memory, and behavior.

IL-1 alpha and IL-1 beta belong to a class of proinflammatory cytokines, along with TNF-α and IL-6 and possibly other cytokines, that act in the brain to cause "sickness behaviors"—symptoms of illness that include fever, hypersomnia, depressed activity, weakness, malaise, inability to concentrate, and profound psychological and behavioral changes (Kelley et al., 2003; Miller, 2003). Depression (Capuron & Dantzer, 2003), hyperalgesia, and memory loss (Maier & Watkins, 2003), along with infection and inflammation (Dantzer et al., 2001), have been directly associated with proinflammatory cytokines. Although intended to be restorative and adaptive, these responses create symptoms that can be prolonged in patients with cancer.

Stress and Psychoneuroimmune Response

The past decade has seen remarkable advances in the medical community's understanding of how stress induces nervous and endocrine responses that affect immunity and how immune challenges, such as infections, vaccinations, and autoimmune diseases, can influence CNS responses (Sheridan, 2003). Several factors influence the ability of stress to regulate immune function. Factors related to the stressors themselves include the cumulative number of stressors, the perceived stressfulness of the event(s), the acuity or chronicity of the stressors, and the timing of onset in relation to other environmental demands. Personal factors include the individual's perception of the event, his or her ability to control or cope effectively with the stressful situation, and concomitant host factors such as age, nutritional status, and existence of comorbid health problems. How the individual responds to the stressors is more important than the stressor itself. The interaction between stress and immune response has implications for cancer risk and survival, as well as for determining interventions that influence quality of life and disease outcomes.

Physiology of the Stress-Immune Response

High emotional distress elevates levels of stress hormones, which impairs T-cell function and immune surveillance. Although overwhelming evidence supports immune suppression in response to stress, reports also show enhancement of immune function, reflecting the complexity of the immune system (Dhabhar & McEwen, 2001; Rabin, 1999). The effects of stress on the immune system are mediated primarily through neuroendocrine and SNS pathways. When the cortex perceives an event as stressful, the amygdala (a neuropeptide-rich area in the limbic system) responds to emotional states by innervating brain-stem catecholaminergic cells that activate the hypothalamus, resulting in corticotropin-releasing hormone. Neuroendocrine responses create a cascade of release of adrenocorticotropic hormone, opioid peptides, and glucocorticoid hormones (cortisol) and catecholamines (epinephrine, norepinephrine [NE]), resulting in modulation of cytokine expression and production of inflammatory mediators (Eskandari & Sternberg, 2002) (see Figure 28-2). Simultaneous SNS activation of noradrenergic pathways results in the secretion of NE by the peripheral SNS and the release of NE and epinephrine from the adrenal medulla. NE is the primary neurotransmitter of the SNS and can enhance or inhibit immune reactivity, suggesting that catecholamines help to balance a rapid immune response to foreign antigens while minimizing destruction of normal tissue (Madden, 2003). The activation of these two neurochemical pathways and the release of hormones and neurotransmitters profoundly influence immune function (Moynihan, 2003).

Neurohormones (e.g., glucocorticoids, catecholamines) that activate the hypothalamic-pituitary-adrenal axis (HPA) in response to stress downregulate Th1 cell-mediated activity and enhance Th2 humoral immune responses, resulting in suppression of natural killer (NK) cells and IL-2 and increased proinflammatory cytokine and antibody production (Elenkov & Chrousos, 1999; Kasprowicz et al., 2000). Catecholamines also modulate lymphocyte proliferation, cytokine and antibody production, cell lysis, and migration (Madden, 2003). Other hormones and neuropeptides selectively inhibit IL-2 and antibody production (vasoactive intestinal peptide), reduce lymphocyte mitosis (somatostatin), contribute to lymphocyte apoptosis (opioids), and contribute to inflammation and mast cell release of histamine (substance P, neuropeptide Y) (Rabin, 1999; Shi et al., 2003). Other hormones enhance immune function, such as growth hormone, insulin-like growth factor, and melatonin, counteracting some of the immune-inhibiting aspects of other hormones (Rabin).

Clinical Implications of Stress-Related Immune Response

All stress hormones influence some aspect of immunity, and immune suppression and infection often accompany increased tumor risk, indicating that a healthy immune system is important for maintaining a tumor-free status (Moynihan, 2003; Shi et al., 2003). Particularly strong support exists for the influence of stress, depression, hostility, and social support on disease outcomes (Kemeny, 2003).

The effect of stressors on immune parameters may result from differential neuroendocrine responses that alter the balance of Th1 to Th2 cells. Stress may contribute to pathogenesis, including cancer, through lymphocyte apoptosis (Shi et al., 2003; Stefanek & McDonald, 2003) and secretion of proinflammatory cytokines in response

Figure 28-2. Psychoneuroimmune Interactions in Response to Stressors

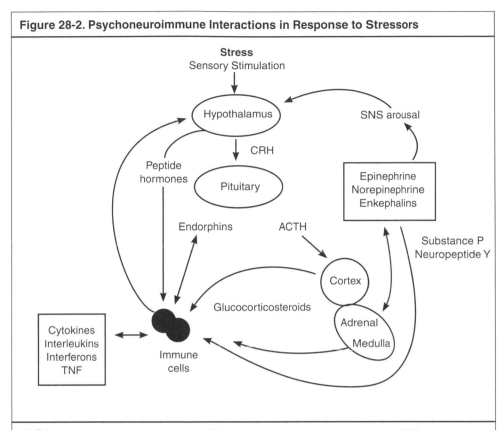

ACTH—adrenocorticotropic hormones; CRH—corticotropin-releasing hormone; SNS—sympathetic nervous system; TNF—tumor necrosis factor

to negative emotions and chronic or recurring infections (Kiecolt-Glaser, McGuire, Robles, & Glaser, 2002b). Immune effects observed in patients with cancer include a shift in Th1 to Th2 (Moynihan, 2003; Yang & Glaser, 2003), changes in HPA axis functioning (Antoni, 2003), and elevation and flattening of the diurnal rhythm of cortisol, which is associated with increased incidence of depression and earlier mortality in breast cancer (Spiegel & Sephton, 2001; Yehuda, 2003). Lymphocytes under oxidative stress are more prone to apoptosis, and some studies have shown that antioxidants block stress-induced lymphopenia (Shi et al.).

The effects of psychological stress on cancer initiation and progression may occur through both stress-induced immune suppression and direct effects on genomic DNA (Yang & Glaser, 2003). Hormonal or immune changes may influence some cancers more than others. Cancers that show a direct relationship between immune suppression and cancer risk include cervical cancer, a virally initiated cancer; malignant melanoma, an example of faulty DNA repair mechanisms and increased lymphocyte apoptosis; and ovarian cancer, in which survival is linked to vascular endothelial growth factor that promotes angiogenesis (Lutgendorf et al., 2003). Other more general immune effects on cancer include the increased potential for metastases following the physical and emotional stress of surgery (Ben-Eliyahu, 2003) and increased rates of second cancers and recurrence following chemotherapy that suppresses NK cells (Antoni, 2003). Although not all tumors are directly responsive to immune control, innate and natural immune resistance is critical to malignant transformation of cells (Sheridan, 2003).

Factors Influencing Stress-Related Immune Response

Increasing evidence supports that different forms of stress and emotional responses may have different CNS pathways and affect physiologic outcomes in different ways (Kemeny, 2003). Factors influencing the stress response include the stressors themselves, the individual's perception of and the response to the stressors, and the vulnerability of the host (see Table 28-1).

Table 28-1. Factors Influencing Stress-Related Immune Response

Stressors	Response to the Stressors	Vulnerability of the Host
Severity, duration, and intensity	Perceived significance and meaning	Personal characteristics: age, gender, socioeconomic status, personality
Acute or chronic	Appraisal and coping	Risk factors: underlying immune function, exposures, circadian rhythm
Control: actual or perceived	Lifestyle changes	Lifestyle factors: smoking habits, social support, nutrition, caregiving, sleep patterns

Stressors: How people respond to individual stressors partly depends on the stressors themselves, including their severity, duration, and intensity, as well as the individual's perceived control over the stressor. Human and animal studies support that perceived or actual control over stressors causes less HPA activation than uncontrolled or helpless situations (Kemeny, 2003). Alternatively, those with HIV who had negative expectancies for the future and feelings of loss of control over self and emotions had accelerated rates of disease progression (Kemeny).

Acute and chronic stress also affects the immune response in different ways. Repeated challenges and cumulative stressors, such as recurrence, multiple complications, and lengthy treatment plans, become more stressful over time. Although acute stress both increases and decreases NK cytotoxicity and delayed-type hypersensitivity (Dhabhar & McEwen, 2001), chronic stress is universally suppressive (Moynihan, 2003). The acute responses may be the result of the classic "fight or flight" stress model, in which catecholamines initially mobilize lymphocytes from the marginal pool and the spleen, resulting in increased circulating lymphocyte numbers and specific increases in NK cells. Following the initial adaptive response, lymphocyte numbers decrease over the next several hours and remain suppressed if the stressor continues.

"Control" is the belief that one has personal responsibility to influence one's health (Nicholas & Webster, 1996). Participating in healthcare decision making, seeking information with which to make decisions, maintaining a sense of normalcy, eating balanced and nourishing meals, getting adequate sleep and exercise, and balancing work and play activities can foster a sense of control. When stressors were controllable, optimism was associated with higher immune parameters. When stressors were uncontrollable, however, optimism was associated with lower immune function because optimistic people were not able to give up (Segerstrom, 2003). Although the stressor itself cannot always be controlled, individuals can modify their response to the stressor to better adapt to the situation.

How one responds to stressors: How an individual responds to stressors is determined by the stressors themselves, their perceived significance and meaning, and the individual's ability to eliminate, adapt to, and cope with the stressors. A common belief in stress and coping theories is that it is not the stressors themselves but how the individual responds to them that influences psychoneuroimmune responses.

Lazarus and Folkman (1984) defined coping as cognitive and behavioral efforts to manage demands that are appraised as taxing or exceeding resources. They described coping strategies as either emotion- or problem-focused. In emotion-focused coping, individuals perceive the situation as one that cannot be managed and try to reduce the intensity of the response to the event rather than directly addressing the stressor. Alternatively, problem-focused coping, a more active coping strategy, increases a sense of participation and is used by individuals who perceive their ability to master the situation and change outcomes. Less emotional distress occurs when patients focus on the positive, rely on social support, and distance themselves from the problem (Dunkel-Schetter, Feinstein, Taylor, & Falke, 1992). Conversely, patients who use cognitive or behavioral escape-avoidance (e.g., fantasizing, wishful thinking, resignation, social withdrawal) experience greater emotional distress and have been shown to have lower suppressor T-cell counts (Fang et al., 2003).

Lifestyle changes affect immune function independently or synergistically with other factors. For example, individuals who cope less effectively or who are lonely and isolated engage in fewer health-promoting behaviors, such as compliance with medical care, exercise, dietary modifications, and avoidance of smoking and use of alcohol and other drugs (Hawkley & Cacioppo, 2003). Caregiving is a lifestyle stressor that creates chronic stress and has been shown to cause a shift in Th1 to Th2 responses (Glaser et al., 2001) and increase IL-6 production (Kiecolt-Glaser et al., 2003).

Vulnerability of the host: Other factors, such as circadian rhythm, sleeping patterns, nutritional state, older age, depression, and underlying immune function also reduce cellular immune function. Circadian rhythm alters gonadal steroid, thymic hormone, and glucocorticoid levels. Chronic sleep deprivation triggers release of IL-1, TNF, and growth hormone and prolactin (Krueger, Majde, & Obal, 2003). Exercise causes transient increases in beta endorphins, catecholamines, and glucocorticoids, and smoking suppresses lymphocyte responses.

The effect of stress on immunity also depends on personality, loneliness, and social isolation (Hawkley & Cacioppo, 2003; Segerstrom, 2003). Personality characteristics determine how an individual interprets and responds to a potential stressor and can lessen or amplify the effects of the stressor (Lutgendorf, 2002). Social support was related to survival in women with ovarian cancer (Lutgendorf et al., 2003), and lower cell-mediated immune responses occurred in individuals who were lonely (Hawkley & Cacioppo; Segerstrom). Older adults with a lower sense of coherence had lower NK cell activity (Lutgendorf, Vitaliano, Tripp-Reimer, Harvey, & Lubaroff,

1999). Of particular importance is that a combination of factors increases the risk for immune-associated disease, such as older age, a genetic predisposition to cancer, or a history of or predisposition to depression. Baseline immune competence at the time of cancer treatment is an independent prognostic factor of recurrence-free survival (Ben-Eliyahu, 2003). All protective and risk factors should be considered in the treatment plan for patients.

The Role of Interventions in Modulating Psychoneuroimmune Responses

Understanding the effects of stress and negative mood states on immune function provides a foundation for current stress-reducing interventions. Interventions that interrupt the perception of stress or the stress response itself potentially can influence health outcomes by modulating immune function. The premise is that if chronic psychological and/or physical stressors have deleterious effects on immune function and health outcomes, then interventions aimed at reducing the stressful experience can have positive effects and improve immunocompetence and health. Interventions aimed at reducing stress responses help by increasing awareness of or changing the perceived significance and meaning of the stressors, facilitating the use of appropriate resources and coping strategies to manage or control the stressors, or reducing physiologic tension through relaxation. A growing body of literature explains the physiologic mechanisms, supports the use of interventions to reduce the negative effects of stress, and improves physical and psychological symptoms and overall quality of life. However, little is known about whether stress-reducing interventions influence health outcomes in humans.

Interventions that modulate psychoneuroimmune responses can be described in two general categories: sensory and cognitive-behavioral-expressive. The common thread for these interventions involves the brain playing a central role in the mechanism of action. Processing of sensory stimulation and thoughts or emotions takes place in several parts of the brain (e.g., cerebral cortex, limbic structures, thalamus, brain stem, hypothalamus) and leads to a complex cascade of neuro-endocrine-immune responses (see previous section). Sensory interventions involve the senses and include massage and other touch interventions, aromatherapy, and music therapy. Cognitive-behavioral-expressive interventions involve the cerebral cortex and include meditation, imagery, expressive writing, support groups, humor, cognitive restructuring, and creative therapies. Figure 28-3 highlights four specific interventions (aromatherapy, imagery, mindfulness meditation [MM], and massage).

Sensory Interventions

Sensory interventions stimulate the body through cranial nerves or peripheral sensory afferent nerve fibers and send information to the brain and spinal cord. The thalamus, located in the center of the brain, acts as a chief traffic relay station for directing sensory signals to a variety of brain structures, thereby initiating neuro-endocrine-immune and other physiologic responses.

Figure 28-3. Interventions in Modulating Psychoneuroimmune Responses

Aromatherapy

Purpose
- The use of scents to induce therapeutic benefit

Format/Process
- Highly concentrated essential oils require just a few drops for therapeutic benefit.
- Pure essential oils can be diluted with or added to skin lotions, body oils, or moist compresses for direct application to the skin, allowing for inhalation of the scent during and after application.
- Essential oil drops can be added to bath water or shampoo.
- Vaporization of essential oil allows for the scent to permeate the room, which can be done by aromatic diffusers, oil burners, lightbulb rings, or a bowl of water with a few drops of oil.
- Put a few drops of essential oil on a cotton ball and place in the clinical area, at patient's bedside.
- Large quantities can be toxic to mucous membranes or skin.
- Do not administer pure, undiluted essential oils directly on the skin because serious skin irritation can occur.

Theory/Mechanisms
- Olfactory nerve (cranial nerve I) is embedded directly into the brain (i.e., limbic structures). Stimulation of the limbic system and cerebral cortex causes bidirectional neuro-endocrine-immune processes via hypothalamus and sympathetic nervous system.

Possible Outcomes
- Decreased anxiety, nausea, pain, respiratory congestion, indigestion, abdominal cramps, headache, and hiccups
- Improvements in sleep, mood, and overall well-being (Buckle, 1999; Lawless, 1995)

Imagery

Purpose
- A technique to cope with difficult circumstances or physical and/or psychological discomfort
- Uses the mind's eye to visualize/imagine/mentally experience, invoking all senses: visual, aural, tactile, olfactory, proprioceptive, kinesthetic
- Heightens psychological insight
  - Manage fears by practicing or desensitizing.
  - Facilitate problem solving or decision making.
  - Access and more deeply experience emotion.
  - Change negative thoughts into positive thoughts.
- Fosters sense of control with active participation and responsibility in health

Format/Process
- Individual or group
- 20–60 minutes of daily practice reinforced by feedback from healthcare professional
- Face-to-face interaction, audio-/videotape, self-imagery
- Music as an optional adjunct
- Deep breathing is essential to achieve relaxed state.
- Invokes all senses

Mechanisms
- Imagined/visualized experience is perceived through thoughts and emotions processed through cerebral cortex and limbic system, leading to bidirectional neuro-endocrine-immune processes via hypothalamus and sympathetic nervous system.

Possible Outcomes
- Lowered levels cortisol and catecholamines
- Decreased heart rate, blood pressure, respiratory rate, and muscle tension
- Increased oxygen saturation
- Less pain, nausea, fatigue, other physical symptoms, anxiety, and depressed mood
- Greater relaxation, positive mood, energy, and quality of life
- Increased sense of control
- Immunologic profile shift from type 1 helper (Th1) cells (proinflammatory) to type 2 helper (Th2) cells (anti-inflammatory)

(Continued on next page)

Figure 28-3. Interventions in Modulating Psychoneuroimmune Responses (Continued)

Mindfulness Meditation
Purpose
- Stress-reducing technique to cultivate full present-moment awareness
- Lets go of past concerns and future worries
- Helps one to fully experience, appreciate, and accept the way things are, right here, right now
  - Without judging or striving
- Heightens psychological insight—self-awareness of thoughts, emotions, and physical reactions
- Fosters gentleness, patience, gratitude, and loving-kindness toward self and others
- Fosters sense of control with active participation and responsibility in health

Format/Process
- Individual or group
- 20–40 minutes of daily practice recommended
- Guided meditation in person or by audiotape or self-practice
- Be quiet and pay attention to physical sensations: the breath, sounds, sights, thoughts, or emotions.
- The breath can be an anchor to remind participant to come back to the present moment.
- Regular practice fosters integration of mindfulness throughout everyday activities.
- Creates awareness that everything changes from one moment to the next, and promotes not clinging

Mechanisms
- Changes perception of stressful circumstances or unpleasant stimuli to be less threatening and less overwhelming via cerebral cortex and limbic system→ bidirectional neuro-endocrine-immune processes via hypothalamus and sympathetic nervous system.

Possible Outcomes
- Lowered cortisol and catecholamines
- Decreased heart rate, blood pressure, respiratory rate, and muscle tension
- Increased oxygen saturation
- Less pain, nausea, fatigue, other physical symptoms, anxiety, and depressed mood
- Greater relaxation, mood, energy, sleep quality, and quality of life
- Increased sense of control
- Greater left anterior brain activity
- Immune shift from Th1 to Th2

Massage
Purpose
- Stress-reducing technique to induce physical and mental relaxation
- Promotes peripheral circulation and lymphatic drainage
- Offers comfort and caring
- Reduces symptoms of anxiety, pain, and fatigue

Format/Process
- Systematic manipulation of soft tissue for therapeutic purposes
- Provided by trained and licensed massage therapist
- Can be taught to parent or caregiver
- Standard technique is head to toe and torso to extremity, but this can vary.
- A variety of techniques and depth of touch may be used (e.g., effleurage is a light gliding touch to relax muscles and ease tension, petrissage is a deeper tissue therapeutic massage to stretch and loosen tense muscles and release trigger points).
- Music facilitates relaxation.
- 45–60 minutes is standard for adults, but children tolerate 20–30 minutes, depending on age.
- Parent-infant massage facilitates bonding and comfort of newborn.

(Continued on next page)

476

Figure 28-3. Interventions in Modulating Psychoneuroimmune Responses (Continued)

Theory/Mechanisms
- Physical touch, offered in a gentle and therapeutic manner, reduces physical and mental tension, promoting relaxation and stress reduction. Reduces sympathetic nervous system activation, resulting in bidirectional neuro-endocrine-immune responses that influence emotional and physical states.

Possible Outcomes
- Lowered cortisol and catecholamines
- Decreased heart rate, blood pressure, respiratory rate, muscle tension, and dyspnea
- Increased oxygen saturation
- Less pain, fatigue, anxiety, and depressed mood
- Greater relaxation, positive mood, energy, sleep quality, and quality of life
- May shift Th1 to Th2 and increase natural killer cells

Massage: Massage use in patients with cancer has been shown to induce relaxation and reduce pain, anxiety, blood pressure, and fatigue (Ahles et al., 1999; Hadfield, 2001; Post-White et al., 2003; Smith, Reeder, Daniel, Baramee, & Hagman, 2003; Wilkinson, Aldridge, Salmon, Cain, & Wilson, 1999), and recent studies also have confirmed the physiologic effects of massage (Diego et al., 2001; Ironson et al., 1996; Wikstrom, Gunnarsson, & Nordin, 2003). A recent nursing study using a two-group experimental design evaluated the effects of a 20-minute therapeutic back massage on spouses of patients with cancer and found significant improvements in mood and perceived stress after massage, in addition to significant inverse relationships between psychological measures (depressed mood and perceived stress) and immune function (NK cytotoxicity) (Goodfellow, 2003).

Aromatherapy: Aromatherapy is the use of scents or smells to trigger a therapeutic response and has become quite popular in recent years (Buckle, 1999; Lawless, 1995). Although anecdotal reports of benefits of aromatherapy are common and can be supported by an understanding of neuroanatomy and PNI physiology, minimal research by acceptable scientific standards has been done to date. Only one large, well-controlled study of aromatherapy involving patients with cancer has been done (N = 313); this study found no anxiety reducing benefit of pure essential oils of lavender, bergamot, and cedarwood in patients undergoing radiotherapy (Graham, Browne, Cox, & Graham, 2003).

Music/music therapy: The effects of music on mood are appreciated ubiquitously. An increasing body of research supports the therapeutic benefits of music and music therapy (a more formal application of specific music techniques performed by a trained therapist, with the goal of improving psychological and/or physical well-being) for individuals with various clinical conditions, including adults and children with cancer (Ezzone, Baker, Rosselet, & Terepka, 1998; Robb, 2000; Standley & Hanser, 1995). Pain, anxiety, nausea, and mood all have been shown to be sensitive to music interventions, although the effects are not consistently effective during invasive hospital procedures (Evans, 2002; Kwekkeboom, 2003). A recent randomized study of music therapy in hospice patients (N = 80) showed improvements in quality of life; however, it identified no effects on survival (Hilliard, 2003).

Cognitive-Behavioral and Expressive Interventions

Cognitive-behavioral and expressive interventions work primarily at the level of the cerebral cortex in the brain. Through control, expression, and modification of thoughts and perceptions (such as perceived stress and fear), an individual's emotional response has system effects that include neuro-endocrine-immune responses (described previously).

Mindfulness meditation: MM is a cognitive-behavioral stress-reducing intervention that involves paying attention to the present moment—physical sensations, the breath, sounds, sights, thoughts, or emotions—without judging or striving (Kabat-Zinn, 1990). It involves acceptance of and openness to what is, not clinging onto the past or worrying about the future, and cultivates stable, nonreactive awareness. Studies over the past 20 years have documented improvements in psychological and physical symptoms and health outcomes, with scientific rigor and PNI outcomes as more recent requisites.

Davidson et al. (2003) conducted a randomized, controlled study of 41 healthy volunteers who participated in an eight-week mindfulness training program. The study included outcomes of anxiety, affect, brain activity, and immune function over a period of six months. Meditators were found to have significant decreases in anxiety and negative affect, increases in influenza antibody titers in response to vaccination, and increases in left-sided anterior brain activation (associated with positive emotional states) compared to nonmeditators. A direct and significant relationship occurred between the magnitude of left-sided brain activation and antibody titers. This is the first documented study of MM demonstrating relationships in brain activity to in vivo immune function and, thus, has important implications for further PNI intervention research.

A randomized, wait-list controlled study of patients with cancer demonstrated significant reduction of total mood disturbance and symptoms of stress in a heterogenous group of 90 outpatients who participated in a seven-week MM program (Speca, Carlson, Goodley, & Angen, 2000). The study found that the average daily time spent meditating predicted improvements in mood disturbance, and the number of sessions attended predicted reduction in symptoms of stress. Two single-arm pre- and postdesign studies of MM (Carlson, Speca, Patel, & Goodley, 2003; Carlson, Ursuliak, Goodley, Angen, & Speca, 2001) demonstrated greater quality of life and reduced stress and a shift from proinflammatory Th1 to anti-inflammatory Th2 profiles in outpatients with cancer. Sleep quality also improved in two studies of women with breast cancer (Carlson et al., 2003; Shapiro, Bootzin, Figueredo, Lopez, & Schwartz, 2003). The use of MM in hospitalized patients with cancer (e.g., undergoing a stem cell or bone marrow transplant) is an important new area of study that has shown promising preliminary results (Bauer-Wu et al., 2004).

Imagery: Imagery involves using the mind's eye to visualize images, scenes, and other sensations. Although not actually experiencing the sensory stimulation, the mind imagines the sensory experience. Imagery, which may be combined with other interventions such as music, progressive muscle relaxation, and group support, has been shown to have positive effects on relaxation, mood, and well-being in studies of patients with cancer (Baider, Peretz, Hadani, & Koch, 2001; Post-White, 1991; Richardson et al., 1997; Sloman, 2002; Syrjala, Donaldson, Davis, Kippes, & Carr, 1995; Troesch, Rodehaver, Delaney, & Yanes, 1993). Studies of the effects of imagery on immune function have had mixed results (Bakke, Purtzer, & Newton, 2002; Gruzelier, 2002; Post-White; Post-White et al., 1996; Richardson et al.). Of the three imagery studies involving breast cancer survivors, no changes in NK cell numbers or activity were identified in two studies (Post-White et al., 1996; Richardson et al.), whereas the other study found an increase in NK cell numbers (consistent with improvements in depressed mood) upon completion of an eight-week imagery training program, although the changes were not maintained three months later (Bakke et al.).

Expressive writing: Expressive writing is a therapeutic technique of writing about personal thoughts and feelings as a means for catharsis, resolution of previous difficulties, and integration of positive and negative experiences (Lepore & Smyth, 2002; Pennebaker, 1997). Pennebaker's model of a brief writing exercise (e.g., 20–30 minutes a day for three to five days) has shown consistent health benefits in noncancer populations (Pennebaker; Smyth, Stone, Hurewitz, & Kaell, 1999). Research findings on expressive writing involving patients with cancer have been mixed yet promising (Bauer-Wu et al., 2003; Rosenberg et al., 2002; Stanton & Danoff-Burg, 2002; Stanton et al., 2002; Walker, Nail, & Croyle, 1999). Given the intensity of the cancer diagnosis, treatment, and associated life changes, very brief writing periods may not be as beneficial as expressive writing over longer periods of time, such as several weeks or months.

Group support: Support groups afford patients with cancer an opportunity to express themselves while at the same time feeling understood by others experiencing a similar situation. Cancer support groups have received considerable attention, with consistent research supporting benefits to psychological well-being and quality of life (Fawzy, Cousins, et al., 1990; Spiegel & Bloom, 1983), although the effects on cancer survival have been inconclusive (Cunningham et al., 1998; Fawzy et al., 1993; Goodwin et al., 2001; Spiegel, Bloom, Kraemer, & Gottheil, 1989). A seminal study by Fawzy, Kemeny, et al. (1990) supported the immune-enhancing effects of a combined psychoeducational support intervention that focused on stress management and coping. In this study of individuals with malignant melanoma, immune effects were not observed immediately following the intervention but were detected six months after the six-week intervention ended (Fawzy, Kemeny, et al.). Increases in NK cell numbers and activity also correlated with less emotional distress (Fawzy, Kemeny, et al.) and recurrence but not longer survival (Fawzy et al., 1993).

Humor: Norman Cousins (1979) popularized therapeutic humor, the use of humor to feel better and improve health, more than 25 years ago in his book *Anatomy of an Illness*. Since then, research in this area has grown, demonstrating consistent psychological and physiologic benefits (Bennett, Zeller, Rosenberg, & McCann, 2003; Berk, Felten, Tan, Bittman, & Westergard, 2001; Martin, 2001; Takahashi et al., 2001). In children, humor contributed to less infection but had no effect on salivary IgA (Dowling, Hockenberry, & Gregory, 2003). Two studies in adults identified significant immune effects (increase in NK activity) associated with laughter in response to watching a humorous video or comedic film (Bennett et al.; Takahashi et al.).

Mind-Body Interventions: Clinical Considerations

These studies demonstrate that mind-body interventions can influence PNI responses in some situations and under some conditions. The many interventions available for adults and children with cancer (Kelly et al., 2000; Phipps, 2002) allow patients to choose those in which they are most interested. Recognizing patients' preferences and individualizing interventions are critical. Assessing patients for appropriateness of interventions should include ascertaining their underlying motivation for learning and practicing the techniques, readiness and willingness to commit to self-learning and regular practice, and expectations for benefits and outcomes, if any. Data validating immune effects and associated health outcomes in patients with cancer are lacking; therefore, the focus for potential benefit should center on positive coping and improved emotional state. Patients with underlying psychiatric or emotional disorders should be referred to psychiatrists or psychologists for evaluation of appropriate interventions. Although most of these interventions are well tolerated, adverse effects have occurred (e.g., drowsiness, confusion, anxiety) and must be monitored (Astin, Shapiro, Eisenberg, & Forys, 2003). Evaluating the use of these interventions in practice requires attention to any negative effects as well as documentation of benefits.

Patients with cancer may be most receptive to using mind-body interventions when they are undergoing diagnostic testing, recently diagnosed, actively making treatment decisions, receiving treatments that cause adverse symptoms, experiencing disease recurrence, or receiving palliative care measures. In some cases, however, the use of mind-body interventions can create additional stress by advocating greater individual responsibility for health at a time when this responsibility can be overwhelming. And, because insurance often does not cover mind-body interventions, patients may have the additional burden of cost, although the cost of these interventions is highly variable. Finally, these interventions can be very helpful for family members who are experiencing related stressors and changes in roles and responsibilities.

Conclusion

Although once considered separate systems, behavioral, neural, endocrine, and immune systems now are known to communicate through direct innervation and indirect signaling by neurotransmitters, hormones, and cytokines. Research in PNI is burgeoning (Kiecolt-Glaser, McGuire, Robles, & Glaser, 2002a), and observations now explain how changes in immune function can result from, as well as induce, behavioral and emotional responses to stressors (Kiecolt-Glaser et al., 2002b). Interventions that reduce acute and chronic stress responses can contribute to an improved sense of well-being and influence psychoneuroimmune responses.

Because psychoneuroimmune interactions are complex and coping responses are individualized, validating these relationships requires scientific rigor, large sample sizes, and replication of results. Nurses have the opportunity to influence the growth of PNI by generating new knowledge concerning mind-body interactions in health and illness and developing strategies that promote mental and physical well-being in people at risk for immune dysfunction (Zeller, McCain, & Swanson, 1996). Nursing has consistently, since its early days, embraced a holistic view of patient care. This is evident in Florence Nightingale's (1969) *Notes on Nursing*, originally published in 1860, in which she eloquently wrote about the healing power of sensory stimulation and personal connection in promoting patients' recovery from illness. Clearly, nurses are well positioned to advance both the science and the art of mind-body interventions.

References

Ader, R. (Ed.). (1981). *Psychoneuroimmunology.* New York: Academic Press.

Ader, R. (1996). On the teaching of psychoneuroimmunology [Commentary]. *Brain, Behavior, and Immunity, 10,* 315–323.

Ader, R. (2003). Conditioned immunomodulations: Research needs and directions. *Brain, Behavior, and Immunity, 17*(Suppl. 1), S51–S57.

Ader, R., & Cohen, N. (1975). Behaviorally conditioned immunosuppression. *Psychosomatic Medicine, 37,* 333–340.

Ader, R., Felten, D.L., & Cohen, N. (Eds.). (1991). *Psychoneuroimmunology* (2nd ed.). New York: Academic Press.

Ader, R., Felten, D.L., & Cohen, N. (Eds.). (2001). *Psychoneuroimmunology* (3rd ed.). San Diego, CA: Academic Press.

Ahles, T.A., Tope, D.M., Pinkson, B., Walch, S., Hann, D., Whedon, M., et al. (1999). Massage therapy for patients undergoing autologous bone marrow transplantation. *Journal of Pain and Symptom Management, 18,* 157–163.

Antoni, M.H. (2003). Psychoneuroendocrinology and psychoneuroimmunology of cancer: Plausible mechanisms worth pursuing? *Brain, Behavior, and Immunity, 17*(Suppl. 1), S84–S91.

Astin, J.A., Shapiro, S.L., Eisenberg, D.M., & Forys, K.L. (2003). Mind-body medicine: State of the science, implications for practice. *Journal of the American Board of Family Practice, 16,* 131–147.

Baider, L., Peretz, T., Hadani, P.E., & Koch, U. (2001). Psychological intervention in cancer patients. *General Hospital Psychiatry, 23,* 272–277.

Bakke, A.C., Purtzer, M.Z., & Newton, P. (2002). The effect of hypnotic-guided imagery on psychological well-being and immune function in patients with prior breast cancer. *Journal of Psychosomatic Research, 53,* 1131–1137.

Banks, W.A. (2001). Cytokines, CVSs, and the blood-brain barrier. In R. Ader, D. Felten, & N. Cohen (Eds.), *Psychoneuroimmunology* (3rd ed., pp. 483–498). San Diego, CA: Academic Press.

Bauer-Wu, S., Healey, M., Rosenbaum, E., Blood, E., Xu, R., Ott, M.J., et al. (2004). Facing the challenges of stem cell/bone marrow transplantation with mindfulness meditation: A pilot study [Abstract]. *Psycho-Oncology, 13*(Suppl. 1), S10–S11.

Bauer-Wu, S.M., Liu, Q., Hsieh, C.C., Laccetti, M., Healey, M., Winer, E., et al. (2003, March). *Expressive writing for metastatic breast cancer patients: Effects on coping, disease status, and healthcare utilization over three months* [Abstract]. Proceedings of the Eastern Nursing Research Society Conference, New Haven, CT.

Ben Eliyahu, S. (2003). The promotion of tumor metastasis by surgery and stress: Immunological basis and implications for psychoneuroimmunology. *Brain, Behavior, and Immunity, 17*(Suppl. 1), S27–S36.

Bennett, M., Zeller, J., Rosenberg, L., & McCann, J. (2003). The effect of mirthful laughter on stress and natural killer cell activity. *Alternative Therapies in Health and Medicine, 9*(2), 38–45.

Berk, L.S., Felten, D.L., Tan, S.A., Bittman, B.B., & Westergard, J. (2001). Modulation of neuroimmune parameters during the eustress of humor-associated mirthful laughter. *Alternative Therapies in Health and Medicine, 7*(2), 74–76.

Besedovsky, H.O., & Del Rey, A. (2001). Cytokines as mediators of central and peripheral immune-neuroendocrine interactions. In R. Ader, D. Felten, & N. Cohen (Eds.), *Psychoneuroimmunology* (3rd ed., pp. 1–20). San Diego, CA: Academic Press.

Bovbjerg, D.H. (2003). Conditioning, cancer, and immune regulation. *Brain, Behavior, and Immunity, 17*(Suppl. 1), S58–S61.

Buckle, J. (1999). Use of aromatherapy as a complementary treatment for chronic pain. *Alternative Therapies in Health and Medicine, 5*(5), 42–51.

Capuron, L., & Dantzer, R. (2003). Cytokines and depression: The need for a new paradigm. *Brain, Behavior, and Immunity, 17*(Supp. 1), S119–S124.

Carlson, S.L. (2001). Neural influences on cell adhesion molecules and lymphocyte trafficking. In R. Ader, D. Felten, & N. Cohen (Eds.), *Psychoneuroimmunology* (3rd ed., pp. 231–240). San Diego, CA: Academic Press.

Carlson, L.E., Speca, M., Patel, K.D., & Goodley, E. (2003). Mindfulness-based stress reduction in relation to quality of life, mood, symptoms of stress, and immune parameters in breast and prostate outpatients. *Psychosomatic Medicine, 65,* 571–581.

Carlson, L.E., Ursuliak, Z., Goodley, E., Angen, M., & Speca, M. (2001). The effects of a mindfulness-based stress reduction program on mood and symptoms of stress in cancer outpatients: 6-month follow-up. *Supportive Care in Cancer, 9,* 112–123.

Castes, M., Palenque, M., Canelones, P., Hagel, I., & Lynch, N. (1998). Classic conditioning and placebo effects in the bronchodilator response of asthmatic children. *Neuroimmunomodulation, 5,* 70.

Cousins, N. (1979). *Anatomy of an illness as perceived by the patient: Reflections on healing and regeneration.* New York: Bantam.

Cunningham, A.J., Edmonds, C.V., Jenkins, G.P., Pollack, H., Lockwood, G.A., & Warr, D. (1998). A randomized controlled trial of the effects of group psychological therapy on survival in women with metastatic breast cancer. *Psycho-Oncology, 7,* 508–517.

Dantzer, R., Bluthe, R.M., Castanon, N., Chauvet, N., Capuron, L., Goodall, G., et al. (2001). Cytokine effects on behavior. In R. Ader, D. Felten, & N. Cohen (Eds.), *Psychoneuroimmunology* (3rd ed., pp. 703–727). San Diego, CA: Academic Press.

Davidson, R.J., Kabat-Zinn, J., Schumacher, J., Rosenkranz, M., Muller, D., Santorelli, S., et al. (2003). Alterations in brain and immune function produced by mindfulness meditation. *Psychosomatic Medicine, 65,* 564–570.

Dhabhar, F.S., & McEwen, B.S. (2001). Bidirectional effects of stress and glucocorticoid hormones on immune function: Possible explanations for paradoxical observations. In R. Ader, D. Felten, & N. Cohen (Eds.), *Psychoneuroimmunology* (3rd ed., pp. 301–338). San Diego, CA: Academic Press.

Diego, M.A., Field, T., Hernandez-Reif, M., Shaw, K., Friedman, L., & Ironson, G. (2001). HIV adolescents show improved immune function following massage therapy. *International Journal of Neuroscience, 106,* 35–45.

Dowling, J.S., Hockenberry, M., & Gregory, R.L. (2003). Sense of humor, childhood cancer stressors, and outcomes of psychosocial adjustment, immune function, and infection. *Journal of Pediatric Oncology Nursing, 20,* 271–292.

Dunkel-Schetter, C., Feinstein, L.G., Taylor, S.E., & Falke, R.L. (1992). Patterns of coping with cancer. *Health Psychology, 11,* 79–87.

Elenkov, I.J., & Chrousos, G.P. (1999). Stress hormones, Th1/Th2 patterns, pro/anti-inflammatory cytokines and susceptibility to disease. *Trends in Endocrinology and Metabolism, 10,* 359–368.

Eskandari, F., & Sternberg, E.M. (2002). Neural-immune interactions in health and disease. *Annals of the New York Academy of Sciences, 966,* 20–27.

Evans, D. (2002). The effectiveness of music as an intervention for hospital patients: A systematic review. *Journal of Advanced Nursing, 37,* 8–18.

Ezzone, S., Baker, C., Rosselet, R., & Terepka, E. (1998). Music as an adjunct to antiemetic therapy. *Oncology Nursing Forum, 25,* 1551–1556.

Fang, C., Miller, S.M., Mills, M., Mangan, C.E., Belch, R., Campbell, D.E., et al. (2003). The effects of avoidance on cytotoxic/suppressor T cells in women with cervical lesions. *Psycho-Oncology, 12,* 590–598.

Fawzy, F.I., Cousins, N., Fawzy, N.W., Kemeny, M.E., Elashoff, R., & Morton, D. (1990). A structured psychiatric intervention for cancer patients: I. Changes over time in methods of coping and affective disturbance. *Archives of General Psychiatry, 47,* 720–725.

Fawzy, F.I., Fawzy, N.W., Hyun, C.S., Elashoff, R., Guthrie, D., Fahey, J.L., et al. (1993). Malignant melanoma. Effects of an early structured psychiatric intervention, coping, and affective state on recurrence and survival 6 years later. *Archives of General Psychiatry, 50,* 681–689.

Fawzy, F.I., Kemeny, M.E., Fawzy, N.W., Elashoff, R., Morton, D., Cousins, N., et al. (1990). A structured psychiatric intervention for cancer patients: II. Changes over time in immunological measures. *Archives of General Psychiatry, 47,* 729–735.

Glaser, R., MacCallum, R.C., Laskowski, B.F., Malarkey, W.B., Sheridan, J.F., & Kiecolt-Glaser, J.K. (2001). Evidence for a shift in the Th-1 to Th-2 cytokine response associated with chronic stress and aging. *Journals of Gerontology Series A: Biological Sciences and Medical Sciences, 56,* 477–482.

Goodfellow, L.M. (2003). The effects of therapeutic back massage on psychophysiologic variables and immune function in spouses of patients with cancer. *Nursing Research, 52,* 318–328.

Goodwin, P.J., Leszcz, M., Ennis, M., Koopmans, J., Vincent, L., Guther, H., et al. (2001). The effect of group psychosocial support on survival in metastatic breast cancer. *New England Journal of Medicine, 345,* 1719–1725.

Graham, P.H., Browne, L., Cox, H., & Graham, J. (2003). Inhalation aromatherapy during radiotherapy: Results of a placebo-controlled double-blind randomized trial. *Journal of Clinical Oncology, 21,* 2372–2376.

Gruzelier, J.H. (2002). A review of the impact of hypnosis, relaxation, guided imagery and individual differences on aspects of immunity and health. *Stress, 5,* 147–163.

Hadfield, N. (2001). The role of aromatherapy massage in reducing anxiety in patients with malignant brain tumors. *International Journal of Palliative Nursing, 7,* 279–285.

Hawkley, L.C., & Cacioppo, J.T. (2003). Loneliness and pathways to disease. *Brain, Behavior, and Immunity, 17*(Suppl. 1), S98–S105.

Hilliard, R.E. (2003). The effects of music therapy on the quality and length of life of people diagnosed with terminal cancer. *Journal of Music Therapy, 40,* 113–137.

Ironson, G., Field, T., Scafidi, F., Hashimoto, M., Kumar, M., Kumar, A., et al. (1996). Massage therapy is associated with enhancement of immune system's cytotoxic capacity. *International Journal of Neuroscience, 84,* 205–217.

Kabat-Zinn, J. (1990). *Full catastrophe living.* New York: Bantam.

Kasprowicz, D.J., Kohm, A.P., Berton, M.T., Chruscinski, A.J., Sharpe, A., & Sanders, V.M. (2000). Stimulation of the B cell receptor, CD86 (B7–2), and the beta 2-adrenergic receptor intrinsically modulates the level of IgG1 and IgE produced per B cell. *Journal of Immunology, 165,* 680–690.

Kelley, K.W., Bluthe, R.M., Dantzer, R., Zhou, J.H., Shen, W.H., Johnson, R.W., et al. (2003). Cytokine-induced sickness behavior. *Brain, Behavior, and Immunity, 17*(Suppl. 1), S112–S118.

Kelly, K.M., Jacobson, J.S., Kennedy, D.D., Braudt, S.M., Mallick, M., & Weiner, M.A. (2000). Use of unconventional therapies by children with cancer at an urban medical center. *Journal of Pediatric Hematology/ Oncology, 22,* 412–416.

Kemeny, M.E. (2003). An interdisciplinary research model to investigate psychosocial cofactors in disease: Application to HIV-1 pathogenesis. *Brain, Behavior, and Immunity, 17*(Suppl. 1), S62–S72.

Kiecolt-Glaser, J.K., McGuire, L., Robles, T.F., & Glaser, R. (2002a). Psychoneuroimmunology and psychosomatic medicine: Back to the future. *Psychosomatic Medicine, 64,* 15–28.

Kiecolt-Glaser, J.K., McGuire, L., Robles, T.F., & Glaser, R. (2002b). Psychoneuroimmunology influences on immune function and health. *Journal of Consulting and Clinical Psychology, 70,* 537–547.

Kiecolt-Glaser, J.K., Preacher, K.J., MacCallum, R.C., Atkinson, C., Malarkey, W.B., & Glaser, R. (2003). Chronic stress and age-related increases in the proinflammatory cytokine IL-6. *Proceedings of the National Academy of Sciences, 100,* 9090–9095.

Krueger, J.M., Majde, J.A., & Obal, F. (2003). Sleep in host defense. *Brain, Behavior, and Immunity, 17*(Suppl. 1), S41–S47.

Kwekkeboom, K.L. (2003). Music versus distraction for procedural pain and anxiety in patients with cancer. *Oncology Nursing Forum, 30,* 433–440.

Lawless, J. (1995). *The illustrated encyclopedia of essential oils.* New York: Barnes & Noble.

Lazarus, R.S., & Folkman, S. (1984). *Stress, appraisal, and coping.* New York: Springer.

Lepore, S.J., & Smyth, J. (Eds.). (2002). *The writing cure: How expressive writing promotes health and emotional well-being.* Washington, DC: American Psychological Association.

Longo, D.L., Duffey, P.L., Kopp, W.C., Heyes, M.P., Alvord, W.G., Sharfman, W.H., et al. (1999). Conditioned immune response to interferon-gamma in humans. *Clinical Immunology, 90,* 173–181.

Lutgendorf, S.K. (2002). Individual differences and immune function: Implications for cancer. *Brain, Behavior, and Immunity, 17*(Suppl. 1), S106–S108.

Lutgendorf, S.K., Johnson, E., Holmes, R., Anderson, B., Sorosky, J.I., Buller, R.E., et al. (2003). Social relationships and tumor angiogenesis factors in ovarian cancer patients. *Cancer, 95,* 808–815.

Lutgendorf, S.K., Vitaliano, P.P., Tripp-Reimer, T., Harvey, J.H., & Lubaroff, D.M. (1999). Sense of coherence moderates the relationship between life stress and natural killer cell activity in healthy older adults. *Psychology and Aging, 14,* 552–563.

Madden, K.S. (2001). Catecholamines, sympathetic nerves, and immunity. In R. Ader, D. Felten, & N. Cohen (Eds.), *Psychoneuroimmunology* (3rd ed., pp. 197–216). San Diego, CA: Academic Press.

Madden, K.S. (2003). Catecholamines, sympathetic innervation, and immunity. *Brain, Behavior, and Immunity, 17*(Suppl. 1), S5–S10.

Maier, S.F., & Watkins, L.R. (2003). Immune-to-central nervous system communication and its role in modulating pain and cognition: Implications for cancer and cancer treatment. *Brain, Behavior, and Immunity, 17*(Suppl. 1), S125–S131.

Martin, R.A. (2001). Humor, laughter, and physical health: Methodological issues and research findings. *Psychological Bulletin, 127,* 504–519.

Miller, A.H. (2003). Cytokines and sickness behavior: Implications for cancer care and control. *Brain, Behavior, and Immunity, 17*(Suppl. 1), S132–S134.

Mosmann, T.R., & Sad, S. (1996). The expanding universe of T-cell subsets: Th1, Th2, and more. *Immunology Today, 17,* 138–146.

Moynihan, J.A. (2003). Mechanisms of stress-induced modulation of immunity. *Brain, Behavior, and Immunity, 17*(Suppl. 1), S11–S16.

Nicholas, P.K., & Webster, A. (1996). A behavioral medicine intervention in persons with HIV. *Clinical Nursing Research, 5,* 391–406.

Nightingale, F. (1969). *Notes on nursing: What it is and what it is not.* New York: Dover Publications. (Original work published 1860)

Pennebaker, J.W. (1997). *Opening up: The healing power of expressing emotions.* New York: Guilford Press.

Phipps, S. (2002). Reduction of distress associated with pediatric bone marrow transplant: Complementary health promotion interventions. *Pediatric Rehabilitation, 5,* 223–234.

Post-White, J. (1991). The effects of mental imagery on emotions, immune function, and cancer outcome. *Dissertation Abstracts International, 52,* 12B. (UMI No. 92–5462)

Post-White, J., Kinney, M.E., Savik, K., Gau, J., Wilcox, C., & Lerner, I. (2003). Therapeutic massage and healing touch improve symptoms in cancer. *Integrative Cancer Therapies, 2,* 332–344.

Post-White, J., Schroeder, L., Hannahan, A., Johnston, M.K., Salscheider, N., & Grandt, N. (1996). Response to imagery/support in breast cancer survivors. *Oncology Nursing Forum, 23,* 355.

Rabin, B.S. (1999). *Stress, immune function, and health: The connection.* New York: Wiley-Liss.

Richardson, M.A., Post-White, J., Grimm, E., Moye, L.A., Singletary, S.E., & Justice, B. (1997). Coping, life attitudes, and immune responses to imagery and group support after breast cancer. *Alternative Therapies in Health and Medicine, 3*(5), 62–70.

Robb, S.L. (2000). The effect of therapeutic music interventions on the behavior of hospitalized children in isolation: Developing a contextual support model of music therapy. *Journal of Music Therapy, 37,* 118–146.

Rosenberg, H.J., Rosenberg, S.D., Ernstoff, M.S., Wolford, G.L., Amdur, R.J., Elshamy, M.R., et al. (2002). Expressive disclosure and health outcomes in a prostate cancer population. *International Journal of Psychiatry in Medicine, 32*(1), 37–53.

Segerstrom, S.C. (2003). Individual differences, immunity, and cancer: Lessons from personality psychology. *Brain, Behavior, and Immunity, 17*(Suppl. 1), S92–S97.

Shapiro, S.L., Bootzin, R.R., Figueredo, A.J., Lopez, A.M., & Schwartz, G.E. (2003). The efficacy of mindfulness-based stress reduction in the treatment of sleep disturbance in women with breast cancer: An exploratory study. *Journal of Psychosomatic Research, 54,* 85–91.

Sheridan, J. (2003). The HPA axis, SNS, and immunity: A commentary. *Brain, Behavior, and Immunity, 17*(Suppl. 1), S17.

Shi, Y., Devadas, S., Greeneltech, K.M., Yin, D., Mufson, R.A., & Zhou, J. (2003). Stressed to death: Implication of lymphocyte apoptosis for psychoneuroimmunology. *Brain, Behavior, and Immunity, 17*(Suppl. 1), S18–S26.

Sloman, R. (2002). Relaxation and imagery for anxiety and depression control in community patients with advanced cancer. *Cancer Nursing, 25,* 432–435.

Smith, M.C., Reeder, F., Daniel, L., Baramee, J., & Hagman, J. (2003). Outcomes of touch therapies during bone marrow transplant. *Alternative Therapies in Health and Medicine, 9*(1), 40–49.

Smyth, J.M., Stone, A.A., Hurewitz, A., & Kaell, A. (1999). Effects of writing about stressful experiences on symptom reduction in patients with asthma and rheumatoid arthritis. *JAMA, 281,* 1304–1329.

Speca, M., Carlson, L.E., Goodley, E., & Angen, M. (2000). A randomized, wait-list controlled clinical trial: The effect of a mindfulness meditation-based stress reduction program on mood and symptoms of stress in cancer outpatients. *Psychosomatic Medicine, 62,* 613–622.

Spiegel, D., & Bloom, J.R. (1983). Group therapy and hypnosis reduces metastatic breast carcinoma pain. *Psychosomatic Medicine, 45,* 333–339.

Spiegel, D., Bloom, J.R., Kraemer, H.C., & Gottheil, E. (1989). Effect of psychosocial treatment on survival of patients with metastatic breast cancer. *Lancet, 2,* 888–891.

Spiegel, D., & Sephton, S.E. (2001). Psychoneuroimmune and endocrine pathways in cancer: Effects of stress and support. *Seminars in Clinical Neuropsychiatry, 6,* 252–265.

Standley, J.M., & Hanser, S.B. (1995). Music therapy research and applications in pediatric oncology treatment. *Pediatric Oncology Nursing, 12,* 3–8.

Stanton, A.L., & Danoff-Burg, S. (2002). Emotional expression, expressive writing, and cancer. In S.J. Lepore & J. Smyth (Eds.), *The writing cure: How expressive writing promotes health and emotional well-being* (pp. 31–51). Washington, DC: American Psychological Association.

Stanton, A.L., Danoff-Burg, S., Sworowski, L.A., Collins, C.A., Branstetter, A.D., Rodriguez-Hanley, A., et al. (2002). Randomized, controlled trial of written emotional expression and benefit finding in breast cancer patients. *Journal of Clinical Oncology, 20,* 4160–4168.

Stefanek, M., & McDonald, P.G. (2003). Biological mechanism of psychosocial effects on disease: Implications for cancer control. *Brain, Behavior, and Immunity, 17*(Suppl. 1), S2–S4.

Syrjala, K.L., Donaldson, G.W., Davis, M.W., Kippes, M.E., & Carr, J.E. (1995). Relaxation and imagery and cognitive-behavioral training reduce pain during cancer treatment: A controlled clinical trial. *Pain, 63,* 189–198.

Takahashi, K., Iwase, M., Yamashita, K., Tatsumoto, Y., Ue, H., Kuratsune, H., et al. (2001). The elevation of natural killer cell activity induced by laughter in a crossover designed study. *International Journal of Molecular Medicine, 8,* 645–650.

Troesch, L.M., Rodehaver, C.B., Delaney, E.A., & Yanes, B. (1993). The influence of guided imagery on chemotherapy-related nausea and vomiting. *Oncology Nursing Forum, 20,* 1179–1185.

Walker, B.L., Nail, M.N., & Croyle, R.T. (1999). Does emotional expression make a difference in reactions to breast cancer? *Oncology Nursing Forum, 26,* 1025–1032.

Wikstrom, S., Gunnarsson, T., & Nordin, C. (2003). Tactile stimulus and neurohormonal response: A pilot study. *International Journal of Neuroscience, 113,* 787–793.

Wilkinson, S., Aldridge, J., Salmon, L., Cain, E., & Wilson, B. (1999). An evaluation of aromatherapy massage in palliative care. *Palliative Medicine, 13,* 409–417.

Yang, E.V., & Glaser, R. (2003). Stress-induced immunomodulation: Implications for tumorigenesis. *Brain, Behavior, and Immunity, 17*(Suppl. 1), S37–S40.

Yehuda, R. (2003). Hypothalamic-pituitary-adrenal alterations in PTSD: Are they relevant to understanding cortisol alterations in cancer? *Brain, Behavior, and Immunity, 17*(Suppl. 1), S73–S83.

Zeller, J.M., McCain, N.L., & Swanson, B. (1996). Psychoneuroimmunology: An emerging framework for nursing research. *Journal of Advanced Nursing, 23,* 657–664.

SECTION V

Special Topics

CHAPTER 29

Psychosocial Aspects of Experimental Therapy: Clinical Trials

ANGELA D. KLIMASZEWSKI, RN, MSN

> *One doesn't discover new lands without consenting to lose sight of the shore for a very long time.*
>
> —Andre Gide

The development of new cytotoxic agents occurs through basic science and clinical trial research. Basic science research involves a lengthy, complex process of preclinical study. It begins with the discovery and identification of agents that may have anticancer activity. The agents are tested on cell cultures and in animals for anticancer activity and stability. Once a human dose may be estimated, the research moves from the laboratory to the clinical setting. The purpose of clinical trial research involving human volunteers is to determine the safety, efficacy, and toxicities of a new agent or combination of agents (Cusack, 1998). It is at this point, when a clinical trial is designed and approved, that patient accrual begins (see Table 29-1).

Factors Affecting Patients' Enrollment

The reason a patient participates in a clinical trial depends on at least three variables: (a) physician factors, (b) patient factors, and (c) protocol factors. Intermingled with these variables are personal feelings that patients with cancer encounter at the time of diagnosis, which, for some, is when enrollment in a clinical trial becomes an option. Ironically, the barriers to clinical trial participation involve the same three variables plus one: the healthcare system.

The benefits of participating in a trial include the following (National Cancer Institute, 2004).

- Trials provide access to promising new approaches that often are not available outside the research setting.

Table 29-1. Phases of Cancer Clinical Trials

Phase	Primary Goals
I	• Establish maximum tolerated dose and dosing schedule. • Evaluate toxicity. • Determine pharmacokinetics.
II	• Determine antitumor activity in specific tumor types. • Evaluate toxicity.
III	• Establish efficacy by assessing survival time to progression. • Obtain quality-of-life data.
IV	• Expand "off-label" use. • Further assess toxicity data.

Note. From "History and Background" (p. 5), by S. Breslin in A.D. Klimaszewski, J.L. Aikin, M.A. Bacon, S.A. DiStasio, H.E. Ehrenberger, and B.A. Ford (Eds.), *Manual for Clinical Trials Nursing,* 2000, Pittsburgh, PA: Oncology Nursing Society. Copyright 2000 by the Oncology Nursing Society. Reprinted with permission.

- The approach being studied may be more effective than the standard approach.
- Participants receive regular and careful medical attention and additional exams and tests from a research team that includes doctors and other healthcare professionals.
- Participants may be the first to benefit from the new method under study.
- Results from the study may help others in the future.

Physician Factors

The trust relationship between a physician and a patient generally is considered sacrosanct. Patients will follow the advice of their physician, including his or her recommendation to participate in a clinical trial (Aungst, Haas, Ommaya, & Green, 2003). Physicians who believe in the goals of the trial, regardless of the phase, are more likely to refer patients to be considered for participation (Meadows, 2000).

However, Aungst et al. (2003) also reported that many physicians are not aware of available clinical trials. Harris Interactive (2001) completed a survey of nearly 6,000 patients with cancer. Results indicated that 85% of the patients were not informed that they could possibly participate in a clinical trial for treatment. Physicians must be aware of the types of trials available for patient referral.

Miller (2002) shared his reluctance to give false hope to patients enrolled in a phase I trial. He reported that few of the patients were told by their primary oncologist that they had less than a 5% chance of achieving a partial response and a 0.5% chance of achieving a complete remission. Miller questioned why patients would believe that there is no hope to improve their condition when the physician contradicts this by presenting a phase I study as a novel treatment or a promising new therapy. Physicians' explanations and consent forms may confuse patients into believing that the study offers more than a small chance for remission or cure.

Conversely, when Schutta and Burnett (2000) studied 22 patients enrolled in phase I trials, they found that patients stressed the importance of how their oncologists' interpersonal skills and positive attitude increased their own trust and confidence in the trial.

Perhaps the major barrier to physicians enrolling—or even referring—patients in clinical trials is a profound lack of resources. Limitations of time, staff, adequate means to handle intense paperwork, and costs associated with data management collectively are referred to by the National Cancer Institute (2001) as "physician bottleneck." The American Society of Clinical Oncology (ASCO) reported in 1999 that a high number of the 3,550 oncologists that were surveyed subsidized the cost of trials to participate.

Patient Factors

Volunteering to participate in a clinical trial is an extremely personal decision. It can be argued that until a patient with cancer is actually approached about participating in a trial, personal views on whether to participate are purely speculative. Yet, studies show that most people would be willing to participate in a clinical trial if they had cancer (Aungst et al., 2003; Comis, Miller, Aldige, Krebs, & Stoval, 2003).

Thirty-two percent of the 1,000 adults aged 18 and older interviewed by Comis et al. (2003) would be very willing to participate in a clinical trial, and 38% would consider participating in a clinical trial if asked. This supports a larger survey of patients with cancer by Harris Interactive (2001) that found that 80% of the public would be willing to participate in a clinical trial for their initial treatment if they were diagnosed with cancer. Similarly, 90% would participate if their initial treatment failed.

According to Harris Interactive (2001), of the 16% of the patients who were aware that a clinical trial might be applicable for their treatment, three-quarters refused to participate. This group cited the following reasons for declining.

- Fear that they would receive medical treatment that is less effective than standard care
- Risk of receiving a placebo
- Fear of being treated "like a guinea pig"
- Concern that their insurance company would not cover costs

Individuals with advanced or aggressive disease who have failed standard therapies may be asked to enroll in a phase I trial designed to determine the toxicity, not the effectiveness, of an agent. For these patients, the two major factors for deciding to participate in a clinical trial were their hope for control of the disease and their present medical condition (Daugherty, 2000; Miller, 2002; Schaeffer et al., 1996). Mack (1999) interviewed 20 patients who met the criteria for participating in phase I trials. She reported an overall theme of a "quest for treatment" that the interviewees expressed. This was viewed as an active process that proceeded along specific steps: taking charge, deciding, living on a trial, and dealing with uncertainty. Participants in Mack's study reported that being involved in a research study provided them with a sense of meaning at a time when their life was nearing the end. Although not often offered, patients on hospice also may qualify for participation in phase I trials (Byock, 2003). Byock and Miles (2003) reported that no clinical or ethical justification exists for denying hospice patients access to these trials.

Schain (1994) related that patients who enroll in phase I trials feel gratification for contributing to the advancement of science, thus meeting a basic altruistic concern for the improvement of care for others when no hope of cure exists for them. The majority of patients studied by Schutta and Burnett (2000) stressed the value and importance of the patient being the one to make the decision to participate in the trial. Patients also cited hope for a therapeutic benefit and a desire to live as reasons to participate in any phase trial (Albrecht, Blanchard, Ruckdeschel, Coovert, & Strongbow, 1999; Schutta & Burnett).

Meadows (2000) identified concerns such as transportation costs and childcare concerns when a daycare center is not available as additional patient factors that will influence decisions about whether to participate in a trial. Unfortunately, patients must make decisions that will affect their health and future during an extremely stressful time (Meadows).

Protocol Factors

Comis et al. (2003) cited the unavailability of an appropriate clinical trial and the disqualification of large numbers of patients because of strict eligibility requirements as the primary reasons for low accrual of adults for clinical trials in the United States. Corrie, Shaw, and Harris (2003) reviewed 1,411 patients from five cancer centers in a descriptive study and found that no suitable trial was available for 561 patients (40%). Additionally, 53% of the 850 patients for whom a clinical trial was available were disqualified because of entry criteria.

Patients may find that a lengthy or complicated protocol that requires additional tests is as unacceptable as one that requires an extended admission (Meadows, 2000). Fatigue, depression, and anxiety may influence patients' willingness to trade quality of life for pain relief or palliation. Meadows noted that "information on clinical trials may not be sought unless it becomes a compelling or desperate issue" (p. 54).

Healthcare System Factors

Patients' concerns for how to pay for study tests, if not covered by their insurance, are an unfortunate reflection on today's healthcare system. Access to clinical trials is impeded for those who lack reimbursement (ASCO, 2003). Certain private insurers will provide coverage, and have done so since 1999, for routine patient costs of specific government-sponsored trials, such as the National Institutes of Health or the U.S. Department of Defense. Similarly, some states, including Maryland, Illinois, and Arizona, have enacted laws mandating insurance coverage for routine care costs associated with clinical trials. The most significant step taken by the federal government occurred when Medicare issued a coverage decision for routine patient care associated with participation in all phases of clinical trials for serious and life-threatening diseases. This is great news, as more than half of all cancers occur in older adults, and the next few decades will see baby boomers enter those ranks *en masse* (ASCO, 2003).

Informed Consent

Informed consent is more than a signed document. It is the ongoing relationship between the patient and the research team (Klimaszewski, Anderson, & Good, 2000).

The process of informed consent ensures that the patient is a willing participant throughout the conduct of a clinical trial. Informed consent has long been addressed in the literature and continues to be the target of ethical scrutiny. Schain (1994) noted that "the ideal balance of frankness and fear-provoking detail is not universally established, nor is it the same for all persons" (p. 2668). The spirit of informed consent is giving information to patients *that they understand* so they may freely choose the best treatment.

Historically, human subjects involved in research were, intentionally, the poor and vulnerable patient populations, including women, minorities, children, older adults, and prisoners (Davis, 2002). The Belmont Report (National Commission for the Protection of Human Subjects of Biomedical and Behavioral Research, 1978) defined three principles for ethical research and the prevention of research subject abuse. **Respect for people** involves recognition of personal dignity and autonomy, or the right of patients to act in their best interest. The goal of the second principle, **beneficence,** is to ensure the well-being of research patients and protect them from harm. An ethical study is considered beneficent if it maximizes possible benefits to the patient and minimizes harm. **Justice,** the third principle, means distributing benefits and burdens fairly among study participants, such as not limiting drug research to one population such as adult males, when it could benefit adult females and children. Similarly, giving a drug to the same populations when it is known to adversely affect only one is not a fair distribution of risks and benefits. Weijer (1998) affirmed that the equitable selection of research subjects is tied to the generalizability of the research. Weijer stated, "It follows that a widely generalizable clinical trial . . . has more scientific value than a narrowly generalizable trial" (p. 4). Vulnerable populations that are currently underrepresented in cancer clinical trials include women, minorities, socioeconomically disadvantaged patients, and older adults (Ehrenberger, Breeden, & Donovan, 2003; Sateren et al., 2002; Underwood & Alexander, 2000).

Vulnerable subjects require additional assistance to protect their rights. For example, a child who possesses the intellectual and emotional ability to understand the concepts of a study needs to be asked to assent, or agree, to receive or discontinue a treatment. However, the parent or guardian actually gives permission to enroll the child in a study (Baylis, Downie, & Kenny, 1999; Broome, 1999). Some institutional review boards require two documents, one with a detailed explanation for parents and a shorter and simpler one for younger children. However, because younger children may not understand the implications of signing their name to a document, it may be more appropriate to have a third party verify, by signature, that the child voluntarily offered assent (U.S. Food and Drug Administration, 1998). Nelson (2002) affirmed that "as a matter of both justice and respect for persons, efforts should be made to conduct research using children capable of assent before enrolling those less able to assent" (p. 387).

Ackerman (1995) questioned the influences of psychosocial constraints (i.e., factors that may impair the ability to evaluate risk/benefit and truly reflect family values [see Figure 29-1]) on the children and parents who consent to participate in phase I pediatric trials. For example, preadolescents generally feel a need to please authority figures; therefore, they may defer decisions about their lives to their parents. Adolescents often elect to control their own lives and refute authority. Progressive disease may make them shift their focus from controlling their lives to feeling helpless

---

Figure 29-1. Psychosocial Constraints Experienced by Parents of Children Who Are Terminally Ill

- Denial that cure will not occur
- Unrealistic hope for extended remission
- Guilt related to causing the cancer
- Helplessness as the disease progresses
- Loss of power to protect the physical well-being of their child
- Increased need for emotional support and interaction with staff

Note. Based on information from Ackerman, 1995.

---

as the disease worsens. As a result, they may not voice their preferences but rather defer decision making to parents (Ackerman).

Miller (2002) suggested that patients enrolled in phase I trials cannot make truly informed decisions because the "morally relevant information is obscured by an overwhelming amount of unnecessary scientific minutiae" (p. 471). He emphasized that clinical research should not be viewed as an extension of medical practice but should be clearly identified as a means of answering scientific questions with the very real probability of not benefiting the patient at all. Conversely, Ackerman (1995) asserted that phase I pediatric drug trials are therapeutic interventions because children will experience some benefit from the treatment. He noted that this type of research should be initiated only after risk/benefit criteria have been fully evaluated and the informed consent process has been accepted and completed. Ackerman noted that the extent to which risk/benefit criteria must be met varies from family to family because different families embrace different values and goals. Thus, one family may willingly enroll a child in a phase I trial, whereas another may find it unacceptable to do so. Family values and beliefs ultimately are the bases of whether a child or adult participates in a clinical trial.

Patients who are mentally ill or impaired and patients with dementia require additional protection. Limitations in patients' ability to provide initial or ongoing consent may occur because of memory, understanding, and reasoning problems (Delano, 2002). Although legislation varies by state, laws delineating guardianship, durable power of attorney for health care, or surrogate consent are most common (Amdur, Bachir, & Stanton, 2002). One alternative is for a healthcare professional to discuss the patient's wishes with the patient before mental incapacitation occurs. Then, the patient can assign durable power of attorney or healthcare proxy to that trusted person. Another alternative is to help the patient to document his or her wishes regarding participation in clinical trials in an advance directive. However, because many people do not have advance directives for end-of-life decision making, participation in a clinical trial after losing mental capacity is less likely to be specifically discussed and documented (High & Doole, 1995).

Older adult patients who have the capacity to make an informed decision about participating in a clinical trial should be encouraged to do so. For patients with poor eyesight or hearing impairments, printing a consent in larger type or using a tape-recorded consent may be all that is needed to facilitate informed decision making.

Nursing Implications in Clinical Trials

Clinical trials are key to making advances in cancer treatment. Patients must deal with a multitude of feelings and emotions while in a study. Whether coping with a new cancer diagnosis or dealing with advanced disease, patients are emotionally vulnerable and require a strong psychosocial support system when they are enrolled in a trial. Nurses can lend support by adhering to the three ethical principles outlined in the Belmont Report.

These three principles are addressed in five values—respectful care, quality of life, competence, collegiality, and fairness—that have been identified in the Oncology Nursing Society's statement of core values (Scanlon & Glover, 1995). Nurses who adopt these values as the foundation of their nursing practice will be best prepared to meet the psychosocial and ethical challenges of patients who are enrolled in clinical trials or receiving experimental therapy.

Nurses provide psychosocial support to patients in clinical trials in many ways. Being available to the patient by phone and during hospitalizations and clinic visits, although time consuming, builds on the underlying trust in the nurse-patient relationship and illustrates that the nurse cares about the patient. Keeping the patient informed of what will happen and new developments in the study and acting as a liaison between the patient and the principal investigator meet the patient's need for information and repetition of information or instruction for symptom management. This also ensures that the principal investigator stays updated on the patient's status. Encouraging the patient to express his or her feelings throughout the study, actively listening, and being sensitive to the patient's cultural and religious beliefs impart empathy while giving the nurse insight about how the patient is coping with the disease and the clinical trial. Being with the patient to share information that is positive (e.g., disease stabilization, remission, cure) or negative (e.g., disease progression) enables nurses to intervene therapeutically when the patient needs emotional support. Being objective and respecting the patient's decisions, although difficult at times, are key ways that nurses can provide psychosocial support to the patient. This can be incredibly challenging, especially when the patient makes a decision that the nurse does not favor, such as going off study or using alternative therapies. Culture, religion, and personal and family values influence the patient's decisions. Fundamentally, it is the patient's disease and the patient's decision. Although these interventions are not unique to clinical trials nursing, they give nurses critical information about the patient's psychosocial status. Nurses, then, may intervene or enlist the assistance of another member of the multidisciplinary team, such as a psychiatric clinical nurse specialist, chaplain, or social worker.

Conclusion

Clinical trials offer patients an opportunity to receive superior care as well as the most up-to-date treatment possible for their disease. Patients come from many age groups, cultures, religions, and psychological profiles and therefore bring a wide range of personal values and beliefs to the clinical trial setting. The nurse's role as patient advocate is maximized as he or she objectively accompanies the patient through the rigors of deciding to participate in a clinical trial, signing a truly informed consent, receiving and completing treatment, and going off study. The nurse's expertise in providing psychosocial support and making appropriate referrals can ease the emotional difficulties that the patient encounters, thereby making the endeavor even more worthwhile.

References

Ackerman, T.F. (1995). The ethics of phase I pediatric oncology trials. *IRB, 17*(1), 1–5.

Albrecht, T.L., Blanchard, C., Ruckdeschel, J.C., Coovert, M., & Strongbow, R. (1999). Strategic physician communication and oncology clinical trials. *Journal of Clinical Oncology, 17,* 3324–3332.

Amdur, R.J., Bachir, N., & Stanton, E. (2002). Selecting a surrogate to consent to medical research. In R.J. Amdur and E.A. Bankert (Eds.), *Institutional review board: Management and function* (pp. 258–264). Sudbury, MA: Jones and Bartlett.

American Society of Clinical Oncology. (1999). *ASCO surveys find cancer clinical trials vastly underfunded.* Retrieved November 9, 2003, from http://www.asco.org

American Society of Clinical Oncology. (2003, March). *Access to clinical trials.* Retrieved November 9, 2003, from http://www.asco.org

Aungst, J., Haas, A., Ommaya, A., & Green, L.W. (Eds.). (2003). *Exploring challenges, progress, and new models for engaging the public in the clinical research enterprise: Clinical Research Roundtable workshop summary.* Washington, DC: National Academies Press. Retrieved November 14, 2003, from http://www.nap.edu/catalog/10757.html

Baylis, F., Downie, J., & Kenny, N. (1999). Children and decisionmaking in health research. *IRB, 21*(4), 5–10.

Broome, M.E. (1999). Consent (assent) for research with pediatric patients. *Seminars in Oncology Nursing, 15,* 96–103.

Byock, I. (2003). Palliative care and the ethics of research: Medicare, hospice and phase I trials. *Journal of Supportive Oncology, 1,* 139–141.

Byock, I., & Miles, S.H. (2003). Hospice benefits and phase I trials. *Annals of Internal Medicine, 138,* 335–337.

Comis, R.L., Miller, J.D., Aldige, C.R., Krebs, L., & Stoval, E. (2003). Public attitudes toward participation in cancer clinical trials. *Journal of Clinical Oncology, 21,* 830–835.

Corrie, P., Shaw, J., & Harris, R. (2003). Rate limiting factors in recruitment of patients to clinical trials in cancer research: Descriptive study. *BMJ, 327,* 320–321.

Cusack, G. (1998). Clinical trials of parenteral antineoplastic agents. *Journal of Intravenous Nursing, 21,* 339–343.

Daugherty, C.K. (2000). Informed consent, the cancer patient, and phase I clinical trials. *Cancer Treatment Research, 102,* 77–89.

Davis, A.L. (2002). The study population: Women, minorities and children. In R.J. Amdur & E.A. Bankert (Eds.), *Institutional review board: Management and function* (pp. 155–159). Sudbury, MA: Jones and Bartlett.

Delano, S.J. (2002). Research involving adults with impairment. In R.J. Amdur & E.A. Bankert (Eds.), *Institutional review board: Management and function* (pp. 389–393). Sudbury, MA: Jones and Bartlett.

Ehrenberger, H.E., Breeden, J.R., & Donovan, M.E. (2003). A demonstration project to increase the awareness of cancer clinical trials among community-dwelling seniors [Online exclusive]. *Oncology Nursing Forum, 30,* E80–E83.

Harris Interactive. (2001). Misconceptions and lack of awareness greatly reduce recruitment for cancer clinical trials. *Health Care News, 1*(3), 1–3. Retrieved November 9, 2003, from http://www.harrisinteractive.com/news/allnewsbydate.asp?NewsID=222

High, D.M., & Doole, M.M. (1995). Ethical and legal issues in conducting research on elderly subjects. *Behavioral Sciences and the Law, 13,* 319–335.

Klimaszewski, A.D., Anderson, S., & Good, M. (2000). Informed consent. In A.D. Klimaszewski, J.L. Aikin, M.A. Bacon, S.A. DiStasio, H.E. Ehrenberger, & B.A. Ford (Eds.), *Manual for clinical trials nursing* (pp. 213–219). Pittsburgh, PA: Oncology Nursing Society.

Mack, C.H. (1999, April). The quest for treatment: Cancer patients' experience of phase I clinical trials [Abstract]. *Oncology Nursing Forum, 26,* 389.

Meadows, B. (2000). Potential accrual base. In A.D. Klimaszewski, J.L. Aikin, M.A. Bacon, S.A. DiStasio, H.E. Ehrenberger, & B.A. Ford (Eds.), *Manual for clinical trials nursing* (pp. 53–55). Pittsburgh, PA: Oncology Nursing Society.

Miller, M. (2002). Phase I oncology trials. In R.J. Amdur & E.A. Bankert (Eds.), *Institutional review board: Management and function* (pp. 465–475). Sudbury, MA: Jones and Bartlett.

National Cancer Institute. (2001, April). *Doctors, patients face different barriers to clinical trials.* Retrieved November 9, 2003, from http://www.cancer.gov/templates/doc.aspx?viewid=E545C73E-6AC6-4CDF-8CC2-8D7D15DE1C69

National Cancer Institute. (2004, January). *Clinical trials: Questions and answers.* Retrieved May 13, 2005, from http://cis.nci.nih.gov/fact/2_11.htm

National Commission for the Protection of Human Subjects of Biomedical and Behavioral Research. (1978). *Belmont report: Ethical principles and guidelines for research involving human subjects.* Washington, DC: Department of Health, Education, and Welfare.

Nelson, R.M. (2002). Research involving children. In R.J. Amdur & E.A. Bankert (Eds.), *Institutional review board: Management and function* (pp. 383–388). Sudbury, MA: Jones and Bartlett.

Sateren, W.B., Trimble, E.L., Abrams, J., Brawley, O., Breen, N., Ford, L., et al. (2002). How sociodemographics, presence of oncology specialists, and hospital cancer programs affect accrual to cancer treatment trials. *Journal of Clinical Oncology, 20,* 2109–2117.

Scanlon, C., & Glover, J. (1995). A professional code of ethics: Providing a moral compass for turbulent times. *Oncology Nursing Forum, 22,* 1515–1521.

Schaeffer, M.H., Krantz, D.S., Wichman, A., Masur, H., Reed, E., & Vinicky, J.K. (1996). The impact of disease severity on the informed consent process in clinical research. *American Journal of Medicine, 100,* 261–268.

Schain, W.S. (1994). Barriers to clinical trials, part II: Knowledge and attitudes of potential participants. *Cancer, 74*(Suppl. 9), 2666–2671.

Schutta, K.M., & Burnett, C.B. (2000). Factors that influence a patient's decision to participate in a phase I cancer clinical trial. *Oncology Nursing Forum, 27,* 1435–1438.

Underwood, S.M., & Alexander, G.A. (Eds.). (2000). Minorities, women and clinical cancer research: The charge, purpose, and challenge. *Annals of Epidemiology, 10*(Suppl. 8), S3–S12.

U.S. Food and Drug Administration. (1998). *Informed consent document content.* Retrieved November 14, 2003, from http://www.fda.gov/oc/ohrt/irbs/faqs.html

Weijer, C. (1998). The IRB's role in assessing the generalizability of non-NIH-funded clinical trials. *IRB, 20*(2–3), 1–5.

CHAPTER 30

Genetic Susceptibility Testing: Issues and Psychosocial Implications

ROBERTA H. BARON, RN, MSN, AOCN®

It has become appallingly obvious that our technology has exceeded our humanity.

—Albert Einstein

The age of genetic susceptibility testing is here. People can be tested for more than 200 diseases by using either direct or indirect DNA analysis (Rieger, 2004). Many of these genetic tests, however, result in unanswered questions, controversies, lessons to be learned, and potential anxieties for patients. Nowhere is this situation more acute than in the emerging field of cancer genetics. Healthcare professionals must have an understanding of the various ethical, psychological, and social issues associated with genetic susceptibility testing so that they may provide appropriate counseling and support to patients and their families.

Ethical Dilemmas of Genetic Testing

As fundamental understanding of genetic susceptibility testing increases, so must the understanding and appreciation of the ethical dilemmas surrounding it. Primary prevention options for many cancers are extremely limited or nonexistent. Because of this, many individuals debate the ethics of commercial testing. Is it fair to provide genetic testing to individuals and then have little to offer them in the way of prevention? In the area of breast cancer genetics, 5%–10% of individuals are likely to have developed their disease as a result of an inherited susceptibility. Mutations in the *BRCA1* and *BRCA2* tumor-suppressor genes are responsible for the majority of cases of hereditary breast cancer in the United States and confer an estimated 55%–87% lifetime risk (birth to age 75) for female carriers to develop the disease compared to

12% in the general population (Ford et al., 1998; Greco & Mahon, 2004). Currently, the only primary preventive options for mutation carriers are bilateral prophylactic mastectomy or the chemopreventive drug tamoxifen. Both of these options have their drawbacks and can lead to difficult decisions for mutation carriers.

Bilateral prophylactic mastectomy is an irreversible measure and remains controversial. Studies have shown that although the procedure may reduce the risk of developing a breast cancer by up to 90%, some residual breast tissue may remain (Hartmann et al., 1999). This remaining tissue leaves patients at risk for subsequent breast cancer development. Undergoing prophylactic mastectomy does not address the risk of developing other cancers for which this population is at risk. In particular, those with a *BRCA1* mutation may have a 28%–44% lifetime risk of developing ovarian cancer, compared to approximately a 1%–2% risk in the general population (Greco & Mahon, 2004). In addition, Borgen et al. (1998) found that women whose physicians initiated the discussion about prophylactic mastectomy more often had regrets about the procedure than women who initiated the discussion themselves.

Although chemoprevention is a new and exciting concept in the field of oncology, it also raises a number of questions. What are the most effective agents? What are the correct dosages in terms of both individual dose and frequency? At what age should chemoprevention start, and how long should it last? Who are the best-suited candidates? Randomized clinical trials are designed to provide answers; however, patient accrual and data analysis take time.

The fundamental issue surrounding chemoprevention concerns the balancing of risk and benefit. In the National Surgical Adjuvant Breast and Bowel Project (NSABP-P1) Breast Cancer Prevention Trial, tamoxifen, a nonsteroidal antiestrogen, was shown to reduce the incidence of breast cancer development by 49% in healthy women who were at an increased risk for developing the disease (Fisher et al., 1998). However, it has a side effect profile that includes postmenopausal symptoms, such as hot flashes and vaginal dryness, and, rarely but more serious, the potential for developing endometrial cancer and blood clots. Drugs whose side effects are tolerable in patients with an invasive cancer may not be acceptable for healthy individuals seeking to lower their risk of a disease. Of particular concern in the NSABP-P1 trial is that the use of tamoxifen did not result in a statistically significant impact on *BRCA*-associated cancer incidence (King et al., 2001). This may be because tamoxifen seemed to prevent only estrogen receptor (ER)-positive cancers, and patients with *BRCA* mutations tend to develop ER-negative cancers.

Before undergoing genetic testing for any hereditary syndrome, individuals at risk and their clinicians must discuss in depth the available treatment options and the efficacy of each option. This will allow individuals to weigh the risks and benefits and make an informed decision.

The subject of eugenics, the improvement of a population by selecting its best specimens for breeding, also has surfaced. Should individuals be allowed to test an unborn fetus for a cancer gene and then have the option to abort if the results are positive? Is it ethical for a woman undergoing in vitro fertilization to have her fertilized embryos individually tested and then select the negative zygote for implantation? These are difficult questions with no easy answers. Although the technology is available, no guidelines currently exist for prenatal testing for cancer syndromes.

Genetic testing of children raises difficult ethical questions. Does a parent have the right to have a child tested without that child understanding the potential implications surrounding the results? A recent policy statement by the American Society of Clinical Oncology (ASCO, 2003) recommended that the testing of children should not be offered when no available risk-reduction strategies exist and the probability of developing a malignancy during childhood is very low.

Psychological Issues

The decision of whether to undergo genetic testing is not a simple one and can have a significant psychological impact, either positive or negative, on the individual considering it. How individuals will react once they receive their actual test results is not always easy to predict. Those individuals from families with known deleterious mutations who receive a negative test result may experience enormous relief from cancer worry for both themselves and their children. A negative test result in a family with no known mutations, however, may result in undue reassurance because of the possibility that existing predisposing genes are yet undetected. Learning that one has a negative test result also may generate feelings of guilt if an individual has family members who did not receive favorable test results. This concept is known as "survivor guilt." Test results may be ambiguous because of the identification of variant forms of genes that may be associated with an increased cancer risk. Such results could lead to feelings of confusion and uncertainty about appropriate screening and treatment.

A positive test result could lead to a variety of reactions. For some, it may act as a motivator to pursue increased surveillance, risk-reducing procedures, or chemo-prevention. For others, it may lead to symptoms of anxiety, depression, and worry. Individuals who are otherwise healthy may now view themselves as vulnerable to developing a life-threatening disease.

As more people participate in genetic testing within a research setting, knowledge about the actual short- and long-term psychological sequelae is increasing. Several studies have examined the short-term psychological effects of genetic testing. Bonadona et al. (2002) interviewed 23 patients with cancer who were identified as mutation carriers for hereditary breast-ovarian or nonpolyposis colorectal cancers one month after they learned about their test results. Eight patients (35%) expressed reactions of distress, and 14 (61%) reported at least one negative feeling, such as unhappiness or worry. Twelve patients (52%), however, expressed no major emotional changes. The majority of patients were worried about their children's risk for the future development of a cancer. Although the sample size is small, this study highlighted the fact that despite having already lived with a diagnosis of cancer, strong emotional reactions still may surface when individuals learn that they harbor a mutation.

Wagner et al. (2000) reported that six to eight weeks after test result disclosure, depression scores on a self-rated depression scale decreased for those who were found to be carriers of a *BRCA* mutation and increased for those found to be noncarriers. Although it is surprising that noncarriers showed an increase in depression, the investigators speculated that they may have had difficulty coping with the effects of the test results within their family unit and may have experienced feelings of survivor guilt. Further investigation is warranted, however, to confirm this suspicion. This study highlighted the importance of providing psychological counseling not only to those identified as carriers but also to those identified as noncarriers.

Another study examined the effect that *BRCA1* test results had among siblings (Smith, West, Croyle, & Botkin, 1999). At a follow-up interview one to two weeks after learning of their test results, male carriers relative to noncarriers experienced significantly more distress if they were the first sibling to be tested than if all of their siblings already tested negative. Noncarrier males whose siblings tested positive had more distress than if siblings tested negative. Female carriers who were tested first and those with no carrier siblings also experienced high levels of distress. This study illustrated how test results within a family can alter levels of distress in both carriers and noncarriers.

Several studies looked at the longer-term psychological effects of genetic testing. Dorval et al. (2000) looked at 65 individuals from *p53* and *BRCA1* testing programs and found that, in general, patients were able to accurately predict their emotional response to the results of genetic testing. The subset of patients who found they were *BRCA1* carriers tended to underestimate their feelings of anger and worry, and this psychological distress persisted at six months' follow-up.

Schwartz et al. (2002), in a large clinic-based testing program (N = 279), found that negative results of genetic testing significantly reduced levels of distress at six months, whereas positive results did not cause an increase in distress or perceived risk.

Broadstock, Michie, and Marteau (2000), in their systematic review of 11 studies, concluded overall that individuals undergoing predictive genetic testing do not experience adverse psychological consequences. No reported levels of increased distress (general and situational distress, anxiety, and depression) occurred in carriers or noncarriers at any point during the 12 months after testing. The studies included genetic testing for Huntington disease, hereditary breast and ovarian cancers, familial adenomatous polyposis, and spinocerebellar ataxia. Both carriers and noncarriers showed decreased distress after testing, although it was greater among noncarriers. Pretest emotional state was predictive of subsequent distress.

Although most of the studies reported favorable psychological outcomes, some reported adverse effects in both carriers and noncarriers. It therefore would be a mistake to make any general assumptions about how an individual may cope after receiving test results. Many of the studies consisted of highly selected participants who were identified from hereditary cancer registries and were already aware that a mutation existed in the family. They may not be representative of individuals who refer themselves to clinic-based genetic counseling programs (Lerman et al., 1996) as in the study done by Schwartz et al. (2002). It therefore is critical to perform a thorough individualized risk assessment along with genetic counseling prior to performing any testing (Greco & Mahon, 2004). Particular attention must be paid to individuals' pretest expectations and emotional state. Relationships with family members also should be explored. The decision to be tested is personal, and each patient and family member must weigh the options, risks, and benefits of testing on an individual basis (Greco & Mahon).

Issues of Confidentiality

Issues of confidentiality and privacy are critical and should be addressed before any testing is initiated. The person who undergoes genetic testing logically should be the one to decide whether to disclose results and, if so, to whom. However, this issue becomes more complicated when others may be affected. Is withholding results from family members who also may be at risk ethical? This brings up a difficult issue of the individual's right to maintain confidentiality versus a family member's right to know. Conversely, it must be anticipated that certain family members might not want to know their relative's test results. A telephone survey was conducted of 200 Jewish women to evaluate their attitudes toward sharing genetic test results with family members (Lehmann, Weeks, Klar, Biener, & Garber, 2000). All of the respondents (100%) believed that an individual should inform at-risk family members if the disease is preventable, compared with 85% who believed so if the disease is nonpreventable. Few believed that a physician should inform a family member against the individual's wishes whether preventable (18%) or not (16%) (Lehmann et al.). ASCO's (2003) position is that healthcare providers should protect the confidentiality of genetic information while also reminding participants during precounseling sessions of the importance of communicating test results to family members. These issues are very complicated and could put a great deal of strain on family relationships.

Individuals considering testing must be informed that there is no guarantee that test results will remain confidential, especially if the goal is to have insurance companies pay for the testing and for possible prophylactic surgery or surveillance. Maintenance of confidentiality is much easier when testing is performed in the context of a research protocol. Research data are not subject to subpoena should discriminatory legal action ensue.

Once confidentiality is breached, a person may be subject to various forms of discrimination. Insurance companies may deny coverage or increase premiums for those who have positive test results. To date, no federal statutes exist to universally protect individuals from genetic discrimination. Congress passed the Health Insurance Portability and Accountability Act in 1996, which prohibits health insurance providers from using genetic information to establish rules for insurance eligibility for people covered by group health insurance. Loopholes in the legislation, however, create the potential for genetic discrimination. Hall and Rich (2000), in a large survey, collected data from multiple states and found no well-documented cases of insurance discrimination. This was true in states with and without laws that prohibited insurers' use of genetic information. Nevertheless, fear of discrimination remains real in the minds of many individuals at high risk and may prevent them from undergoing testing.

In a recent survey of 184 individuals who were eligible for testing based on a family history suggestive of a hereditary breast-ovarian cancer syndrome, 78 declined testing. Of those who declined, 48 cited concerns about cost and insurance discrimination (Peterson, Milliron, Lewis, Goold, & Merajver, 2002). In another survey, 163 cancer genetic counselors were asked to predict hypothetically whether they would submit charges to their insurance company if they decided to undergo genetic testing. Sixty-eight percent of the providers would not submit the charges because of fears of discrimination for both themselves and their children (Matloff et al., 2000).

A potential for discrimination in the workplace also exists. Individuals may receive unfair treatment or lose a job or employment opportunities. Social stigmatization may occur. As no law currently exists that protects all individuals, ASCO (2003) strongly supports a federal statute to prohibit genetic discrimination by all health insurance providers and employers.

A more subtle form of discrimination may exist in a person's private life (Surbone, 2001). An individual may decide not to marry or have a family with a partner who is predetermined to be at high risk for developing cancer. Patients who carry a cancer susceptibility mutation have reported feelings of vulnerability or guilt about the possibility of passing the mutation onto their children (Greco & Mahon, 2004).

Social Issues

Costs Associated With Genetic Testing

A major social concern involves the cost of genetic testing. Who will pay for genetic testing and the services that relate to it? Individuals who underwent *BRCA* testing through Myriad Genetics Laboratories in Salt Lake City, UT, were charged anywhere from $395 for analysis of a single mutation to $2,400 for full sequencing of the *BRCA1* and *BRCA2* genes (Peterson et al., 2002). Although progress is occurring, still no universal coverage exists for genetic testing, screening, counseling, and implementation of surveillance and prevention strategies.

Finally, as genetic testing becomes incorporated into our society, the need for more healthcare professionals to develop expertise in this area will increase. How will the educational programs be funded, and who should cover the cost of the education? Opportunities for oncology nurses to become educated in genetics previously have been limited in the academic setting; however, credentialing in genetics is available at the baccalaureate and master's level, and a scope and standards of genetics and clinical nursing practice has been established (Calzone & Masny, 2004). Access to and the costs of these resources remain of concern as oncology nurses are being asked to answer the genetic questions and concerns of patients with cancer.

Knowledge, Attitudes, and Willingness to Undergo Testing

Genetic testing presents a new and promising method for obtaining knowledge of one's individual risk. With the discovery of more predisposition genes, the number of individuals seeking testing likely will increase. Because of the potential substantial demand for genetic susceptibility testing, increased awareness of people's knowledge, attitudes, and willingness to undergo testing is important. Bottorff et al. (2002) conducted a telephone survey of 260 women with breast cancer and 761 women without breast cancer (randomly selected from the general population) to ascertain their interest in genetic testing for breast cancer risk. Of the women with breast cancer, 30.8% reported an interest in getting tested or already had been tested, compared to 28.5% of women without breast cancer. Among the women with breast cancer, the two most common reasons for wanting testing were "curiosity" and "to warn the family." Women without breast cancer reported "curiosity" and "to take preventative action" as their most common reasons. Women with at least one first- or second-degree relative with breast cancer were 2.3 times more likely to express interest in genetic testing than those with no family history. Young women without breast cancer and well-educated women with breast cancer were the most likely candidates to be interested in testing. In general, women with and without breast cancer demonstrated limited knowledge of genetic testing.

Several studies have focused on race/ethnicity and culture as predictors of interest to undergo genetic counseling and testing. Thompson et al. (2002) interviewed 76 African American women with a positive family history of breast cancer. Women who declined genetic counseling (n = 17) had significantly less knowledge of breast cancer genetics and higher perceived "barrier" scores than those who underwent both counseling and testing (n = 40). Barriers included a high concern about stigmatization and greater anticipation of negative emotional reactions to positive test results. Those who declined counseling or who underwent counseling but declined testing demonstrated strong anticipation of guilt about family members if they were found to be mutation carriers. Women who chose to undergo counseling regardless of their decision to be tested reported having more intrusive thoughts about breast cancer than those who declined counseling.

Another study surveyed 426 first-degree relatives of patients diagnosed with colon cancer to ascertain their interest in genetic counseling and colorectal cancer susceptibility testing. The participants were Japanese (n = 336), Hawaiian/part-Hawaiian (n = 50), and Caucasian (n = 40). Overall, 45% of the participants were interested in genetic counseling, and 26% were interested in pursuing testing. The most important predicators for interest in counseling included cancer worry, family social support, education, and Hawaiian ethnicity. The most important predictors for interest in genetic testing included cancer worry, perceived risk, and older age. The Japanese participants were markedly less interested in obtaining genetic testing (Glanz, Grove, Lerman, Gotay, & Le Marchand, 1999).

A 1999 study examined the attitudes about and interest in genetic testing for breast and ovarian cancers in women with a family history of breast cancer who were white (n = 307) (main study group), African American (n = 36), lesbian/bisexual (n = 87), and Ashkenazi Jewish (n = 113) (Durfy, Bowen, McTiernan, Sporleder, & Burke, 1999). Interest in getting tested was high (> 80%) in all four groups, although the majority of women knew very little about genetic testing. African American women were the least likely to have heard about genetic testing. Interest dropped among all groups if they had to pay for the test themselves, with the biggest drop occurring in the African American group (51.6%). Significant predictors of interest in testing included cancer worry, perceived risk, and beliefs about access to testing. It is of interest that the mean perceived risk in all the groups was 3.7–4.5-fold higher than the mean actual risk as calculated by the Gail model, with the highest perceived risk being in the main study group. Most women in all the groups reported that if they learned that they had a gene mutation, they would undergo more frequent screening, including breast self-examination, clinical breast examination, and mammography. The majority of women would not consider prophylactic surgery.

The aforementioned studies begin to elucidate why some individuals are interested in genetic testing, whereas others are not. Interest in undergoing testing varied greatly, ranging from 26% to more than 80%. Many factors could have influenced this variance, including the level of cancer risk of the individual, which differed among the study participants; the cultural background; and the individual's perceived risks and benefits. In general, knowledge about genetic testing among study participants was low. These studies reinforced an ongoing need to increase knowledge of the issues surrounding genetic testing. They highlighted the importance of developing programs that not only provide basic genetic information but also are sensitive to the individual's cultural, demographic, and psychological makeup.

Implications for Practice

With the rapid advancement in genetic technology and the numerous ethical, psychological, and social dilemmas surrounding it, several large and prestigious organizations including ASCO (2003), the Oncology Nursing Society (ONS, 2004b), and the Society of Surgical Oncology (Klimberg et al., 1999) have developed position statements setting forth guidelines and recommendations to address many of these complex issues. Highlighted among these statements is the importance of informed consent prior to testing, pre- and post-test counseling from someone who is knowledgeable in the field of genetics, regulation of laboratories that provide genetic testing, protection from insurance and employment discrimination, and provision of educational resources for healthcare professionals, individuals at high risk, and the lay public. The organizations agreed that genetic testing should be performed in the context of long-term outcome studies and endorsed continued support of patient-oriented research to analyze all aspects of cancer genetics (e.g., efficacy of surveillance programs, psychological impact of testing).

Oncology nurses are in a strategic position to educate and support patients in a variety of ways throughout this difficult process. To be effective educators, nurses first must gain a basic knowledge of cancer genetics. ONS's (2004a) position is that both general- and advanced-practice oncology nurses should be educated in genetics principles. In 1995, 25 professional specialty organizations (representing more than 500,000 nurses) met at the National Institutes of Health to make recommendations for the training needed to prepare nurses to incorporate genetics knowledge into practice (Jenkins, Calzone, Dimond, & Fraser, 1996). Since that time, a variety of educational resources have become available to help to disseminate information and expand knowledge, including educational seminars, journal articles, textbooks, and Web sites. Several examples include a toolkit developed by ONS (2002) titled *Genetics and Cancer Care: A Guide for Oncology Nurses* (www.ons.org/clinical/documents/pdfs/Kit.pdf). ONS also offers a Genetics Short Course for Cancer Nurses (http://onsopcontent.ons.org/Meetings/GeneticsSC/geneticshome.html), which will be conducted through 2007. Another resource is a textbook titled *Genetics in Oncology Practice: Cancer Risk Assessment,* published by ONS (Tranin, Masny, & Jenkins, 2003). Table 30-1 identifies Web sites that contain information on genetics and cancer for healthcare professionals, and Hutson and Loud (2004) published a comprehensive resource guide that is applicable to both nurses and patients.

Course work on crosscultural counseling must become part of training programs to meet the needs of the increasing number of immigrants and ethnic groups in the United States. Programs must be devised to overcome potential barriers to screening, such as geographic isolation, poverty, and a lack of knowledge concerning genetic risk. One way to bridge potential cultural and religious barriers may be to recruit and train healthcare professionals from diverse ethnic backgrounds.

Depending on their level of expertise, some oncology nurses can provide full genetic counseling services to their patients, whereas others may feel more comfortable

Table 30-1. Cancer Genetics Resources on the Web

Organization	Web Site
American Society of Clinical Oncology	www.asco.org
Genetics Education Center, University of Kansas Medical Center	www.kumc.edu/gec
International Society of Nurses in Genetics	www.isong.org
National Cancer Institute (NCI)	www.nci.nih.gov
National Human Genome Research Institute, NCI	www.nhgri.nih.gov
Oncology Nursing Society	www.ons.org

referring them to appropriate specialists (e.g., oncologist, clinical nurse specialist, genetic counselor) when indicated. Even if the nurses' knowledge base is limited, an awareness of available resources that they could provide to their patients would be very helpful. Nurses with more knowledge in the field can discuss the risks, benefits, and potential limitations of genetic testing and ensure that patients not only receive the information but also comprehend it. Nurses must tailor the information to the cultural background and literacy level of the individual. Differences may exist in the awareness of, understanding of, and access to genetic testing in minority populations (Vadaparampil, Wey, & Kinney, 2004). A person who proceeds with testing without fully understanding the implications potentially could be devastated after receiving the results. Nurses must ensure that patients across all cultures are competent to make voluntary and informed decisions.

Nurses also are excellent candidates to participate in a variety of genetics-related research. Numerous topics need further exploration, including continued assessment of short- and long-term psychological sequelae, reasons for opting for or declining testing, and the influence of culture/ethnicity on decision making.

Conclusion

The age of genetic susceptibility testing for cancer is here, and education programs for patients, nurses, and physicians must accompany its arrival. Nurses, with their long history as patient advocates, can play central roles in ensuring informed consent and assisting patients through this difficult process. They must be considered integral members of the genetic counseling team in both research endeavors and the clinical arena.

References

American Society of Clinical Oncology. (2003). American Society of Clinical Oncology policy statement update: Genetic testing for cancer susceptibility. *Journal of Clinical Oncology, 21,* 2397–2406.

Bonadona, V., Saltel, P., Desseigne, F., Mignotte, H., Saurin, J.C., Wang, Q., et al. (2002). Cancer patients who experienced diagnostic genetic testing for cancer susceptibility: Reactions and behavior after the disclosure of a positive test result. *Cancer Epidemiology, Biomarkers and Prevention, 11,* 97–104.

Borgen, P.I., Hill, A.D., Tran, K.N., Van Zee, K.J., Massie, M.J., Payne, D., et al. (1998). Patient regrets after bilateral prophylactic mastectomy. *Annals of Surgical Oncology, 5,* 603–606.

Bottorff, J.L., Ratner, P.A., Balneaves, L.G., Richardson, C.G., McCullum, M., Hack, T., et al. (2002). Women's interest in genetic testing for breast cancer risk: The influence of sociodemographics and knowledge. *Cancer Epidemiology, Biomarkers and Prevention, 11,* 89–95.

Broadstock, M., Michie, S., & Marteau, T. (2000). Psychological consequences of predictive genetic testing: A systematic review. *European Journal of Human Genetics, 8,* 731–738.

Calzone, K.A., & Masny, A. (2004). Genetics and oncology nursing. *Seminars in Oncology Nursing, 20,* 178–185.

Dorval, M., Patenaude, A.F., Schneider, K.A., Kieffer, S.A., DiGianni, L., Kalkbrenner, K.J., et al. (2000). Anticipated versus actual emotional reactions to disclosure of results of genetic tests for cancer susceptibility: Findings from p53 and BRCA1 testing programs. *Journal of Clinical Oncology, 18,* 2135–2142.

Durfy, S.J., Bowen, D.J., McTiernan, A., Sporleder, J., & Burke, W. (1999). Attitudes and interest in genetic testing for breast and ovarian cancer susceptibility in diverse groups of women in western Washington. *Cancer Epidemiology, Biomarkers and Prevention, 8,* 369–375.

Fisher, B., Costantino, J.P., Wickerham, D.L., Redmond, C.K., Kavanah, M., Cronin, W.M., et al. (1998). Tamoxifen for prevention of breast cancer: Report of the National Surgical Adjuvant Breast and Bowel Project P-1 study. *Journal of the National Cancer Institute, 90,* 1371–1388.

Ford, D., Easton, D.F., Stratton, M., Narod, S., Goldgar, D., Devilee, P., et al. (1998). Genetic heterogeneity and penetrance analysis of the BRCA1 and the BRCA2 genes in breast cancer families. *American Journal of Human Genetics, 62,* 676–689.

Glanz, K., Grove, J., Lerman, C., Gotay, C., & Le Marchand, L. (1999). Correlates of intentions to obtain genetic counseling and colorectal cancer gene testing among at-risk relatives from three ethnic groups. *Cancer Epidemiology, Biomarkers and Prevention, 8,* 329–336.

Greco, K.E., & Mahon, S. (2004). Common hereditary cancer syndromes. *Seminars in Oncology Nursing, 20,* 164–177.

Hall, M.A., & Rich, S.S. (2000). Laws restricting health insurers' use of genetic information: Impact on genetic discrimination. *American Journal of Human Genetics, 66,* 293–307.

Hartmann, L.C., Schaid, D.J., Woods, J.E., Crotty, T.P., Myers, J.L., Arnold, P.G., et al. (1999). Efficacy of bilateral prophylactic mastectomy in women with a family history of breast cancer. *New England Journal of Medicine, 340,* 77–84.

Health Insurance Portability and Accountability Act of 1996, Public Law No. 104-191. Retrieved May 16, 2005, from http://aspe.hhs.gov/admnsimp/pl104191.htm

Hutson, S.P., & Loud, J.T. (2004). Cancer genetic resources: A guide for nurses and patients. *Seminars in Oncology Nursing, 20,* 213–215.

Jenkins, J., Calzone, K., Dimond, E., & Fraser, M. (1996). Ongoing meetings promote the integration of genetics education into nursing practice. *ONS News, 11*(11), 3.

King, M.C., Wieand, S., Hale, K., Lee, M., Walsh, T., Owens, K., et al. (2001). Tamoxifen and breast cancer incidence among women with inherited mutations in BRCA1 and BRCA2. *JAMA, 286,* 2251–2256.

Klimberg, V.S., Galandiuk, S., Singletary, E.S., Cohen, A., Sener, S., Talamonti, M.S., et al. (1999). Society of Surgical Oncology: Statement on genetic testing for cancer susceptibility. *Annals of Surgical Oncology, 6,* 507–509.

Lehmann, L.S., Weeks, J.C., Klar, N., Biener, L., & Garber, J.E. (2000). Disclosure of familial genetic information: Perceptions of the duty to inform. *American Journal of Medicine, 109,* 705–711.

Lerman, C., Narod, S., Schulman, K., Hughes, C., Gomez-Caminero, A., Bonney, G., et al. (1996). BRCA1 testing in families with breast-ovarian cancer. *JAMA, 275,* 1885–1892.

Matloff, E.T., Shappell, H., Brierley, K., Bernhardt, B.A., McKinnon, W., & Peshkin, B.N. (2000). What would you do? Specialists' perspectives on cancer genetic testing, prophylactic surgery, and insurance discrimination. *Journal of Clinical Oncology, 18,* 2484–2492.

Oncology Nursing Society. (2002). *Genetics and cancer care: A guide for oncology nurses.* Pittsburgh, PA: Author.

Oncology Nursing Society. (2004a, October). *Cancer predisposition genetic testing and risk assessment counseling.* Pittsburgh, PA: Author. Retrieved May 16, 2005, from http://www.ons.org/publications/positions/CancerPredisposition.shtml

Oncology Nursing Society. (2004b, October). *The role of the oncology nurse in cancer genetic counseling.* Pittsburgh, PA: Author. Retrieved May 16, 2005, from http://www.ons.org/publications/positions/CancerGeneticCounseling.shtml

Peterson, E.A., Milliron, K.J., Lewis, K.E., Goold, S.D., & Merajver, S.D. (2002). Health insurance and discrimination concerns and BRCA1/2 testing in a clinic population. *Cancer Epidemiology, Biomarkers and Prevention, 11,* 79–87.

Rieger, P.T. (2004). The biology of cancer genetics. *Seminars in Oncology Nursing, 20,* 145–154.

Schwartz, M.D., Peshkin, B.N., Hughes, C., Main, D., Isaacs, C., & Lerman, C. (2002). Impact of BRCA1/BRCA2 mutation testing on psychologic distress in a clinic-based sample. *Journal of Clinical Oncology, 20,* 514–520.

Smith, K.R., West, J.A., Croyle, R.T., & Botkin, J.R. (1999). Familial context of genetic testing for cancer susceptibility: Moderating effect of siblings' test results on psychological distress one to two weeks after BRCA1 mutation testing. *Cancer Epidemiology, Biomarkers and Prevention, 8,* 385–392.

Surbone, A. (2001). Ethical implications of genetic testing for breast cancer susceptibility. *Critical Reviews in Oncology/Hematology, 40,* 149–157.

Thompson, H.S., Valdimarsdottir, H.B., Duteau-Buck, C., Guevarra, J., Bovbjerg, D.H., Richmond-Avellaneda, C., et al. (2002). Psychosocial predictors of BRCA counseling and testing decisions among urban African-American women. *Cancer Epidemiology, Biomarkers and Prevention, 11,* 1579–1585.

Tranin, A.S., Masny, A., & Jenkins, J. (Eds.). (2003). *Genetics in oncology practice: Cancer risk assessment.* Pittsburgh, PA: Oncology Nursing Society.

Vadaparampil, S.T., Wey, J.P., & Kinney, A.Y. (2004). Psychosocial aspects of genetic counseling and testing. *Seminars in Oncology Nursing, 20,* 186–195.

Wagner, T.M., Moslinger, R., Langbauer, G., Ahner, R., Fleischmann, E., Auterith, A., et al. (2000). Attitude towards prophylactic surgery and effects of genetic counseling in families with BRCA mutations. Austrian Hereditary Breast and Ovarian Cancer Group. *British Journal of Cancer, 82,* 1249–1253.

CHAPTER 31

Psychosocial Aspects of Hematopoietic Stem Cell Transplantation

CATHERINE H. KELLEY, RN, MSN

The paradox of courage is that a man must be a little careless of his life even in order to keep it.

—G.K. Chesterton

Hematopoietic stem cell transplantation (HSCT) (also referred to as bone marrow and peripheral blood stem cell transplantation) is a widely accepted treatment for malignant and nonmalignant diseases. With advances in autologous and allogeneic stem cell transplants, umbilical cord blood transplant, and improved biomedical support therapies, the need to evaluate the impact of technology on patients and families continues to be an important aspect of medical and nursing research.

HSCT has been described as a procedure associated with isolation of the patient, prolonged hospitalizations, rapid fluctuations in medical condition, frequent and often life-threatening infections, and graft-versus-host disease (GVHD). Although some patients encounter such difficult experiences during recovery and a significant mortality rate is associated with the procedure, other patients experience rapid recovery with minimal risk of serious complications and a shortened length of hospitalization (Blume & Thomas, 2000; Dansey & Baynes, 2001; Little & Storb, 2002; Tallman et al., 2003). Most HSCT units use high-efficiency particulate-arresting filtration, which allows the patient freedom of movement and frequent family and staff contact. Other patients are treated as outpatients using clinic visits and hotel living, whereas some remain in their own home environment during recovery (Svahn et al., 2002). Issues related to caregiver availability and caregiver burden become more important considerations in these aggressive outpatient settings.

Psychosocial Impact of Hematopoietic Stem Cell Transplantation on Recipients

The early HSCT literature, which described valuable clinical observations, case histories, and suggestions for psychosocial management of patients and families, provided a foundation for more scientific study into the stressors and responses of patients. Brown and Kelly (1976) presented one of the earliest reports of the psychological impact of HSCT. They described eight characteristic stages of HSCT with associated psychological reactions as patients progressed through the medical treatment, beginning with their admission to the hospital and ending with their adaptation outside of the hospital.

The decision to proceed with transplant involves significant pretransplant activities, including reviewing and understanding informed consent for the protocol and admission to the hospital for the conditioning treatment. Stressors for patients during these initial stages included significant anxiety, fear of dying, and psychiatric symptoms caused by prescribed medications (e.g., antiemetics, steroids, cytotoxic agents). Brown and Kelly (1976) described the actual day of marrow infusion as uneventful, with many patients expressing gratitude for the donor. Feelings of anxiety, anger, frustration, and depression complicate the recovery period as patients experience a lengthy engraftment period and deal with issues related to prolonged isolation. Development of GVHD also contributes to the frustration and depression. Preparation for hospital discharge includes issues such as separation anxiety from the treatment team and ambivalence and concern about reintegration into the patient's usual activities and roles. Brown and Kelly described adaptation out of the hospital as the final stage of this process. For the small number of patients who survived HSCT in the early 1970s, the stressors identified were body-image changes, feelings of indebtedness to the donor and others, and concerns about being remembered by staff upon leaving the transplant center.

Contemporary authors, such as Andrykowski and McQuellon (1999), also divide the transplant experience into stages. Stage 1 is the decision to undergo transplantation. Stage II is pretransplant preparation. Stage III is the post-transplant hospitalization. Stage IV covers hospital discharge and post-transplant recovery. Stage V is long-term recovery. The psychosocial issues for patients during each stage are similar to the descriptions by Brown and Kelly (1976). Despite the fact that hospitalization is shorter or that, in some cases, patients may remain in an outpatient setting during treatment and recovery, patients' psychological needs and concerns remain connected to the various medical stages of HSCT (Packman, 1999).

Several researchers have assessed patients at specific times during the transplant trajectory. In a prospective study, Syrjala, Chapko, Vitaliano, Cummings, and Sullivan (1993) followed 67 patients undergoing allogeneic HSCT with a variety of self-assessment instruments pretransplant and at 90 days and one year post-transplant. Physical functioning was most impaired at 90 days but returned to pretransplant levels by one year for most areas assessed. By two years, 68% of patients had returned to full-time work. Impaired physical recovery was associated with more severe chronic GVHD. Results of mean levels of anxiety and depression indicated that patients showed little change in their response over the course of a year. Pretransplant, 27% of patients reported experiencing depression, and 41% reported feeling anxiety. Patients who were at the highest risk for emotional distress at one year had pretransplant family conflict, were not married, or had developed less severe chronic GVHD. Overall, the majority of patients returned to full-time employment with normal physical and psychosocial functioning.

In another study, Andrykowski et al. (1995) investigated 172 disease-free adult HSCT survivors from five different transplant centers with pretransplant and post-transplant questionnaires and interviews. Patients receiving both autologous (n = 95) and allogeneic (n = 77) transplants were included. Researchers compared patients' pre-HSCT outcome expectations, their actual post-transplant outcomes, and patients' perceptions of whether they had "returned to normal" post-HSCT. Results indicated that 47% expected to return to normal, but physical and psychosocial functioning often did not return to normal following HSCT. Only 19% of patients reported that they had anticipated difficulties in returning to normal. Specific problem areas included working outside the home, sexual activity, and vigorous physical activity. The optimistic attitude of most of the patients, despite signing lengthy consent forms, may indicate a type of coping strategy pretransplant. However, patients who had not met their own post-transplant expectations were more distressed than patients who had expected some problems. Study results implied that realistic information about post-transplant recovery may influence post-transplant psychological adjustment.

Lee, Fairclough, Antin, and Weeks (2001) described discrepancies in expectations for transplant outcomes between physicians and patients. Three hundred and thirteen patients and their physicians responded to a questionnaire assessing expectations of HSCT. Results were compared to actual outcomes. Results showed that physicians' and patients' estimates of outcomes were similar if the actual risk of death was less than 30%. However, patients in high-risk transplant categories (e.g., allogeneic, advanced disease) were found to be considerably more optimistic than their physicians. Researchers concluded that those patients either did not fully appreciate their situation, or the medical team withheld or minimized prognostic estimates. This suggests that more realistic discussions of prognosis and risk may be warranted to allow patients and families time to prepare for a possible poor outcome or death.

Several authors have explored the inpatient phase of transplantation and its psychosocial impact. An early study by Steeves (1992) used a hermeneutic approach whereby six men undergoing HSCT were assessed for their quest for meaning during the process. The men clearly tried to negotiate a social position for themselves in that setting. They established new social relationships by identifying who had power in the system (i.e., physicians and nurses), learning their own position in the system (i.e., noting those who were worse off than themselves), establishing and maintaining feelings of love and friendship (e.g., feelings of attachment to nurses), and normalizing social relationships and behavior. They expressed belief in luck, identified their odds of success, and related to a higher power (e.g., helping others, religion) in their search for meaning of the transplant experience. In another study, Shuster, Steeves, and Richardson (1996) interviewed 11 patients at several intervals during their transplant hospitalization and identified five themes or patterns of meaning that represented the way in which the patients coped during transplant.

1. **Physiologic:** Dealing with symptoms such as pain, nausea, fevers, and itching
2. **Alertness:** Escape through sleep, drug-induced sleep, and pretending not to be alert

3. **Attitude:** Realizing they could alter their experience through attitude (e.g., ignoring things, use of television programs to alter mood, managing time with schedules)
4. **Social relationships:** Attachment to others on the HSCT unit and dealing with physical changes
5. **Spirituality:** Reference to organized religion and seeking the meaning of their experience

The study results emphasized that nurses must view their patients in a holistic way and recognize that patients undergoing transplant find meaning in their experiences in different ways. More recently, Cohen and Ley (2000) used a hermeneutic phenomenology approach to report on 20 patients post–autologous HSCT. Patient interviews revealed four common themes, the most prevalent of which was fear of dying during the transplant. Participants were concerned about their outcome but felt certain that they would die of their disease without transplant. Subjects felt unprepared for the intensity, both physically and emotionally, of the experience. This "fear of the unknown," the second theme, included minor invasive procedures. Feelings of loss of control, the third theme, related to the previous theme of fear of the unknown but included loss of control over physical changes and function. The final theme was related to hospital discharge. Participants reported feeling ambivalent as they prepared to leave a protected hospital environment and return home. Major concerns associated with discharge were fear of cancer recurrence and the loss of trust in one's body.

Many researchers consider patients undergoing HSCT to be at risk for depressive symptoms. Murphy, Jenkins, and Whittaker (1996) prospectively evaluated 56 patients for a median follow-up time of 82 months post-transplant. Thirty-seven percent of the women and 17% of the men had significant depressive illness post-transplant. The authors strongly recommended involvement of a psychiatrist during the transplant process. Loberiza et al. (2002) prospectively evaluated 193 HSCT patients for depressive syndrome. They reported that 35% of the patients who were alive six months post-transplant had symptoms of depressive syndrome and were at a three-fold higher risk for death during the following 6–12 months. They strongly supported the need for psychological/pharmacologic intervention for patients exhibiting signs of depressive syndrome.

For children undergoing HSCT, hospitalization is a necessary but difficult disruption in their young lives. Children's ability to cope with the psychosocial aspects of HSCT depends on their age, developmental stage, intellectual ability, personality, and available support systems. Nursing care throughout each phase of transplant should reflect age-specific needs. Play therapy, parental involvement, attention to daily routines, and an age-appropriate environment contribute to children's happiness during the transplant hospitalization. The realization that a child's behavior often is indicative of feelings related to fear and anxiety may help nurses to plan care that is responsive to behavioral cues. Loss of control is a common experience for patients of all ages during transplantation. However, allowing children to make appropriate choices within their daily routine can be beneficial to their psychological response and coping (Abramovitz & Senner, 1995).

Kupst et al. (2002) performed a prospective, longitudinal study of cognitive and psychosocial functioning of pediatric patients undergoing HSCT. They found that children and adolescents with higher pretransplant cognitive functioning did better post-transplant in cognitive, academic, and psychosocial functioning. Other factors that seemed to contribute to better post-transplant adjustment were higher socioeconomic status and age older than one year.

Psychosocial Impact of Hematopoietic Stem Cell Transplantation on the Family

Patenaude, Szymanski, and Rappeport (1979) described HSCT's impact on the family. They identified several key factors that affected the family with a child undergoing transplantation: previous illness (e.g., the length of time that the family member had been ill, siblings' previous illness or death, especially when dealing with genetic diseases), geographic dislocation of the patient from his or her home and family, and other serious family emotional problems, such as marital conflict, separation or divorce, financial concerns, and concerns about other children in the family. Patenaude et al. emphasized the value of including a psychologist or psychiatrist as an integral part of the HSCT team to provide needed support to both the patient and the family.

Heiney, Neuberg, Myers, and Bergman (1994) identified that parental support and involvement are key for the psychological well-being of a child undergoing HSCT. However, parents may experience considerable distress (e.g., feelings of helplessness, loss of control, fear of the unknown, anger, guilt, fear of death) during the transplant process. These feelings may result in post-traumatic stress disorder (PTSD) in parents of children undergoing HSCT. Parental perceptions of the degree of life threat (for the child), duration of the trauma (length of transplant recovery), bereavement (deaths of other children on the unit), displacement from home and community, potential for recurrence, role of the parent in the trauma (caregiving activities), and exposure to death and destruction (side effects) were key risk factors for developing PTSD.

A small quantitative study by Stevens and Pletsch (2002) described similar emotional turmoil. They found that a mother's ability to provide informed consent on behalf of her child for transplant clinical trials was compromised by the emotional trauma of having a child with a life-threatening illness. They recommended that the process of informed consent should not end with pretransplant enrollment into a clinical trial but should be a continuous dialogue with the parents throughout treatment.

Evidence has shown that nondonor siblings of pediatric transplant recipients undergo mild to moderate levels of traumatic stress reactions, which Packman (1999) reported after interviewing siblings (donors and nondonors) three months to six years after HSCT. Findings suggested that the nondonor sibling experiences the additional stress of having two family members involved in medical procedures related to the transplant (the sibling donor and the sibling recipient). The implication, for both professionals and parents, is to direct more emotional support to siblings and address concerns and feelings early and often throughout the transplant process.

Researchers also have described the psychosocial impact of HCST on the recipient's spouse or partner. Because spouses or partners often are key support people, they are confronted with demands from the patient, the rest of the family, and their own jobs or role responsibilities. Often, they take a leave of absence from work or from child-rearing responsibilities and suffer from fatigue as they remain at the patient's bedside for long hours. As the patient progresses through the transplant process, feelings of fear, anger, and ambivalence frequently occur. Little support is available to the spouse, as other friends and family members may have remained at home, away from the transplant center. Changes in roles and responsibilities between the patient and spouse may add to the already significant stress of transplantation. Conflicts may occur when caregivers begin to expect a return to a normal couple relationship and a reduced need for the caregiver role (Langer, Abrams, & Syrjala, 2003).

Zabora, Smith, Baker, Wingard, and Curbow (1992) determined that families often reported feelings of physical and emotional exhaustion six months post-transplant. Most of these feelings were related to the families' expectation that the patient would resume previous roles and responsibilities. Zabora et al. reported that financial concerns were an increasing cause of distress six months post-transplant, although the majority of patients returned to work. Patients who were unable to regain employment post-transplant suffered from chronic GVHD, lower social functioning, and greater job discrimination (Wingard, Curbow, Baker, & Piantadosi, 1991). HSCT survivors and their families identified insurance discrimination and changes in both personal and professional relationships as significant long-term problems (Belec, 1992).

As the model of care for patients undergoing HSCT changes, so do the needs of the caregivers. In a study by Stetz, McDonald, and Compton (1996), 19 adult family caregivers whose family members had undergone inpatient or outpatient HSCT participated in focus groups. Interview questions focused on informational needs, the caregiver role, the impact of illness and treatment on the family's coping, and strategies used by the family members to meet demands. Five major themes evolved from the interviews.

1. **Preparing for caregiving:** Seeking information and evaluating the validity of the information
2. **Managing the care:** Providing physical care, protecting and maintaining the patient's connection with life, and advocating
3. **Facing challenges:** Personal and interpersonal stress, communication barriers with staff, and healthcare barriers
4. **Developing supportive strategies:** Personal and self-care strategies and healthcare system facilitators
5. **Discovering unanticipated rewards and benefits:** Personal growth and family cohesion

Overall, the findings showed that caregivers face considerable personal and interpersonal stress as patients move through transplantation (Stetz et al., 1996). A consistent theme demonstrated by the family was the difficulty in seeking effective communication with the healthcare team. It was clear that the caregiver's need for information was significant and related to areas such as learning complex skills (e.g., managing ambulatory pumps, obtaining supplies, identifying and reporting symptoms). Families responded to many challenges by developing their own self-care strategies and identifying those members of the system who could facilitate their needs. Finally, the families interviewed identified positive feelings of personal growth and closeness among family members.

The issue of financial burden for patients undergoing HSCT and their families is an important problem that may affect psychosocial recovery. Downs (1994) stated that as much as 60% of the total cost of HSCT might be personal expenses for the family, including lodging, transportation, child care, housekeeping, special foods, and home modification. The family also may suffer from the loss of income from the patient or spouse or both. Insurance coverage for out-of-pocket expenses is inconsistent. Frey et al. (2002) found that by moving the transplant setting from inpatient to outpatient, the medical cost savings were more than $14,000. However, the outpatient setting resulted in an estimated out-of-pocket and lost opportunity costs to the caregiver of $2,520. Out-of-pocket costs included expenses such as meals, parking, child care, lawn care, and dog walking. Lost opportunity costs were equated to the time involved in caregiving that would otherwise be used for work, school, or homemaking. The psychosocial impact of financial burden requires continued investigation.

Psychosocial Impact of Hematopoietic Stem Cell Transplantation on the Donor

In HSCT, the donor often is key to the success of the transplant. In fact, it is well documented that the donor type has an impact on recipient outcomes (Filipovich et al., 2001; Henslee-Downey & Gluckman, 1999; Mogul, 2000). The type of donor needed and the method for collection (i.e., bone marrow harvest, apheresis, umbilical cord blood) often are based on medical necessity and donor availability. Potential donors include the recipient (autologous), the recipient's sibling (allogeneic matched related), other relatives (mismatched related), individuals from the National Marrow Donor Program (NMDP) (unrelated), or neonates upon delivery (umbilical cord blood).

Research continues to try to determine the psychosocial impact of HSCT on the donor. Early transplant literature reflects medical practice and the common use of matched sibling donors in allogeneic transplant. These donors—even to-day—commonly undergo a bone marrow harvest procedure for stem cell collection. One unique issue that affects families with a child undergoing transplantation is the selection of a sibling for the donor. For example, if more than one sibling is a "match" for the child, selection of one sibling over another may suggest to the nondonor sibling that the donor is more valued in the family. The relationship between the patient and donor sibling also may change as the donor becomes the "hero." The patient also may be concerned that the sibling donor may die during the harvest procedure. Patenaude et al. (1979) stated that the sibling donor is under considerable psychological stress because of issues related to informed consent and ambivalence about undergoing the harvest procedure. In addition, if the patient's outcome is poor, the sibling donor may experience guilt, fear, and anxiety (Heiney, Bryant, Godder, & Michaels, 2002).

Futterman and Wellisch (1990) identified similar themes of feelings between sibling donors and recipients, even when the siblings were adults. They found, on follow-up, that 20% of the sibling donors had psychological problems directly related to the HSCT. In some cases, problems were related to the death of the patient, but problems also were apparent when the patient experienced complications such as GVHD. Adult siblings with a prior history of relationship conflict seemed to compound their psychological problems when the transplant was unsuccessful or complicated. MacLeod, Whitsett, Mash, and Pelletier (2003) reported similar findings. They compared the psychosocial experience of sibling donors of either successful or unsuccessful HSCT. Siblings who participated in successful transplants reported the experience to be a positive influence on relationships, feelings about self, and their understanding of their sibling's experience. In contrast, donors for unsuccessful transplants reported feelings of guilt and blame over time for the sibling's outcome. Siblings in both groups felt that they had little choice in the decision to donate, and many felt that they needed more information about the procedure than they received from family or healthcare providers. Williams, Green, Morrison, Watson, and Buchanan (2003) reiterated such concerns after interviewing sibling donors undergoing apheresis. They found that donors had little opportunity to refuse to donate because most were asked by the sibling recipient or another family member.

Christopher (2000) described a small sample of adult sibling donors who were interviewed an average of 9.25 months following donation. Her findings were similar to previous reports. Donors reported that the opportunity to donate provided a sense of satisfaction and pride and a sense of responsibility for the transplant outcome. Several donors were concerned that should they become ill themselves, it could jeopardize their sibling's outcome. Donor-recipient relationships became stronger, but the process affected other family relationships negatively. Some conflicts occurred between the recipient's spouse and the birth family.

Researchers have interviewed volunteer donors recruited through NMDP about their decision to donate. Switzer et al. (2003) queried 426 newly recruited donors. They assessed several areas: decision to donate, intrinsic commitment, knowledge about donation, and concerns about donation. Surprisingly, 7% had not yet made the decision to donate. One-third of the group admitted ambivalence about donating. Ambivalence was highest in individuals who perceived a lack of information about the process or who had external pressure to join the registry.

As the number of methods of donation increases, so does the need to evaluate the impact of these technologies on the donor. Rowley, Donaldson, Lilleby, Bensinger, and Appelbaum (2001) compared traditional bone marrow harvest and the newer apheresis procedure using hematopoietic cytokines precollection. They examined 69 donors who were randomized to one or the other collection method. The researchers found that the symptom burden and level of pain for the two groups were similar. In the apheresis group, the filgrastim used to mobilize the cells prior to collection caused the majority of somatic toxicity. Donors who underwent bone marrow harvest reported symptoms associated with anesthesia and multiple needle punctures. Return to baseline measurements (with regard to physical symptoms) was faster for the apheresis group. Neither group reported any significant changes in emotional status pre- or postdonation.

Umbilical cord blood donation and banking have been topics of legal and ethical discussion. Concerns about donation for the "common good" versus storage for potential self-need have been examined. Ethics surrounding intentional pregnancy and donation at birth for a sibling also have stirred comment (Burgio, Gluckman, & Locatelli, 2003; Snyder, 1999). Cord blood donation has many advantages: no risk to the donor, a potential lowered risk of GVHD to the recipient, availability of cells, and low risk of infection transmittal (Barker & Wagner, 2003; Rocha et al., 2000).

However, little research has been conducted regarding the mother's feelings following donation to a cord blood bank. Danzer et al. (2003) prospectively questioned 131 women six months post–cord blood donation. Seventy-eight women returned the questionnaire. The women had a high acceptance of the banking procedure. More than 90% said they would consent to a donation in the future. Forty-six percent of the women were interested in knowing who had received their donation, and 52% thought the recipient should know who had donated the cord blood for them. Sugarman, Kurtzberg, Box, and Horner (2002) reported similar findings. They conducted telephone interviews with 170 women who had agreed to donate cord blood to a public bank. The researchers cited some deficits in the informed consent process related to the women's understanding of the donation process. For example, although generally a positive experience, only 32.9% understood that they had the option of not donating umbilical cord blood, and only 55% were aware that they had an alternative option of private storage (rather than donating to the public bank). The researchers recommended that healthcare professionals, as part of informed consent, emphasize that cord blood banking is considered research, and parents should know how to contact the bank, if needed, following donation.

Quality-of-Life Issues

HSCT, particularly allogeneic transplant, is associated with significant delayed complications that can occur even after 100 days of recovery. It is well documented that recipients are at risk for opportunistic infections, ocular complications, central nervous system sequelae, dental problems, and urologic, skeletal, gonadal, and endocrine complications. Risk for secondary malignancies and relapse of disease are significant concerns for these patients (Antin, 2002; Leiper, 2002). The complexity of the transplant procedure mandates a more comprehensive evaluation of quality of life (QOL) for these patients and their families.

Ferrell et al. (1992a) developed a conceptual model to measure QOL in four key domains: physical well-being and symptoms, social well-being, psychological well-being, and spiritual well-being. This model goes beyond simple evaluation of psychosocial impact to evaluate the interrelationships among domains, providing a more comprehensive method of evaluating QOL for patients undergoing HSCT. Findings were consistent with previous research in that health was a major factor in perception of QOL and that actual physical problems and fear of recurrence had a negative impact on QOL. Many respondents felt that HSCT had a positive effect because it provided a second chance for life.

Other authors have attempted to define QOL post-transplant. Chao et al. (1992) evaluated QOL of 58 patients every 90 days for the first year following autologous HSCT. They found that one year post-transplant, 78% of the patients were employed, 14% reported difficulties with sexual activity, and only 5% reported difficulty sleeping or experienced frequent colds. Overall, 88% reported above-average to excellent QOL. Haberman, Bush, Young, and Sullivan (1993) reported that 74% of 125 patients evaluated stated that their current QOL was the same or better than pretransplant, 9% reported their life to be worse, and 19% gave ambiguous responses. Baker et al. (1994) reported high levels of QOL with regard to major life domains; areas related to physical recovery, strength, and sexual difficulties rated the lowest in satisfaction. Watson et al. (1999) compared findings between patients undergoing HSCT (n = 168) and patients receiving intensive consolidation chemotherapy (n = 311) for acute myeloid leukemia. Significantly more patients undergoing HSCT reported a decreased interest in sex (48% versus 24%), decreased sexual activity (53% versus 35%), decreased pleasure from sex (36% versus 18%), and a decreased ability to have sex (38% versus 18%). Worel et al. (2002) found that 73% (N = 106) of survey respondents reported good to very good QOL within five years of HSCT. However, patients with chronic GVHD experienced significant physical, role, and social impairment. Only 60% of that group were able to return to work.

Hensel, Egerer, Schneeweiss, Goldschmidt, and Ho (2002) evaluated QOL in patients post–autologous transplant. Sixty-seven percent of the 304 responders rated global QOL as good to excellent, and 64% reported their physical status to be good to excellent. Only 5% of the patients rated global QOL or health status as poor. In addition, in patients who were employed prior to transplant, the majority (68% full time and 32% part time) resumed their previous occupation post-transplant.

Molassiotis, Boughton, Burgoyne, and van den Akker (1995) compared QOL of 50 long-term survivors of autologous and allogeneic HSCT. Overall, autologous transplant recipients reported more difficulty with psychosocial adjustment, whereas allogeneic transplant recipients reported more physical problems. They noted a 20% incidence of anxiety and a 10% incidence of clinical depression in autologous transplant recipients. Allogeneic transplant recipients had a 10% incidence of anxiety but no reported incidence of clinical depression. A quarter of both groups had failed to return to work or school, and up to 10% had difficulty carrying out daily tasks. Family relationships were more integrated and lower in conflict when compared to normal families. Overall, patients described their QOL as good to excellent.

Gruber, Fegg, Buchmann, Kolb, and Hiddemann (2003) described the long-term effects of HSCT in 163 patients. They found that the total distress score was the same for patients who had an autologous or allogeneic transplant. Most patients had regained their pretransplant QOL level within two years. The most distressing reported symptoms were fitness (24%), pain (17%), and fear/emotional stress (14%). Patients who did not return to work (31%) had higher scores for pain, anxiety, sleep problems, depression, and impairment in relationships.

Hacker and Ferrans (2003), in a prospective, longitudinal study, examined QOL in patients post–autologous or allogeneic HSCT. Because recovery tends to be faster for patients using mobilized stem cells obtained through apheresis rather than bone marrow harvest, these researchers looked at QOL immediately after transplant and again after the transition from hospital to home. The findings for this small sample were as expected: Patients reported a decrease in global QOL and function immediately after the conditioning regimen. However, improvement, with a return to pretransplant baseline, occurred within two to six weeks.

Phipps, Dunavant, Garvie, Lensing, and Rai (2002) assessed 153 children undergoing HSCT in a prospective, longitudinal study. Their findings showed that children begin the transplant trajectory with a high level of distress that increases and peaks one week after conditioning. However, the distress rapidly returns to admission levels within four or five weeks and returns to preadmission baseline in four to six months. They noted that children undergoing unrelated donor transplant had the highest levels of distress, followed by those undergoing a matched sibling transplant compared to autologous transplant. Also, younger children had lower levels of distress and higher health-related QOL measurements.

King, Ferrell, Grant, and Sakurai (1995) evaluated nurses' perceptions of the impact of HSCT on survivors' QOL using the conceptual model developed by Ferrell et al. (1992a). Nurses were able to describe the negative and positive sequelae of HSCT but perceived patients as having a poorer QOL than the patients themselves reported. This discrepancy is significant because it implies that nursing care for survivors may be inadequate or may not focus on the needed domains.

QOL continues to be an important aspect of HSCT. Many studies have been small, nonrandomized, or retrospective. Assessment tools used in research vary among studies, so it is difficult to make comparisons between them (Hacker, 2003). Research has only begun to suggest using QOL findings to enhance transplant-related treatment decision making (Lee et al., 2002; Mounier et al., 2000; Sung, Buckstein, Doyle, Crump, & Detsky, 2003; Watson et al., 1999, 2004). Research that is prospective, is longitudinal, or shows validation and improvement in QOL tools continues to be necessary for better understanding of the impact of HSCT on QOL domains.

Cultural Influences

Cultural influences on the psychosocial needs of patients and their families are not well delineated in the HSCT literature. Yet, nurses frequently care for patients and families from a variety of cultural, religious, and ethnic backgrounds. The HSCT trajectory demands tremendous amounts of communication, interchange of information, and responsiveness on the part of all involved—the healthcare team, patients, and families. Many issues arise when patients and family members must confront the prospect of HSCT and begin to learn of its risks. Language differences, even when an interpreter is present, can pose a significant barrier to informed consent and treatment decisions. The literature clearly identifies the need for patients to understand the short- and long-term sequelae of transplantation. HSCT nurses are obligated to provide supportive information and to ensure patients' comprehension. However, the ongoing process of informed consent and patient and family education remains a challenge when cultural differences exist. Nurses must use creativity in these cases (e.g., a multimedia approach to patient education to facilitate understanding of key issues) (see Chapter 6).

Donor search and selection may be more problematic, depending on the cultural background and belief system of the patient or potential donor. Misunderstanding of the risks of collection procedures and lack of information on the challenge of tissue typing as related to ethnic groups have been cited as reasons that contribute to the lack of minority donors. Religious beliefs surrounding the body also pose barriers to donation for many cultures (Yancy, Coppo, & Kawanishi, 1997). Donor availability through the NMDP is somewhat limited for patients within ethnic genetic groups. This can be distressing for patients and families who cannot find the ideal match. Efforts directed toward recruitment of minority donors have been a priority for the NMDP. Aggressive marketing to ethnic groups and communities has resulted in an increase of volunteer minority donors, improving the likelihood of a minority patient finding a matched donor. Since 1987, the NMDP (2004) has facilitated more than 20,000 unrelated marrow transplants, of which more than 3,500 have been for minority patients. This reflects significant progress for these patients and emphasizes the need for continued efforts in minority donor recruitment.

During recovery, issues related to nutrition and self-care become more important as patients begin preparation for discharge. Dietary restrictions and cultural variations in diet may impede a patient's ability to return to normal eating. Education related to food preparation and elimination of foods that may pose a health risk for the patient (e.g., raw seafood or meat) are areas that may need considerable attention. Culture also influences role expectations among family members and issues related to caregiving. Nurses must carefully assess expectations among family members. Not all family members want to provide physical care to their loved one; some do not feel that high-tech care is appropriate in the home. Sensitivity to these issues enables nurses to discuss the plan of care with patients and families and use necessary resources to allow patients to achieve success in the outpatient or homecare setting.

Finally, response to serious illness or death is very much a part of the individual's culture, beliefs, and ethnic background. Nurses caring for patients undergoing HSCT and their families need to interact with each individual in a caring and respectful manner. Nurses must allow patients and families to express grief in a way that is consistent with their values and beliefs. Understanding cultural differences enables nurses to care for patients and families in a holistic manner (Brant et al., 2000).

Nursing Implications

Managing patients and families through transplant and the associated stressors remains a challenge for oncology nurses. The psychosocial issues that Brown and Kelly originally described in 1976 continue to be relevant for many patients experiencing allogeneic HSCT—particularly those at significant risk for complications, such as those receiving matched but unrelated transplants. Several authors have identified interventions for patients and caregivers undergoing HSCT to help them to cope with the process of transplantation. Many interventions, such as hypnosis, relaxation techniques, massage therapy, biofeedback, and music therapy, have been used successfully with patients with cancer and are relevant for patients undergoing HSCT. In addition, a pretransplant psychosocial assessment done by a psychologist, advanced practice nurse, or social worker may help to identify preexisting problems that could affect the patient's recovery (Bishop, Rodrigue, & Wingard, 2002; Caudell, 1996; Ferrell et al., 1992b; Hymovich, 1995; Rexilius, Mundt, Megel, & Agrawal, 2002; Rhodes, McDaniel, & Johnson, 1995; Winters, Miller, Maracich, Compton, & Haberman, 1994).

To facilitate early recognition of patients at risk for psychosocial morbidity, Futterman and Wellisch (1990) developed a model of care that describes three levels of psychosocial adjustment based on characteristics of the patient, family, and previous life experiences. The levels range from mild difficulties (level 1), to moderate difficulties (level 2), to severe difficulties (level 3). Recommendations for clinical interventions were based on the level of adjustment after evaluating the patient's history of prior coping, ability to cope with the disease and treatment, quality of affect, mental status, support systems, prior psychiatric history, and ability to anticipate problems. Futterman and Wellisch recommended pharmacologic intervention for some patients during the transplant process. However, careful attention to the risk of side effects and drug interactions is warranted. This model still reflects assessment and interventions that are relevant in both inpatient and outpatient transplant settings.

Another way to assess the psychosocial needs of patients and families is to conduct interviews with them in the home prior to transplant. Homecare nurse involvement at this early stage, although not common, provides the nurse with an opportunity to assess families' dynamics and interactions, as well as to assess potential caregivers' needs. The home health nurse can assess the home environment for safety and infection prevention, which is relevant for early discharge transplant recipients. Identification of problems during this assessment, whether they are related to the actual physical environment or to caregiver issues, affords patients and families, along with the healthcare team, time to resolve the problems prior to HSCT (Kelley, Randolph, & Leum, 2000).

Pretransplant support may be available to patients and families through community or hospital-based groups or Internet chat rooms. Community support and informational resources for transplant recipients and their families are numerous. Identification of community resources is important information that patients and families can use throughout the transplant process (Kapustay & Buchsel, 2000).

During the hospitalization phase of transplantation, regular support for patients and families has been identified as an important component of care. Inclusion of other professionals, such as psychiatrists and psychiatric liaison nurses, chaplains, or social workers, is appropriate. Ersek (1992) identified the importance of maintaining hope during transplantation and the use of hope as an effective coping strategy for patients. She cautioned clinicians that patients must be able to deal with negative information or events in such a way that allows them to maintain hope. She recommended that healthcare professionals create an interactive environment that enables patients to manage information in ways that allow them to cope effectively.

Physical symptoms related to the conditioning regimen and the transplant process, such as nausea, vomiting, anorexia, mucositis, diarrhea, fatigue, and skin breakdown, clearly are associated with distress for patients (Cohen & Ley, 2000; Kapustay & Buchsel, 2000). Nurses must assess the patients' perceptions of their experience and work collaboratively to achieve maximum relief. The nurse's ability to anticipate symptoms and act accordingly to relieve perceived distress is one of the many challenges in HSCT nursing.

Winters et al. (1994) developed a five-concept framework for delineating psychosocial needs of patients and families and for designing nursing therapeutics.

1. **Discovering the lived reality:** The nurse attempts to define the transplant experience through the patient's and family's perceptions.
2. **Managing the flow:** The nurse considers actions taken within the patient's social network that structure interpersonal interactions.
3. **Emerging awareness:** The nurse becomes intuitively aware of relationships within the setting.
4. **Keeping watch:** The nurse monitors the quality of interactions between the patient and family.
5. **Behind closed doors:** The nurse considers interactions between the nurse and patient that are not fully documented in the medical record.

The study results suggested that preparation of HSCT nurses should include education in specific psychosocial strategies, documentation, and coping with personal implications of practice in this unique setting (Winters et al., 1994).

Post-transplant care of patients has dramatically changed. Reinfusion of mobilized peripheral stem cells has decreased significantly the length and severity of neutropenia following the administration of high-dose chemotherapy. This has resulted in a decreased length of hospitalization, earlier hospital discharge, and earlier return of the patient to the referring physician. The use of recombinant colony-stimulating factors pre- and post-transplant and the administration of oral and IV prophylactic drugs (e.g., antimicrobials) have facilitated the management of these patients in the outpatient setting. More frequently, patients receiving peripheral stem cells are managed totally as outpatients through clinic visits, hotel living, and home care.

Early discharge and outpatient programs result in cost reductions. Obviously, evaluating good clinical outcomes is necessary. Caregiver responsibilities include monitoring and documenting vital signs and fluid balances, administering multiple medications by ambulatory pump, documenting medications given, and assisting with activities of daily living (Carter, 2003; Compton, McDonald, & Stetz, 1996; Ezzone, 2000). In other words, much of the care delivered by the caregiver in this setting mimics traditional high-tech inpatient nursing care. Stetz et al. (1996) described the challenges that caregivers face during transplantation. The need to participate in the delivery of high-tech care compounds the traditional problems experienced by caregivers—disruptions of daily life, loss of free time for socialization, childcare issues, housekeeping needs, alteration of employment, and financial concerns. In addition to the supportive strategies suggested by McDonald, Stetz, and Compton (1996), classroom instruction and support groups for the caregiver also are essential (see Table 31-1).

Interestingly, home nursing care is an underutilized resource for patients and families in outpatient settings. Potentially, the homecare nurse can provide the much-needed technical support for therapy administration for families who feel overwhelmed by such tasks. The homecare nurse can supervise administration of the therapies and reinforce education for both patients and caregivers. The nurse can assess the physical and psychosocial needs of patients and caregivers, whether the setting is a nearby hotel, an apartment at the transplant center, or the home. In fact, the homecare nurse can assist in the transition of care as patients and families return to their referring physicians and communities (Kelley et al., 2000).

Conclusion

Care of patients undergoing HSCT represents a challenge for oncology nurses from both a technical and a psychosocial perspective. As nurses continue to evaluate the clinical outcomes and QOL of patients undergoing transplantation and their families, they need to cautiously and proactively identify the impact of medical advancements in this setting. Although aggressive discharge and outpatient management of transplant recipients and their families may be beneficial in many ways, nurses must examine carefully the psychosocial impact and provide resources needed for support. As medical and nursing care evolves from the traditional inpatient setting to the outpatient arena,

Table 31-1. Educational Strategies for Caregivers in the Bone Marrow Transplant Setting

Caregiver Issues	Educational Strategies
Preparing the caregiver • Accessing health care • Acquiring information • The learning process	• Provide written information about the center. • Provide contact person for questions. • Provide accurate, consistent information related to the transplant experience for both the patient and caregiver. • Develop a network of caregivers. • Provide information related to area resources. • Provide a flow sheet of the transplant process. • Identify best methods of teaching based on learning needs.
Managing the care • Gaining needed skills • Becoming homecare managers • Reorganizing the structure of life	• Provide skill education (e.g., written materials, classroom instruction, one-on-one demonstration). • Provide education for management of symptoms and decision making. • Identify resources (at transplant center and in community). • Teach coping skills.
Facing the challenges • Dealing with the stress of information • Communicating with healthcare providers	• Identify clear roles of the caregiver for each phase of transplant. • Divide information into more manageable segments. • Provide new information as needed.
Developing supportive strategies • Using self-care strategies • Participating as a member of the healthcare team	• Provide information about self-care of the caregiver (e.g., rest, proper diet, relaxation). • Review information on additional resources available. • Include caregivers in decision-making process; acknowledge caregiver contributions.

Note. From "Educational Interventions for Family Caregivers During Marrow Transplantation," by J.C. McDonald, K.M. Stetz, and K. Compton, 1996, *Oncology Nursing Forum, 23,* pp. 1434–1437. Copyright 1996 by the Oncology Nursing Society. Adapted with permission.

the stressors that patients undergoing transplantation and their families experience also may be changing. Continued nursing research is needed to evaluate the impact of this treatment modality on the psychosocial outcomes for patients, donors, families, and caregivers and to provide evidence-based nursing interventions.

References

Abramovitz, L.Z., & Senner, A.M. (1995). Pediatric bone marrow transplantation update. *Oncology Nursing Forum, 22,* 107–115.

Andrykowski, M.A., Brady, M.J., Greiner, C.B., Altmaier, E.M., Burish, T.G., Antin, J.H., et al. (1995). 'Returning to normal' following bone marrow transplantation: Outcomes, expectations and informed consent. *Bone Marrow Transplantation, 15,* 573–581.

Andrykowski, M.A., & McQuellon, R.P. (1999). Psychological issues in hematopoietic cell transplantation. In E.D. Thomas, K.G. Blume, & S.J. Forman (Eds.), *Hematopoietic cell transplantation* (2nd ed., pp. 398–406). Malden, MA: Blackwell Science.

Antin, J.H. (2002). Long-term care after hematopoietic-cell transplantation in adults. *New England Journal of Medicine, 347*, 36–42.

Baker, F., Wingard, J.R., Curbow, B., Zabora, J., Jodrey, D., Fogarty, L., et al. (1994). Quality of life of bone marrow transplant long-term survivors. *Bone Marrow Transplantation, 13*, 589–596.

Barker, J.N., & Wagner, J.E. (2003). Umbilical-cord blood transplantation for the treatment of cancer. *Nature Reviews: Cancer, 3*, 526–532.

Belec, R.H. (1992). Quality of life: Perceptions of long-term survivors of bone marrow transplantation. *Oncology Nursing Forum, 19*, 31–37.

Bishop, M.M., Rodrigue, J.R., & Wingard, J.R. (2002). Mismanaging the gift of life: Noncompliance in the context of adult stem cell transplantation. *Bone Marrow Transplantation, 29*, 875–880.

Blume, K., & Thomas, E. (2000). A review of autologous hematopoietic cell transplantation. *Biology of Blood and Marrow Transplantation, 6*, 1–12.

Brant, J., Ishida, D., Itana, J., Kagawa-Singer, M., Palos, G., Phillips, J., et al. (2000). Multicultural outcomes: Guidelines for cultural competence. Pittsburgh, PA: Oncology Nursing Society.

Brown, J.N., & Kelly, M.J. (1976). Stages of bone marrow transplantation: A psychiatric perspective. *Psychosomatic Medicine, 38*, 439–446.

Burgio, G., Gluckman, E., & Locatelli, F. (2003). Ethical reappraisal of 15 years of cord-blood transplantation. *Lancet, 361*, 250–252.

Carter, P. (2003). Family caregivers' sleep loss and depression over time. *Cancer Nursing, 26*, 253–259.

Caudell, K.A. (1996). Psychoneuroimmunology and innovative behavioral interventions in patients with leukemia. *Oncology Nursing Forum, 23*, 493–502.

Chao, N.J., Tierney, D.K., Bloom, J.R., Long, G.D., Barr, T.A., Stallbaum, B.A., et al. (1992). Dynamic assessment of quality of life after autologous bone marrow transplantation. *Blood, 80*, 825–830.

Christopher, K. (2000). The experience of donating bone marrow to a relative. *Oncology Nursing Forum, 27*, 693–700.

Cohen, M., & Ley, C.D. (2000). Bone marrow transplantation: The battle for hope in the face of fear. *Oncology Nursing Forum, 27*, 473–480.

Compton, K., McDonald, J.C., & Stetz, K.M. (1996). Understanding the caring relationship during marrow transplantation: Family caregivers and healthcare professionals. *Oncology Nursing Forum, 23*, 1428–1432.

Dansey, R., & Baynes, R. (2001). Nonablative allogeneic hematopoietic stem cell transplantation. *Current Opinion in Oncology, 13*, 27–32.

Danzer, E., Holzgreve, W., Troeger, C., Kostka, U., Steimann, S., Bitzer, J., et al. (2003). Attitudes of Swiss mothers toward unrelated umbilical cord blood banking 6 months after donation. *Transfusion, 43*, 604–608.

Downs, S. (1994). Ethical issues in bone marrow transplantation. *Seminars in Oncology Nursing, 10*, 58–63.

Ersek, M. (1992). The process of maintaining hope in adults undergoing bone marrow transplantation for leukemia. *Oncology Nursing Forum, 19*, 883–889.

Ezzone, S.A. (2000). Patient and family caregiver teaching. In P.C. Buchsel & P.M. Kapustay (Eds.), *Stem cell transplantation: A clinical textbook* (pp. 6.3–6.12). Pittsburgh, PA: Oncology Nursing Society.

Ferrell, B., Grant, M., Schmidt, G.M., Rhiner, M., Whitehead, C., Fonbuena, P., et al. (1992a). The meaning of quality of life for bone marrow transplant survivors. Part 1: The impact of bone marrow transplant on quality of life. *Cancer Nursing, 15*, 153–160.

Ferrell, B., Grant, M., Schmidt, G.M., Rhiner, M., Whitehead, C., Fonbuena, P., et al. (1992b). The meaning of quality of life for bone marrow transplant survivors. Part 2: Improving quality of life for bone marrow transplant survivors. *Cancer Nursing, 15*, 247–253.

Filipovich, A., Stone, J., Tomany, S., Ireland, M., Kollman, C., Petz, C., et al. (2001). Impact of donor type on outcome of bone marrow transplantation for Wiskott-Aldrich syndrome: Collaborative study of the International Bone Marrow Transplant Registry and the National Marrow Donor Program. *Blood, 97*, 1598–1603.

Frey, P., Stinson, T., Siston, A., Knight, S.J., Ferdman, E., Traynor, A., et al. (2002). Lack of caregivers limits use of outpatient hematopoietic stem cell transplant program. *Bone Marrow Transplantation, 30*, 741–748.

Futterman, A.D., & Wellisch, D.K. (1990). Psychodynamic themes of bone marrow transplantation: When I becomes thou. *Hematology/Oncology Clinics of North America, 4*, 699–709.

Gruber, U., Fegg, M., Buchmann, M., Kolb, H.J., & Hiddemann, W. (2003). The long-term psychosocial effects of haematopoetic stem cell transplantation. *European Journal of Cancer Care, 12,* 249–256.

Haberman, M., Bush, N., Young, K., & Sullivan, K.M. (1993). Quality of life of adult long-term survivors of bone marrow transplantation: A qualitative analysis of narrative data. *Oncology Nursing Forum, 20,* 1545–1553.

Hacker, E.D. (2003). Quantitative measurement of quality of life in adult patients undergoing bone marrow transplant or peripheral blood stem cell transplant: A decade in review. *Oncology Nursing Forum, 30,* 613–630.

Hacker, E.D., & Ferrans, C.E. (2003). Quality of life immediately after peripheral blood stem cell transplantation. *Cancer Nursing, 26,* 312–322.

Heiney, S.P., Bryant, L.H., Godder, K., & Michaels, J. (2002). Preparing children to be bone marrow donors. *Oncology Nursing Forum, 29,* 1485–1489.

Heiney, S.P., Neuberg, R.W., Myers, D., & Bergman, L.H. (1994). The aftermath of bone marrow transplant for parents of pediatric patients: A post-traumatic stress disorder. *Oncology Nursing Forum, 21,* 843–847.

Hensel, M., Egerer, G., Schneeweiss, A., Goldschmidt, H., & Ho, A.D. (2002). Quality of life and rehabilitation in social and professional life after autologous stem cell transplantation. *Annals of Oncology, 13,* 209–217.

Henslee-Downey, J., & Gluckman, E. (1999). Allogeneic transplantation from donors other than HLA-identical siblings. *Hematology/Oncology Clinics of North America, 13,* 1017–1035.

Hymovich, D.P. (1995). The meaning of cancer to children. *Seminars in Oncology Nursing, 11,* 51–58.

Kapustay, P.M., & Buchsel, P.C. (2000). Process, complications, and management of peripheral stem cell transplantation. In P.C. Buchsel & P.M. Kapustay (Eds.), *Stem cell transplantation: A clinical textbook* (pp. 5.3–5.28). Pittsburgh, PA: Oncology Nursing Society.

Kelley, C.H., Randolph, S.R., & Leum, E. (2000). Home care of peripheral stem cell transplantation recipients. In P.C. Buchsel & P.M. Kapustay (Eds.), *Stem cell transplantation: A clinical textbook* (pp. 13.3–13.16). Pittsburgh, PA: Oncology Nursing Society.

King, C.R., Ferrell, B.R., Grant, M., & Sakurai, C. (1995). Nurses' perceptions of the meaning of quality of life for bone marrow transplant survivors. *Cancer Nursing, 18,* 118–129.

Kupst, M.J., Penati, B., Debban, B., Camitta, B., Pietryga, D., Margolis, D., et al. (2002). Cognitive and psychosocial functioning of pediatric hematopoietic stem cell transplant patients: A prospective longitudinal study. *Bone Marrow Transplantation, 30,* 609–617.

Langer, S., Abrams, J., & Syrjala, K. (2003). Caregiver and patient marital satisfaction and affect following hematopoietic stem cell transplantation: A prospective longitudinal investigation. *Psycho-Oncology, 12,* 239–253.

Lee, S.J., Fairclough, D., Antin, J.H., & Weeks, J.C. (2001). Discrepancies between patient and physician estimates for the success of stem cell transplantation. *JAMA, 285,* 1034–1038.

Lee, S.J., Zahrieh, D., Alyea, E.P., Welter, E., Ho, V.T., Antin, J.H., et al. (2002). Comparison of T-cell-depleted and non-T-cell-depleted unrelated donor transplantation for hematologic diseases: Clinical outcomes, quality of life, and costs. *Blood, 100,* 2697–2702.

Leiper, A.D. (2002). Non-endocrine late complications of bone marrow transplantation in childhood. Part II. *British Journal of Haematology, 118,* 23–43.

Little, M.T., & Storb, R. (2002). History of haematopoietic stem-cell transplantation. *Nature Reviews: Cancer, 2,* 231–238.

Loberiza, F.R., Rizzo, J.D., Bredeson, C.N., Antin, J.H., Horowitz, M.M., Weeks, J.C., et al. (2002). Association of depressive syndrome and early deaths among patients after stem-cell transplantation for malignant diseases. *Journal of Clinical Oncology, 20,* 2118–2126.

MacLeod, K., Whitsett, S., Mash, E., & Pelletier, W. (2003). Pediatric sibling donors of successful and unsuccessful hematopoietic stem cell transplants: A qualitative study of their psychosocial experience. *Journal of Pediatric Psychology, 28,* 223–231.

McDonald, J.C., Stetz, K.M., & Compton, K. (1996). Educational interventions for family caregivers during marrow transplantation. *Oncology Nursing Forum, 23,* 1432–1439.

Mogul, M.J. (2000). Unrelated cord blood transplantation vs. matched unrelated donor bone marrow transplantation: The risks and benefits of each choice. *Bone Marrow Transplantation, 25*(Suppl. 2), S58–S60.

Molassiotis, A., Boughton, B.J., Burgoyne, T., & van den Akker, O.B. (1995). Comparison of the overall quality of life in 50 long-term survivors of autologous and allogeneic bone marrow transplantation. *Journal of Advanced Nursing, 22,* 509–516.

Mounier, N., Haioun, C., Cole, B., Gisselbrecht, C., Sebban, C., Morel, P., et al. (2000). Quality of life-adjusted survival analysis of high-dose therapy with autologous bone marrow transplantation versus sequential chemotherapy for patients with aggressive lymphoma in first complete remission. *Blood, 95,* 3687–3692.

Murphy, K.C., Jenkins, P.L., & Whittaker, J.A. (1996). Psychosocial morbidity and survival in adult bone marrow transplant recipients—A follow-up study. *Bone Marrow Transplantation, 18,* 199–201.

National Marrow Donor Program. (2004, December). *Facts and figures.* Minneapolis, MN: Author. Retrieved July 10, 2005, from http://www.marrow.org/MEDIA/facts_figures.pdf

Packman, W.L. (1999). Psychosocial impact of pediatric HSCT on siblings. *Bone Marrow Transplantation, 24,* 75–80.

Patenaude, A.F., Szymanski, L., & Rappeport, J. (1979). Psychological costs of bone marrow transplantation in children. *American Journal of Orthopsychiatry, 49,* 409–422.

Phipps, S., Dunavant, M., Garvie, P.A., Lensing, S., & Rai, S.N. (2002). Acute health-related quality of life in children undergoing stem cell transplant: I. Descriptive outcomes. *Bone Marrow Transplantation, 29,* 425–434.

Rexilius, S.J., Mundt, C., Megel, M.E., & Agrawal, S. (2002). Therapeutic effects of massage therapy and healing touch on caregivers of patients undergoing autologous hematopoietic stem cell transplant [Online exclusive]. *Oncology Nursing Forum, 29,* E35–E44. Retrieved May 18, 2005, from http://www.ons.org/publications/journals/ONF/Volume29/Issue3/290335.asp

Rhodes, V.A., McDaniel, R.W., & Johnson, M.H. (1995). Patient education: Self-care guidelines. *Seminars in Oncology Nursing, 11,* 298–304.

Rocha, V., Wagner, J., Sobocinski, K., Klein, J., Zhang, M., Horowitz, M., et al. (2000). Graft-versus-host disease in children who have received a cord-blood or bone marrow transplant from an HLA-identical sibling. *New England Journal of Medicine, 342,* 1846–1854.

Rowley, S.D., Donaldson, G., Lilleby, K., Bensinger, W.I., & Appelbaum, F.R. (2001). Experiences of donors enrolled in a randomized study of allogeneic bone marrow or peripheral blood stem cell transplantation. *Blood, 97,* 2541–2548.

Shuster, G.F., Steeves, R.H., & Richardson, B. (1996). Coping pattern among bone marrow transplant patients: A hermeneutical inquiry. *Cancer Nursing, 19,* 290–297.

Snyder, D.S. (1999). Ethical issues in hematopoietic cell transplantation. In E.D. Thomas, K.G. Blume, & S.J. Forman (Eds.), *Hematopoietic cell transplantation* (2nd ed., pp. 398–406). Malden, MA: Blackwell Science.

Steeves, R.H. (1992). Patients who have undergone bone marrow transplantation: Their quest for meaning. *Oncology Nursing Forum, 19,* 899–905.

Stetz, K.M., McDonald, J.C., & Compton, K. (1996). Needs and experiences of family caregivers during marrow transplantation. *Oncology Nursing Forum, 23,* 1422–1427.

Stevens, P.E., & Pletsch, P.K. (2002). Ethical issues of informed consent: Mothers' experiences enrolling their children in bone marrow transplantation research. *Cancer Nursing, 25,* 81–87.

Sugarman, J., Kurtzberg, J., Box, T., & Horner, R. (2002). Optimization of informed consent for umbilical cord blood banking. *American Journal of Obstetrics and Gynecology, 187,* 1643–1646.

Sung, L., Buckstein, R., Doyle, J., Crump, M., & Detsky, A. (2003). Treatment options for patients with acute myeloid leukemia with a matched sibling donor. *Cancer, 97,* 592–600.

Svahn, B.M., Remberger, M., Myrback, K.E., Holmberg, K., Eriksson, B., Hentschke, P., et al. (2002). Home care during the pancytopenic phase after allogeneic hematopoietic stem cell transplantation is advantageous compared with hospital care. *Blood, 100,* 4317–4324.

Switzer, G., Myaskovsky, L., Goycoolea, J., Dew, M.A., Confer, D., & King, R. (2003). Factors associated with ambivalence about bone marrow donation among newly recruited unrelated potential donors. *Transplantation, 75,* 1517–1523.

Syrjala, K.L., Chapko, M.K., Vitaliano, P.P., Cummings, C., & Sullivan, K.M. (1993). Recovery after allogeneic marrow transplantation: Prospective study of predictors of long-term physical and psychosocial functioning. *Bone Marrow Transplantation, 11,* 319–327.

Tallman, M., Gray, R., Robert, N., LeMaistre, C., Osborne, K., Vaughan, W., et al. (2003). Conventional adjuvant chemotherapy with or without high-dose chemotherapy and autologous stem-cell transplantation in high-risk breast cancer. *New England Journal of Medicine, 349,* 17–26.

Watson, M., Buck, G., Wheatley, K., Homewood, J.R., Goldstone, A.H., Rees, J.K., et al. (2004). Adverse impact of bone marrow transplantation on quality of life in acute myeloid leukaemia patients: Analysis of the UK Medical Research Council AML 10 Trial. *European Journal of Cancer, 40,* 971–978.

Watson, M., Wheatley, K., Harrison, G., Zittoun, R., Gray, R., Goldstone, A., et al. (1999). Severe adverse impact on sexual functioning and fertility of bone marrow transplantation, either allogeneic or autologous, compared with consolidation chemotherapy alone. *Cancer, 86,* 1231–1239.

Williams, S., Green, R., Morrison, A., Watson, D., & Buchanan, S. (2003). The psychosocial aspects of donating blood stem cells: The sibling donor perspective. *Journal of Clinical Apheresis, 18,* 1–9.

Wingard, J.R., Curbow, B., Baker, F., & Piantadosi, S. (1991). Health, functional status, and employment of adult survivors of bone marrow transplantation. *Annals of Internal Medicine, 114,* 113–118.

Winters, G., Miller, C., Maracich, L., Compton, K., & Haberman, M.R. (1994). Provisional practice: The nature of psychosocial bone marrow transplant nursing. *Oncology Nursing Forum, 21,* 1147–1154.

Worel, N., Biener, D., Kalhs, P., Mitterbauer, M., Keil, F., Schulenburg, A., et al. (2002). Long-term outcome and quality of life of patients who are alive and in complete remission more than two years after allogeneic and syngeneic stem cell transplantation. *Bone Marrow Transplantation, 30,* 619–626.

Yancy, A.K., Coppo, P., & Kawanishi, Y. (1997). Progress in availability of donors of color: The National Marrow Donor Program. *Transplantation Proceedings, 29,* 3760–3765.

Zabora, J.R., Smith, E.D., Baker, F., Wingard, J.R., & Curbow, B. (1992). The family: The other side of bone marrow transplantation. *Journal of Psychosocial Oncology, 10*(1), 35–46.

CHAPTER 32

Complementary and Alternative Medicine: Moving Toward Integrative Cancer Care

DIANE M. FLETCHER, MA, RN, OCN®

Say not "I have found the truth," but rather, "I have found a truth."
—Kahlil Gibran

Despite the continuing medical advances, cancer remains a terrifying disease that is not uniformly treatable or curable (American Cancer Society [ACS], 2005a; Jemal et al., 2005). In their quest for an easy and certain cure, patients with cancer and their families often consider and may use therapies that are outside the realm of standard care. With patients' growing interest in complementary and alternative medicine (CAM), myriad psychosocial issues arise that can create unique professional concerns for oncology nurses.

Definition of Terms

CAM encompasses a wide range of healing philosophies and approaches (ACS, 2005b; Eisenberg et al., 1998). As defined by the National Institutes of Health's National Center for Complementary and Alternative Medicine (NCCAM, 2002), CAM is "a group of diverse medical and healthcare systems, practices, and products that are not presently considered to be part of conventional medicine." CAM therapies range from dangerous, outright frauds to methods that may enhance physical and psychological well-being (Cassileth, 1999). Generally, a therapy is **complementary** when it is used in conjunction with standard care, often either to enhance the conventional therapy or to maintain wellness during the mainstream treatment. Conversely, the purpose of an **alternative** therapy is to replace or substitute for standard care; it is used independently of conventional medical practice. Table 32-1 defines CAM-related terms and shows how these methods

Table 32-1. Types of Cancer Care

Type	Other Terms	Definition/Distinguishing Characteristics	Examples
Standard	Orthodox, conventional, traditional, allopathic, mainstream, proven, Western biomedicine, regular	• Scientifically demonstrated to be safe and effective in curing or controlling cancer (American Cancer Society [ACS], 2005b) • Evidence-based treatments approved by the U.S. Food and Drug Administration (ACS, 2005b)	Surgery, chemotherapy, radiation therapy, hormonal therapy, some biotherapy
Investigational[a]	Research, experimental, protocols	• New and unproven methods under scientific investigation; systematic evaluation with patients enrolled in clinical trials with informed consent and close monitoring (ACS, 2005b; Fletcher, 1992)	New chemotherapy or hormonal agents, antioxidants, gene therapy, some biotherapy
Alternative[a]	Unproven, unconventional, nontraditional, unorthodox, irregular	• Practices, beliefs, or remedies in popular use that are under study or otherwise scientifically unproven • Therapies used in place of standard care • Lacking documentation in the United States for safety and effectiveness against specific diseases (ACS, 2005b) • Interventions not in conformity with medical standards, not taught widely at U.S. medical schools, or not generally available at U.S. hospitals (Eisenberg et al., 1993) • Health therapy initiated or prescribed by patients, their family or friends, or an alternate care healer who operates outside of mainstream biomedicine (Montbriand, 1994)	Homeopathy, naturopathy, Ayurveda, traditional Oriental medicine, Native American medicine, herbal medicine, reflexology, megavitamins
Complementary[a]	Any "alternative" terms	• Treatments used to supplement, or in conjunction with, conventional treatments, generally with scientifically unknown/unproven effects on disease course but may be proved to improve quality of life, maintain wellness, or minimize symptoms/side effects (ACS, 2005b)	Mental imagery for relaxation or prevention of side effects, chiropractic for musculoskeletal pain and tension, changes in nutrition or lifestyle for symptom management, acupuncture for pain or nausea, prayer to reduce stress, massage for fatigue

(Continued on next page)

Table 32-1. Types of Cancer Care *(Continued)*

Type	Other Terms	Definition/Distinguishing Characteristics	Examples
Integrative	Combination, holistic	• Combined evidence-based standard and complementary therapies (ACS, 2005b; National Center for Complementary and Alternative Medicine [NCCAM], 2002) • Holistic approach with multidimensional focus on healing rather than disease (Rees & Weil, 2001)	Guided imagery with chemotherapy, acupuncture after surgery, prayer during conventional treatment, acupuncture with emetic chemotherapy, Chinese herbs with radiation therapy, nutrition/lifestyle counseling with standard therapy
Disproven	Quackery, questionable	• Methods promoted for the prevention, diagnosis, or treatment of cancer that, on scientific and clinical review, are found lacking evidence of value; may cause physical, emotional, or financial harm (ACS, 2005b)	Immuno-augmentive therapy (National Cancer Institute, 1999); Laetrile (ACS, 2004b); nutritional/metabolic therapies used to cure cancer: vitamin C megadoses (Moertel et al., 1985; Weiger et al., 2002), Livingston-Wheeler therapy (ACS, 1998), macrobiotic diet (BC Cancer Agency, 2000a), Gerson therapy (ACS, 2004b), Di Bella therapy (ACS, 2004b); electromagnetic therapy (NCCAM, 2004); psychic surgery (BC Cancer Agency, 2000b)

[a]Methods currently classified as "alternative" or "complementary" also may be considered "investigational" while under study by the National Institutes of Health or other reputable investigators.

differ from standard treatments; as the table shows, they may be difficult to distinguish from one another. The categories are imprecise and not mutually exclusive; some methods may fit into more than one category or may shift from one group to another. What is considered CAM is fluid because methods may move into conventional care once they have been scientifically validated (NCCAM, 2002). Labeling a therapy as disproven may help to distinguish methods known to be worthless. The newer term **integrative medicine** involves selectively combining standard care with CAM therapies, ideally with a multidimensional approach focused on health and healing (Hughes, 2001; NCCAM, 2002; Rees & Weil, 2001). NCCAM (2000, 2002), the key federal agency for CAM research, has developed a classification system to facilitate scientific investigation of CAM (see Figure 32-1).

Figure 32-1. National Center for Complementary and Alternative Medicine Classification of Major Types of Complementary and Alternative Medicine (CAM)

1. **Alternative Medical Systems**
   Alternative medical systems are built upon complete systems of theory and practice that have evolved independently of conventional biomedicine. Examples include Ayurveda (traditional medicine of India), homeopathic medicine, Native American medicine, naturopathic medicine, and traditional Oriental medicine.

2. **Mind-Body Interventions**
   Mind-body interventions employ a variety of techniques designed to enhance the mind's capacity to affect bodily function and symptoms. Some techniques that were considered CAM in the past have become mainstream (for example, patient support groups and cognitive-behavioral therapy). Other mind-body techniques still are considered CAM, including meditation, prayer, mental healing, and therapies that use creative outlets such as art, music, or dance.

3. **Biologically Based Therapies**
   Biologically based therapies in CAM use include natural and biologically based practices, interventions, and products, many of which overlap with conventional medicine's use of dietary supplements. Included are herbal, special dietary, orthomolecular, and individual biological therapies. Examples include Gerson therapy, macrobiotic diet, megavitamins, Laetrile, shark cartilage, herbal remedies, and metabolic therapies.

4. **Manipulative and Body-Based Methods**
   Manipulative and body-based methods in CAM use manipulation or movement of the body. Examples include acupressure, Alexander technique, chiropractic medicine, massage therapy, and osteopathic medicine.

5. **Energy Therapies**
   Energy therapies involve the use of energy fields. They consist of two types.
   - Biofield therapies aim to affect energy fields that purportedly surround and penetrate the human body. The existence of such fields has not yet been scientifically proved. Some forms of energy therapy manipulate biofields by applying pressure and/or manipulating the body by placing the hands in, or through, these fields. Examples include Qi gong, Reiki, and therapeutic touch.
   - Bioelectromagnetic-based therapies involve the unconventional use of electromagnetic fields, such as pulsed fields, magnetic fields, or alternating current or direct current fields.

Note. From "What Is Complementary and Alternative Medicine (CAM)?" by the National Center for Complementary and Alternative Medicine, 2002. Retrieved May 19, 2005, from http://nccam.nci.nih.gov/health/whatiscam

Prevalence and Disclosure of Use

Statistics for use of CAM vary, largely because of the imprecise definitions and categorizations of these therapies. Despite these limitations, recent studies have confirmed the widespread and growing use of CAM. Eisenberg et al.'s (1998) follow-up to the group's landmark 1993 survey (Eisenberg et al., 1993) revealed that CAM use among Americans had increased from 36% to 46%. Visits to CAM practitioners exceeded total visits to all primary care physicians, and out-of-pocket expenditures for CAM increased by 45%. Alarmingly, the rate of disclosure of CAM use remained low; patients disclosed less than 40% of the CAM therapies used to physicians in both 1990 and 1997. In a more recent nationwide survey, Kessler et al. (2001) found that 68% of respondents had used at least one CAM therapy. They noted the growing trend of increased CAM use since the 1950s.

Among people with cancer worldwide, a review of 26 prevalence studies revealed a broad range of CAM use, from 7%–64%, with the average prevalence across all adult studies at 31% (Ernst & Cassileth, 1998). Again, discrepancies arise because of varied definitions and methodologies. Several recent studies in the United States and Canada have shown more than 25% of patients using CAM across cancer types, ages, and the continuum of illness (see Table 32-2).

Table 32-2. Complementary and Alternative Medicine (CAM) Use in Patients With Cancer in the United States and Canada

Population	% Using CAM	% Not Disclosing CAM Use to Physicians	Author(s)
Women with breast cancer	72	50	Adler & Fosket, 1999
Patients concurrently on conventional cancer treatment	29	Not assessed	Kumar et al., 2002
Men with prostate cancer	39	24	Nam et al., 1999
Patients with head and neck cancer	39	73	Warrick et al., 1999
Oncology outpatients (breast, thoracic, head and neck, gastrointestinal, gynecologic, prostate, melanoma, urologic, sarcoma, and lymphoma)	83	60	Richardson et al., 2000
Breast cancer survivors	49–87	Not assessed	Ganz et al., 2002
Patients with breast and other malignancies	75	37–47	Morris et al., 2000
Children with cancer	84	50	Kelly et al., 2000
Patients with HIV/AIDS	53	33	Hsiao et al., 2003
Multiethnic adult inpatients with cancer	80	Not assessed	Bernstein & Grasso, 2001
Patients in National Institutes of Health–sponsored cancer clinical trials	63	62% stated that "talking with physician" was important; specific disclosure not assessed	Sparber et al., 2000
Pediatric outpatients with cancer	47	41	McCurdy et al., 2003

Of note are two important consistencies across nearly all studies. First, patients overwhelmingly used complementary, not alternative, therapies, and second, higher rates of CAM use occurred in younger, more educated, female, nonminority, more affluent, and more ill populations. These statistics translate into large numbers of people and confirm for oncology nurses that patients and their loved ones commonly explore CAM options.

Because of the potential physical or psychosocial risks of some CAM therapies, nurses must be aware of patients' use of CAM. Patients usually do not offer this information to their physicians, and it is not known how often they discuss CAM use with nurses or other healthcare professionals. Common reasons why patients choose not to disclose their CAM use to physicians include anticipation of physician disinterest or negative response, belief that their doctor will be unwilling or unable to contribute useful information, perception that use of CAM is irrelevant to conventional care, desire for privacy, and personal views regarding integration/coordination of disparate healing strategies. For many patients, it simply is that "the doctor never asked" (Adler & Fosket, 1999; Eisenberg et al., 2001; Nam et al., 1999). Not all CAM users anticipated a negative interaction with physicians. Sparber et al. (2000) found that a majority of users would have welcomed the opportunity to discuss CAM with their physicians, and Warrick et al. (1999) found that CAM users viewed conventional physicians as a knowledgeable source for CAM information. However, even those individuals who believed a discussion with their doctor would have been useful did not offer information about their CAM use.

Potential Risks and Benefits

Standard medical treatments have undergone thorough investigation, which allows healthcare professionals to anticipate, monitor, and, ideally, prevent or minimize adverse effects. In contrast, although promoters may label CAM therapies as "natural" and "nontoxic," potential risks largely are unknown. Lethal toxicities and interactions have occurred, particularly with certain dietary (botanical) supplements used in conjunction with conventional cancer treatments (Antman et al., 2001; Burstein, 2000; De Smet, 2002; Kumar et al., 2002; Weiger et al., 2002). Without objective information, evaluating the safety and efficacy of specific CAM therapies is impossible, and patients may face real risks.

Lack of information leads to another risk for patients—the threat of being deluded and given false hope. Patients may become burdened with guilt, especially if they believe that cure is ultimately within their control (Burstein, 2000; Richardson, Sanders, Palmer, Greisinger, & Singletary, 2000; Zollman & Vickers, 1999).

If a patient elects to use CAM as an alternative and avoids or discontinues potentially effective treatment, the cancer may advance to a stage where standard treatment no longer is beneficial (ACS, 2004c; Ernst, 2002). Loss of time may cause permanent loss of opportunities for cure, control, or even symptom palliation. Finally, costs of alternative care may be substantial, which insurance typically does not cover. This may cause financial strain and further emotional stress (ACS, 2004c; NCCAM, 2000; Zollman & Vickers, 1999).

As with potential risks, possible benefits of CAM are not always clearly identified. Certain approaches may have a positive effect on a patient's quality of life. CAM may relieve adverse symptoms and side effects associated with cancer or its conventional treatment or may generally improve well-being. Improvements in various adverse conditions, such as pain, fatigue, anxiety and emotional distress, muscle tension, nausea, mucositis, lymphedema, skin reactions, and anorexia, have occurred when patients use CAM interventions. Methods that patients have used include therapeutic massage (Greene, 2000; Weiger et al., 2002), relaxation/mental imagery (Rossman & Bresler, 2000; Sultanoff & Zalaquett, 2000; Weiger et al.), hypnotherapy (Saichek, 2000), faith/prayer/meditation (Astin, Shapiro, & Schwartz, 2000; Koenig, 2000), acupuncture (Dean, Mullins, & Yuen, 2000; Weiger et al.), diet and lifestyle modifications (Block, 2000; Weiger et al.), yoga (Quigley & Dean, 2000), and tai chi (Liu & Morgan, 2000). Patients with cancer typically use combinations of these interventions as an adjunct to standard treatment (Antman et al., 2001).

Human data relating CAM therapies to direct antitumor effect and prolonged survival remain limited and inconsistent. However, the evidence from cancer cell line studies, animal research, observational human studies, and a few clinical trials is especially promising in showing certain botanical supplements as having the potential to prevent or inhibit development or progression of neoplasia (Antman et al., 2001; Kumar et al., 2002; National Cancer Institute [NCI], Office of Cancer Complementary and Alternative Medicine [OCCAM], 2004; Weiger et al., 2002). The hope is that provocative preclinical data revealing a direct effect on cancer cells will lead to well-designed clinical trials in the future.

A critical need exists for rigorous scientific research to confirm the safety and efficacy of CAM. This is, in fact, the mission of NCCAM (2000, 2002) and NCI's OCCAM (2004). Proponents of any cancer treatments, conventional or CAM, must bear the burden of proof of antitumor effect or improved quality of life (ACS, 2004a, 2004c; Antman et al., 2001; Jacobson, Workman, & Kronenberg, 2000; Mason, Tovey, & Long, 2002; NCCAM, 2000; Weiger et al., 2002).

Why Patients Choose Complementary and Alternative Therapies

Nature of Cancer, Impact of Diagnosis, and Limits of Standard Biomedical Approach

The fundamental appeal of CAM is a result of cancer's prevalence and unpredictable nature (Jarvis, 1986). Cancer strikes often, and standard medical care currently cannot cure all cancers in all people. Thus, to most people, cancer is mysterious and frightening. The diagnosis evokes anxiety, fear, and a sense of vulnerability (Gorman, 1998); cancer threatens one's life and integrity (Rowland, 1990b). The desires to regain control and to maintain hope are two of the most frequently given reasons for considering and using CAM (Truant & McKenzie, 1999).

Standard biomedical care has not aggressively addressed all aspects of healing (e.g., psychosocial, emotional, spiritual), whereas CAM therapies and philosophies often embrace a more holistic approach (Novey, 2000). Patients may use CAM as a means to improve their chance of survival, as well as to prevent or manage symptoms or side effects (Jacobson et al., 2000). Of those patients surveyed at a major comprehensive cancer center, Richardson et al. (2000) found that patients expected CAM to improve their quality of life (77%), boost their immune system (71%), prolong life (63%), or relieve symptoms (44%). However, approximately one-third of the patients (38%) expected CAM therapies to cure their disease. Fear of suffering and death, unmet psychosocial needs, and hope for a simple cure may lead patients to desperate thoughts and actions.

American Social Influence

The use of CAM frequently reflects the norms of one's social environment. The common belief in the power of the individual and individual rights influences patients' decisions in the United States (Fletcher, 1992; Holland, Geary, & Furman, 1990). Other underlying social trends include consumerism, the mind-body connection, self-care and fitness, dissatisfaction and mistrust of organized health care and its providers, and an aggressive proactive approach to illness (Ernst, 2000).

Personal, Family, and Cultural Values

Each patient and family holds a unique value system. Values and responses to cancer often are enmeshed in individuals' ethnic background. The appeal of various treatment options and the decisions made reflect these individual, family, and cultural values.

Individuals define "unconventional" based on their own cultural norms (i.e., what is nontraditional for one may be the norm for another). Native Americans typically will consult a traditional healer before seeking a physician's advice and often will combine both types of care (Nauman, 2000). African Americans may distrust organized medicine and hesitate to pursue standard care for cancer. Fear and fatalism are two common culture-related attitudes (Phillips & Smith, 2004). African American women with breast cancer were far more likely to choose spiritual healing than other ethnic groups (Lee, Lin, Wrensch, Adler, & Eisenberg, 2000). Herbs and acupuncture are an integral part of traditional Chinese and Japanese culture and health care (Dean et al., 2000; Lee et al.; Parker, 2000). Asian American women traditionally suppress emotions, are nonassertive, and often make decisions out of a sense of stoicism, believing that they must endure illness alone (Ishida, 2004). Caucasian Americans of Anglo-Saxon European heritage frequently use a direct, problem-solving approach when deciding among treatment options (Danielson, Hamel-Bissel, & Winstead-Fry, 1993). Many Hispanic/Latino Americans concurrently use Western biomedicine along with an ancient Latin American folk-healing system practiced by traditional healers called *curanderos* (Padilla, Gomez, Biggerstaff, & Mehler, 2001). Decisions about CAM also may reflect lifestyle preferences, as well as personal and cultural beliefs (Kelly-Powell, 1997; Montbriand, 1995).

Spiritual beliefs and traditions are entwined into the fabrics of all cultures and contribute to an individual's perceptions and responses (Taylor, 1998). Age, developmental stage, and gender are interrelated with one's ethnicity and help to establish norms and values (Gorman, 1998; Rowland, 1990a). A patient may be unaware of the sometimes subtle influence of his or her values on treatment choices.

Psychosocial Needs and Issues of Patients and Families

Each patient with cancer has a unique psychosocial perspective when facing the disease. An individual's diagnosis, stage of disease, and treatment options, as well as physical and psychological status, age, developmental phase, ethnicity, and value systems, all set him or her apart from others. How and why a particular patient seeks to use CAM is as unique as the patient.

Choosing CAM therapy may be the expression of an acute need. For example, a fearful and desperate patient may need to blame conventional medical care for his or her diagnosis (Ernst, 2000). Ernst identified the needs for philosophical congruence, empathy, "high-touch, low-tech" care, and control over treatment as other psychosocial factors that influence CAM decisions. Henderson and Donatelle (2003) demonstrated that patients with cancer with a higher perception of control over their disease were predictably more likely to use CAM. CAM may "offer patients a participatory experience of empowerment, authenticity, and enlarged self-identity when illness threatens their sense of intactness and connection to the world" (Kaptchuk & Eisenberg, 1998, p. 1061). Astin's (1998) large national survey revealed that the majority of CAM users generally are satisfied with conventional medicine, but they find that CAM practices often are congruent with their personal philosophies about life and health. Moschen et al. (2001) concluded that CAM therapies fulfill an important psychological need for a substantial proportion of patients with cancer. They found that CAM users generally had a more active style of coping with illness; interestingly, however, those patients using more than three CAM therapies had a more depressive coping style than those patients using less than three.

Family dynamics significantly may sway patients' thoughts and decisions. Families have their own power hierarchies, communication styles, and role delineations, as well as entrenched traditions, beliefs, coping mechanisms, and lifestyles (Danielson et al., 1993; Gorman, 1998). The family structure, as well as the larger cultural system, ultimately may determine patients' decisions.

Professional, Legal, and Ethical Considerations

When patients consider or use CAM, nurses may face professional, legal, and ethical dilemmas. Nurses perform responsibilities within the framework of each state's nurse practice act and standards of care established by national organizations. Standards developed by the American Nurses Association (ANA), the Joint Commission on Accreditation of Healthcare Organizations (JCAHO), and the Oncology Nursing Society (ONS) contribute to the definition of oncology nursing practice but do not entirely define it (Fletcher, 1998; ONS, 2004).

As licensed professionals, nurses are legally accountable for their actions. Courts of law determine malpractice or negligence based on each state's board of nursing code of professional and vocational standards, as well as on ANA and JCAHO standards (Loeb, 1992). Nurses also follow ethical principles outlined in the ANA and International Council of Nurses codes (Loeb; Scanlon & Glover, 1995).

If a patient is considering or electing to use CAM, nurses must support the patient's autonomy and right to self-determination, privacy, and freedom of choice (Husted & Husted, 1995; Kaler & Ravella, 2002). However, nurses are equally obligated to educate patients and facilitate informed consent, provide safe and effective care, and protect vulnerable patients from exploitation, deception, and physical, psychological, or emotional harm (Husted & Husted; Kaler & Ravella). Patients' choices can lead to conflicts of nursing principles, obligations, and responsibilities. Also, children with cancer often create distinct challenges. Assessing a child's needs and wishes and parents' goals and expectations, determining what types of care are in the child's best interest, and balancing parental rights and obligations with professional responsibilities may be difficult (Enskar, 1995; Kemper, 2001; Kemper & Wornham, 2001; McCurdy, Spangler, Wofford, Chauvenet, & McLean, 2003).

Patients may notify nurses of their interest in CAM and may ask for information and/or recommendations about CAM therapies. Again, because of the lack of consensus on CAM's safety and efficacy, providing education or recommendations has professional implications. It may be unethical to withhold information about potentially beneficial CAM therapies, such as acupuncture for pain (Adams, Cohen, Eisenberg, & Jonsen, 2002; Ernst & Cohen, 2001; Kaler & Ravella, 2002). Conversely, recommendation of CAM or referral to a CAM provider may carry liability risks in certain situations, especially if the patient incurs harm as a result of the CAM (Studdert et al., 1998). Adams et al. presented a useful tool for risk-benefit analysis of CAM versus conventional medical treatment. Some institutions include a verbal and written disclaimer even when professionals simply are providing information about CAM therapies (see Figure 32-2 for an example). The challenge is to provide information about the known risks and benefits of CAM while respecting patients' values (Adams et al.) and always maintaining one's own professional integrity.

Nurses always must provide care within the confines of established laws and standards. Some CAM therapies are not drugs or specific medical therapies and therefore are not regulated by law. Examples of these include vitamins, relaxation and mental imagery, and diet and lifestyle recommendations. Because these therapies are unregulated and may have potential benefits, nurses may incorporate these methods if patients desire them. However, if nurses practice any type of CAM, they must be acutely aware of their state's licensing or credentialing requirements. A number of state boards of nursing permit nurses to practice certain, but not all, CAM therapies (Cady, 2002; Lorenzo, 2003), but nurses may be held liable for patients' well-being (Fletcher, 1992; Lorenzo). Employers may

---

Figure 32-2. University of Pittsburgh Medical Center Cancer Centers/University of Pittsburgh Cancer Institute Integrative Medicine Program Disclaimer

Disclaimer

The information and resources provided by the University of Pittsburgh Medical Center (UPMC) Cancer Centers/University of Pittsburgh Cancer Institute (UPCI) Integrative Medicine Program may not be complete. The UPMC Cancer Centers, the UPCI, and UPMC do not make endorsements or recommendations of the therapies in this information, and make no guarantees about their value or use.

The information and resources provided are by definition outside the scope of conventional medicine standards of care. Information discussed may fall under the classification of unconventional, alternative, complementary, or integrative therapies. Some of the treatments may have scientific evidence of safety and effectiveness, while there may be as yet limited or no research data for others. The extent of supporting and refuting data will be discussed with all information given.

The information and resources provided by the Integrative Medicine Program are for educational purposes only. This information is not meant to provide diagnoses or prescriptions. As with conventional medicine, indiscriminate use of some of these therapies without medical supervision may be harmful. Please discuss your interest in these therapies with your doctor.

Note. Figure courtesy of Diane Fletcher, MA, RN, OCN®. Reprinted with permission.

---

further limit the scope of practice. Many legal and professional liability issues often are unclear because CAM-related law currently is a novel and evolving field (Weintraub, 1999).

Clinical Guidelines

With preparation, insight, and practice, oncology nurses can address the challenging psychosocial and professional issues surrounding CAM therapies. The following guidelines can provide direction.

Personally Evaluate and Educate

Before interacting with patients, nurses must recognize their own personal, family, and cultural values and beliefs (Fletcher, 1992). They need to contemplate their biases and assumptions and determine how these influence their judgment of CAM. Self-awareness may help to prevent nurses from imposing their values and attitudes onto patients (Cauffield, 2000; Fitch et al., 1999; Husted & Husted, 1995).

To inform patients accurately, nurses first must educate themselves and use the same critical thinking about CAM as they do about conventional cancer therapies (Koretz, 2002; Smith, 1998). Weiger et al. (2002) offered an objective method for critiquing the safety and efficacy of CAM therapies. Nurses cannot know everything about the vast array of CAM methods, but credible information sources are available (see Figure 32-3). Web sites of reputable organizations often have the most current information in this rapidly evolving field.

Nurses and physicians alike increasingly are recognizing their need for at least basic education on CAM therapies (Fitch et al., 1999; Wetzel, Kaptchuk, Haramati, & Eisenberg, 2003; Winslow & Shapiro, 2002). Schools of nursing and medicine are responding by adding formal CAM courses to their curricula (Pepa & Russell, 2000; Richardson, 2001; Wetzel et al.). Continuing education opportunities also are increasingly available. As they learn more about CAM, nurses must strive to keep an open mind and remember that today's CAM treatment may become tomorrow's standard of care.

Anticipate and Communicate

Because the use of CAM is well established and growing, nurses can anticipate that many patients are likely to be interested in CAM practices. However, in one survey of nurse practitioners (Hayes & Alexander, 2000), only 10% of the 202 respondents reported that they "usually" asked about their patients' use of CAM. Eisenberg (1997) suggested that all healthcare professionals should proactively discuss "other therapies" that patients may be investigating or using. Using a non-threatening approach, nurses should attempt to discover why *this method* appeals to *this patient* at *this time*. The most effective approach may be using open-ended questions and normalizing CAM use. For example, the nurse could say, "Many people with cancer use other methods to help them feel better during treatment, such as following special diets, seeing a chiropractor, or taking supplements. What

---

Figure 32-3. Resources for Information About Complementary and Alternative Medicine (CAM) in Cancer Care

Organizations/Web Sites

American Cancer Society
1599 Clifton Road, NE
Atlanta, GA 30329
800-ACS-2345
www.cancer.org
Complementary and alternative therapies:
    http://www.cancer.org/docroot/ETO
    /ETO_5.asp

National Center for Complementary and Alternative Medicine (NCCAM), National Institutes of Health (NIH)
NCCAM Clearinghouse
P.O. Box 7923
Gaithersburg, MD 20898
888-644-6226
http://nccam.nih.gov
E-mail: info@nccam.nih.gov

Office of Cancer Complementary and Alternative Medicine (OCCAM), NIH
6116 Executive Plaza North, Suite 609, MSC 8339
Bethesda, MD 20852
www.cancer.gov/cam
For health professionals with research inquires, contact OCCAM via e-mail at ncioccam1-r@mail.nih.gov
For public/patient inquires, please see http://cancer.gov/contact

U.S. Food and Drug Administration
5600 Fishers Lane
Rockville, MD 20857
888-INFO-FDA (888-463-6332)
www.fda.gov
Information for health professionals:
    www.fda.gov/oc/oha/default.htm

U.S. National Library of Medicine and NIH, MedlinePlus Health Information: Cancer Alternative Therapy
www.nlm.nih.gov/medlineplus/
    canceralternativetherapy.html

Books With Overviews of Common CAM Therapies

American Cancer Society. (2000). *American Cancer Society's guide to complementary and alternative cancer methods.* Atlanta, GA: Author.
Novey, D.W. (Ed.). (2000). *Clinician's complete reference to complementary/alternative medicine.* St. Louis, MO: Mosby.

Note. A vast number of Internet sites offer diverse and widely available information on CAM therapies. Monitoring or evaluating the accuracy of such information is impossible. Lay people and professionals alike may find reliable, accurate, state-of-the-art findings as well as fraudulent promotional material. Thus, electronic information is best evaluated with the same critical thinking as any other unvalidated source.

---

kinds of things do you do to help you feel well?" To protect patients from harm and to facilitate informed consent, it is the nurse's ethical and legal responsibility to elicit information about CAM use (Cady, 2002; Kaler & Ravella, 2002). Documentation of CAM use should be part of routine assessment for all patients with cancer (Richardson et al., 2000).

As previously noted, many patients are reluctant to disclose their use of CAM. In light of this, nurses must assess and address possible reasons for the patient's hesitancy. Again, normalizing patients' thoughts and feelings may make them more comfortable in revealing CAM use. Nurses always should encourage patients to discuss their interest in CAM with their physicians and should facilitate open communication.

To identify critical needs, nurses first must assess the patient's and family's psychosocial status. Assessment includes personal, family, and cultural perceptions of cancer and treatment options. Nurses need to communicate openly with patients and families and acknowledge common fears and responses to having cancer. They should assist patients in exploring and clarifying their values, family dynamics, and views regarding CAM care. Through initial and ongoing discussion, nurses can convey empathy, nonjudgmental acceptance, and respect for the patient (ACS, 2004a; Canales & Geller, 2003). This alone may help to meet the patient's need for support, hope, and trust in healthcare professionals.

Advocate

Nurses act as patient advocates. They are intermediaries who guide patients through complicated healthcare systems (Ades & Yarbro, 2000) and help them to understand and decide about treatment. Nurses play a central role in teaching patients about cancer and the worth of standard care, in clarifying misconceptions, and in empathizing with overwhelming and confusing choices (Danielson et al., 1993).

Nurses must facilitate a patient's understanding of his or her right to truly informed consent (Cady, 2002; Husted & Husted, 1995; Kaler & Ravella, 2002; Loeb, 1992). If patients are not aware of the potential risks and benefits of a CAM method, they cannot judge its value and safety. NCCAM's (2003) first recommendation to individuals considering CAM is to be an informed consumer, and nurses can play a vital role in guiding patients. Patients may need particular assistance in evaluating Web sites proclaiming CAM cancer cures because this information can be especially misleading and dangerous (Ernst & Schmidt, 2002). Together, nurses, patients, and family members can investigate specific CAM interventions and attempt to evaluate their possible values or dangers.

Throughout this process, nurses must balance appreciation of patient autonomy and self-determination with protecting the patient from physical, psychological, or financial harm. Nurses should try to understand patients' expectations from using CAM (e.g., do they expect CAM to cure cancer or to relieve symptoms?). Again, a curious, nonbiased, open attitude is essential. Ultimately, the patient's choice must be respected (ACS, 2004a; Kaler & Ravella, 2002).

Integrate

With each patient and family, nurses need to consider how to incorporate potentially beneficial aspects of CAM into the treatment plan (Eisenberg, 2002; Fletcher, 1992). Rees and Weil (2001) described integrative treatment as that which selectively incorporates the best of CAM with proven standard biomedicine. Integrated medicine focuses on "health and healing rather than disease and treatment. It views patients as whole people with minds and spirits, as well as bodies, and includes these dimensions into diagnosis and treatment. It also involves patients and doctors working to maintain health by paying attention to lifestyle factors . . . " (Rees & Weil, p. 119). Within their scope of practice, nurses routinely can discuss diet, stress reduction, exercise and activity, lifestyle changes, and support systems with their patients. They may be able to merge specific cultural healing approaches (e.g., acupuncture, prayer) with standard biomedical care.

Ideally, each patient's care should integrate methods that not only cure or control cancer but also maintain or improve quality of life (e.g., nutritional status, sense of control, peace of mind and spirit, physical comfort). As Burstein (2000) noted, "The use of complementary health-related practices is an opportunity to discuss the meanings that lie behind these practices, to share further in the experience of illness and well-being, and to focus clinicians on the genuine needs of cancer patients that neither surgery nor radiation nor chemotherapy can satisfy" (p. 2504). In addition, nurses can find ways to incorporate the support and hopefulness, provider availability, and marketing tactics that alternative therapy promoters and the lay literature have used successfully (Eisenberg, 2002). Healthcare professionals must accurately and completely document any discussion or provision of CAM.

Multidisciplinary colleagues are valuable sources of information and support for patients and nurses alike (Yaramus, Fletcher, & Baum, 2003). When facing CAM therapy choices, other members of the healthcare team—pharmacists, nutritionists, physicians, psychologists, social workers, and spiritual leaders—can help nurses to resolve complex dilemmas and provide optimal patient care.

As integrative care is becoming more common (Burstein, 2000; Eisenberg et al., 2001; Eisenberg, 2002; Markman, 2001; Snyderman & Weil, 2002), reputable CAM practitioners can be rich sources for CAM information. To better address the issues surrounding CAM methods, nurses should welcome the opportunity to participate in CAM research and develop innovative clinical approaches (Antman et al., 2001; Eisenberg et al., 2001). The oncology care of the future holds the promise of offering the best of all therapies to provide safe and effective yet individualized and truly holistic patient care.

Conclusion

No type of cancer care offers easy answers or a single or absolute truth. A variety of therapies is available, and a patient's choices may bring to light a number of psychosocial and professional issues. Interest in complementary and alternative therapies is growing, so oncology nurses must be aware of the challenging and exciting issues associated with the use of these therapies. By increasing their understanding and maintaining open communication with patients, nurses can better assist patients while maintaining professional integrity. Patients, their families, and healthcare professionals must work together to continue to search for truths.

References

Adams, K.E., Cohen, M.H., Eisenberg, D., & Jonsen, A.R. (2002). Ethical considerations of complementary and alternative medical therapies in conventional medical settings. *Annals of Internal Medicine, 137,* 660–664.

Ades, T., & Yarbro, C.H. (2000). Alternative and complementary therapies in cancer management. In C.H. Yarbro, M.H. Frogge, M. Goodman, & S.L. Groenwald (Eds.), *Cancer nursing: Principles and practice* (5th ed., pp. 616–630). Sudbury, MA: Jones and Bartlett.

Adler, S.R., & Fosket, J.R. (1999). Disclosing complementary and alternative medicine use in the medicinal encounter: A qualitative study in women with breast cancer. *Journal of Family Practice, 48,* 453–458.

American Cancer Society. (1998, July). *Another view of healing.* Retrieved May 18, 2005, from http://www.cancer.org/docroot/NWS/content/NWS_1_1X_Another_view_of_healing.asp

American Cancer Society. (2004a, December). *American Cancer Society operational statement on complementary and alternative methods of cancer management.* Retrieved May 18, 2005, from http://www.cancer.org/docroot/ETO/content/ETO_5_3x_American_Cancer_Society_Operational_Statement_on_CAM.asp

American Cancer Society. (2004b, August). *Are 'alternatives' good medicine?* Retrieved May 18, 2005, from http://www.cancer.org/docroot/NWS/content/NWS_2_1X_Are_alternatives_good_medicine.asp

American Cancer Society. (2004c, December). *Making treatment decisions: Guidelines for using complementary and alternative methods.* Retrieved May 18, 2005, from http://www.cancer.org/docroot/ETO/content/ETO_5_3x_Guidelines_For_Using_Complementary_and_Alternative_Methods.asp

American Cancer Society. (2005a). *Cancer facts and figures, 2005.* Atlanta, GA: Author.

American Cancer Society. (2005b). *Making treatment decisions: Complementary and alternative therapies.* Retrieved May 18, 2005, from http://www.cancer.org/docroot/ETO/ETO_5.asp

Antman, K., Benson, M.C., Chabot, J., Cobrinik, D., Grann, V.R., Jacobson, J.S., et al. (2001). Complementary and alternative medicine: The role of the cancer center. *Journal of Clinical Oncology, 19*(Suppl. 18), 55S–60S.

Astin, J.A. (1998). Why patients use alternative medicine: Results of a national survey. *JAMA, 279,* 1548–1553.

Astin, J.A., Shapiro, S.L., & Schwartz, G.E.R. (2000). Meditation. In D.W. Novey (Ed.), *Clinician's complete reference to complementary/alternative medicine* (pp. 73–85). St. Louis, MO: Mosby.

BC Cancer Agency. (2000a, February). *Unconventional therapies—Macrobiotic diets/Zen macrobiotics.* Retrieved June 14, 2005, from http://www.bccancer.bc.ca/PPI/UnconventionalTherapies/MacrobioticDietsZenMacrobiotics.htm

BC Cancer Agency. (2000b, February). *Unconventional therapies—Psychic surgery.* Retrieved June 14, 2005, from http://www.bccancer.bc.ca/PPI/UnconventionalTherapies/PsychicSurgery.htm

Bernstein, B.J., & Grasso, T. (2001). Prevalence of complementary and alternative medicine use in cancer patients. *Oncology, 15,* 1267–1272.

Block, K.I. (2000). Nutritional oncology and integrative cancer care: A rational, mechanism-based approach. In D.W. Novey (Ed.), *Clinician's complete reference to complementary/alternative medicine* (pp. 618–636). St. Louis, MO: Mosby.

Burstein, H.J. (2000). Discussing complementary therapies with cancer patients: What should we be talking about? *Journal of Clinical Oncology, 18,* 2501–2504.

Cady, R. (2002). Are there legal issues of concern for nurses when patients use complimentary and alternative medicine? *MCN: The American Journal of Maternal/Child Nursing, 27,* 119.

Canales, M.K., & Geller, B.M. (2003). Surviving breast cancer: The role of complementary therapies. *Family and Community Health, 26,* 11–24.

Cassileth, B. (1999). Complementary therapies: Overview and state of the art. *Cancer Nursing, 22,* 85–90.

Cauffield, J.S. (2000). The psychosocial aspects of complementary and alternative medicine. *Pharmacotherapy, 20,* 1289–1294.

Danielson, C.B., Hamel-Bissel, B., & Winstead-Fry, P. (1993). *Families, health, and illness: Perspectives on coping and intervention.* St. Louis, MO: Mosby.

De Smet, P.A. (2002). Herbal remedies. *New England Journal of Medicine, 347,* 2046–2056.

Dean, C.F.A., Mullins, M., & Yuen, J. (2000). Acupuncture. In D.W. Novey (Ed.), *Clinician's complete reference to complementary/alternative medicine* (pp. 191–202). St. Louis, MO: Mosby.

Eisenberg, D.M. (1997). Advising patients who seek alternative medical therapies. *Annals of Internal Medicine, 127,* 61–69.

Eisenberg, D.M., Davis, R.B., Ettner, S.L., Appel, S., Wilkey, S., Van Rompay, M.I., et al. (1998). Trends in alternative medicine use in the United States, 1990–1997: Results of a follow-up national survey. *JAMA, 280,* 1569–1575.

Eisenberg, D.M., Kessler, R.C., Foster, C., Norlock, F.E., Calkins, D.R., & Delbanco, T.L. (1993). Unconventional medicine in the United States. *New England Journal of Medicine, 328,* 246–252.

Eisenberg, D.M., Kessler, R.C., Van Rompay, M.I., Kaptchuk, T.J., Wilkey, S.A., Appel, S., et al. (2001). Perceptions about complementary therapies relative to conventional therapies among adults who use both: Results from a national survey. *Annals of Internal Medicine, 135,* 344–351.

Eisenberg, L. (2002). Complementary and alternative medicine: What is its role? *Harvard Review of Psychiatry, 10,* 221–230.

Enskar, K. (1995). Ethical aspects of judging the alternative treatment of children with cancer. *Nursing Ethics, 2,* 51–62.

Ernst, E. (2000). The role of complementary and alternative medicine. *BMJ, 321,* 1133–1135.

Ernst, E. (2002). The dark side of complementary and alternative medicine. *International Journal of STD and AIDS, 13,* 797–800.

Ernst, E., & Cassileth, B.R. (1998). The prevalence of complementary/alternative medicine in cancer: A systematic review. *Cancer, 83,* 777–782.

Ernst, E., & Cohen, M.H. (2001). Informed consent in complementary and alternative medicine. *Archives of Internal Medicine, 161,* 2288–2292.

Ernst, E., & Schmidt, K. (2002). 'Alternative' cancer cures via the Internet [Editorial]? *British Journal of Cancer, 87,* 479–480.

Fitch, M.I., Gray, R.E., Greenberg, M., Douglas, M.S., Labrecque, M., Pavlin, P., et al. (1999). Oncology nurses' perspectives on unconventional therapies. *Cancer Nursing, 22,* 90–96.

Fletcher, D.M. (1992). Unconventional cancer treatments: Professional, legal, and ethical issues. *Oncology Nursing Forum, 19,* 1351–1354.

Fletcher, D.M. (1998). Alternative and complementary therapies. In R.M. Carroll-Johnson, L.M. Gorman, & N.J. Bush (Eds.), *Psychosocial nursing care along the cancer continuum* (pp. 413–425). Pittsburgh, PA: Oncology Nursing Society.

Ganz, P.A., Desmond, K.A., Leedham, B., Rowland, J.H., Meyerowitz, B.E., & Belin, T.R. (2002). Quality of life in long-term, disease-free survivors of breast cancer: A follow-up study. *Journal of the National Cancer Institute, 94,* 39–49.

Gorman, L.M. (1998). The psychosocial impact of cancer on the individual, family, and society. In R.M. Carroll-Johnson, L.M. Gorman, & N.J. Bush (Eds.), *Psychosocial nursing care along the cancer continuum* (pp. 3–25). Pittsburgh, PA: Oncology Nursing Society.

Greene, E. (2000). Massage therapy. In D.W. Novey (Ed.), *Clinician's complete reference to complementary/alternative medicine* (pp. 338–348). St. Louis, MO: Mosby.

Hayes, K.M., & Alexander, I.M. (2000). Alternative therapies and nurse practitioners: Knowledge, professional experience, and personal use. *Holistic Nursing Practice, 14*(3), 49–58.

Henderson, J.W., & Donatelle, R.J. (2003). The relationship between cancer locus of control and complementary and alternative medicine use by women diagnosed with breast cancer. *Psycho-Oncology, 12,* 59–67.

Holland, J.C., Geary, N., & Furman, A. (1990). Alternative cancer therapies. In J.C. Holland & J.H. Rowland (Eds.), *Handbook of psychooncology: Psychological care of the patient with cancer* (pp. 508–515). New York: Oxford University Press.

Hsiao, A.F., Wong, M.D., Kanouse, D.E., Collins, R.L., Liu, H., Andersen, R.M., et al. (2003). Complementary and alternative medicine use and substitution for conventional therapy by HIV-infected patients. *Journal of Acquired Immune Deficiency Syndromes, 33,* 157–165.

Hughes, E.F. (2001). Overview of complementary, alternative, and integrative medicine. *Clinical Obstetrics and Gynecology, 44,* 774–779.

Husted, G.L., & Husted, J.H. (1995). *Ethical decision making in nursing* (2nd ed.). St. Louis, MO: Mosby.

Jacobson, J.S., Workman, S.B., & Kronenberg, F. (2000). Research on complementary/alternative medicine for patients with breast cancer: A review of the biomedical literature. *Journal of Clinical Oncology, 18,* 668–683.

Jarvis, W. (1986). Helping your patients deal with questionable cancer treatments. *CA: A Cancer Journal for Clinicians, 36,* 293–301.

Jemal, A., Murray, T., Ward, E., Samuels, A., Tiwari, R., Ghafoor, A., et al. (2005). Cancer statistics, 2005. *CA: A Cancer Journal for Clinicians, 55,* 10–30.

Ishida, D. (2004). Asian women and breast cancer. In K.H. Dow (Ed.), *Contemporary issues in breast cancer: A nursing perspective* (2nd ed., pp. 299–310). Sudbury, MA: Jones and Bartlett.

Kaler, M.M., & Ravella, P.C. (2002). Staying on the ethical high ground with complementary and alternative medicine. *Nurse Practitioner, 27*(7), 38–42.

Kaptchuk, T.J., & Eisenberg, D.M. (1998). The persuasive appeal of alternative medicine. *Annals of Internal Medicine, 129*, 1061–1065.

Kelly, K.M., Jacobson, J.S., Kennedy, D.D., Braudt, S.M., Mallick, M., & Weiner, M.A. (2000). Use of unconventional therapies by children with cancer at an urban medical center. *Journal of Pediatric Hematology/Oncology, 22*, 412–416.

Kelly-Powell, M.L. (1997). Personalizing choices: Patients' experiences with making treatment decisions. *Research in Nursing and Health, 20*, 219–227.

Kemper, K.J. (2001). Complementary and alternative medicine for children: Does it work? *Western Journal of Medicine, 174*, 272–276.

Kemper, K.J., & Wornham, W.L. (2001). Consultations for holistic pediatric services for inpatients and outpatient oncology patients at a children's hospital. *Archives of Pediatric and Adolescent Medicine, 155*, 449–454.

Kessler, R.C., Davis, R.B., Foster, D.F., Van Rompay, M.I., Walters, E.E., Wilkey, S.A., et al. (2001). Long-term trends in the use of complementary and alternative medical therapies in the United States. *Annals of Internal Medicine, 135*, 262–268.

Koenig, H.G. (2000). Spiritual healing and prayer. In D.W. Novey (Ed.), *Clinician's complete reference to complementary/alternative medicine* (pp. 130–140). St. Louis, MO: Mosby.

Koretz, R.L. (2002). Is alternative medicine alternative science? *Laboratory and Clinical Medicine, 139*, 329–333.

Kumar, N.B., Hopkins, K., Allen, K., Riccardi, D., Besterman-Dahan, K., & Moyers, S. (2002). Use of complementary/integrative nutritional therapies during cancer treatment: Implications in clinical practice. *Cancer Control, 9*, 236–243.

Lee, M.M., Lin, S.S., Wrensch, M.R., Adler, S.R., & Eisenberg, D. (2000). Alternative therapies used by women with breast cancer in four ethnic populations. *Journal of the National Cancer Institute, 92*, 42–47.

Liu, Y., & Morgan, T.M. (2000). Tai chi. In D.W. Novey (Ed.), *Clinician's complete reference to complementary/alternative medicine* (pp. 219–230). St. Louis, MO: Mosby.

Loeb, S. (Ed.). (1992). *Nurse's handbook of law and ethics*. Springhouse, PA: Springhouse.

Lorenzo, P. (2003). Complementary therapies—They're not without risk. *RN, 66*(1), 65–68.

Markman, M. (2001). Interactions between academic oncology and alternative/integrative medicine: Complex but necessary. *Journal of Clinical Oncology, 19*(Suppl. 18), 52S–53S.

Mason, S., Tovey, P., & Long, A.F. (2002). Evaluating complementary medicine: Methodological challenges of randomized controlled trials. *BMJ, 325*, 832–834.

McCurdy, E.A., Spangler, J.G., Wofford, M.M., Chauvenet, A.R., & McLean, T.W. (2003). Religiosity is associated with the use of complementary medical therapies in pediatric oncology patients. *Journal of Pediatric Hematology/Oncology, 25*, 125–129.

Moertel, C.G., Fleming, T.R., Creagan, E.T., Rubin, J., O'Connell, M.J., & Ames, M.M. (1985). High-dose vitamin C versus placebo in the treatment of patients with advanced cancer who have had no prior chemotherapy: A randomized double-blind comparison. *New England Journal of Medicine, 312*, 137–141.

Montbriand, M.J. (1994). An overview of alternate therapies chosen by patients with cancer. *Oncology Nursing Forum, 21*, 1547–1554.

Montbriand, M.J. (1995). Decision tree model describing alternate health care choices made by oncology patients. *Cancer Nursing, 18*, 104–117.

Morris, K.T., Johnson, N., Homer, L., & Walts, D. (2000). A comparison of complementary therapy use between breast cancer patients and patients with other primary tumor sites. *American Journal of Surgery, 179*, 407–411.

Moschen, R., Kemmler, G., Schweigkofler, H., Holzner, B., Dunser, M., Richter, R., et al. (2001). Use of alternative/complementary therapy in breast cancer patients—A psychological perspective. *Supportive Care in Cancer, 9*, 267–274.

Nam, R.K., Fleshner, N., Rakovitch, E., Klotz, L., Trachtenberg, J., Choo, R., et al. (1999). Prevalence and patterns of the use of complementary therapies among prostate cancer patients: An epidemiological analysis. *Journal of Urology, 161*, 1521–1524.

National Cancer Institute. (1999, October). *Immuno-augmentative therapy*. Retrieved June 14, 2005, from http://cis.nci.nih.gov/fact/9_15.htm

National Cancer Institute, Office of Cancer Complementary and Alternative Medicine. (2004, December). *Clinical trials*. Retrieved May 19, 2005, from http://www.cancer.gov/cam/clinicaltrials_intro.html

National Center for Complementary and Alternative Medicine. (2000). *Expanding horizons of healthcare: Five-year strategic plan, 2001–2005*. Retrieved October 19, 2003, from http://nccam. nih.gov/about/plans/fiveyear/index.htm

National Center for Complementary and Alternative Medicine. (2002, May). *What is complementary and alternative medicine (CAM)?* Retrieved October 19, 2003, from http://nccam.nci.nih.gov/ health/whatiscam

National Center for Complementary and Alternative Medicine. (2003). *Are you considering using complementary and alternative medicine (CAM)?* Retrieved October 29, 2003, from http://nccam. nih.gov/health/decisions/index.htm

National Center for Complementary and Alternative Medicine. (2004, May). *Questions and answers about using magnets to treat pain*. Retrieved June 14, 2005, from http://nccam.nih.gov/health/ magnet/magnet.htm

Nauman, E. (2000). Native American medicine. In D.W. Novey (Ed.), *Clinician's complete reference to complementary/alternative medicine* (pp. 293–300). St. Louis, MO: Mosby.

Novey, D.W. (2000). Basic principles of complementary/alternative therapies. In D.W. Novey (Ed.), *Clinician's complete reference to complementary/alternative medicine* (pp. 5–7). St. Louis, MO: Mosby.

Oncology Nursing Society. (2004, October). *The use of complementary and alternative therapies in cancer care*. Retrieved May 19, 2005, from http://www.ons.org/publications/positions/ ComplementaryTherapies.shtml

Padilla, R., Gomez, V., Biggerstaff, S.L., & Mehler, P.S. (2001). Use of curanderismo in a public health care system. *Archives of Internal Medicine, 161,* 1336–1340.

Parker, M.J. (2000). Traditional Chinese herbal medicine. In D.W. Novey (Ed.), *Clinician's complete reference to complementary/alternative medicine* (pp. 203–218). St. Louis, MO: Mosby.

Pepa, C., & Russell, C.A. (2000). Introducing complementary/alternative strategies in a baccalaureate curriculum. *Nursing and Health Care Perspectives, 21,* 127–129.

Phillips, J.M., & Smith, E. (2004). African American women and breast cancer. In K.H. Dow (Ed.), *Contemporary issues in breast cancer: A nursing perspective* (2nd ed., pp. 283–298). Sudbury, MA: Jones and Bartlett.

Quigley, D., & Dean, C.F.A. (2000). Yoga. In D.W. Novey (Ed.), *Clinician's complete reference to complementary/alternative medicine* (pp. 141–151). St. Louis, MO: Mosby.

Rees, L., & Weil, A. (2001). Integrated medicine: Imbues orthodox medicine with the values of complementary medicine [Editorial]. *BMJ, 322,* 119–120.

Richardson, J. (2001). Integrating complementary therapies into health care education: A cautious approach. *Journal of Clinical Nursing, 10,* 793–798.

Richardson, M.A., Sanders, T., Palmer, J.L., Greisinger, A., & Singletary, S.E. (2000). Complementary/alternative medicine use in a comprehensive cancer center and the implications for oncology. *Journal of Clinical Oncology, 18,* 2505–2514.

Rossman, M.L., & Bresler, D.E. (2000). Interactive guided imagery. In D.W. Novey (Ed.), *Clinician's complete reference to complementary/alternative medicine* (pp. 64–72). St. Louis, MO: Mosby.

Rowland, J.H. (1990a). Developmental stage and adaptation: Adult model. In J.C. Holland & J.H. Rowland (Eds.), *Handbook of psychooncology: Psychological care of the patient with cancer* (pp. 25–43). New York: Oxford University Press.

Rowland, J.H. (1990b). Intrapersonal resources: Coping. In J.C. Holland & J.H. Rowland (Eds.), *Handbook of psychooncology: Psychological care of the patient with cancer* (pp. 44–57). New York: Oxford University Press.

Saichek, K.I. (2000). Hypnotherapy. In D.W. Novey (Ed.), *Clinician's complete reference to complementary/alternative medicine* (pp. 53–63). St. Louis, MO: Mosby.

Scanlon, C., & Glover, J. (1995). A professional code of ethics: Providing a moral compass for turbulent times. *Oncology Nursing Forum, 22,* 1515–1521.

Smith, M. (1998). Researching integrative therapies: Guidelines and application. *Journal of Emergency Nursing, 24,* 609–613.

Snyderman, R., & Weil, A.T. (2002). Integrative medicine: Bringing medicine back to its roots. *Archives of Internal Medicine, 162,* 395–397.

Sparber, A., Bauer, L., Curt, G., Eisenberg, D., Levin, T., Parks, S., et al. (2000). Use of complementary medicine by adult patients participating in cancer clinical trials. *Oncology Nursing Forum, 27,* 623–630.

Studdert, D.M., Eisenberg, D.M., Miller, F.H., Curto, D.A., Kaptchuk, T.J., & Brennan, T.A. (1998). Medical malpractice implications of alternative medicine. *JAMA, 280,* 1610–1615.

Sultanoff, B.A., & Zalaquett, C.P. (2000). Relaxation therapies. In D.W. Novey (Ed.), *Clinician's complete reference to complementary/alternative medicine* (pp. 114–129). St. Louis, MO: Mosby.

Taylor, E.J. (1998). Spirituality and the cancer experience. In R.M. Carroll-Johnson, L.M. Gorman, & N.J. Bush (Eds.), *Psychosocial nursing care along the cancer continuum* (pp. 71–82). Pittsburgh, PA: Oncology Nursing Society.

Truant, T., & McKenzie, M. (1999). Discussing complementary therapies: There's more than efficacy to consider. *Canadian Medical Association Journal, 160,* 351–352.

Warrick, P.D., Irish, J.C., Morningstar, M., Gilbert, R., Brown, D., & Gullane, P. (1999). Use of alternative medicine among patients with head and neck cancer. *Archives of Otolaryngology—Head and Neck Surgery, 125,* 573–579.

Weiger, W.A., Smith, M., Boon, H., Richardson, M.A., Kaptchuk, T.J., & Eisenberg, D.M. (2002). Advising patients who seek complementary and alternative medical therapies for cancer. *Annals of Internal Medicine, 137,* 889–903.

Weintraub, M.I. (1999). Legal implications of practicing alternative medicine. *JAMA, 281,* 1698–1699.

Wetzel, M.S., Kaptchuk, T.J., Haramati, A., & Eisenberg, D.M. (2003). Complementary and alternative medical therapies: Implications for medical education. *Annals of Internal Medicine, 138,* 191–196.

Winslow, L.C., & Shapiro, H. (2002). Physicians want education about complementary and alternative medicine to enhance communication with their patients. *Archives of Internal Medicine, 162,* 1176–1181.

Yaramus, M.B., Fletcher, D.M., & Baum, A. (2003, April). *An innovative oncology integrative medicine informatics and consultative service.* Paper presented at the Comprehensive Cancer Care Conference, Washington, DC. Retrieved October 29, 2003, from http://www.cmbm.org/conferences/SummerSessions.pdf

Zollman, C., & Vickers, A. (1999). Complementary medicine and the patient. *BMJ, 319,* 1486–1489.

CHAPTER 33

Ethical Issues Along the Cancer Continuum

LIBBY BOWERS, RN, MSN, CHPN, CCRN

We do not act rightly because we have virtue or excellence, but rather we have those because we have acted rightly.

—Aristotle

The contemporary context of oncology nursing is filled with a plethora of ethical challenges. Attention to the ethical dimensions of cancer care is central to nursing practice and the well-being of patients, families, and the community. Nurses assume a prominent role in the care of people throughout the cancer trajectory and therefore possess a responsibility to model, guide, and provide ethically sound care.

Unprecedented advances in medical science have created great promise for individual health but also rivet oncology care with new and complex ethical quandaries. Among the most perplexing ethical challenges confronting the cancer care continuum are distinctions between medical paternalism and autonomy, withholding and withdrawing treatment, ordinary and extraordinary means of preserving life, intentionally causing or allowing death, and equal distribution of healthcare resources versus rationing of care and services. This chapter focuses on the ethical dilemmas that challenge nurses, patients, and the greater healthcare community related to prevention, detection, education, treatment options and outcomes, and palliation in cancer care.

Defining Ethics

"Ethics" is concerned with systematically evaluating varying viewpoints related to what is morally "right or wrong" or "good or bad." The study of ethics as it intersects with health care is termed "bioethics." The evolution of bioethics was a natural extension of the move away from a mechanistic model to a holistic approach toward caring for ill people. Over time, a myriad of ethical theories and methodologies has arisen, shaped by the gender, socioeconomic strata, and culture of philosophers.

However, foundational ethical principles construct frameworks that are common to many of the ethical theories.

Four primary ethical principles traditionally define ethical decision making and consequential actions: autonomy, beneficence, nonmaleficence, and justice (see Table 33-1 for complete definitions) (Beauchamp & Childress, 1994). Ethical dilemmas emerge across the spectrum of care as nurses endeavor to provide the best possible care while responding to threats to their personal, professional, or community value structure. One's beliefs about what is "right" or "wrong" or "good" or "bad" largely are embedded in the individual's beliefs, values, societal norms, and past experiences.

In the healthcare arena, professionals are expected to apply ethical principles to a wide array of healthcare encounters to aid them in determining how they are morally obligated to respond. Often, a clash occurs between the ethical principles, requiring that they be weighed against one another to determine which one obliges. The most complex ethical choices, those embracing both the good and bad, are the actions and omissions that generate the great controversies in ethics (Devettere, 2000).

In the clinical setting, a bioethics consultation typically is requested when a clinical case presents competing values, which often are articulated as opinions regarding the appropriate direction or options of treatment, and none is clearly or irrefutably the overriding value (Dalinis, 2004).

Table 33-1. Definitions of Ethical Principles

Principle	Definition
Autonomy	The individual's freedom from controlling interferences by others and from personal limitations that prevent meaningful choices, such as adequate understanding
Beneficence	Actions performed that contribute to the welfare of others
Nonmaleficence	An obligation not to inflict harm intentionally. It forms the framework for the standard of due care to be met by any professional.
Justice	The fair, equitable, and appropriate treatment in light of what is due or owed to a person. Distributive justice refers to fair, equitable, and appropriate distribution in society determined by justified norms that structure the terms of social cooperation.

Scopes and Standards for Ethical Nursing Practice

The many ethical challenges that confront the nursing profession have propelled the formation of several professional statements articulating its shared values. The American Nurses Association's (ANA's, 2001) *Code of Ethics for Nurses With Interpretive Statements* reflects a framework of ethical standards for the nursing profession. This code of ethics for nurses outlines the ethical obligations and duties of every individual who enters the nursing profession, represents the profession's nonnegotiable ethical standards, and expresses nursing's own understanding of its commitment to society.

Similarly, the Oncology Nursing Society (ONS) published the *Statement on the Scope and Standards of Oncology Nursing Practice* (Brant & Wickham, 2004), which states that oncology nurses' decisions and actions are portrayed in an ethical manner. Oncology nurses need to examine their personal philosophy, discuss ethical issues with colleagues, address advance directives with patients and families, serve as patient advocates, maintain sensitivity to patients' cultural differences, find resources to examine issues, engage in ethical decision making, and preserve patient autonomy, dignity, and rights. The profession's ethical statements provide a starting point for ethical discernment; however, they do not provide explicit answers to the troubling ethical realities that confront nurses in practice.

Ethical Issues in Nursing Care

The nomenclature of ethical theories and principles gives way to the practical necessity of determining "right or wrong" or "good or bad" in the daily activities and varied settings of nursing care. By virtue of their distinct relationship with patients and their families and their central role as coordinators of care, nurses bring a unique perspective to understanding and evaluating the ethical dimensions of cancer care (Scanlon, 1998).

Autonomy: Informed Consent, Truth Telling, and Advance Directives

In recent decades, the assertion of autonomous decision making has challenged the longstanding model of paternalism, in which one person determines what is good for another person instead of facilitating the other's self-determined good. For instance, in the past, the majority of physicians elected not to discuss a diagnosis of cancer with a patient (Oken, 1961). Under a paternalistic model, the medical practitioner operated independently in determining which information to communicate and choosing the course of disease management. However, research over the past 40 years has indicated that patients want to be informed of their diagnosis and prognosis as well as be active participants in care-related decision making (Auvinen et al., 2004; Samp & Curreri, 1957). The rise of the consumer-rights era disrupted the paternalistic paradigm that dominated health care (Angelos, 1999). Autonomy, the ability to govern oneself, became a central paradigm resulting in shared healthcare information and decision making.

The doctrine of informed consent (i.e., the right to accept or reject treatment) is a cornerstone of the ethical and legal rights of individuals to make autonomous healthcare decisions. The philosophic, sociologic, and legal doctrine of informed consent prevents forced, coerced, or manipulated decision making. However, at times, healthcare interventions occur without a patient's informed consent; this results when the individual's capacity for decision making is lost, in emergencies when there is not enough time for complete disclosure, and when patients waive their right to give informed consent (Devettere, 2000).

Disease-related or treatment-induced alterations in patients' capacity for autonomous decision making may occur along the cancer continuum. Nurses, because of their enduring relationship with patients over time, play a vital role in clarifying patients' decisional capacity. Written or verbal advance care directives are paramount to the preservation of self-determination when decisional capacity is absent. Advance directives afford patients the opportunity to provide treatment instructions and/or appoint a decision maker, called a healthcare power of attorney or surrogate. In 1991, Congress enacted the Patient Self-Determination Act into legislation, mandating that all patients be informed of their prerogative to accept or refuse treatment and to execute advance directives (Omnibus Reconciliation Act of 1990). Unfortunately, despite formalized legislation granting the right and privilege to each person to make known his or her healthcare preferences, the rate of advance directive completion is low (Kish, Martin, & Price, 2000). Further, no studies to date have confirmed that advance directives facilitate decision making or truly direct care (Teno, Licks, et al., 1997; Teno, Lynn, et al., 1997).

In situations where an individual has lost the capacity for self-determination of care and treatment preferences and an advance directive is not present, the responsibility for healthcare decision making generally is assigned to family members, particularly the next of kin. In the absence of oral or written advance directives, the surrogate decision maker attempts to use substituted judgment, making the decision the patient would have made if he or she were capable. The role of the surrogate decision maker is legally recognized in the United States (Hayes, 2003).

Ongoing Ethical Challenges to Autonomy

Despite the transition from medical paternalism to shared decision making and the introduction of informed consent and advance directives, ethical challenges still surround the promotion of patient autonomy. Although it is generally accepted that healthcare decision making should be shared, the issue remains of how much information should be given to patients. An imbalance of power exists between the patient and the healthcare team. The ability of patients to enact autonomous decision making is wholly dependent upon the range of choices presented by the healthcare team; these choices are dependent upon the divulgence of the healthcare team members and the healthcare system (Drought & Koenig, 2002). Disparities persist in the cancer care arena between the amount of information patients wish to receive to inform their decision making and the amount of information the healthcare team divulges. According to Jefford and Tattersall (2002), patients with cancer prefer to receive as much information as possible about their condition, regardless of whether the information is good or bad. However, oncology care providers continue to remain hesitant to provide prognostic information that has the potential to threaten patients' hope (Gordon & Daugherty, 2003). Several studies have shown that the healthcare team is only moderately better than chance at identifying patients' wishes (Mattimore et al., 1997; Weeks et al., 1998; Wilson et al., 1997). The cornerstone of communication about difficult issues in cancer care is maintenance of a therapeutic relationship between caregivers and patients.

Hastened Death: Assisted Suicide and Euthanasia

The ability to exercise autonomy in healthcare decision making has extended into the arena of self-determination over the events that will lead to one's death.

Few issues in health care remain as controversial as assisted suicide and euthanasia (see Table 33-2 for definitions of terms). The focus of ethical scrutiny as it relates to assisted suicide and euthanasia is on the patient–healthcare provider relationship as the ethical principles of autonomy, beneficence, and nonmaleficence collide.

Table 33-2. Glossary of Terms Related to Termination of Life

Term	Definition
Suicide	One takes his or her own life.
Assisted suicide	Someone else provides the means by which one takes his or her life (i.e., a physician prescribes a lethal dose of medication with the understanding that the patient intends to use it to commit suicide).
Voluntary euthanasia	The healthcare provider, with the consent of the terminally ill patient, intentionally causes death.
Involuntary euthanasia	The healthcare provider, without the consent of the terminally ill patient, intentionally causes death.

The experience of facing a potentially life-limiting illness, such as cancer, is a common catalyst for the contemplation of one's mortality. Fears of living or dying with distressing symptoms, being stripped of dignity, becoming a burden to family and friends, and losing control may provoke an individual with cancer to consider suicide. In fact, the rate of suicide among patients with cancer is at least twice that of the general population (Chochinov, Wilson, Enns, & Lander, 1998). The incidence of suicide among patients with cancer appears to be greatest in the advanced stages of illness and for those with uncontrolled symptoms.

At the center of one's desire to hasten death often is a hope of avoiding or curtailing suffering, maintaining control over potentially frightening and unknown circumstances, forgoing burdening family members with care needs, and avoiding the financial implications of treatment (Ersek, 2004). Patients may request that healthcare team members, as a result of their enduring relationships with patients throughout the cancer continuum, actively aid them in ending their life. A national survey of physicians indicated that 18% had received requests for hastened death, and a similar study of nurses indicated that 30% of oncology nurses received requests for assisted dying (Matzo & Emanual, 1997; Meier et al., 1998).

Actively assisting a patient to die is different from withholding or withdrawing life-sustaining treatment or administering high doses of pain-relieving medication that may hasten death. The differences between the active and passive participation in one's death are the principles that fuel the ethical debate over assisted dying. Proponents of assisted dying argue that the ability to choose death is a moral extension of autonomy, and violation of one's autonomy infringes upon patients' rights (Devettere, 2000). Additionally, advocates of assisted dying argue that a compassionate and merciful response to one's suffering at the end of life is assisted dying. Other advocates for assisted dying propose that assisted dying is consistent with the legitimate medical desire to prevent suffering and exercise beneficence in aiding in the achievement of a "good death" (Angell, 1997).

Opponents of hastened death counter the arguments of those favoring assisted suicide point by point. First, opponents refute patient autonomy, self-determination, and the right to choose freely with the argument that solely because an individual has a *right* to choose something does not mean that what one chooses is morally justified (Devettere, 2000). The task of ethics is to determine whether one's choice is morally good and contributes to the welfare of the one choosing it. The argument that hastened death relieves suffering is countered by the adoption of aggressive palliative care that advocates extraordinary means to offset physical, psychosocial, and spiritual suffering (Stanley & Zoloth-Dorfman, 2001). Palliative care professionals may use palliative sedation to induce somnolence while patients are awaiting an inevitable death when symptoms cannot be controlled any other way (Rousseau, 2004). Palliative sedation generally is viewed as ethically and legally acceptable in appropriate situations (Hospice and Palliative Nurses Association, 2003). Rousseau reported that it is not associated with hastened death. Finally, those opposing hastened death do not find this practice to be a normal, beneficent part of their healthcare practices and vehemently proclaim that it violates the Hippocratic oath, finding evidence that it in fact opposes "normal" healthcare practices.

Hastened Death: Legal Matters

Although the practice of hastened death is a widely debated topic, the actual incidence of occurrence is unknown. Euthanasia, both voluntary and involuntary, is illegal in the United States. Assisted suicide, with the aid of a physician prescribing a lethal dose of barbiturate, is legal only in the state of Oregon. In 1994, Oregon voters narrowly passed Measure 16, the Death With Dignity Act, legitimizing physician-assisted suicide (PAS) for terminally ill adults. A court injunction immediately blocked its implementation. The U.S. Supreme Court heard the case on appeal and determined that patients do not have a constitutional right to PAS. However, it left the opportunity open at a state level for the adoption of affirmative legislation (*Vacco v. Quill*, 1997). In 1997, after debate about the reliability of the method used for hastening death, the Oregon legislature returned the vote to the citizens, and the measure once again passed and became available to the residents of the state.

Despite the legalization of PAS in Oregon, a large utilization of this intervention has not occurred. In the first two years following its legalization, only 42 persons died by PAS. The majority of the patients seeking PAS have a cancer diagnosis (Chin, Hedberg, Higginson, & Fleming, 1999; Sullivan, Hedberg, & Fleming, 2000). Nurses caring for patients requesting PAS retain the prerogative to continue or discontinue involvement in care as they feel morally inclined.

Response of Professional Organizations to Hastened Death

Many professional organizations have formulated responses to the ethical, legal, and social debates arising in response to assisted suicide. ANA, the largest professional body representing nursing, took a strong stance in opposition to hastening death: "The nurse does not act deliberately to terminate the life of any person" (ANA, 2001, p. 3). In 1995, ONS endorsed the position of the ANA and in 2004 adopted a strong position of support, nonabandonment, and advocacy (ONS, 2004). The medical oncology community has not taken a distinct stand, resolving "to neither condone nor condemn" assisted suicide (American Society of Clinical Oncology, 1998, p. 1987). Although professional societies formalize responses for those they represent, it remains necessary for each individual professional to morally examine and formulate a response that will guide his or her delivery of health care.

Medically Inappropriate Treatment: Determining Life and Death

Remarkable advances in medical technology are responsible for the prolongation of life. The broad publicity of these advances in science fosters an expectation of continuing growth of treatment choices or a cure that is on the horizon. At times, the extension of life may lead to the meaningful attainment of goals and the return of functional capacity. However, there remain times when the application of advanced treatment interventions will never achieve the return of functional capabilities or the potential for life independent of applied life-sustaining interventions. Therapies that prolong life despite outcomes that are both ethically and medically unacceptable are inappropriate and often described as being futile (Rivera, Kim, Garone, Morgenstern, & Mohsenifar, 2001). Serious ethical, medical, and societal dilemmas result from the application of medically inappropriate treatment (also referred to as nonbeneficial medical treatment).

Patients with advanced cancer and their families experience many difficult emotions in the face of an often-bleak prognosis. The conflict between hope and reality can exacerbate the stress a patient and family are experiencing, and these emotions may obscure their ability to make informed and calculated decisions about treatment. Many patients and families experiencing a cancer diagnosis are blitzed with information from healthcare professionals, well-meaning acquaintances, news headlines, and the Internet. Patients, well-versed in the ethical premise of autonomy, desire to be informed and involved in the determination of their health care. However, the ethical principle of autonomy is central to the dilemma of nonbeneficial medical treatment. How far does patient autonomy extend? Do patients and family members have the right to sway the hand of healthcare professionals with requests for certain interventions or treatment? Are healthcare professionals obligated to provide interventions requested by patients and families even when they may be medically unreasonable, might incur greater harm, or have little chance of achieving the desired outcome? Society is concerned about the denial of treatment based upon economic interests and outcomes-based standards.

Conversely, are representatives of the healthcare profession obligated to make patients and families aware of all available treatment options? Is it within the domain of health care to withhold or withdraw therapies deemed to be inappropriate without subjecting such a decision to the patient's approval? Ethically, what is the deciding principle when conflicts arise between a healthcare professional's duty to do good and prevent harm and the patient's and family's right to self-determination? The long-established orientation of healthcare personnel is toward the preservation of life, an attitude that potentially overshadows realistic medical expectations.

Ethically, the argument of medically inappropriate treatment or futility arises when values collide. Futility is a concept that does not stand well alone and is situationally dependent. Rubin (1998) proposed that futility exists when the treatment under consideration does not achieve the patient's intended goals. The appropriateness of an intervention is seeded in two important features. First, for the patient under consideration, the harms of the intervention are not indisputably greater than the harms eliminated, relieved, or prevented (Shapiro, 1999). Second, the therapy has a reasonable probability of meeting the therapeutic goals of the patient (Shapiro). How the patient ranks the benefits and harms of that treatment ultimately determines the appropriateness of a treatment.

The crux of the futility debate is the distinction between causing death and letting die. The California Superior Court has ruled that the withdrawal of life-sustaining treatment is neither homicide nor suicide (*Barber v. Superior Court*, 1983; *Bartling v. Superior Court*, 1984). Some of the most difficult and distressing decisions in health care are whether to withdraw treatment. However, at times, the limits of technology prevent medical professionals from curing and permit them to venture beyond their limits of doing good and preventing harm.

When conflicts arise, as they inevitably do, over the withholding or withdrawal of therapies, collaborative practice, institutional policies, and ethics committees can help healthcare professionals to navigate resources. The University of Texas M.D. Anderson Cancer Center has proposed a systemwide policy that methodically reviews and makes recommendations for situations in which medically inappropriate treatment is being given (see Figure 33-1). Perhaps one of the most important roles of nursing surrounding the time of decision making involves the withdrawal of treatment; the nurse has a valuable role in communicating nonabandonment. Oncology nurses often are a liaison between patients and families and the medical team. Principle

---

Figure 33-1. Seven-Step Process for Evaluating Medically Inappropriate Treatments

- The healthcare provider outlines to the patient or surrogate decision maker the nature of the illness, the prognosis, alternatives, and the reasons why he or she believes the requested intervention is medically inappropriate.
- The healthcare provider gives the options of transferring the patient to another physician or institution and obtaining an independent opinion on the appropriateness of the intervention in question.
- The patient or surrogate decision maker is offered other resources within the healthcare system, ranging from chaplaincy and social services to patient care representatives and the clinical ethics committee.
- The attending physician obtains an opinion from a second physician who examines the patient and then prepares to present the case, with clinical and scientific evidence that the intervention is inappropriate, for review by an institutional interdisciplinary body.
- The healthcare provider informs the patient or decision maker of the time, site, and possible outcomes of the review; the patient still can choose to be transferred during this process.
- The institutional review is conducted in the presence of the physician and patient or surrogate decision maker.
- The review committee arrives at a finding. If it determines the requested intervention to be inappropriate, the intervention is halted and replaced by a care plan designed to provide comfort to the patient and preserve his or her dignity.

Note. Based on information from Norwood, 1997.

---

roles of oncology care providers include clarifying information, practicing advocacy, and providing nurturing care throughout the continuum of care.

The Injustice of Health Disparities

Another ethical conundrum common to cancer care is the vast disparities in care. Throughout the entire cancer continuum, from prevention to palliation, inequalities exist. Despite the progress of medical science resulting in increased longevity and improved quality of life, some groups carry a heavier burden, particularly the poor and minorities. The unequal burden of disease in American society is a challenge to science, as well as a moral and ethical dilemma for the world. In the words of Freeman (2000), "Racial distinctions in science can provide us with evidence of significant variation in health and disease, but this evidence must be interpreted, by examining the social, economic, cultural, and environmental factors in order to understand the underlying causes of the unequal burden of disease among groups."

One of the major goals of the U.S. Department of Health and Human Services' (2000) Healthy People 2010 initiative is to eliminate health disparities. The first step toward eliminating health disparities is to recognize the disparities within the cancer care arena. Disparities in cancer care are recognized among socioeconomic, racial, and environmental clusters. A study conducted in Kentucky revealed that for the four most common types of malignancies, uninsured individuals demonstrated lower cancer survival rates than those with insurance or state or federal healthcare support (McDavid, Tucker, Sloggett, & Coleman, 2003).

A 1999 study that evaluated the racial differences in the treatment of early-stage lung carcinoma uncovered disparities between the care and consequent outcomes of African American and Caucasian patients with cancer (Bach, Cramer, Warren, & Begg, 2003). Non-small cell lung cancer, if discovered at an early stage, potentially is curable through surgical resection. The study revealed that African Americans were less likely to receive surgical treatment than Caucasians and were likely to die sooner than Caucasians from this condition. The study further concluded that those African American patients who did receive the surgical resection had a survival rate similar to Caucasian patients. African Americans have a higher overall incidence of cancer and a higher rate of death from cancer than any other racial or ethnic group. Further, racial and ethnic disparities in pain perception, assessment, and treatment were found in all settings and across all types of pain. The literature suggests that the sources of pain disparities among racial and ethnic minorities are complex, involving patients, healthcare providers, and the healthcare system (Green et al., 2003).

Finally, environmental factors as measured by sanitary conditions and environmental exposure are worse in many of the world's developing countries as compared with the industrialized world; this inequality results in higher mortality, lower cancer survival rates, and a significantly shorter life expectancy in developing countries than in industrialized countries (Boffetta, Matisane, Mundt, & Dell, 2003; Sudakin, 2003; Tomatis, 1997). Society as a whole, and the healthcare profession specifically, has a responsibility to recognize injustices in the division of cancer prevention, screening, education, treatment, and palliation.

Justice and the Allocation of Health Resources

The 20th century was fraught with healthcare costs escalating beyond control. Expensive, state-of-the-art medical facilities, rising costs of medical education, advancement of novel technologies, new and expensive medications, and increasing morbidity among an aging population were factors that directly increased healthcare costs. The fee-for-service system of healthcare reimbursement offered no incentive for reducing healthcare expenditures and, in fact, conspired to escalate the price tag for health services; reform was needed.

Managed care was the primary response to the dilemma of rising healthcare costs; one of its chief aims is to manage costs. Several models of managed care organizations exist, but in general, managed care both insures patients and manages the care that patients receive through shifting some of the financial risk to the healthcare provider. The creation of shared risk by both the managed care organization and the healthcare professional invokes dual responsibility for cost containment and the allocation of healthcare resources. In the words of Hellman (1999), "There is a tense triad in medical care as we attempt to achieve superior, economical care that is equitably distributed" (p. 92). Healthcare providers share a dual and seemingly incompatible role of honoring the principles of beneficence and nonmaleficence in caring for patients while satisfying the needs of the managed care organization in controlling costs. In reality, the ethical principle of justice may be violated as the healthcare provider is asked to serve two potentially differing interests.

Managed care is not inherently unethical, but it does introduce some ethical conundrums. Healthcare professionals, who share responsibility for managing and conserving resources, may succumb to financial pressures from the managed care organization and make poor treatment choices (Devettere, 2000). Trust between healthcare professionals and their patients may diminish as patients learn that their care providers are interested in potentially withholding care to reduce costs. Treatment protocols may not cover or permit the use of expensive or novel therapies (e.g., hematopoietic stem cell transplant); this is particularly troublesome for cancer care. Finally, managed care tends to find that prescribing a medication is more cost effective than offering counseling for mental or emotional anguish. In the oncology setting, the use of individual or group therapy is well established and complements the use of medication when indicated (Lovejoy, Tabor, Matteis, & Lillis, 2000; Pirl & Roth, 1999). The evolution of managed care has resulted in a shift away from the primacy of the provider-patient relationship and has created new ethical challenges.

The managed care marketplace is changing the delivery of cancer care. Treatment for cancer is undergoing much scrutiny as case managers require detailed reviews of treatment plans to provide initial verification and recertification for the provider's recommended course of therapy. Therapies that are expensive, new on the market, or investigational undergo particular inquiry. Managed care also has resulted in shorter hospital stays, which has led to sicker patients being sent into the community, where families have an increasing responsibility to provide care. Oncology nurses must remain aware of the impact that managed care has on patients and families—clinically, fiscally, and practically.

Guidelines for Addressing Ethical Dilemmas

Healthcare professionals experience ethical dilemmas when one or more of their personal beliefs, professional values, or societal mandates are in conflict (Hayes, 2004). Cultural, sociologic, and political contexts color the lens through which one views ethical conflicts. ANA (2001) and other professional organizations have established ethical statements elevating the pivotal role that nurses play in recognizing, articulating, and resolving ethical conflicts in the healthcare arena. Figure 33-2 proposes a systematic framework for appraising and resolving ethical dilemmas within the care environment.

Figure 33-2. A Systematic Process for Managing Ethical Conflicts

1. Clarify the need for an immediate decision versus the consequences of delaying a decision.
2. Gather together those directly involved in the conflict; in addition to the person receiving care and/or his or her proxy, this might include various health care providers, family members, and administrators.
3. If necessary, choose a person not involved in the conflict to facilitate discussions. It is imperative that this person be acceptable to all those involved and have the skills to facilitate open discussion and decision-making.
4. Identify and agree on the points of agreement and disagreement. While ensuring confidentiality, share among those involved all relevant medical and personal information, interpretations of the relevant facts, institutional policies, and professional norms and laws.
5. Establish the roles and responsibilities of each participant in the conflict.
6. Offer the person receiving care, or his or her proxy, access to institutional, agency or community resources for support in the conflict resolution process, e.g., a patient representative, chaplain or other resource person.
7. Determine if the group needs outside advice or consultation. For example, a second opinion, use of an ethics committee or other resource.
8. Identify and explore all options and determine a time line for resolving the conflict. Ensure that all participants have the opportunity to express their views.
9. If, after reasonable effort, agreement or compromise cannot be reached through dialogue, accept the decision of the person with the right or responsibility for making the decision. If it is unclear or disputed who has the right or responsibility to make the decision, seek mediation, arbitration or adjudication.
10. If the person receiving care or his or her proxy is dissatisfied with the decision, and another care provider, facility or agency is prepared to accommodate the person's needs and preferences, provide the opportunity for transfer.
11. If a healthcare provider cannot support the decision that prevails as a matter of professional judgment or personal morality, allow him or her to withdraw without reprisal from participation in carrying out the decision, after ensuring that the person receiving care is not at risk of harm or abandonment.

Note. From "Joint Statement on Preventing and Resolving Ethical Conflicts Involving Health Care Providers and Persons Receiving Care," by the Canadian Healthcare Association, Canadian Medical Association, Canadian Nurses Association, and Catholic Health Association of Canada, 1999. Retrieved November 24, 2004, from http://www.cha.ca/documents/joint.htm. Copyright 1999 by the Canadian Healthcare Association, Canadian Medical Association, Canadian Nurses Association, and Catholic Health Association of Canada. Reprinted with permission.

Conclusion

The distinctions of "good" and "bad" and "right" and "wrong" increasingly are blurred by the ethical complexity of care in today's healthcare delivery system. Oncology nurses face a new taxonomy of ethical challenges propagated by scientific advancement, new legislation, and fewer resources with which to accomplish the privilege of providing adequate care for those living with cancer. The ethical principles of autonomy, beneficence, nonmaleficence, and justice are the catalysts that proliferate dissent in the ethics of health care on topics such as paternalism and self-determination, ordinary versus extraordinary means of preserving life, delaying death and extending life, and rationing versus good stewardship. Oncology nurses have an invaluable role in the discussion of ethical issues in the arena of cancer care; they serve as patient advocates, a liaison between the provider and the patient, and representatives of the community and the healthcare system. As such, oncology nurses have a voice in ethical deliberation.

References

American Nurses Association. (2001). *Code of ethics for nurses with interpretive statements.* Washington, DC: Author.

American Society of Clinical Oncology. (1998). Cancer care during the last phase of life. *Journal of Clinical Oncology, 16,* 1986–1996.

Angell, M. (1997). The Supreme Court and physician-assisted suicide—The ultimate right. *New England Journal of Medicine, 336,* 50–53.

Angelos, P. (1999). Physicians and cancer patients: Communication and advance directives. In P. Angelos (Ed.), *Ethical issues in cancer patient care* (pp. 1–11). Norwell, MA: Kluwer Academic.

Auvinen, A., Hakama, M., Ala-Opas, M., Vornanen, T., Leppilahti, M., & Salminen, P. (2004). A randomized trial of choice of treatment in prostate cancer: The effect of intervention on the treatment chosen. *British Journal of Urology International, 93,* 52–56.

Bach, P.B., Cramer, L.D., Warren, J.L., & Begg, C.B. (2003). Racial differences in the treatment of early-stage lung cancer. *New England Journal of Medicine, 341,* 1198–1205.

Barber v. Superior Court, 147 Cal. App.3d 1006, 195 Cal. Rptr. 484. (Cal. Ct. App., 2nd Dist. 1983).

Bartling v. Superior Court, 163 Cal. App.3d 186, 209 Cal. Rptr. 220 (1984).

Beauchamp, T.L., & Childress, J.F. (1994). *Principles of biomedical ethics* (4th ed.). New York: Oxford University Press.

Boffetta, P., Matisane, L., Mundt, K.A., & Dell, L.D. (2003). Meta-analysis of studies of occupational exposure to vinyl chloride in relation to cancer mortality. *Scandinavian Journal of Work, Environment and Health, 29,* 220–229.

Brant, S.M., & Wickham, R.S. (Eds.). (2004). *Statement of the scope and standards of oncology nursing practice* (3rd ed.). Pittsburgh, PA: Oncology Nursing Society.

Chin, A.E., Hedberg, K., Higginson, G.K., & Fleming, D.W. (1999). Legalized physician-assisted suicide in Oregon—The first year's experience. *New England Journal of Medicine, 340,* 577–583.

Chochinov, H.M., Wilson, K.G., Enns, M., & Lander, S. (1998). Depression, hopelessness, and suicidal ideation in the terminally ill. *Psychosomatics, 39,* 366–370.

Dalinis, P.M. (2004). Bioethics consultation: Appropriate uses in end-of-life care. *Journal of Hospice and Palliative Nursing, 6,* 117–122.

Devettere, R.J. (2000). *Practical decision making in health care ethics: Cases and concepts* (2nd ed.). Washington, DC: Georgetown University Press.

Drought, T.S., & Koenig, B.A. (2002). "Choice" in end-of-life decision making: Researching fact or fiction? *Gerontologist, 42*(Spec. No. 3), 114–128.

Ersek, M. (2004). The continuing challenge of assisted death. *Journal of Hospice and Palliative Nursing, 6,* 46–59.

Freeman, H. (2000, September). *Ethnic minority disparities in cancer treatment: Why the unequal burden?* Testimony presented before the House Committee on Government Reform, Washington, DC.

Gordon, E.J., & Daugherty, C.K. (2003). 'Hitting you over the head': Oncologists' disclosure of prognosis to advanced cancer patients. *Bioethics, 17,* 142–168.

Green, C.R., Anderson, K.O., Baker, T.A., Campbell, L.C., Decker, S., Fillingim, R.B., et al. (2003). The unequal burden of pain: Confronting racial and ethnic disparities in pain. *Pain Medicine, 4,* 277–294.

Hayes, C.M. (2003). Surrogate decision-making to end life-sustaining treatments for incapacitated adults. *Journal of Hospice and Palliative Nursing, 5,* 91–102.

Hayes, C.M. (2004). Ethics and end-of-life care. *Journal of Hospice and Palliative Nursing, 6,* 36–43.

Hellman, S. (1999). The ethical lessons of managed care applied to clinical trials. In P. Angelos (Ed.), *Ethical issues in cancer patient care* (pp. 91–98). Norwell, MA: Kluwer Academic.

Hospice and Palliative Nurses Association. (2003). *Palliative sedation at end of life* [Position paper]. Pittsburgh, PA: Author.

Jefford, M., & Tattersall, M.H. (2002). Informing and involving cancer patients in their own care. *Lancet Oncology, 3,* 629–637.

Kish, S.K., Martin, C.G., & Price, K.J. (2000). Advance directives in critically ill cancer patients. *Critical Care Nursing Clinics of North America, 12,* 373–383.

Lovejoy, N.C., Tabor, D., Matteis, M., & Lillis, P. (2000). Cancer-related depression: Part I—Neurologic alterations and cognitive-behavioral therapy. *Oncology Nursing Forum, 27,* 667–678.

Mattimore, T.J., Wenger, N.S., Desbiens, N.A., Teno, J.M., Hamel, M.B., Liu, H., et al. (1997). Surrogate and physician understanding of patients' preferences for living permanently in a nursing home. *Journal of the American Geriatrics Society, 45,* 818–824.

Matzo, M.L., & Emanuel, E.J. (1997). Oncology nurses' practices of assisted suicide and patient-requested euthanasia. *Oncology Nursing Forum, 24,* 1725–1732.

McDavid, K., Tucker, T.C., Sloggett, A., & Coleman, M.P. (2003). Cancer survival in Kentucky and health insurance coverage. *Archives of Internal Medicine, 163,* 2135–2144.

Meier, D.D., Emmons, C.A., Wallenstein, S., Quill, T., Morrison, R.S., & Cassell, C.K. (1998). A national survey of physician-assisted suicide and euthanasia in the United States. *New England Journal of Medicine, 338,* 1193–1201.

Norwood, D. (1997, January/March). Handling requests for medically inappropriate interventions. *OncoLog, 42*(1). Retrieved January 10, 2004, from http://www3.mdanderson.org/~oncolog/futilecare.html

Oken, D. (1961). What to tell cancer patients: A study of medical attitudes. *JAMA, 175,* 1120–1128.

Omnibus Reconciliation Act of 1990, Public Law No. 101-508, Sections 4206, 4751.

Oncology Nursing Society. (2004, July). *Oncology Nursing Society position on the nurse's responsibility to the patient requesting assisted suicide.* Retrieved May 24, 2005, from http://www.ons.org/publications/positions/AssistedSuicide.shtml

Pirl, W.F., & Roth, A.J. (1999). Diagnosis and treatment of depression in cancer patients. *Oncology, 13,* 1293–1302.

Rivera, S., Kim, D., Garone, S., Morgenstern, L., & Mohsenifar, Z. (2001). Motivating factors in futile clinical interventions. *Chest, 119,* 1944–1947.

Rousseau, P. (2004). Palliative sedation in the management of refractory symptoms. *Journal of Supportive Oncology, 2,* 181–186.

Rubin, S. (1998). *When doctors say "no": The battleground of medical futility.* Bloomington, IN: Indiana University Press.

Samp, R.J., & Curreri, A.R. (1957). Questionnaire survey on public cancer education obtained from cancer patients and their families. *Cancer, 10,* 382–384.

Scanlon, C. (1998). Unraveling ethical issues in palliative care. *Seminars in Oncology Nursing, 14,* 137–144.

Shapiro, G.R. (1999). Are there limits to oncology care (futility)? In P. Angelos (Ed.), *Ethical issues in cancer patient care* (pp. 49–63). Norwell, MA: Kluwer Academic.

Stanley, K.J., & Zoloth-Dorfman, L. (2001). Ethical considerations. In B.R. Ferrell & N. Coyle (Eds.), *Textbook of palliative nursing* (pp. 663–681). New York: Oxford University Press.

Sudakin, D.L. (2003). Dietary aflatoxin exposure and chemoprevention of cancer: A clinical review. *Journal of Toxicology: Clinical Toxicology, 41,* 195–204.

Sullivan, A.D., Hedberg, K., & Fleming, D.W. (2000). Legalized physician-assisted suicide in Oregon—The second year. *New England Journal of Medicine, 342,* 598–604.

Teno, J., Licks, S., Lynn, J., Wenger, N., Connors, A.F., Jr., Phillips, R.S., et al. (1997). Do advance directives provide instructions that direct care? *Journal of the American Geriatrics Society, 45,* 508–512.

Teno, J., Lynn, J., Wenger, N., Phillips, R.S., Murphy, D.P., Connors, A.F., et al. (1997). Advance directives for seriously ill hospitalized patients: Effectiveness with the Patient Self-Determination Act and the SUPPORT intervention. *Journal of the American Geriatrics Society, 45,* 500–507.

Tomatis, L. (1997). Poverty and cancer. *IARC Scientific Publications, 138,* 25–39.

U.S. Department of Health and Human Services. (2000). *Healthy People 2010: Volume I: With understanding and improving health and objectives for improving health* (2nd ed.). Washington, DC: Government Printing Office.

Vacco v. Quill, 117 S. Ct. 2293 (1997).

Weeks, J.C., Cook, E.G., O'Day, S.J., Peterson, L.M., Wenger, N., Reding, D., et al. (1998). Relationship between cancer patients' predictions of prognosis and their treatment preferences. *JAMA, 279,* 1709–1714.

Wilson, I.B., Green, M.L., Goldman, L., Tsevat, J., Cook, E.F., & Phillips, R.S. (1997). Is experience a good teacher? How interns and attending physicians understand patients' choices for end-of-life care. *Medical Decision Making, 17,* 217–227.

CHAPTER 34

Substance Abuse

PEGGY COMPTON, RN, PHD

Wine is only sweet to happy men.

—John Keats

Substance abuse and addiction are chronic diseases that can complicate the nursing care of patients with cancer in subtle yet challenging and important ways. They may affect patients' ability to comply with treatment protocols, affect physiologic responses to therapy and surgery, and complicate responses to pain and analgesia. Effective treatments for these diseases exist, and recovery brings improvements in multiple aspects of the individual's life. Substance abuse and addiction are not uncommon comorbidities in patients with cancer, and, at least in the case of alcohol, play a demonstrated role in the etiology of oncologic disease. Assessment for and management of addiction in patients with cancer are necessary to provide optimal nursing care.

Epidemiology

Alcohol use is an extremely common behavior in American society. Approximately half (51%) of Americans age 12 or older (an estimated 120 million people) reported having at least one alcoholic drink in the past 30 days in 2002, according to the National Survey on Drug Use and Health (NSDUH) (Substance Abuse and Mental Health Services Administration [SAMHSA], 2004). More than one-fifth (22.9%) of people age 12 or older participated in binge drinking (drinking five or more drinks on one occasion) at least once in 30 days, 6.7% reported engaging in heavy drinking (five or more drinks on five or more occasions during the past 30 days).

Furthermore, the use of illicit drugs also is widespread in the United States. In 2002, an estimated 19.5 million Americans age 12 or older had used an illicit drug in the month prior to the NSDUH, representing 8.3% of the population older than the age of 11 (SAMHSA, 2004). Marijuana is the most commonly used illicit drug; in 2002, it was used by 75% of the current illicit drug users. Illicit drug use also was associated with the level of alcohol use. Among youths who were heavy drinkers, 67% also were current illicit drug users, whereas among nondrinkers, the rate was only 5.6%.

With repeated use, some alcohol and drug users can develop the neuropsychological diseases known as "substance abuse" and "substance dependence," classified as "substance use disorders" in the *Diagnostic and Statistical Manual of Mental Disorders (DSM-IV-TR)* (American Psychiatric Association [APA], 2000) (see Figure 34-1). The diagnostic criteria for these disorders are largely behavioral in nature (e.g., inability to control use, continued use despite consequences, failure to fulfill role obligations) and are based on alcohol- and drug-induced changes to both the reward and behavioral systems of the brain (described later in this chapter). An estimated 9.4% of Americans age 12 or older were diagnosed with substance dependence or abuse in 2002 (SAMSHA, 2004). Of these, 3.2 million were classified with abuse or dependence of both alcohol and illicit drugs, 3.9 million were dependent on or abused illicit drugs but not alcohol, and 14.9 million were dependent on or abused alcohol but not illicit drugs. Of the 22 million people with a substance use disorder in 2002, approximately half (11.5 million) met the criteria for substance dependence.

At any one point in time, almost 1 out of 10 Americans meets the diagnostic criteria for substance use disorder, making it one of the most common chronic diseases in the United States. It is also one of the most expensive, costing Americans more

---

Figure 34-1. Diagnostic Criteria for Substance Dependence

A maladaptive pattern of substance use, leading to clinically significant impairment or distress, as manifested by three (or more) of the following, occurring at any time in the same 12-month period:
(1) tolerance, as defined by either of the following:
    (a) a need for markedly increased amounts of the substance to achieve intoxication or desired effect
    (b) markedly diminished effect with continued use of the same amount of the substance
(2) withdrawal, as manifested by either of the following:
    (a) the characteristic withdrawal syndrome for the substance
    (b) the same (or a closely related) substance is taken to relieve or avoid withdrawal symptoms
(3) the substance is often taken in larger amounts or over a longer period than was intended
(4) there is a persistent desire or unsuccessful efforts to cut down or control substance use
(5) a great deal of time is spent in activities necessary to obtain the substance (e.g., visiting multiple doctors or driving long distances), use the substance (e.g., chain-smoking), or recover from its effects
(6) important social, occupational, or recreational activities are given up or reduced because of substance use
(7) the substance use is continued despite knowledge of having a persistent or recurrent physical or psychological problem that is likely to have been caused or exacerbated by the substance (e.g., current cocaine use despite recognition of cocaine-induced depression, or continued drinking despite recognition that an ulcer was made worse by alcohol consumption)

Note. From *Diagnostic and Statistical Manual of Mental Disorders* (4th ed., text rev., p. 197), by the American Psychiatric Association, 2000, Washington, DC: Author. Copyright 2000 by American Psychiatric Association. Reprinted with permission.

than $250 billion in 1999 (see Table 34-1). In addition, substance abuse significantly contributes to population morbidity by instances of unintentional injury (especially motor vehicle accidents), fetal exposure, domestic violence, sexual assault, suicide, and homicide. Of the estimated $166 billion of societal costs of alcohol abuse in the United States, $16 billion is directly attributed to healthcare expenditures (National Institute on Drug Abuse, 1998). The White House Office of National Drug Control Policy estimated that between 1995 and 1998, Americans spent $57.3 billion on illicit drugs, representing a clear loss to the U.S. gross national product (National Institute on Drug Abuse, 2005).

Table 34-1. Cost Estimates for Adjusted Costs of Alcohol and Drug Abuse for 1995 (In Billions of 1999 Dollars)

Category	Alcohol	Drugs
Specialty alcohol and drug services	6,660	5,258
Medical consequences	15,830	6,623
Lost earnings—premature death	34,921	16,247
Lost earnings—illness	77,150	17,481
Lost earnings—crime/victims	7,231	43,829
Crashes, fires, criminal justice, etc.	24,752	20,407
Total	166,544	109,845

Note. Based on information from National Institute on Drug Abuse, 2005.

Addictive Disease

As with all chronic diseases, addiction has identifiable risk factors and a demonstrated pathophysiologic basis, can be diagnosed according to a well-described cluster of signs and symptoms, follows a predictable pattern of progression, and can be managed and treated with interventions of known efficacy. Also, as with other diseases, its expression in individual patients is unique and varied, and its negative effects protract onto psychological and social domains. Treatment approaches include pharmacotherapy, cognitive-behavioral skill training, group support, and lifestyle changes.

Addiction is clearly a disease of the brain, much like Parkinson disease, schizophrenia, and depression. All drugs of abuse, including alcohol and nicotine, activate two key pathways in the brain, which are believed to underlie their "addictive" properties (see Figure 34-2). First, drugs and alcohol activate so-called "reward" pathways in subcortical areas extending from the ventral tegmental area (VTA) to

Figure 34-2. Brain Pathways Involved in Addictive Disease

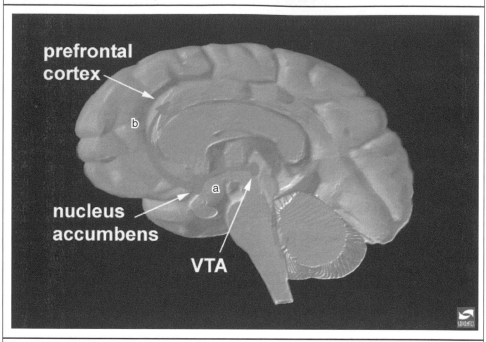

a: The mesolimbic dopaminergic pathway, which provides the rewarding feelings associated with alcohol and drugs of abuse

b: Ascending fibers from the nucleus accumbens to the prefrontal cortex, which lay down powerful behavioral memories in the frontal lobe

VTA—ventral tegmental area

Note. From "The Neurobiology of Drug Addiction," by the National Institute of Drug Abuse, 2002. Retrieved November 24, 2004, from http://www.drugabuse.gov/pubs/teaching/Teaching2/ Teaching3.html

the nucleus accumbens, providing very reinforcing or pleasurable feelings. Next, this reward lays down very strong memories that drive subsequent behaviors to repeat the rewarding experience. Over time, the drug-induced memorized behaviors take over more volitional behaviors to become the predominant behavior state of the diseased individual, and he or she meets the diagnostic criteria of addictive disease.

The term "addiction," as it has thus far been used in this chapter, corresponds to what was previously described as substance dependence, a "maladaptive pattern of substance use, leading to clinically significant impairment or distress" as specified in the *DSM-IV-TR* (APA, 2000, p. 197) (see Figure 34-1). Note that these criteria identify addiction across classes of drugs, provide a temporal context for the disease (symptoms must be present for at least a year), and require the presence of any three indicators to arrive at the diagnosis of substance dependence or addictive disease. It is of diagnostic significance that the first two criteria refer to neurophysiologic consequences, tolerance, and physical dependence (see Table 34-2). Tolerance to and

Table 34-2. Definition of Terms Related to Substance Abuse

Term	Definition
Addiction	An acquired, chronic disease of subcortical brain structures; equivalent to substance dependence as defined in the *Diagnostic and Statistical Manual of Mental Disorders (DSM-IV-TR)* (American Psychiatric Association [APA], 2000). Characterized by a persistent pattern of dysfunctional drug use and aberrant behavior involving loss of control over use and continued use despite adverse physiologic, psychological, and/or social consequences.
Chemical dependence	Physical dependence on a drug or medication (see below).
"Drug seeking"	A set of behaviors in which an individual makes a directed and concerted effort to obtain a drug or medication, which may at times be illegal (e.g., calling for frequent refills of medication, hoarding medication, using multiple providers, augmenting physical complaints, prescription forgery). Appropriate drug seeking may present as pseudoaddiction (Weissman & Haddox, 1989) or therapeutic dependence (Portenoy, 1994). These behaviors do not, in themselves, constitute addiction.
Narcotic	Legal, not pharmacologic, term used in reference to all substances covered by the Single Convention on Narcotic Drugs (1961), including synthetic and naturally occurring opioids and cocaine. Because the term covers a variety of substances with abuse potential, it is considered an obsolete term in the fields of addiction and pain management.
Opioid	Generic term used to refer to all agents, natural or synthetic, endogenous or exogenous, that bind to opioid receptor sites in the central and peripheral nervous system. A broader and increasingly preferred term to *opiate*, which is a pharmacologic term used in reference to substances produced from the poppy plant, specifically, such as codeine and morphine.
Physical dependence	A neuroadaptive state resulting from chronic drug administration in which abrupt cessation of the drug, or administration of an antagonist to the drug, results in a drug-specific withdrawal syndrome. Physical dependence is an expected physiologic occurrence in all individuals in the presence of continuous use of certain drugs for therapeutic or non-therapeutic purposes. It does not, in and of itself, imply addiction.
Substance abuse	The *DSM-IV-TR* (APA, 2000) term for a less severe form of, and often a predecessor to, addiction or substance dependence, distinguished by a shorter duration of impairment and the absence of neurophysiologic symptoms.
Substance dependence	The *DSM-IV-TR* (APA, 2000) term for addiction to a drug or medication defined as a "maladaptive pattern of substance use, leading to clinically significant impairment or distress" (p. 110).
Tolerance	A neuroadaptive state resulting from chronic drug administration that results in diminution of drug effect over time, resulting in the need for increasing amounts of the drug to induce the same effect as obtained with the original dose. Tolerance is an expected physiologic occurrence in all individuals in the presence of continuous use of certain drugs for therapeutic or nontherapeutic purposes. It does not, in and of itself, imply addiction.

physical dependence on drug exposure also may occur in the absence of addiction (i.e., chronic opioid use for analgesia).

The *DSM-IV-TR* (APA, 2000) also recognizes an earlier or less severe form of addictive disease, termed "substance abuse" (defined in Table 34-2). Substance abuse is distinguished from substance dependence by the shorter duration of impairment and the absence of neurophysiologic symptoms. Evident in the diagnostic criteria for both substance abuse and addiction is the multidimensionality of the syndrome. Like cancer, addiction has manifestations in the biologic, psychological, social, and spiritual life of the individual.

Beyond having standardized diagnostic criteria, the nature and course of addictive disease have been well characterized. Specifically, the sufferer of addictive disease also commonly suffers from a concurrent psychiatric illness or disorder. The NSDUH (SAMHSA, 2004) found that serious mental illness (defined as having at some time during the past year a diagnosable mental, behavioral, or emotional disorder that met *DSM-IV-TR* criteria [APA, 2000] and resulted in functional impairment that substantially interfered with or limited one or more major life activities) was highly correlated with substance dependence or abuse. Among adults with substance dependence or abuse, 20.4% had a serious mental illness. In 2002, 23.2% of adults with serious mental illness were dependent on or abused alcohol or illicit drugs, whereas the rate among adults without serious mental illness was only 8.2%. An estimated four million adults met the criteria for both serious mental illness and substance dependence or abuse in 2002 (SAMHSA).

Addiction also is a familial disease. A positive family history of substance abuse, whether for alcohol or other prescribed or illicit drugs, is a risk factor for addictive disease in all clinical populations. Best studied is the case of alcoholism (alcohol being a particularly prevalent drug of abuse across populations and generations). Large surveys of adoptees and twins reared apart from their biologic family of origin have indicated that heredity is a stronger predictor of alcoholism than is environment (Tyndale, 2003). Children of alcoholics and members of certain ethnic groups demonstrated patterned differences in their physiologic responses to alcohol (Evans & Levin, 2003). However, the importance of the family environment in predicting adult drug and alcohol dependence cannot be minimized. First exposure to a drug that might be only mildly rewarding in a neutral or comfortable environment becomes highly rewarding when the individual is experiencing significant or chronic stress, conditions that are likely to be present among families experiencing alcoholism or addiction (Bjarnason et al., 2003).

With respect to the course of addictive disease, relapse is a relatively common occurrence, especially early in the course (i.e., within the first 90 days) of recovery or during times of undue stress (Cami & Farre, 2003; Shalev, Grimm, & Shaham, 2002). Although often considered as a failure or an end point in the treatment of addictive disease, relapse increasingly is considered an exacerbation of a chronic disease or a disease state not under good control. In working with an addicted patient who has relapsed, healthcare professionals must try to minimize the extent of the relapse episode and help the patient to reframe it as a "slip" and a learning opportunity. If relapse is viewed as "part-and-parcel" of recovery as opposed to a treatment failure, positive outcomes are more likely (O'Brien, 2003).

Stress is a primary precipitator of relapse (Lu, Shepard, Hall, & Shaham, 2003; Marlatt & Gordon, 1985); strong psychological reliance on drug use in addicted individuals functions to maintain the behavior. As people become increasingly dependent upon drugs and alcohol, their repertoire of adaptive coping responses to stress narrows, with drug use eventually becoming their primary coping response. Drug- and alcohol-induced memory-driven behaviors are extremely resistant to degradation and, unless the individual has developed alternate behaviors via coping strategies, supports, pharmacologic adjuncts, resources, or skills, drug and alcohol use will resume under stressful situations.

Alcohol and Cancer

The paucity of health studies of self-identified regular illicit drug users over time precludes making conclusions on the role between illicit drugs and cancer. Growing epidemiologic evidence, however, shows that marijuana smoking may put individuals at increased risk for head and neck cancers (Hashibe, Ford, & Zhang, 2002); cannabis smoke contains many of the same carcinogens as tobacco smoke, is mutagenic in microbial assays, and was shown to be carcinogenic in some animal tests (Hall & MacPhee, 2002; Tashkin, Baldwin, Sarafian, Dubinett, & Roth, 2002).

The U.S. Department of Health and Human Services (2005) identified alcoholic beverages as a known human carcinogen in its *Report on Carcinogens, Eleventh Edition.* Considerable evidence suggests that heavy alcohol consumption results in increased risks for cancer (Marmot & Brunner, 1991), with an estimated 2%–4% of all cancer cases thought to be caused either directly or indirectly by alcohol. Oncology nurses, therefore, likely will encounter in their practice some patients who are alcohol abusers or addicts.

The strongest link between alcohol and cancer involves cancers of the upper digestive tract, including the esophagus, the mouth, the pharynx, and the larynx. Chronic heavy drinkers have a higher incidence of esophageal cancer than that of the general population. The risk appears to increase as alcohol consumption increases. An estimated 75% of esophageal cancers in the United States are attributable to chronic, excessive alcohol consumption. Nearly 50% of cancers of the mouth, pharynx, and larynx are associated with heavy drinking. People who drink large quantities of alcohol over time have an increased risk of these cancers as compared to abstainers (National Institute on Alcohol Abuse and Alcoholism [NIAAA], 1993).

Less-consistent data link alcohol consumption to cancers of the liver, breast, and colon. Prolonged, heavy drinking has been associated with primary liver cancer; however, it is liver cirrhosis, whether caused by alcohol or another factor, that is thought to induce cancer. Chronic alcohol consumption has been associated with a small (approximately 10%) increase in women's risk of breast cancer. According to NIAAA (1993), the risk appears to increase as the quantity and duration of alcohol consumption increase. Epidemiologic studies have found a small but consistent dose-dependent association between alcohol consumption and colorectal cancer, even when controlling for fiber and other dietary factors. Despite the large number of studies, however, causality cannot be determined from the available data. Together, the cancers linked to heavy alcohol use kill more than 125,000 people annually in the United States (NIAAA).

Alcohol as a Cocarcinogen

In addition to its role as a carcinogen, alcohol may act as a cocarcinogen by enhancing the carcinogenic effects of other chemicals. For example, studies indicate that alcohol enhances tobacco's ability to stimulate tumor formation in rats (NIAAA, 1993). In humans, the risk for oral, tracheal, and esophageal cancers is 35 times greater for people who both smoke and drink than for people who neither smoke nor drink, implying a cocarcinogenic interaction between alcohol and tobacco-related carcinogens. At least in the case of alcohol addiction, substance abuse and dependence are causative factors in the development of oncologic disease (NIAAA).

Treatment Compliance

The care plan of a patient receiving treatment for oncologic disease typically includes recommendations for adequate activity and rest, good nutrition and water intake, the adding of new medications to daily regimens, and the scheduling of multiple appointments with multiple specialists—a number of new behavioral changes that the patient must integrate into his or her daily life. The behavioral repertoire of the actively addicted patient is relatively narrow, as "a great deal of time is spent in activities necessary to obtain the substance . . . , use the substance . . . , or recover from its effects" (APA, 2000, p. 197). The patient may not have the ability to integrate new treatment-related behaviors into a substance-using lifestyle, may not take medications as scheduled, or may miss appointments. Drug and alcohol use may continue at the expense of adequate nutritional intake and restful sleep. Ongoing drug and alcohol addiction precludes optimal adherence to the cancer treatment plan, which ultimately results in poorer outcomes.

Surgical Outcomes

Often, the treatment of oncologic disease includes surgical intervention. Alcohol exerts chronic toxic effects on immune, cardiac, and hematopoietic function, and rates of postoperative morbidity and mortality resulting from infection, cardiopulmonary insufficiency, or bleeding disorders are two to five times greater in alcohol-dependent patients than in the general surgical population. Accordingly, alcoholics require prolonged intensive care unit treatment and overall hospital stays (Spies, Tonnesen, Andreasson, Helander, & Conigrave, 2001) related to preoperative immune suppression, preoperative subclinical cardiomyopathy, and preoperative altered coagulation, in addition to common comorbidities such as nicotine and illicit drug abuse, coronary artery disease, nutritional deficiencies, and liver disease. The high prevalence of alcohol abuse in surgical patients and the significant morbidity associated with chronic alcohol ingestion require that nurses assess for the presence of alcohol abuse and dependence in all surgical patients with cancer (Compton, 2002). Less is known about the surgical outcomes of illicit drug users specifically.

Interactions With Immunosuppressive Therapies

With respect to the effects of drugs and alcohol on the immune system, the effects of alcohol have been the most studied. Both stimulant and opioid abuse appear to have immunosuppressant effects, but it is difficult to rule out the effects of the drug-abusing lifestyle in human models. Some experimental evidence supports that cannabinol suppresses T-cell function and cell-mediated immunity (Tashkin et al., 2002).

Alcoholism has clearly been associated with suppression of the human immune system; therefore, chronic alcohol abusers who are receiving immunosuppressive therapy are more susceptible to various infections. Alcohol abusers have been shown to be more susceptible than nonabusers to septicemia, most commonly originating from pneumonia, urinary tract infections, or bacterial peritonitis. Alcoholics appear to be more susceptible than nonalcoholics to several less common infections, such as lung abscess, empyema, spontaneous bacterial peritonitis, diphtheria, cellulitis, and meningitis.

Parenteral drug use brings with it a host of other immunologic considerations. Injection of infectious particulates can cause inflammation and infection proximate to (cellulitis) or distant to (infective endocarditis) the site of injection. Repeat injection drug users commonly present with immunologic abnormalities, viral hepatitis and liver disease, and HIV infection. They also often present with pneumonia and sexually transmitted diseases. Although beyond the scope of this chapter, people in a severely immunocompromised state as a result of their addictive disease will need carefully managed immunosuppressive therapy.

Assessment for Addiction in Patients With Cancer

Because of the impact of addictive disease on cancer and cancer treatment, assessment for its presence in patients with cancer is an important aspect of nursing practice. The first goal is to determine whether the patient has a history of substance abuse, and then to determine whether he or she is actively abusing, is in drug-free recovery, or is being medically maintained (e.g., methadone) in recovery. Assessment should begin at diagnosis with the CAGE screening tool, a simple and easily administered four-item instrument with excellent reliability, validity, and specificity (see Figure 34-3). A "yes" response to one question is cause for suspicion of a current alcohol or drug problem; more than one "yes" is a strong indication that a problem exists.

When taking a patient's history, nurses should use a matter-of-fact approach and explain that drinking alcohol or using certain medications or drugs can influence responses to cancer medications and treatment. In addition to the medical history,

---

Figure 34-3. The CAGE Questionnaire
• Have you ever felt you could **Cut** down on your drinking (drug use)?   • Have people **Annoyed** you by criticizing your drinking (drug use)?   • Have you ever felt bad or **Guilty** about your drinking (drug use)?   • Have you ever had an **Eye-opener** first thing in the morning to steady your nerves or get rid of a hangover?
Note. Based on information from Ewing, 1984.

patients need to answer questions regarding substance use patterns (e.g., onset, frequency, types, amounts, circumstances of use). Current use, including the last episode, needs to be explored. A family history that explores the presence of addiction is necessary. Questions regarding legal problems, employment, and social and sexual history must be asked. Nurses must inquire about psychiatric history, including prior treatment for addiction, depression, and suicide attempts, and also should note obvious signs of intoxication or withdrawal. Other signs of substance abuse disorders, such as the medical sequelae of abuse (e.g., liver dysfunction), can aid in identification of chemically dependent patients.

With patients who are in drug-free recovery, nurses should ask them for how long and under what circumstances they have been drug free. The primary substance of abuse should be noted, as well as any current relationship with a support/recovery group and/or sponsor. Patients' concerns about exposure to potentially addicting pain medications over the course of treatment should be explored. For patients who are taking methadone for the treatment of opioid addiction, nurses should note the daily dose of methadone the patient receives and, with the patient's permission, initiate contact with the methadone clinic nurse. Patients should be assured that methadone therapy for the treatment of addiction will continue throughout cancer treatment and will not interfere with the provision of adequate analgesia as needed.

One of the most difficult challenges for clinicians is identifying patients who currently are addicted and are either in denial about the problem or do not want to disclose the behavior to healthcare personnel. Vague or inconsistent responses to specific questions about substance abuse should be explored. Red flags on history include trauma in higher frequency than expected, single-vehicle accidents, seizures with onset between ages 10 and 30, family history of addictive disease, sexual abuse as a child, prior history of addictive disease, and a psychiatric history. Laboratory markers, such as mean corpuscular volume, gamma-glutamyl-transferase, and, increasingly, carbohydrate-deficient transferrin, provide evidence of the toxic effects of chronic alcohol abuse on body tissues and function but do not prove that the patient is physically dependent on alcohol (Compton, 2002). As noted, immunologic abnormalities may be noted in parenteral drug users.

One of the surest ways to determine whether a patient's social or recreational drug or alcohol use constitutes a disorder is to ask the patient to limit or curtail his or her use of the substance for a given period of time (e.g., limit intake of alcohol to one glass of wine per evening for two weeks). If the patient is unable to control his or her use, a substance use disorder should be considered.

Pain-Related Drug Seeking

Individuals seek and obtain drugs for myriad reasons, only one of which is because they are addicted. Although clear in the case of drugs that have no psychoactive effect (e.g., antibiotics, nonopioid analgesics), the distinction between appropriate drug seeking and addiction becomes less apparent when a patient seeks a drug with a known abuse potential (e.g., an opioid analgesic), regardless of the apparent validity of the complaint. The confusion is exemplified in the case of opioid analgesic–seeking by a person who is in pain, as the severity of pain suffered cannot be objectively quantified but only subjectively reported (Compton & Athanasos, 2003).

Patients with pain may take what appear to be extraordinary steps to ensure adequate medication supply, but, rather than indicating addictive disease, these may, in fact, be appropriate responses to either under-relieved or well-relieved pain. In the case of the former, drug-seeking behaviors arise when a patient cannot obtain tolerable relief with the prescribed dose of analgesic and seeks alternate sources or increased doses, a phenomenon called "pseudoaddiction" (Weissman & Haddox, 1989). Alternatively, patients receiving good pain relief may demonstrate drug-seeking behaviors because they fear not only the reemergence of pain but also, perhaps, the emergence of withdrawal symptoms. Rather than indicating addictive disease, such behaviors, termed "therapeutic dependence" (Portenoy, 1994), are actually the efforts of an anxious patient to maintain a tolerable level of comfort. Clearly, even in the case of highly addictive drugs, drug seeking may not indicate addiction. Unfortunately, some healthcare professionals continue to view such behaviors as abuse or addiction in patients without considering that they may be seeking opioid analgesics for pain relief (Compton, Darakjian, & Miotto, 1998; Compton & Estepa, 2000).

Approaches to Addiction in Patients With Cancer

The treatment of addictive disease is beyond the scope of oncology nursing practice, but the ongoing nature of the relationship between oncology nurses and patients provides an ideal therapeutic setting to support recovery efforts. First, via assessment and case identification strategies discussed previously, oncology nurses initiate the addiction treatment process by referring patients for a formal addiction evaluation. Many oncology groups and clinics have psychiatrists and psychologist affiliates to whom such referrals are made; in other settings, referrals are made to community mental health centers or clinics. As shown in Figure 34-4, self-help groups and outpatient rehabilitation are the most common types of treatment provided for substance abusers, and payment for treatment is fairly evenly divided between insurance providers and patients' savings (see Figures 34-5 and 34-6).

The diagnosis of cancer may be enough to motivate some individuals to enter drug or alcohol treatment, but this is not always the case. In some cases, it is necessary, before nurses refer a patient to drug treatment, that the patient acknowledges that drug use has become problematic and that treatment is necessary. A powerful strategy that oncology nurses can use to prepare patients for drug treatment, as well as to support their efforts at recovery, is an interpersonal technique known as "motivational interviewing" (Miller & Rollnick, 1991) (see Figure 34-7). Motivational interviewing consists of a set of formalized, theory-based, and empirically evaluated interpersonal communication techniques designed to help patients to identify and acknowledge substance-abusing behaviors and to move toward cessation of these behaviors (Beich, Thorsen, & Rollnick, 2003; Compton, Monahan, & Simmons-Cody, 1999).

Motivational interviewing relies on nonconfrontational approaches, which ideally result in patients, rather than nurses, eliciting concerns about alcohol or drug use and expressing the need to reduce or cease substance intake. Using these techniques, the reality of relapse in addictive disease is acknowledged and,

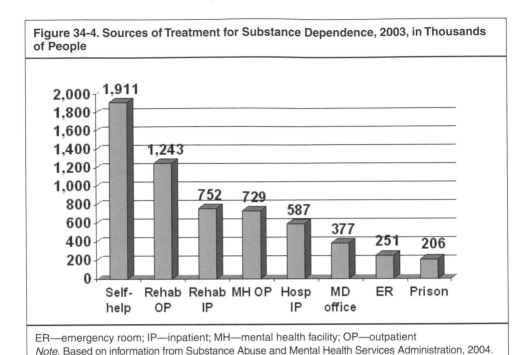

Figure 34-4. Sources of Treatment for Substance Dependence, 2003, in Thousands of People

ER—emergency room; IP—inpatient; MH—mental health facility; OP—outpatient
Note. Based on information from Substance Abuse and Mental Health Services Administration, 2004.

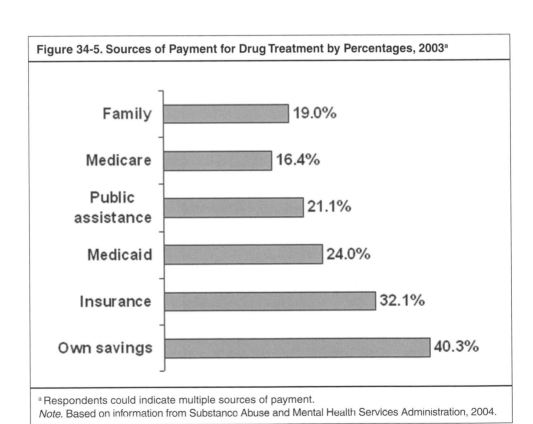

Figure 34-5. Sources of Payment for Drug Treatment by Percentages, 2003[a]

[a] Respondents could indicate multiple sources of payment.
Note. Based on information from Substance Abuse and Mental Health Services Administration, 2004.

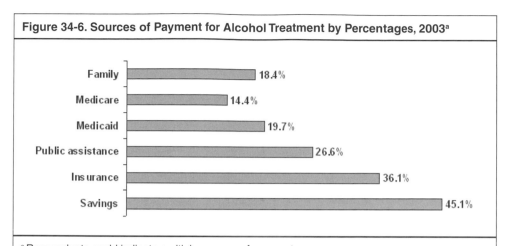

Figure 34-6. Sources of Payment for Alcohol Treatment by Percentages, 2003[a]

Family — 18.4%
Medicare — 14.4%
Medicaid — 19.7%
Public assistance — 26.6%
Insurance — 36.1%
Savings — 45.1%

[a] Respondents could indicate multiple sources of payment.
Note. Based on information from Substance Abuse and Mental Health Services Administration, 2004.

rather than considered a failure, is viewed as a potential opportunity to move patients toward more healthful outcomes. Further, the techniques central to motivational interviewing are consistent with those demonstrated to be effective in brief intervention settings, making motivational interviewing an ideal intervention for the relatively short and episodic patterns of care that are characteristic of oncologic nursing (Burke, Arkowitz, & Menchola, 2003; Miller & Johnson, 2001).

Figure 34-7. Eight Motivational Interviewing Strategies

A. Giving **A**dvice
B. Removing **B**arriers
C. Providing **C**hoice
D. Decreasing **D**esirability
E. Practicing **E**mpathy
F. Providing **F**eedback
G. Clarifying **G**oals
H. Active **H**elping

Note. Based on information from Miller & Rollnick, 1991.

Motivational interviewing techniques take into account what is known about the stages of behavioral change as described by Prochaska and DiClemente (1982). Acknowledging that people proceed through a predictable sequence of stages (see Table 34-3) in achieving and maintaining a behavioral change, Miller and Rollnick (1991) conceptualized a "wheel of change" illustrating the steps individuals go through toward changing problematic drug or alcohol use. In this conceptualization, five stages are shown on the wheel, with a sixth, the precontemplation stage, lying outside the wheel as the entry point to change. The circular nature of these stages reflects the revolving nature of change and the fact that people typically have to go around the wheel multiple times (average is between four and seven times) before maintaining the change. Thus, relapse to alcohol or drug use is recognized as a distinct stage of change, not a failure to change; if approached appropriately, relapse can result in a renewed and refined change effort.

Nurses must understand that different nursing skills and interpersonal techniques are required at different stages; patients just beginning to accept that they may have a problem with alcohol intake (in the precontemplation or contemplation stages) require different motivational approaches from nurses than people engaging in

Table 34-3. Motivational Tasks by Stages of Change

Client Stage	Definition	Clinician's Motivational Tasks
Precontemplation	The entry stage to the process of change; the patient may not even recognize that his or her use of alcohol or drugs is problematic and thus is not considering a behavioral change. A patient in this stage needs information and feedback to be delivered in a nonconfrontational manner to raise his or her awareness of a problem and the possibility of change.	Raise doubt—increase the client's perception of risks and problems with current behavior.
Contemplation	The first stage of change; the patient is willing to consider that his or her use of drugs or alcohol may constitute a problem and that changing this behavior may be necessary. Characterized by ambivalence.	Tip the balance—evoke reasons to change and explain the risks of not changing; strengthen the client's self-efficacy for change of current behavior.
Determination	Occurs when the patient expresses a commitment to take action and decides to take steps to stop the problem behavior. May be transient, and, if not capitalized upon, the patient can slip back into the contemplation stage.	Help the client to determine the best course of action to take in seeking change.
Action	The agreed-upon change strategy is implemented, and the role of the clinician is to enhance or maintain the patient's sense of self-efficacy, praise accomplishments, and attribute successes to the capabilities of the patient. The action stage usually lasts three to six months with most addicted patients.	Help the client to take steps toward change.
Maintenance	Once the new behavior patterns initiated in the action stage become firmly established, the patient is described as having entered the maintenance stage. To maintain the change, the patient must adopt a new set of skills and behavior patterns, which are different from those needed to initiate a change. To be successful, these behaviors must include strategies to prevent relapse.	Help the client to identify and use strategies to prevent relapse.
Relapse	Relapses are normal and expected as individuals attempt to change a long-standing behavior to which they have multiple and powerful attachments.	Help the client to renew the processes of contemplation, determination, and action, without becoming stuck or demoralized because of relapse.

Note. Based on information from Miller & Rollnick, 1991.

activities to bring about change (action stage). If interventional techniques that are appropriate for one stage are applied at another, the likely patient response is resistance to change, commonly interpreted as a "lack of motivation." In fact, if resistance is encountered, the stage of change likely has been misidentified by the nurse and requires reassessment. By recognizing what stage patients are in with respect to changing their addictive behavior, oncology nurses can use interactions with patients as opportunities to enhance their motivation for change. For example, for an actively using patient in the precontemplation stage, the nurse can show the patient altered liver enzyme laboratory reports, whereas for the newly diagnosed patient in the maintenance stage, the nurse can help the patient to intensify recovery supports.

Substance Abuse and Palliative Care

As patients reach the end of life, it is hoped that the disease of addiction is under control and that their palliative care experience includes recovery, bringing with it improved familial relationships, functionality, and insight. Adequate comfort without undue sedation is another desired outcome for the palliative care of patients with addictive disease, and the use of potentially addicting drugs (e.g., opioids) poses special consideration in patients with cancer. The remainder of this chapter will discuss the principles of pain management for palliative care patients with addictive disease.

Pain and Addiction

For more than 25 years, researchers have known that the parts of the brain that mediate pain and pleasure overlap neuroanatomically and neurophysiologically via endogenous and exogenous opioids, suggesting that individuals who have altered opioid-related reward pathways because of addictive disease may have altered pain pathways as well. In other words, the substance abuser's experience of pain may be different from that of a nonabuser.

In particular, evidence supports that the presence of addiction worsens the pain experience. Savage and Schofferman (1995) wrote that addiction results in a "syndrome of pain facilitation," in which discomfort is augmented by subtle withdrawal syndromes, intoxication or withdrawal-related sympathetic arousal or muscular tension, sleep disturbance, affective changes, or functional changes. Experimental pain data support decreased pain tolerance in males currently using opioids or cocaine as compared to patients in recovery and matched normal controls (Compton, 1994; Compton, Charuvastra, Kintaudi, & Ling, 2000). It may be that addictive disease decreases one's ability to endure discomfort.

In the case of opioid addiction, clear effects on pain systems and pain management are evident. With respect to the provision of opioid analgesics, the effects of opioid tolerance (see Table 34-2) must be considered. Several factors are involved in the development of tolerance. The liver attempts to adapt by increasing hepatic enzyme activity for detoxification. Tolerance of this type is called pharmacokinetic tolerance. Cellular adaptation is a type of functional tolerance that takes place when changes occur in neurotransmitters as a result of repeated use of a substance. Behavioral tolerance develops in substance-dependent individuals over time as their behavior adapts so they can remain functional. Patients who are actively abusing opioids or who are participating in a methadone maintenance program will have some degree of pharmacokinetic and functional tolerance and, apparently, analgesic tolerance. The abused or prescribed opioid provides little, if any, pain relief. Patients on methadone typically need analgesic doses slightly higher than nonaddicted patients, in addition to their daily methadone dose, to manage pain.

It appears that as tolerance for morphine (or other full μ agonists) develops in the absence of pain, as would be the case for opioid addiction, an appreciable degree of opioid-induced hyperalgesia also develops. In other words, people with an opioid addiction are more sensitive to pain than they were prior to opioid exposure, a finding that has been repeatedly demonstrated in animal models and correlated with methadone maintenance in human samples. As theorized mechanisms of tolerance and opioid-induced hyperalgesia merge, what was previously defined as "analgesic tolerance" may become recognized as the opponent process of hyperalgesia (Compton & Anthanasos, 2003). It is possible that the pain an opioid-dependent patient with cancer experiences is complicated by such hyperalgesic states.

Pain Treatment and Addiction

As previously discussed, the presence of addiction might alter the pain experience of patients with cancer, and untreated alcohol or drug abuse or dependence likely complicates the pain experience. How might the treatment of the substance abuser's pain with opioids actually protect the patient from addiction? First, as previously mentioned, one of the best known precipitators for relapse of addictive disease, regardless of the substance, is stress. Poorly or inadequately treated pain is a significant stressor that easily can lead the individual to seek relief or comfort with the substance that provided relief and comfort before. Likewise, unmanaged stress, anxiety, and depression in patients with cancer increase the risk of relapse.

Also, the fact that palliative care patients are taking opioids while in states of moderate to severe pain actually may protect them from some of the so-called "addictive" qualities of opioid medications. The nervous system of a person in pain does not appear to respond to opioids in quite the same way as the nervous system of a person not in pain (i.e., the state in which an addict would use it). Under conditions of acute pain, animals developed significantly less morphine analgesic tolerance and significantly less morphine physical withdrawal symptoms (Vaccarino et al., 1993), and humans reported significantly less opioid reward or euphoria (Zacny et al., 1996) than pain-free models. Under chronic pain conditions, patients who abruptly stopped taking opioids evidenced little physical dependence or withdrawal with ongoing pain (Brown, Glass, & Park, 2002). Taking opioids in the presence of pain appears to mitigate their addictive potential.

Managing Pain in Substance Abusers

Managing the pain of substance abusers has historically been complicated by several factors, but thankfully less so in the realm of palliative care. Prescribing opioids to people with addiction has been restricted by a generalized "opiophobia" because of the addictive potential of the opioids, regulatory sanctions for opioid prescribing practices, punitive moral and social views of addiction, and clinician concerns about being "duped" into providing an opioid to an addict. Palliative care nurses must remember to consider an addicted patient like any other patient with a coexisting medical condition; specific interventions may have to be modified while still working toward the goal of providing adequate pain relief.

For an actively addicted patient, it is important to first build trust. Openly acknowledge the patient's history of addiction, and allow the patient to discuss fears about how this may affect pain management from and treatment by staff. Respect and believe the patient's report of pain, keeping in mind that a person with active addictive disease is likely to be less tolerant of pain than nonaddicted patients. Aggressively treat reports of pain; remember that provision of adequate analgesia in this population carries the additional benefit of averting relapse and, although not the priority during acute pain periods, makes the patient more receptive to addiction treatment interventions. If opioids will be self-administered, the treatment plan should be broadened to include an opioid treatment contract that enables careful monitoring of opiate use, including the use of a single provider, urine toxicology screens, and methods of obtaining rescue doses. Consultation from an addiction medicine specialist should be initiated if possible, and analgesic use and response should be documented carefully.

With respect to providing opioid analgesics to palliative care patients with a history of addictive disease, many principles are the same as with other patients. Choose long-acting opioids with gradual onset of action, administered around the clock. Consider patient-controlled analgesia; not only does it decrease total opioid requirements, but it also decreases drug-seeking behaviors and is not abused by substance abusers (Paige, Preble, Watrous, Kaalaas-Sittig, & Compton, 1994). Intervene to prevent physically dependent people from going through withdrawal. During opioid withdrawal, opioid-induced hyperalgesia is most pronounced; thus, patients will be very pain-sensitive during withdrawal (Compton & Athanasos, 2003). If the patient is physically dependent on opioids or is on methadone, do not administer mixed opioid agonist/antagonist analgesics, as this will precipitate opioid withdrawal. If the patient is physically dependent on opioids, alcohol, or sedative hypnotics, provide long-acting substitute medications to prevent withdrawal. If substitution therapy is provided, monitor for emergence of withdrawal symptoms at least every four hours, and treat aggressively and symptomatically. Remember that it is illegal to provide opioids to a known opioid addict for the treatment of addiction but not for the treatment of pain. If pain states improve, taper opioids slowly to minimize the emergence of withdrawal symptoms.

If patients are methadone-maintained, continue their daily methadone dose for the treatment of the addictive disease, and provide opioids for pain control as you would for any other patient, titrating to effect. It is helpful to maintain contact with the methadone clinic nurse and coordinate care as end-of-life needs change. Studies are lacking on the treatment of pain in patients maintained on alternate opioid agonist therapies (levo-alpha-acetylmethodol, buprenorphine); at this point, it is recommended that patients be transferred to an equivalent dose of methadone under the supervision of a certified addiction medicine specialist and maintained on methadone.

For patients in recovery, it also is very important to build trust. Openly acknowledge their history of addiction, and allow patients, families, and staff to discuss fears of relapse. Explain any intent to use opioids or other psychoactive medications, and respect patients' rights to decide whether to take opioids for pain relief. It is important to educate patients about the health risks associated with unrelieved pain, including the risk of relapse, and to reassure them that the known risk for addiction to opioids in the context of pain appears to be low, informing that if they decide against opioid analgesia now, they can always opt for this treatment in the future.

During this stressful time, oncology nurses should broaden the treatment plan to support patients' recovery efforts and include their recovery program or sponsor in patients' care when possible. Stress relief interventions should be offered. Again, an addiction medicine specialist and the use of support groups (12-step or otherwise) may assist in patients' recovery. Keep in mind that a relapse may occur during this stressful time period, but the goal of the palliative care nurse is to minimize the extent of the lapse and get the patient back to the determination stage of the wheel of change.

Conclusion

Addiction is a chronic, relapsing disease that affects up to 10% of the general population and a somewhat higher rate of patients with cancer. Untreated symptoms or exacerbations of the disease have health implications ranging from bleeding disorders to family violence and motor vehicle accidents. The effects of addiction certainly complicate the course of cancer treatment in multiple domains, specifically with patients' ability to comply with prescribed regimens and to achieve good surgical or immunosuppressive therapeutic outcomes. For these reasons, oncology nurses must take a leadership role in assessing for and identifying addictive disease in patients with cancer and work to be a motivational force in patients' process of changing their addictive behavior. With an understanding that pain and addiction systems are interrelated, palliative care nurses can provide aggressive and appropriate pain care to individuals with addictive disease in the manner most likely to control its symptoms.

Special thanks to Christine Rodemich, RN, MS, CSPMH, CSFNP, CARN, who served as the author of this chapter in the first edition.

References

American Psychiatric Association. (2000). *Diagnostic and statistical manual of mental disorders* (4th ed., text rev.). Washington, DC: Author.

Beich, A., Thorsen, T., & Rollnick, S. (2003). Screening in brief intervention trials targeting excessive drinkers in general practice: Systematic review and meta-analysis. *BMJ, 327,* 536–542.

Bjarnason, T., Andersson, B., Choquet, M., Elekes, Z., Morgan, M., & Rapinett, G. (2003). Alcohol culture, family structure and adolescent alcohol use: Multilevel modeling of frequency of heavy drinking among 15–16 year old students in 11 European countries. *Journal on the Study of Alcohol, 64,* 200–208.

Brown, S.C., Glass, J.M., & Park, D.C. (2002). The relationship of pain and depression to cognitive function in rheumatoid arthritis patients. *Pain, 96,* 279–284.

Burke, B.L., Arkowitz, H., & Menchola, M.J. (2003). The efficacy of motivational interviewing: A meta-analysis of controlled clinical trials. *Consulting Clinical Psychology, 71,* 843–861.

Cami, J., & Farre, M. (2003). Drug addiction. *New England Journal of Medicine, 349,* 975–986.

Compton, M. (1994). Cold pressor pain tolerance in opiate and cocaine abusers: Correlates of drug type and use status. *Journal of Pain and Symptom Management, 9,* 462–473.

Compton, P. (2002). Caring for an alcohol-dependent patient. *Nursing, 32,* 58–64.

Compton, P., & Athanasos, P. (2003). Chronic pain, substance abuse and addiction. *Nursing Clinics of North America, 38,* 525–537.

Compton, P., Charuvastra, V.C., Kintaudi, K., & Ling, W. (2000). Pain responses in methadone-maintained opioid abusers. *Journal of Pain and Symptom Management, 20,* 237–245.

Compton, P., Darakjian, J., & Miotto, K. (1998). Screening for addiction in patients with chronic pain with "problematic" substance use: Evaluation of a pilot assessment tool. *Journal of Pain and Symptom Management, 16,* 355–363.

Compton, P., & Estepa, C. (2000). Differential diagnosis: Addiction in patients with chronic pain. *Lippincott's Primary Care Practice, 4,* 254–272.

Compton, P., Monahan, G., & Simmons-Cody, H. (1999). Motivational interviewing: An effective brief intervention for alcohol and drug abuse patients. *Nurse Practitioner, 24*(11), 27–47.

Evans, S.M., & Levin, F.R. (2003). Response to alcohol in females with a paternal history of alcoholism. *Psychopharmacology, 169,* 10–20.

Ewing, J.A. (1984). Detecting alcoholism: The CAGE questionnaire. *JAMA, 252,* 1905–1907.

Hall, W., & MacPhee, D. (2002). Cannabis use and cancer. *Addiction, 97,* 243–252.

Hashibe, M., Ford, D.E., & Zhang, Z.F. (2002). Marijuana smoking and head and neck cancer. *Journal of Clinical Pharmacology, 42*(Suppl. 11), 103S–107S.

Lu, L., Shepard, J.D., Hall, F.S., & Shaham, Y. (2003). Effect of environmental stressors on opiate and psychostimulant reinforcement, reinstatement and discrimination in rats: A review. *Neuroscience and Biobehavior Reviews, 27,* 457–491.

Marlatt, G.A., & Gordon, J.R. (1985). *Relapse prevention.* New York: Guilford Press.

Marmot, M., & Brunner, E. (1991). Alcohol and cardiovascular disease: The status of the U shaped curve. *BMJ, 303,* 565–568.

Miller, C.E., & Johnson, J.L. (2001). Motivational interviewing. *Canadian Nurse, 97*(7), 32–33.

Miller, W.R., & Rollnick, S. (1991). *Motivational interviewing: Preparing people to change addictive behavior.* New York: Guilford Press.

National Institute on Alcohol Abuse and Alcoholism. (1993, July). *Alcohol and cancer* (Alcohol alert No. 21 PH 345). Bethesda, MD: Author.

National Institute on Drug Abuse. (1998, September). *The economic costs of alcohol and drug abuse in the United States, 1992* (NIH Publication No. 98-4327). Bethesda, MD: Author.

National Institute on Drug Abuse. (2005, March). *The economic costs of alcohol and drug abuse in the United States, 1992.* Retrieved June 30, 2005, from http://www.nida.nih.gov/EconomicCosts/Table1_4.html

O'Brien, C.P. (2003). Research advances in the understanding and treatment of addiction. *American Journal of Addiction, 12*(Suppl. 2), S36–S47.

Paige, D., Preble, L., Watrous, G., Kaalaas-Sittig, J., & Compton, P. (1994). PCA use in cocaine abusing patients. *American Journal of Pain Management, 4,* 101–105.

Portenoy, R.K. (1994). Opioid therapy for chronic non-malignant pain: Current status. In H.L. Fields & J.C. Liebskind (Eds.), *Progress in pain research and management* (pp. 247–287). Seattle, WA: IASP Press.

Prochaska, J.O., & DiClemente, C.C. (1982). Transtheoretical therapy: Toward a more integrative model of change. *Psychotherapy: Theory, Research and Practice, 19,* 276–288.

Savage, S.R., & Schofferman, J. (1995). Pharmacological therapies of pain in drug and alcohol addictions. In N.S. Miller & M.S. Gold (Eds.), *Pharmacological therapies for drug and alcohol addiction* (pp. 373–409). New York: Marcel Decker.

Shalev, U., Grimm, J.W., & Shaham, Y. (2002). Neurobiology of relapse to heroin and cocaine seeking: A review. *Pharmacology Review, 54,* 1–42.

Spies, C., Tonnesen, H., Andreasson, S., Helander, A., & Conigrave, K. (2001). Perioperative morbidity and mortality in chronic alcoholic patients. *Alcoholism, Clinical and Experimental Research, 25*(5 Suppl. ISBRA), 164S–170S.

Substance Abuse and Mental Health Services Administration. (2004). *Results from the 2003 National Survey on Drug Use and Health* (NSDUH Series H-25, DHHS Publication No. SMA 04-3964). Rockville, MD: Author. Retrieved June 30, 2005, from http://oas.samhsa.gov/nsduh.htm#NSDUH

Tashkin, D.R., Baldwin, G.C., Sarafian, T., Dubinett, S., & Roth, M.D. (2002). Respiratory and immunologic consequences of marijuana smoking. *Journal of Clinical Pharmacology, 42*(Suppl. 11), 71S–81S.

Tyndale, R.F. (2003). Genetics of alcohol and tobacco use in humans. *Annals of Internal Medicine, 35,* 94–121.

U.S. Department of Health and Human Services. (2005, January). *Report on carcinogens, eleventh edition.* Research Triangle Park, NC: National Toxicology Program.

Vaccarino, A.L., Marek, P., Kest, B., Ben-Eliyahu, S., Couret, L.C., Jr., Kao, B., et al. (1993). Morphine fails to produce tolerance when administered in the presence of formalin pain in rats. *Brain Research, 627,* 287–290.

Weissman, D.E., & Haddox, J.D. (1989). Opioid pseudoaddiction—An iatrogenic syndrome. *Pain, 36,* 363–366.

Zacny, J.P., McKay, M.A., Toledano, A.Y., Marks, S., Young, C.J., Klock, P.A., et al. (1996). The effects of a cold-water immersion stressor on the reinforcing and subjective effects of fentanyl in healthy volunteers. *Drug and Alcohol Dependence, 42,* 133–142.

SECTION VI

Caring for the Caregiver

CHAPTER 35

Stress Management for Oncology Nurses: Finding a Healing Balance

DALE G. LARSON, PHD, AND NANCY JO BUSH, RN, MN, MA, AOCN®

> *We are shaped and fashioned by what we love.*
>
> —Goethe

> *Joan, my patient with ovarian cancer, had a fistula. It was so upsetting to her to have constant drainage of stool from her vagina. She was spending most of her time in the bathroom. She was filled with anxiety and tears. I went into the bathroom with her and sat on the floor in front of her and we cried together. "How could this happen to me?" she asked. I responded, "I don't know, but I'm with you, and I care." And she knew it. It was beautiful.* (Larson, 1992)

This inspiring vignette shared by an oncology nurse captures both the challenges and rewards of oncology nursing. It also raises important issues. How can this nurse continue to be emotionally involved with Joan and other patients without burning out? How will the nurse cope with Joan's death if treatment fails? And how can this experience contribute to the nurse's personal growth, strengthening connections with others and appreciation of life?

This chapter will address these questions while examining two related aspects of oncology nursing: the adaptive demands of the work and the rewards it can offer. The chapter begins with a look at oncology nurses and some of the key stressors in their work. Then, it explores the variety of emotional experiences that can result from frequent confrontations with loss and trauma. It concludes by offering strategies for enhancing stress management and promoting personal growth.

Stress, Coping, and Oncology Nurses

Oncology nursing often attracts individuals who seek a sense of purpose in their work. The nature of the work acts as a powerful screening device that selects idealistic, altruistic, committed, and empathic individuals. For these individuals, helping others expresses deep values and personal goals and contributes to the sense of purpose and significance in their lives.

These personal qualities are a double-edged sword. In an early study investigating stress in nurse caregivers, Stotland, Mathews, Sherman, Hansson, and Richardson (1978) found that beginning nurses who scored highest on a measure of empathic capacity were the first to leave the rooms of patients who were dying. However, after receiving support and advice on how to relate to patients more effectively, these same nurses eventually spent the greatest amounts of time with patients and were highly successful. The psychological impact of caring for patients with cancer can be overwhelming, especially for beginning nurses who are acclimating to their new roles. If the appropriate and needed emotional and social support is not in place, the oncology nurse may never learn the coping skills necessary for personal and professional survival (Medland, Howard-Ruben, & Whitaker, 2004). The availability of this support is especially crucial because the idealism and altruism that fuel caregiving often are compounded by a sense of invulnerability, with caregivers not recognizing the implications their work has for their own health and welfare (Alexander & Klein, 2001).

As the Stotland et al. (1978) study illustrates, a high level of empathy is simultaneously a great asset and a point of real vulnerability. To be truly effective and emotionally present, caregivers must put their empathy to work, but they also must acknowledge their weaknesses (Alexander & Klein, 2001; Saakvitne & Pearlman, 1996). They face the challenge of finding a way to use this deep empathy and powerful commitment to help others without burning out. The greater one's commitment, the more vulnerable one is to psychological stress in the area of that commitment (Lazarus & Folkman, 1984). Therefore, highly motivated oncology nurses are more susceptible to burnout if they perceive that they are not moving toward their care goals and do not see a way to do so. For these reasons, idealistic, highly motivated, and highly empathic helpers often are the first to burn out, as does a bright flame by virtue of its intensity (Larson, 1993a).

Stressors in Health Care and Oncology Nursing

Oncology nurses must try to meet the challenges of caring in a rapidly changing, increasingly stressful healthcare environment. Consumer demands for zero-defect and hassle-free care, the ever-increasing complexity of high-technology medicine, cost-containment efforts that lead to increased workloads, and a proliferation of complex ethical dilemmas that strain interdisciplinary teams are just some of the stressors affecting oncology nurses. These escalating demands make it more important than ever for oncology nurses to have good personal stress management programs firmly in place.

When we think about stress in oncology nursing, the emotional demands of the work usually are first to come to mind. However, as the previous list of stressors suggests, events indirectly related to patient care may play an equal—or even greater—role as stressors for oncology nurses. In a study of caregivers working with critically ill, dying, and bereaved populations, the most frequently cited stressors were related to team communication problems, not direct patient care (Vachon, 1987). A review of research on factors related to nursing burnout (Duquette, Kerouac,

Sandhu, & Beaudet, 1994) concluded that stressors related to the workplace were more influential than stressors related to patients. The two organizational stressors with the greatest impact were role ambiguity and workload. A recent study (Payne, 2001) aimed at identifying predictors of burnout in a sample of hospice nurses supports the findings of Duquette et al., showing that burnout is strongly related to interpersonal stressors at work, such as conflicts with staff. Medland et al. (2004) noted that failure of the workplace environment to support the "human side of work" places caregivers at risk for developing burnout.

Confrontations With Loss and Trauma

Repeated exposure to loss certainly is a major stressor in oncology work. After analyzing interviews with oncology nurses, Cohen (1995) noted that the rewards nurses found in their work often were paradoxically also the sources of challenge and difficulties. For example, nurses can experience a connectedness to others and to life through sharing the personal experiences of patients and families, yet this connectedness presents risks. Hill (1991) eloquently conveyed this dilemma: "One cannot remain in this work for long without being wounded. Caregivers who function only as technicians, who do not instinctively offer their souls, hands, and hearts, will not thrive. Therefore, by serving well, they, by definition, operate from a position of tenderness and vulnerability" (pp. 107–108). Vachon (2001) also described oncology caregivers as "wounded" healers. Hill went on to say, "Learning how to manage the accumulated sadness in growth-enhancing rather than destructive ways may be the central task for long-term oncology workers" (p. 110).

Personal losses: One kind of loss to which oncology nurses must adapt is the loss of patients when treatments are not successful. Caring, empathic involvement with people in distress naturally leads to the development of relationships with significant personal meaning for the nurse, and when these relationships end with death, the nurse suffers real, personal loss. Several factors can deepen the personal meanings that relationships with patients hold for the nurse (Larson, 2000). First, the relationship may span a long period. For example, pediatric oncology nurses often will care for a child for several years, experiencing along with the family the child's remissions, recurrences, and, sometimes, death. Second, nurses often become more deeply emotionally involved with certain patients. As Lederberg (1998) noted, greater involvement (sometimes overinvolvement) with "special patients" is common, and it can lead to more intense and, sometimes, unexpected grief reactions in oncology workers when these patients die.

Oncology nurses who work in palliative care are especially at risk for multiple losses that can result in chronic grief (Vachon, 2001). These caregivers experience the deaths of multiple patients within a short time of one another or even simultaneously. Vachon (2001) pointed out that the associated grief and loss can lead to depression and chronic grief reactions.

Vicarious traumatization: Perhaps even more stressful than the personal losses endured by oncology nurses are the ongoing exposures to the losses and traumas of patients and their family members. These exposures include, for example, the cumulative effects of repeatedly empathizing with mothers of dying children, giving people bad medical news, and listening to the anger and pain of family members struggling to cope with the impending loss of a loved one.

Recent research and theory on vicarious traumatization in rescue workers and therapists who treat victims of trauma and disaster may shed light on the dynamics and cumulative impact of such exposures. Pearlman and Mac Ian (1995) described vicarious traumatization as a "transformation that occurs within the . . . trauma worker . . . as a result of empathic engagement with clients' trauma experiences and their sequelae" (p. 558). Figley (1995, 2002) used the terms "compassion fatigue" and "secondary traumatic stress disorder" to describe these same phenomena. The essential idea is that repeated exposure to the processing of traumatic events, while empathically engaged with patients, can lead to psychological distress and disrupted cognitive schemata, or basic theories about the world, in the areas of safety, trust, intimacy, self-esteem, and power (Figley, 2002; Larson, 2000; Pearlman, 1999).

The role these phenomena play in oncology nursing is still largely unknown. What is known is that some of the same strong emotional reactions occur in both trauma and oncology workers. With exposure to traumatic events or stressful patient encounters, these nurses may experience symptoms of vicarious trauma for several weeks, months, or longer (Badger, 2001) and may meet the diagnostic criteria for acute stress disorder or post-traumatic stress disorder (PTSD) as defined by the *Diagnostic and Statistical Manual of Mental Disorders (DSM-IV-TR)* (American Psychiatric Association, 2000). Nurses who have experienced trauma or grief and loss in their personal lives are at greater risk for developing symptoms of secondary traumatic stress (Badger). The symptoms may range from "emotional numbing" to psychological "intrusive responses" such as experiencing involuntary flashbacks of the traumatic event.

The long-term effects of vicarious trauma include the risk of nurses suppressing their emotions over time and refusing to acknowledge their intense emotional reactions for fear of being negatively judged as incompetent (Badger, 2001). These behaviors have a negative effect on patient care as nurses may attempt to distance themselves from emotionally tinged or traumatic patient situations (Badger). More than a decade ago, Massie, Holland, and Straker (1990) made essentially the same point concerning oncology workers, suggesting that in response to the complex psychological stressors of oncology, caregivers can get caught in the dynamics of rescue (emotional overinvolvement) and withdrawal (emotional distancing).

Vicarious traumatization has been described as an experience deeper than the emotional and psychological effects of simple empathy (Blair & Ramones, 1996) and as a state that not only incorporates changes in cognitive schemata and memory but also one that includes symptoms of burnout and countertransference. Countertransference (the process when one sees something that is not there or does not see something that is there) often occurs when feelings of fear, grief, and helplessness are evoked within the professional caregiver (Blair & Ramones; Larson, 2000). It is a pathway to ineffective helping and personal distress because helpers are relating most strongly to their own thoughts and feelings, not to those of the patient, and cannot maintain a balanced position.

The Continuum of Emotional Involvement

Extremes of closeness and distance are the end points of a continuum of emotional involvement along which all nurses constantly move back and forth. At one end of the continuum is emotional overinvolvement, and at the other extreme is emotional distance, or burnout. In the middle of the continuum is balanced empathy, what

Lief and Fox (1963) described as "detached concern"—a state of being emotionally involved and yet able to maintain a certain emotional distance. At both ends of the continuum, nurses will experience personal distress, and their connections with patients can become weak or even nonexistent as they focus their attention on their own pain, feelings of failure, and other difficult emotional reactions (Thompson, Cowan, & Rosenhan, 1980).

High levels of arousal can result in personal distress. For example, if empathic sadness becomes too great, overarousal can occur, and a more self-oriented, distressed response will ensue. If the nurse believes that he or she will have to continue to witness the other person's suffering—a scenario not uncommon in oncology care—and that it will not be significantly eased by future interventions, overarousal is particularly likely to occur. Increased awareness of PTSD has stimulated researchers to examine and understand the effects of these and other powerful stressors affecting caregivers (Lederberg, 1998). Table 35-1 lists some of the stressors that oncology caregivers encounter in their work with patients.

Table 35-1. Stresses at the Caregiver-Patient Interface

Variable	Patient and Family Challenges	Caregiver Reactions/ Challenges
Patient's reactions to severe illness	Numbness and inappropriate denial	Judicious confrontation
	Panic and grief	Patience and understanding
	Propitiation and bargaining	Recognition and gentle discouragement
	Disappointment and anger	Enduring without altering care
The "difficult" patient	Emotional chaos	Angry, unempathic, guilty
The "special" patient	Caregiver becomes deeply involved with a particular patient because of personal feelings or experiences	Overinvolvement, impaired judgment, unresolved grief
Responses to severe disfigurement/debilitation	Pain and sadness; fear and revulsion	Shame, guilt with avoidance
Responses to death and dying	Grief and fear	Painful awareness of mortality, fear of death, survivor guilt
Responses to suicidal ideation	Fear and frustration	Fear, negativity, confusion
Responses to poor outcomes	Patient and family desperation	Coming to terms with reality
Injustice of human suffering	–	Existential crisis, spirituality, cynicism, hopefulness

Note. Based on information from Lederberg, 1998.

Burnout

The hazards of empathic involvement with distressed and often traumatized people are extensively documented in the literature on burnout in the helping professions. The hallmarks of burnout are emotional exhaustion (chronic fatigue and feeling emotionally drained, frustrated, and used-up), diminished caring (feeling apathetic; not wanting to take on new patients and families), and a profound sense of demoralization or reduced personal accomplishment (a feeling of "I cannot do well at doing good; I cannot make a difference") (Maslach, 1993). In nurses experiencing burnout, the feelings of guilt, self-reproach, frustrated idealism, and failure to move successfully toward important personal goals combine to create a downward spiral, deepening nurses' distress and exhaustion.

The construct of burnout has been well researched over the past 25 years (Maslach, Schaufeli, & Leiter, 2001). The literature on burnout shows that committed caregivers begin to practice with empathic engagement, characterized by energy, involvement, and efficacy. These three dimensions of empathic engagement then are gradually replaced by their direct opposites: "Energy turns into exhaustion, involvement turns into cynicism, and efficacy turns into ineffectiveness" (Maslach et al., p. 416). Exhaustion is viewed as the main component of the burnout syndrome, and the anxiety and fatigue experienced by oncology caregivers contribute to a vicious circle that drains self-esteem and exacerbates the nurse's fear of failure (Lederberg, 1998).

Strategies for Stress Management

Given the many stressors potentially affecting oncology nurses, burnout may seem to be an inevitable outcome of this work. Fortunately, it is not. In this area, patients with cancer can teach nurses a great deal. Every oncology nurse has learned something about courage and resilience from patients who somehow transform adversity into a challenge and find hope in "hopeless" situations. Researchers studying how people cope with cancer and other stressful encounters found that individuals' responses in these situations play an enormous role in determining the outcomes they experience (Beckham, Burker, Lytle, Feldman, & Costakis, 1997; Fredrickson, Tugade, Waugh, & Larkin, 2003; Livneh, 2000).

Which coping strategies can maximize positive outcomes for oncology nurses? The key recommendations can be distilled into a single word: balance. When demands (internal and external) exceed the resources available to cope with them, the stress response occurs and the body tries to preserve its homeostasis, or balance, through a number of adjustments: increased perspiration, higher respiratory and heart rates, higher blood pressure, the release of cortisol and other stress hormones, and suppression of the immune system. This "fight or flight" physiology, particularly when chronic or of high intensity, eventually can lead to stress-related symptoms and illnesses. If, instead, a state of balance exists between demands and resources, the stress cycle will not initiate. In this scenario, which Csikszentmihalyi (1990) called a flow experience, nurses' actions almost can be effortless, and feelings of exhilaration and fulfillment can overtake them.

Dispositional coping styles that reflect individual personality differences have been found to play an important role in determining coping outcomes. Stress-prone individuals tend to have low self-esteem, an external locus of control, an avoidant coping style, and low levels of hardiness (Maslach et al., 2001). Vachon (1998) noted that interpersonal threats to one's sense of mastery and self-esteem may underlie the interpretation of events as stressful and overwhelming.

A review of stressors in oncology nursing identified some key external demands (e.g., work overload, team and organizational stressors, high-technology care, confrontations with loss and trauma) and internal demands (e.g., idealism, a quest for personal significance) that oncology nurses must negotiate. The recommendations that follow are designed to reduce these demands or to strengthen nurses' available resources and coping strategies to deal with them.

Set Limits

The first line of attack in stress management is to reduce external demands. In an era of increasing workloads, this often is difficult to accomplish. However, nurses easily can lose sight of their own needs, particularly when they know that if they are not there for the patient, nobody will be. Think of the vignette at the beginning of this chapter. If Joan's nurse had experienced a similar encounter the day before, she might have been unable to assist Joan without exceeding her personal coping limits. The principle, again, is that nurses should keep a dynamic balance between the demands they face and their available resources.

Take Charge

The most important principle of stress management is, perhaps, to take charge. Nurses must change their environment or change themselves and cannot fall into the trap of believing that they are powerless against the stress in their work. They must ask, "What can I do to change this stressful situation?" and allow some creative options to emerge, and then actively pursue one or more of these alternative behaviors. Research strongly confirms the overall adaptive advantage of approach over avoidance in coping with stressful events (Moos & Schaefer, 1993). Avoidant and passive forms of coping, such as social withdrawal, increased drinking or smoking, or wishful thinking, can lead to demoralization and increased stress. In contrast, approach coping includes behaviors such as seeking guidance and support, performing cognitive reappraisal, and engaging in active problem solving. Nurses can take charge by discussing a situation with a team member, concentrating on something good that could come out of the experience, or by looking for some small way in which they can influence the course of events.

Practice the Art of the Possible

Highly motivated, idealistic nurses are likely to have unrealistic self-expectations. Although they are more difficult to see and measure than some of the external stressors discussed previously, these unrealistic expectations can be a major source of stress. The best antidote is for nurses to practice the "art of the possible" and work consistently toward the goals that matter to them. In other words, they should develop realistic self-expectations without losing hold of the vision that inspires and guides them. If nurses can make even small progress toward their goals and not place unrealistic demands on themselves, their work-related stress will decrease. Remember that although each act of caring might seem insignificant in a given context, significant results usually accrue from repeatedly doing whatever seems to have the best chance of making a difference (Weisman, 1981).

Practice Self-Care

Nurses must balance giving to others with giving to oneself. Welsh (1999) called this "practicing responsible selfishness." Engage in activities that are restoring and rejuvenating. Figure 35-1 outlines a list of activities that trauma therapists endorse as being most helpful in coping with the demands of their work, beginning with the most effective strategies. Notice that some of these activities, such as teaching and doing community service, involve giving to others but take place in a setting other than work. Volunteering to work with healthy populations to broaden one's world view and perspective can provide a hopefulness that often is distorted by vicarious trauma (Pearlman, 1999). The notion of additional helping as a form of self-care makes sense if one believes that caring and helping are natural and good. When demands and resources are in balance, helping is a natural expression of a healthy human heart, and caring connections with others, in turn, sustain one's health (Larson, 1993a).

Exercise deserves special emphasis as a stress-management technique. Because stress is unavoidable, some stress-management interventions need to be employed at a more downstream point in the stress cycle. Once stress hormones have been released into one's body, the best thing an individual can do is get them out of one's system, and exercise is probably the best way to do this. Walking, swimming, running, jogging, hiking, bicycling, playing racquetball, or engaging in any other form of exercise that burns 200 or more calories an hour three to four times a week will lead to dramatic changes. People who exercise regularly are much less susceptible to burnout and are better prepared to deal with stress. Good nutrition and adequate sleep also are important elements of any effective stress management strategy or program.

Figure 35-1. Self-Care Activities

- Discuss cases with colleagues.
- Attend workshops.
- Spend time with family or friends.
- Take a vacation, engage in a hobby, or go to the movies.
- Talk with colleagues between staff support meetings.
- Socialize.
- Exercise.
- Limit one's caseload.
- Develop a spiritual life.
- Receive supervision.
- Teach.
- Give supervision.
- Perform community service.
- Receive bodywork/massage.

Note. Based on information from Pearlman, 1999.

Develop a Strong Support System

Different forms of social support have been identified as important for creating a healing work environment. These include emotional and affirmational support, informational support, and instrumental support. An environment that creates a "climate of care" cannot always prevent the personal factors that contribute to burnout (e.g., dispositional coping styles, existential fears), but a supportive organizational structure can lessen the impact of stressors on caregivers (Alexander & Klein, 2001; Medland et al., 2004) and can help to strengthen their engagement with patients and peers.

Self-doubt, fears, and other uncomfortable feelings are an unavoidable part of oncology nurses' experiences. Embarrassment may lead nurses to conceal these reactions from coworkers (Larson, 1987, 1993b). When these difficult feelings and experiences are shared, normalized, and worked through, the bias toward self-blame can be corrected, and one can direct his or her energies toward developing better coping skills and strategies (Larson & Chastain, 1990). Peer support in the form of assistance with problem solving can enhance the caregiver's sense of control and coping skills (Lyon, 2001). Participation in a staff support group or regular support meetings with a trusted colleague can be an excellent resource for coping with these internal stressors. It may be helpful for nurses to share their feelings with those who will listen, empathize, understand, and help them to problem solve (Welsh, 1999). Finally, affirmational support is feedback that recognizes the contributions of the caregiver. Affirmational support translates as "you are appreciated" and "you belong" (Lyon).

Coworkers can be an invaluable source of support, but, as the earlier review of stressors revealed, they also can be a tremendous source of stress. Stress-free teams do not exist, but high-functioning teams, in contrast to low-functioning teams, maximize the benefits to team members. High-functioning teams are characterized by support, interdependent collaboration, shared leadership, a sense of shared mission (commitment to a worthy purpose) and vision (what the team will do to fulfill its mission), and a willingness by team members to change their behaviors to make the team more successful (Connor, Egan, Kwilosz, Larson, & Reese, 2002; Larson, 1993a). Helping the team to move in these directions might have short-term costs, such as taking the time for a retreat or a review of the team's functioning, but these efforts can yield long-term gains in stress reduction.

The Schwartz Center Rounds (Lintz et al., 2002) at Massachusetts General Hospital is an example of a monthly multidisciplinary forum that provides caregivers with the opportunity to discuss issues related to the care of patients and families and to explore how these situations are affecting them personally. Often, the support and feedback from colleagues serve the simple yet profound function to reassure the staff that they are doing all that can be done as professionals and as compassionate caregivers (Lintz et al.; Vachon, 1998).

Emotional and affirmational support also can come from relationships with family and friends. Maintaining a positive self-image is important when working with traumatized people and can be accomplished by building and nourishing relationships apart from the work setting. Enjoying time with loved ones, reaching out for emotional support, and expressing one's emotions (e.g., laughing and crying openly) can reinforce a positive sense of self. Balancing work, play, rest, and time with family and friends can help caregivers to feel grounded in their many identities (e.g., parent, friend, spouse), not just their identity as a caregiver (Pearlman, 1999).

The remaining forms of social support exist in the workplace and include informational and instrumental support. Informational support includes providing caregivers with realistic expectations of their work and clearly defining what situations are within their control and what situations are not. This kind of support prevents caregivers from feeling powerless to effect change and helps to reduce the burnout-related feelings of anxiety, anger, and guilt (Lyon, 2001). Instrumental support within the work environment is the support given for learning and maintaining the skills that are necessary to feel competent and effective. This type of support can occur through mentorship and orientation programs and should include self-care skills for both physical and psychological safety (Lyon). Instrumental support is important in preventing the feelings of reduced personal accomplishment that are part of the burnout experience.

Strive for Balanced Empathy

Working in high-mortality settings, in which the presence and awareness of suffering and pain are pervasive, requires a balanced, empathic engagement with both immediate and more universal dimensions of loss. Rogers (1957) wrote, "To sense the client's private world as if it were your own, but without ever losing the *as if* quality—this is empathy" (p. 99). If one's empathy loses the "as if" quality, that individual is subject to a host of countertransferential and personal distress experiences that can severely limit effectiveness and lead to burnout.

Maintaining a balanced sense of empathy requires developing an internal sense of the optimal level of empathic arousal. Some nurses are able to empathically engage with extremely distressed people frequently without becoming personally distressed; others can do so less often. All oncology nurses must find a way to be emotionally involved with the people they care for, not just for the welfare of patients but for themselves as well. As Hill (1991) noted, if one functions only as a technician, he or she will not thrive as a caregiver.

How can nurses know whether they are experiencing personal distress or are just experiencing intense emotional involvement with the person for whom they are caring? Strong emotions are a natural and necessary part of helping people to cope with grief and life-threatening illness. Almost every veteran oncology nurse has been visibly moved and has shed a tear with someone, as did the nurse in the chapter's opening vignette. This display of deep feeling almost always strengthens, not weakens, the nurse-patient relationship because it shows the patient that the nurse truly cares. However, an enormous difference exists between crying and sobbing. When one sobs, attention has shifted to his or her own distress, and empathy and helping are derailed.

Develop a Stress-Hardy Outlook

How nurses view themselves and the events in their worlds has an enormous impact on the amount of stress they experience. Certain characteristics appear to differentiate high-stress/healthy people from high-stress/unhealthy groups. People who manage stress better and have fewer illnesses are more likely to have an attitude of hardiness. The defining characteristic of hardiness is a sense of challenge, control, and commitment (Ouellette, 1993).

A stress-hardy person tends to see a challenge where others see a threat and, thus, avoids many unnecessary stress reactions. If people are open to change and can see potentially stressful events as opportunities for growth rather than as threats, they are likely to better cope with the demands confronting them. For example, one who is always "waiting for things to settle down" is going to have more stress than the person who knows that change will never cease.

A sense of control is the second component of stress hardiness. Believing and acting as if life experiences were controllable and predictable can—within certain limits—markedly decrease stress. This sense of control includes the belief that one can perform successfully in a given situation (i.e., an optimistic outlook) and a sense that one's world and its demands are manageable. In one study of oncology nurses, a sense of personal control over the things that happen in life and in the work environment protected nurses from all three dimensions of burnout (i.e., emotional exhaustion, depersonalization, and a lack of personal accomplishment) (Papadatou, Anagnostopoulos, & Monos, 1994).

However, as a coping strategy, nourishing one's sense of control might seem at odds with the many aspects of the work environment that are beyond one's control, such as the recovery of patients, decisions by physicians and the hospital administration, and confrontations with death and dying (Buunk & Schaufeli, 1993). Here, nurses can learn an important lesson from their patients. Taylor (1983) studied the reactions of women with a diagnosis of breast cancer and found that one of the ways in which these women gained mastery over their circumstances was to create illusions of control. These "healthy illusions" proved to be highly adaptive and allowed the patients to manage this potentially overwhelming life event. Assuming that the demands of the world *can* be met might help to increase the likelihood that they *will* be met.

Although nurses cannot control every outcome, they can always choose a meaning-ful response to whatever occurs. Look for the possible, and try to focus on things that can be changed now. In this regard, many stress experts have recognized the powerful wisdom of theologian Reinhold Neibuhr's serenity prayer, "God, give us the serenity to accept what cannot be changed; give us the courage to change what should be changed; give us the wisdom to distinguish one from the other" (Fox, 1985, p. 290).

The third component of stress hardiness is commitment. Stress-hardy individuals are fully involved in life and life's activities (e.g., work, family, friendships). They have a sense of meaning and purpose in life and the capacity for a deep commitment to whatever they undertake. One can hypothesize that a sense of commitment and purpose in the work can be a tremendous stress buffer for oncology nurses. Oncology workers probably would not say that patient contact is their major source of burnout, precisely because this also is the greatest source of meaning and the reason they chose this career in the first place. A review of research on burnout in nursing (Duquette et al., 1994) revealed that stress hardiness, social support in the workplace, and the use of action-oriented versus avoidance-oriented coping strategies all acted as buffers against stress. Among challenge, commitment, and control, commitment levels were the best buffers, with the more-committed nurses experiencing less burnout.

In a study of 645 hospital nurses, "high commitment" nurses, who endorsed statements such as "I like nursing too well to give it up" and "If I could do it all over again, I would choose to work in the nursing profession" reported less burnout overall (Reilly, 1994). However, Reilly also found that these same nurses showed a stronger relationship between stressors and burnout than the less-committed nurses. It was not that the more-committed nurses were more burned out, per se, but that they reported a stronger connection between stressful events and burnout. Reilly inferred that the more-committed nurses may not "sweat the little stuff" but may have a breaking point. When helping goals are seriously threatened, more-committed helpers suffer the most. Thus, being a committed nurse may reduce overall levels of burnout, but when the "way it is" does not match "the way it should be," the nurse is more likely to feel emotionally drained and burned out.

Do Not Mislabel "Caring" as "Codependence"

In the struggle to maintain a sense of commitment and purpose and to meet the needs of patients, self-doubts concerning one's motivations as a helper are common. With the proliferation of the concept of the "codependent helper" (i.e., the helper who satisfies his or her own needs through the people he or she cares for) (Mellody, 1989), many nurses have identified themselves as codependent.

The codependence model has several problems. First, because no valid and reliable testing instruments exist for measuring codependency, codependent people cannot be differentiated from anyone else. Second, one of the unintended and negative consequences of labeling people and care methods as codependent is that considering difficulties in providing care to be symptoms of a disorder is an unhealthy, self-defeating approach to these problems. It heightens self-blame and shifts attention away from the situational determinants of stress. Third, the codependence model makes people doubt themselves—their altruistically inspired helping becomes, instead, a product of emotional instability. These doubts about one's motivations can erode one of the best buffers against stress in nursing—the sense of purpose in the work. Finally, perhaps the most destructive consequence, the codependence model undermines support for performing work that is neither easy nor distress free.

Although these unintended and harmful consequences accompany the concept of codependence, there is wisdom in the idea that oncology nurses need to set limits for themselves as helpers, as discussed previously. All nurses must determine whether they are overly controlling and ensure that they are not setting boundaries, are not vicariously living through the lives of the people they care for, and are not generally "giving" in a way that has become "taking."

Stress, Coping, and Personal Growth

Oncology nurses know firsthand that stress can lead to personal growth. As Haan (1993) stated, "Stress benefits people, making them more tender, humble, and hardy" (p. 259). Hill (1991) commented that thriving, tenderness, and vulnerability are inseparable elements in the oncology nursing experience. The adaptive challenges that individuals face as oncology nurses can make them feel more resilient and alive, but vulnerability and a kind of personal grief are inescapable companions to this growth.

Klein (2004) discussed the essential rewards that most nurses are searching for in their professional work: (a) to deepen their sense of meaning and passion, (b) to express their true gifts and talents, (c) to have a compelling career purpose, and (d) to develop relationships that support them in learning and growing. To gain these rewards, one's work must align with one's true core values, unique gifts, and chosen legacy. When one's work is fundamental to realizing one's higher purpose, it can become transformational (Klein).

Nurses need to have purpose and meaning in their lives, and helping others is one of the important ways they can achieve this. Becker (1973) said that the "only real problem in life" is discovering one's unique talent, and then finding a way to express it and "dedicate it to something beyond" oneself (p. 82). Altruistically inspired helping is not a product of emotional instability or codependent strivings (Larson, 1992). Indeed, most developmental theorists agree that a caring extension of self toward others is the capstone of human development.

Conclusion

Oncology nursing affords an opportunity to combine profound personal growth with professional accomplishment. To take full advantage of this opportunity, nurses need to construct a personal philosophy of life that can make sense of the losses they encounter. In difficult times, they will need a wellspring of caring that they can draw upon and an inner voice that can reaffirm a higher purpose to which they have committed themselves. Most of all, they will have to find balance between the demands they face and the resources they have to meet them and between giving to others and giving to themselves.

References

Alexander, D.A., & Klein, S. (2001). Caring for others can seriously damage your health. *Hospital Medicine, 62*, 264–267.

American Psychiatric Association. (2000). *Diagnostic and statistical manual of mental disorders* (4th ed., text rev.). Washington, DC: Author.

Badger, J.M. (2001). Understanding secondary traumatic stress. *American Journal of Nursing, 101*(7), 26–32.

Becker, E. (1973). *The denial of death.* New York: Free Press.

Beckham, J.C., Burker, E.J., Lytle, B.L., Feldman, M.E., & Costakis, M.J. (1997). Self-efficacy and adjustment in cancer patients: A preliminary report. *Behavioral Medicine, 23*, 138–142.

Blair, D.T., & Ramones, V.A. (1996). Understanding vicarious traumatization. *Journal of Psychosocial Nursing, 34*(11), 24–30.

Buunk, B.P., & Schaufeli, W.B. (1993). Burnout: A perspective from social comparison theory. In W.B. Schaufeli, C. Maslach, & T. Marek (Eds.), *Professional burnout: Recent developments in theory and research* (pp. 53–69). Washington, DC: Taylor and Francis.

Cohen, M.Z. (1995). The meaning of cancer and oncology nursing: Link to effective care. *Seminars in Oncology Nursing, 11*, 59–67.

Connor, S.R., Egan, K., Kwilosz, D., Larson, D.G., & Reese, D. (2002). Interdisciplinary approaches to assisting with end-of-life care and decision making. *American Behavioral Scientist, 46*, 340–356.

Csikszentmihalyi, M. (1990). *Flow: The psychology of optimal experience.* New York: Harper & Row.

Duquette, A., Kerouac, S., Sandhu, B.K., & Beaudet, L. (1994). Factors related to nursing burnout: A review of empirical knowledge. *Issues in Mental Health Nursing, 15,* 337–358.

Figley, C.R. (1995). Compassion fatigue as secondary traumatic stress disorder: An overview. In C.R. Figley (Ed.), *Compassion fatigue: Coping with secondary traumatic stress disorder in those who treat the traumatized* (pp. 1–20). New York: Brunner/Mazel.

Figley, C.R. (2002). Introduction. In C.R. Figley (Ed.), *Treating compassion fatigue* (pp. 1–14). New York: Brunner-Routledge.

Fox, R.W. (1985). *Reinhold Neibuhr: A biography.* New York: Pantheon.

Fredrickson, B.L., Tugade, M.M., Waugh, C.E., & Larkin, G.R. (2003). What good are positive emotions in crises? A prospective study of resilience and emotions following the terrorist attacks on the United States on September 11th, 2001. *Journal of Personality and Social Psychology, 84,* 365–376.

Haan, N. (1993). The assessment of coping, defense, and stress. In L. Goldberger & S. Breznitz (Eds.), *Handbook of stress: Theoretical and clinical aspects* (2nd ed., pp. 258–273). New York: Free Press.

Hill, H.L. (1991). Point and counterpoint: Relationships in oncology care. *Journal of Psychosocial Oncology, 9*(2), 97–112.

Klein, E. (2004). Missing something in your career? *Reflections on Nursing Leadership, 30*(1), 41–42.

Larson, D.G. (1987). Helper secrets: Internal stressors in nursing. *Journal of Psychosocial Nursing and Mental Health Services, 25*(4), 20–27.

Larson, D.G. (1992, May). *The challenge of caring in oncology nursing.* Paper presented at the annual Oncology Nursing Society Congress, San Diego, CA.

Larson, D.G. (1993a). *The helper's journey: Working with people facing grief, loss, and life-threatening illness.* Champaign, IL: Research Press.

Larson, D.G. (1993b). Self-concealment: Implications for stress and empathy in oncology care. *Journal of Psychosocial Oncology, 11*(4), 1–16.

Larson, D.G. (2000). Anticipatory grief: Challenges for professional and volunteer caregivers. In T. Rando (Ed.), *Clinical dimensions of anticipatory mourning: Theory and practice in working with the dying, their loved ones, and caregivers* (pp. 379–395). Champaign, IL: Research Press.

Larson, D.G., & Chastain, R.L. (1990). Self-concealment: Conceptualization, measurement, and health implications. *Journal of Social and Clinical Psychology, 9,* 439–455.

Lazarus, R.A., & Folkman, S. (1984). *Stress, appraisal, and coping.* New York: Springer.

Lederberg, M.S. (1998). Oncology staff stress and related interventions. In J.C. Holland (Ed.), *Psycho-oncology* (pp. 1035–1048). New York: Oxford University Press.

Lief, H.I., & Fox, R.C. (1963). Training for "detached concern" in medical students. In H.I. Lief, V.F. Lief, & N.R. Lief (Eds.), *The psychological basis of medical practice* (pp. 12–35). New York: Harper & Row.

Lintz, K.C., Penson, R.T., Cassem, N., Harmon, D.C., Chabner, B.A., & Lynch, T.J. (2002). A staff dialogue on aggressive palliative treatment demanded by a terminally ill patient: Psychosocial issues faced by patients, their families, and caregivers. *Oncologist, 7*(Suppl. 2), 23–29.

Livneh, H. (2000). Psychosocial adaptation to cancer: The role of coping strategies. *Journal of Rehabilitation, 66*(2), 40–49.

Lyon, B.L. (2001). Social support as TLC: The great elixir. *Reflections on Nursing Leadership, 27*(4), 36–37.

Maslach, C. (1993). Burnout: A multidimensional perspective. In W.B. Schaufeli, C. Maslach, & T. Marek (Eds.), *Professional burnout: Recent developments in theory and research* (pp. 19–32). Washington, DC: Taylor and Francis.

Maslach, C., Schaufeli, W.B., & Leiter, M.P. (2001). Job burnout. *Annual Review of Psychology, 52,* 397–422.

Massie, M.J., Holland, J.C., & Straker, N. (1990). Psychotherapeutic interventions. In J.C. Holland & J.H. Rowland (Eds.), *Handbook of psychooncology: Psychological care of the patient with cancer* (pp. 455–469). New York: Oxford University Press.

Medland, J., Howard-Ruben, J., & Whitaker, E. (2004). Fostering psychosocial wellness in oncology nurses: Addressing burnout and social support in the workplace. *Oncology Nursing Forum, 31,* 47–54.

Mellody, P. (1989). *Facing codependence.* San Francisco: Harper & Row.

Moos, R.H., & Schaefer, J. (1993). Coping resources and processes: Current concepts and measures. In L. Goldberger & S. Breznitz (Eds.), *Handbook of stress: Theoretical and clinical aspects* (2nd ed., pp. 234–257). New York: Free Press.

Ouellette, S. (1993). Inquiries into hardiness. In L. Goldberger & S. Breznitz (Eds.), *Handbook of stress: Theoretical and clinical aspects* (2nd ed., pp. 77–100). New York: Free Press.

Papadatou, D., Anagnostopoulos, F., & Monos, D. (1994). Factors contributing to the development of burnout in oncology nursing. *British Journal of Medical Psychology, 67,* 187–199.

Payne, N. (2001). Occupational stressors and coping as determinants of burnout in female hospice nurses. *Journal of Advanced Nursing, 33,* 396–405.

Pearlman, L.A. (1999). Self-care for trauma therapists: Ameliorating vicarious traumatization. In B.H. Stamm (Ed.), *Secondary traumatic stress: Self-care issues for clinicians, researchers, and educators* (pp. 51–64). Lutherville, MD: Sidran Press.

Pearlman, L.A., & Mac Ian, P.S. (1995). Vicarious traumatization: An empirical study of the effects of trauma work on trauma therapists. *Professional Psychology: Research and Practice, 26,* 558–565.

Reilly, N.P. (1994). Exploring a paradox: Commitment as a moderator of the stressor-burnout relationship. *Journal of Applied Social Psychology, 24,* 397–414.

Rogers, C.R. (1957). The necessary and sufficient conditions of therapeutic personality change. *Journal of Consulting Psychology, 21,* 95–103.

Saakvitne, K.W., & Pearlman, L.A. (1996). *Transforming the pain: A workbook on vicarious traumatization.* New York: W.W. Norton.

Stotland, E., Mathews, K.E., Sherman, S.E., Hansson, R.O., & Richardson, B.Z. (1978). *Empathy, fantasy, and helping.* Beverly Hills, CA: Sage.

Taylor, S.E. (1983). Adjustment to threatening events: A theory of cognitive adaptation. *American Psychologist, 38,* 1161–1173.

Thompson, W., Cowan, C., & Rosenhan, D. (1980). Focus of attention mediates the impact of negative affect on altruism. *Journal of Personality and Social Psychology, 38,* 291–300.

Vachon, M.L. (1987). *Occupational stress in the care of the critically ill, the dying, and the bereaved.* Washington, DC: Hemisphere.

Vachon, M.L. (1998). Caring for the caregiver in oncology and palliative care. *Seminars in Oncology Nursing, 14,* 152–157.

Vachon, M.L. (2001). The nurse's role: The world of palliative care nursing. In B.R. Ferrell & N. Coyle (Eds.), *Textbook of palliative nursing* (pp. 647–662). New York: Oxford University Press.

Weisman, A.D. (1981). Understanding the cancer patient: The syndrome of caregiver's plight. *Psychiatry, 44,* 161–168.

Welsh, D.J. (1999). Caring for the caregiver: Strategies for avoiding "compassion fatigue." *Clinical Journal of Oncology Nursing, 3,* 183–184.

CHAPTER 36

Caring for the Family Caregiver

SHEILA M. FERRALL, RN, MS, AOCN®

Behold, I am going to send an angel before you to guard you along the way.

—Exodus

Cancer is widely considered to be a disease of both individuals and their families. Spouses, children, parents, and significant others are profoundly affected by the diagnosis. Family members have always played a role in the care of patients with cancer. However, changes in health care have served to significantly increase demands on these caregivers. Technologic advances allow for the management of cancers that were previously considered untreatable. With an eye toward cost savings, patients are being discharged earlier from inpatient settings. Treatments once provided only during an inpatient hospitalization now are given on an outpatient basis and often at home. The increasing availability of oral chemotherapy further contributes to the shift from managing care in a medical setting to the home. In light of these changes, family caregivers are assuming increasing responsibility for the care of loved ones, often with little preparation.

The range of potential caregivers for patients with cancer is wide. Family members such as spouses, parents, children, siblings, and others are all possible caregivers. Likewise, people not related to the individual in the traditional sense but designated by the patient may function as caregivers. Friends, neighbors, lovers, or partners may play a significant caregiving role.

One in three Americans voluntarily provides unpaid care each year to ill or disabled family members or friends (U.S. Department of Health and Human Services, 1998). According to statistics compiled by the National Family Caregivers Association (2002), the value of services provided by family caregivers is estimated to be $257 billion a year. People assuming the caregiver role experience unique challenges. Accurate and thorough assessment of these challenges will allow oncology nurses to structure interventions to support this diverse group of vital individuals.

Assessment of Caregiver Challenges

Regardless of the type of cancer or stage at diagnosis, caregivers must cope with inevitable changes. A roller coaster analogy aptly depicts both patients' and caregivers' feelings during this time, with highs and lows throughout the illness. Patients' and caregivers' quality of life can be affected by their responses to the situation. This area requires assessment by the healthcare team and offers oncology nurses an opportunity to facilitate caregiver coping.

Diagnosis

In 1991, Sales reviewed literature on the psychosocial impact of cancer on the family and presented the information within a framework of six phases of cancer. During the initial or diagnosis phase of illness, caregivers face many of the same feelings of anxiety, anger, and helplessness as patients. Caregivers may feel ignored or excluded by medical personnel who attend to the patient and may have difficulty communicating their questions and information needs. Caregivers of hospitalized patients find themselves in the position of helping patients to cope with the physical and emotional traumas of surgery, radiation, and chemotherapy. In addition to visiting and providing emotional support, caregivers often must assume multiple roles vacated by the patient during hospitalization, resulting in feelings of overload and exhaustion. As the patient leaves the hospital, caregivers face a new problem: how to deal with the patient's day-to-day challenges of living with cancer. If the patient has physical limitations, the caregiver has the task of adapting his or her preexisting lifestyle to the patient's needs. Direct caregiving tasks may take priority over the caregiver's usual activities. The economic realities of treatment become clear and may involve significant financial burden. Family disagreement over treatment decisions may further complicate this difficult period (Zhang & Siminoff, 2003).

Treatment

During the adjuvant treatment phase, patients and caregivers again find themselves interacting repeatedly with healthcare providers. Frequent visits for treatments pose scheduling and transportation problems. Caregivers must coordinate treatment visits for the patient while maintaining some connection to their own work or personal commitments. Both caregivers and patients may feel unprepared to manage treatment effects (Harden et al., 2002).

Recurrence and Advanced Cancer

Recurrence creates emotional distress rivaling that created by the initial diagnosis. Options for treatment may be restricted to more aggressive, higher risk modalities that require closer monitoring and more caregiver involvement. Progressive deterioration and physical decline are hallmarks of the terminal phase. As the disease interferes with normal functioning, caregivers, by necessity, assume added responsibilities.

As cancer progresses, the caregiving burden increases. Home care of patients with advanced cancer can have a negative impact on caregivers' health, schedule, anxiety, and energy (Aranda & Hayman-White, 2001). Weitzner, McMillan, and Jacobsen (1999) compared the impact of cancer caregiving in curative and palliative settings on caregiver quality of life. Not surprisingly, caregivers of patients receiving palliative care had significantly lower quality-of-life scores and lower scores on physical health.

Likewise, a significant relationship exists between caregiver stressors and caregiver outcomes. Redinbaugh, Baum, Tarbell, and Arnold (2003) examined caregiver stressors, coping, and caregiver strain in a sample of 31 family caregivers and their terminally ill loved ones enrolled in home hospice programs. Data collection occurred in the patients' homes. Patient questionnaires were administered in an interview format, and caregivers completed their questionnaires in a separate room. Higher levels of caregiver strain were noted when patients had greater physical needs, greater psychological distress, and poorer existential quality of life. Caregivers who believed that their families accepted the patient's illness, defined problems related to the illness in a more manageable way, and felt more capable of managing and resolving illness-related stressors reported lower levels of strain.

Caregiver Quality of Life

Assessment of caregiver quality of life is essential, given the significant impact of a cancer diagnosis in a loved one. Deeken, Taylor, Mangan, Yabroff, and Ingham (2003) conducted a comprehensive review of self-report instruments developed to measure the burden, needs, and quality of life of informal caregivers. After extensive literature review, the researchers identified 28 instruments, which they evaluated in terms of development, content, and psychometric properties. Deeken et al. concluded that a number of instruments are available to both clinicians and researchers to evaluate caregiver burden, quality of life, and, to a lesser extent, needs.

Likewise, Edwards and Ung (2002) reviewed the psychometric properties of quality-of-life instruments of caregivers of patients with cancer. According to those authors, quality-of-life instruments developed specifically to measure the quality of life of patients with cancer had the best psychometric properties. They identified one instrument, the Quality of Life Index—Cancer Scale, among the four reviewed that met or exceeded minimum psychometric criteria for reliability and validity. The authors of both articles (Deeken et al., 2003; Edwards & Ung) agreed that use of these tools is paramount to adequate caregiver assessment.

Psychological distress for caregivers may rival, and in some cases exceed, that of patients. Matthews (2003) evaluated role (caregiver or survivor), gender, and psychological distress in 135 caregiver-patient dyads. The researcher found significantly higher overall distress levels for caregivers than cancer survivors. Caregiver scores were significantly higher than survivors' on distress for diagnosis and fear of cancer recurrence. Pitceathly and Maguire (2003), in a review of the psychological impact of cancer on patients' partners and other key relatives, suggested that certain caregivers are particularly vulnerable to stresses associated with the caregiver role. Specifically, those in conflicted relationships and those who have a negative view of illness-related events or of the impact of the caring role on their life are more likely to experience problems. Additionally, Matthews reported that female caregivers scored higher than their male counterparts on cancer-related anxiety, future uncertainties, fear of recurrence, and future diagnostic tests.

Caregivers often report significant issues related to depression and sleep. Carter and Chang (2000) administered the Center for Epidemiological Studies—Depression and the Pittsburgh Sleep Quality Index to 51 caregivers of patients with cancer. Their purpose was to describe sleep problems and depression levels of caregivers and explore the relationship between those two variables. Caregivers in this descriptive study primarily were white, female spouses. More than half of the caregivers were experiencing depressive symptoms at a level that suggested a risk for clinical depression, and 95% reported severe sleep problems. Caregivers who reported higher levels of sleep problems reported higher levels of depression.

Carter (2002) sought to describe caregiver sleep problems and depression levels using narratives. Forty-seven caregivers of patients with advanced cancer were interviewed in person or via the phone. Carter reported that caregivers described significant fluctuations in sleep patterns over time. Caregivers also described how chronic sleep loss set into motion the downward movement toward depressive symptoms. Emanuel, Fairclough, Slutsman, and Emanuel (2000) conducted a national study looking at a number of factors impacting patients (50% with cancer). They found that caregivers of patients with advanced and terminal illnesses were significantly more depressed. Of terminally ill patients with high care needs, 15% gave serious thought to euthanasia/physician-assisted suicide because of the burden created by their illness. Financial burden also was significant for patients with terminal illness.

Spiritual Assessment

Caregivers have been observed to have spiritual needs similar to those of patients (Taylor, 2003), yet this is an area that oncology nurses may overlook. Kuuppelomaki (2002) studied 166 nurses from five hospitals in Finland. Although the majority of the participating nurses agreed that the patient's family should be given spiritual support, half of the nurses were not willing to offer that support. The nurses identified a number of obstacles to providing spiritual support, including family members turning to other experts with their spiritual needs, the lack of time, and family members being unable to express their spiritual needs (see Chapter 7).

Cultural Assessment

Finally, healthcare providers must consider crosscultural issues when assessing caregiver needs and structuring interventions. Patterns of resource utilization, lack of trust in social services providers, and varying interpretations of pain are just a few areas where culture may influence the role of the caregiver (Glajchen, 2004) (see Chapter 6).

Strategies to Facilitate Caregiver Coping

Oncology nurses hold key positions in terms of assessing caregiver coping and developing interventions to support them in their roles. Interventions vary according to the specific issues for each caregiver, but they generally fall into one of four categories: providing information, providing psychological support, providing physical support, and mobilizing resources.

Providing Information

Studies repeatedly have identified information or cognitive needs as a primary area of concern for caregivers (Friesen, Pepler, & Hunter, 2002; Fukui, 2002; Harrington, Lackey, & Gates, 1996; Rees & Bath, 2000; Steele & Fitch, 1996; Stetz, McDonald, & Compton, 1996). During the initial phase of illness, obtaining information about the disease and its treatment can serve as a useful coping strategy for caregivers and patients. However, some patients and families may prefer limited information initially, delaying negative information that they have not asked for and are not prepared to hear (Wideheim, Edvardsson, Pahlson, & Ahlstrom, 2002).

As the disease progresses, caregivers want to know what symptoms to expect, the underlying cause of the symptoms, and how to manage the changes at home (Ferrall, 1998). For example, caregivers of patients with brain tumors or brain metastases need to be informed about the potential development of seizures and what measures to take if they occur. Caregivers want to know what the future holds and may ask questions such as "What will happen as things get worse?" and "Will you let me know when it gets close to the end?" Some caregivers will need information about how to deal with the physical demands of caring for the patient at home. Questions about nutrition, activity restrictions, medications, and treatment effects are common.

Given, Given, and Kozachik (2001) suggested that interventions such as family conferences, skills training, problem-solving strategies, caregiver training, help sheets, and books, videos, compact discs, and Web pages will address the information needs of family caregivers. In this era of increasing outpatient treatments and fewer hospital admissions, caregiver interactions with the healthcare team often are limited. However, allowing time for specific questions is critical. Asking the caregiver to identify specific information needs will help to ensure that the areas of greatest concern are addressed. Encouraging appropriate decision making, providing advance care planning, and supporting home care are ways in which healthcare providers can be of service to caregivers as patients approach the end of life (Rabow, Hauser, & Adams, 2004).

Providing Psychological Support

As professional caregivers become more involved in the high-tech aspect of cancer care, the potential to neglect psychological needs of family caregivers exists. Caregivers indicate that they have considerable psychological needs (Blanchard, Albrecht, & Ruckdeschel, 1997); an estimated 20%–30% of partners suffer from psychological and mood disturbances. One randomized clinical trial sought to determine the impact of a structured supportive nursing intervention on the depressive symptoms among caregivers of patients with cancer (Kozachik et al., 2001). Based on their findings, the investigators concluded that the "intervention appeared to be more effective in slowing the rate of deterioration of depressive symptoms than in decreasing the levels of depression in this sample of caregivers" (p. 1149). More randomized clinical trials are needed to evaluate specific nursing interventions aimed at caregivers (Petrie, Logan, & DeGrasse, 2001).

Telephoning patient caregivers rather than waiting for them to initiate contact is one way to convey support. Scheduled contact via the telephone allows caregivers to ventilate and discuss problems as they arise. Offering caregivers the opportunity for individual, group, or peer counseling may help them to identify and resolve issues. Oncology nurses can provide caregivers with ongoing information about stress management, coping with role changes, anxiety, and depression.

As with identifying information needs, asking caregivers to talk about their stressors allows specific concerns to be addressed. Isolating some time alone with the caregiver during an outpatient visit or on the telephone may provide an opportunity for catharsis. Asking questions such as "How are you coping with this situation?", "What do you find most difficult to deal with?", and "How are you taking care of yourself?" gives caregivers permission to discuss issues that they might otherwise feel guilty mentioning. Finally, recognizing depressive symptoms that require further intervention and making appropriate referrals will further support caregivers.

Providing Physical Support

Caregivers may need assistance with the physical demands of caring for a patient with cancer at home. In a study of family caregivers of hospice patients (Steele & Fitch, 1996), participants identified time away from the house, time for personal needs, time for rest, and adequate sleep as significant needs. Caregivers of patients in the terminal phase may demonstrate a need for overnight respite to prevent exhaustion. Patients receiving the Medicare hospice benefit may have access to short-term respite care in a skilled nursing facility so that caregivers can have some time away from caring for the patient. Nurses should work with the caregivers and team members to determine whether hired caregivers are needed. Although often not covered by insurance, this may be necessary to keep the patient out of the hospital at any stage of the illness.

In addition to evaluating the physical demands of caregiving, oncology nurses should assess the availability of appropriate equipment in the home. Harrington et al. (1996) studied the needs of 55 caregivers of clinic and hospice patients. The caregivers of hospice patients ranked equipment to help with patient care as a top need. Routine assessment of the home environment will ensure that required equipment is available to meet the patient's changing needs.

Mobilizing Resources

Exploring avenues of support for caregivers is an important intervention for oncology nurses. Caregivers today are more sophisticated than ever in terms of seeking information via the Internet and other resources. Despite this level of sophistication, caregivers may be unaware of resources available in their own communities. Maintaining a current list of community aids and distributing it to caregivers will make them aware of resources. Likewise, keeping track of local support group meetings for caregivers may be helpful.

In addition to seeking community resources, caregivers should explore their personal resources for support. Extended family, friends, and church members are a few examples of people who can offer support after a cancer diagnosis. Encourage caregivers to identify specific ways in which these people can help, such as providing transportation one or two days a week for radiation treatments, light housekeeping duties, preparing meals, shopping, and spending time with the patient. Oncology nurses should seize the opportunity to have frank discussions about personal resources with caregivers and encourage them to ask for help (see Appendix).

Conclusion

An increasing number of lay individuals are caring for patients with cancer throughout their illness. Assuming this role as a caregiver entails myriad challenges. Yet, caregivers take on this burden without question and often with little help. Adequate assessment of caregiver needs is central to identifying appropriate interventions. Further research is required to help to define which interventions would be most effective for this important group. Oncology nurses can play a vital role in supporting caregivers as they make this difficult journey with their loved one.

References

Aranda, S.K., & Hayman-White, K. (2001). Home caregivers of the person with advanced cancer: An Australian perspective. *Cancer Nursing, 24,* 300–307.

Blanchard, C.G., Albrecht, T.L., & Ruckdeschel, J.C. (1997). The crisis of cancer: Psychological impact on family caregivers. *Oncology, 11,* 189–194.

Carter, P.A. (2002). Caregivers' descriptions of sleep changes and depressive symptoms. *Oncology Nursing Forum, 29,* 1277–1283.

Carter, P.A., & Chang, B.L. (2000). Sleep and depression in cancer caregivers. *Cancer Nursing, 23,* 410–415.

Deeken, J.F., Taylor, K.L., Mangan, P., Yabroff, R., & Ingham, J.M. (2003). Care for the caregivers: A review of self-report instruments developed to measure the burden, needs, and quality of life of informal caregivers. *Journal of Pain and Symptom Management, 26,* 922–953.

Edwards, B., & Ung, L. (2002). Quality of life instruments for caregivers of patients with cancer: A review of their psychometric properties. *Cancer Nursing, 25,* 342–349.

Emanuel, E.J., Fairclough, D.L., Slutsman, J., & Emanuel, L.L. (2000). Understanding economic and other burdens of terminal illness. The experience of patients and their caregivers. *Annals of Internal Medicine, 132,* 451–459.

Ferrall, S.M. (1998, May). *Caregiver burden and caregiver needs in brain tumor patients.* Paper presented at the Oncology Nursing Society 23rd Annual Congress, San Francisco, CA.

Friesen, P., Pepler, C., & Hunter, P. (2002). Interactive family learning following a cancer diagnosis. *Oncology Nursing Forum, 29,* 981–987.

Fukui, S. (2002). Information needs and the related characteristics of Japanese family caregivers of newly diagnosed patients with cancer. *Cancer Nursing, 25,* 181–186.

Given, B.A., Given, C.W., & Kozachik, S. (2001). Family support in advanced cancer. *CA: A Cancer Journal for Clinicians, 51,* 213–231.

Glajchen, M. (2004). The emerging role and needs of family caregivers in cancer care. *Journal of Supportive Oncology, 2,* 145–155.

Harden, J., Schafenacker, A., Northouse, L., Mood, D., Smith, D., Pienta, K., et al. (2002). Couples' experience with prostate cancer: Focus group research. *Oncology Nursing Forum, 29,* 701–709.

Harrington, V., Lackey, N.R., & Gates, M.F. (1996). Needs of caregivers of clinic and hospice cancer patients. *Cancer Nursing, 19,* 118–125.

Kozachik, S.L., Given, C.W., Given, B.A., Pierce, S.J., Azzouz, F., Rawl, S.M., et al. (2001). Improving depressive symptoms among caregivers of patients with cancer: Results of a randomized clinical trial. *Oncology Nursing Forum, 28,* 1149–1157.

Kuuppelomaki, M. (2002). Spiritual support for families of patients with cancer: A pilot study of nursing staff assessments. *Cancer Nursing, 26,* 209–218.

Matthews, B.A. (2003). Role and gender differences in cancer-related distress: A comparison of survivor and caregiver self-reports. *Oncology Nursing Forum, 30,* 493–499.

National Family Caregivers Association. (2002). *Caregiving statistics.* Retrieved June 16, 2005, from http://www.thefamilycaregiver.org/who/stats.cfm

Petrie, W., Logan, J., & DeGrasse, C. (2001). Research review of the supportive care needs of spouses of women with breast cancer. *Oncology Nursing Forum, 28,* 1601–1607.

Pitceathly, C., & Maguire, P. (2003). The psychological impact of cancer on patients' partners and other key relatives: A review. *European Journal of Cancer, 39,* 1517–1524.

Rabow, M.W., Hauser, J.M., & Adams, J. (2004). Supporting family caregivers at the end of life. *JAMA, 291,* 483–491.

Redinbaugh, E.M., Baum, A., Tarbell, S., & Arnold, R. (2003). End-of-life caregiving: What helps family caregivers cope? *Journal of Palliative Medicine, 6,* 901–909.

Rees, C.E., & Bath, P.A. (2000). Exploring the information flow: Partners of women with breast cancer, patients, and healthcare professionals. *Oncology Nursing Forum, 27,* 1267–1275.

Sales, E. (1991). Psychosocial impact of the phase of cancer on the family: An updated review. *Journal of Psychosocial Oncology, 9*(4), 1–18.

Steele, R.G., & Fitch, M.I. (1996). Needs of family caregivers of patients receiving home hospice care for cancer. *Oncology Nursing Forum, 23,* 823–828.

Stetz, K.M., McDonald, J.C., & Compton, K. (1996). Family caregivers and the marrow transplant experience. *Oncology Nursing Forum, 23,* 1421–1427.

Taylor, E.J. (2003). Nurses caring for the spirit: Patients with cancer and family caregiver expectations. *Oncology Nursing Forum, 30,* 585–590.

U.S. Department of Health and Human Services. (1998, June). *Informal caregiving: Compassion in action.* Washington, DC: Author.

Weitzner, M.A., McMillan, S.C., & Jacobsen, P.B. (1999). Family caregiver quality of life: Differences between curative and palliative cancer treatment settings. *Journal of Pain and Symptom Management, 17,* 418–428.

Wideheim, A., Edvardsson, T., Pahlson, A., & Ahlstrom, G. (2002). A family's perspective on living with a highly malignant brain tumor. *Cancer Nursing, 25,* 236–244.

Zhang, A.Y., & Siminoff, L.A. (2003). The role of the family in treatment decision making by patients with cancer. *Oncology Nursing Forum, 30,* 1022–1028.

Appendix

Psychosocial Support Programs and Resources for People Surviving Cancer and Their Families

ROBIN M. LALLY, PHD(c), RN, MS, AOCN®, CNS,
AND JUDI JOHNSON, PHD, RN, FAAN

Cancer survivors and their families may need help when dealing with the emotional aspects of living with cancer. This appendix lists organizations and services that provide information, support, and wellness activities. All of them, in the literature they provide, indicate that their primary goal is to offer support to people touched by cancer. Some cancer survivors want to connect with other survivors in person or via the Internet to share information and encouragement. Others want to learn about wellness retreats or camps that they or a family member can attend. Additionally, some patients may seek organizations that are devoted to a specific type of cancer; others may benefit from the support of people from various cultural, age, or sexual-preference groups. This resource listing is intended to be a guide to help nurses and other healthcare professionals to fulfill these types of requests. Information about each organization as it relates to the support of cancer survivors, families, and caregivers is provided along with a Web site and other contact information as available. Abbreviations have been used to indicate the type of service offered: "E" for education, "S" for support, and "W" for wellness.

This resource list is by no means a comprehensive guide of all organizations that offer psychosocial services. And, although the supportive aspect of these resources is highlighted here, each may offer other services as well. Many other resources exist that are limited to a local area through hospitals and clinics, places of worship, and social groups. Nurses also should familiarize themselves with these resources. If you have a specific need and do not find it in this listing of organizations, you can embark on your own investigation by using an Internet search engine like Google (www.google.com) or Yahoo (www.yahoo.com).

Selection criteria for inclusion in this listing of psychosocial services include organizations that appear to offer services that reach outside the local area and whose major goal is to provide support, education (beyond written information), or wellness activities. Each of the resources was determined to have programs and services that offer people ways to discover how to enjoy living in the present, to avoid carrying unnecessary burdens, to know they are not alone in their cancer journey, and to learn a different meaning for hope and healing. Some organizations charge a fee for their services, whereas other services are free. This information, of course, is subject to change over time as the funding and needs of the organizations change.

The information provided in this list is current as of the time of publication. Inclusion in this list is not intended to be an endorsement of any organization or program.

Appendix. Psychosocial Support Programs and Resources for People Surviving Cancer and Their Families

Program	Purpose	Fees[a]/Sponsor	Duration/ Frequency	Focus	Cancer Populations
Bone Marrow Transplant					
Blood & Marrow Transplant Information Network Highland Park, IL 847-433-3313 www.bmtnews.org	E, S	Fee varies as applicable	Ongoing	Quarterly newsletter; resource directory; 24-hour patient-survivor telephone link	Bone marrow and stem cell transplant and cord blood recipients
National Bone Marrow Transplant Link Southfield, MI TF 800-546-5268 www.nbmtlink.org	S	Free	Ongoing	"Resource Guide for Bone Marrow/Stem Cell Transplant: Friends Helping Friends"; telephone support groups	Patients, friends, and families affected by bone marrow transplant
Brain Tumors					
American Brain Tumor Association Des Plains, IL TF 800-886-2282 www.abta.org	E, S	Fee varies as applicable	Ongoing	Assistance with access to support groups; education	People surviving brain tumors and their families
Brain Tumor Society Watertown, MA TF 800-770-8287 www.tbts.org	E, S	Fee varies as applicable	Ongoing	Telephone support network; assistance connecting with support groups nationally	Patients, parents of children surviving brain tumors, and their families
National Brain Tumor Foundation San Francisco, CA TF 800-934-CURE www.braintumor.org	E, S	Fee varies as applicable	Ongoing	Patient and caregiver support networks; international listing of support groups; assistance with starting local groups	People surviving brain tumors and their caregivers

(Continued on next page)

614

Appendix. Psychosocial Support Programs and Resources for People Surviving Cancer and Their Families (Continued)

Program	Purpose	Fees[a]/Sponsor	Duration/Frequency	Focus	Cancer Populations
Breast Cancer					
Adelphi NY Statewide Breast Cancer Hotline and Support Program Garden City, NY TF 800-877-8077 www.adelphi.edu/nysbreastcancer/index.html	E, S	Free; donations accepted	Ongoing	Education and support	Women surviving breast cancer
African American Breast Cancer Alliance, Inc. (AABCA) Minneapolis, MN 612-825-3675 www.geocities.com/aabcainc	S	Fee varies as applicable	Ongoing	Support groups	African American women and men and their families affected by breast cancer
Breast Friends Atlanta, GA Local 404-843-0677 TF 888-718-3523 www.breastfriends.org	E, S	Fee varies as applicable	Ongoing	24-hour telephone peer support; face-to-face support and visits in Atlanta area	Women surviving breast cancer
Dragon Boat Racing Teams Edmonton, Alberta, Canada www.cbcn.ca/breastfriends/	W	Fee varies as applicable	Ongoing	Races throughout North America; 95 international teams, including many in New Zealand, Australia, the United States, and Canada, train in a specialized program to reduce the risk of arm lymphedema and race in dragon boat (50-foot boats with 20 paddlers) competitions	Women surviving breast cancer

(Continued on next page)

Appendix. Psychosocial Support Programs and Resources for People Surviving Cancer and Their Families *(Continued)*

Program	Purpose	Fees[a]/Sponsor	Duration/ Frequency	Focus	Cancer Populations
Las Isabelas San Jose, CA 408-287-4890 www.lasisabelas.org	S	Fee varies as applicable	Contact for group meeting times	Support group	Latinas surviving breast cancer
Living Beyond Breast Cancer Ardmore, PA TF 888-753-5222 www.lbbc.org	E, S	Free; donations accepted	Ongoing	Serving unmet needs, online support, quarterly newsletter (available by mail), volunteer help line	Women surviving breast cancer, especially young women and those with advanced disease
Male Breast Cancer Awareness Group Legacy Good Samaritan Hospital and Medical Center Portland, OR See www.malecare.org/support_groups.htm for program information	S	Fee varies as applicable	First Thursday of each month	Support group	Men surviving breast cancer
Me Again Breast Completion Kit Cinta Latina Research Red Bank, NJ 732-213-3954 http://cintalatina.org meagain@cintalatina.org	S, W	Fee varies as applicable	Ongoing	Stencil and colorant kit that can be self-applied or done by technician to simulate appearance of nipple-areola	Women following a mastectomy who have faded areola tattoos
Men Against Breast Cancer Adamstown, MD TF 866-547-6222 www.menagainstbreastcancer.org	S	Fee varies as applicable	Group early in its development, frequency of offerings variable	Goal is to provide programs nationally: "Survival Guide for Men" and "Partners in Survival"	Men supporting women experiencing breast cancer

(Continued on next page)

Appendix. Psychosocial Support Programs and Resources for People Surviving Cancer and Their Families *(Continued)*

Program	Purpose	Fees[a]/Sponsor	Duration/ Frequency	Focus	Cancer Populations
Mothers Supporting Daughters With Breast Cancer Chestertown, MD 410-778-1982 www.mothersdaughters.org	S	Free; donations accepted	Ongoing	Developed by cancer survivor and nurse Lillie Shockney and her mother; one-tc-one support from mothers in 18 states	Mothers of daughters surviving breast cancer
SHARE: Self-Help for Women With Breast or Ovarian Cancer New York City and throughout New Jersey Peer hot line TF 866-891-2392 www.sharecancersupport.org	E, S, W	Fee varies as applicable	Ongoing	Wellness workshops, support groups, and educational programs	Women surviving breast and/or ovarian cancer and their families
Sharsheret Nationwide, based in Hackensack, NJ Peer link TF 866-474-2774 www.sharsheret.org	S	Fee varies as applicable	Ongoing	Provides links to peers; online newsletter	Young Jewish women surviving breast cancer
Sisters Network, Inc. Houston, TX 866-781-1808 www.sistersnetworkinc.org	S	Fee varies as applicable	Ongoing	Support chapters in 25 states; *The National Network* quarterly newsletter ($10)	African American women surviving breast cancer

(Continued on next page)

Appendix. Psychosocial Support Programs and Resources for People Surviving Cancer and Their Families (Continued)

Program	Purpose	Fees[a]/Sponsor	Duration/ Frequency	Focus	Cancer Populations
Y-ME National Breast Cancer Organization Chicago, IL TF 800-221-2141 (English) TF 800-986-9505 (Español) www.y-me.org	E, S	Fee varies as applicable	Ongoing	24-hour hot line for patients or caregivers with translators in 150 languages; "Men's Match Program" connects men with volunteers for support; one-hour monthly teleconferences with volunteers matching participants profiles; quarterly newsletter, *Lifeline*	Women with breast cancer and their friends and family
Young Survival Coalition New York, NY 212-206-6610 www.youngsurvival.org	S	Free; donations accepted	Ongoing	International with chapters in 13 states; connects young patients with peer survivors; assistance with finding local support groups; newsletter	Women 40 years of age and younger surviving breast cancer
YWCA (Young Women's Clubs of America) TF 800-95-EPLUS Contact your local YWCA	E, S, W	Fee varies as applicable	Ongoing	ENCORE Plus program of support for low-cost early detection, peer support, and exercise during treatment	Women in need of screening services and those surviving breast cancer
Gastrointestinal/Colorectal Cancers					
Colon Cancer Alliance TF hot line 877-422-2030 www.ccalliance.org	E, S	Fee varies as applicable	Ongoing	"Buddy program" of support; scheduled topical online chats	People surviving colon cancer, their families, friends, and caregivers

(Continued on next page)

Appendix. Psychosocial Support Programs and Resources for People Surviving Cancer and Their Families (Continued)

Program	Purpose	Fees[a]/Sponsor	Duration/ Frequency	Focus	Cancer Populations
Colorectal Cancer Network (International) Kensington, MD 301-879-1500 www.colorectal-cancer.net	S	Fee varies as applicable	Ongoing	International support network; "SemiColon Club" and "SemiColon Friends" support networks for patients and caregivers; adventure retreat	People surviving colon cancer and their caregivers
The Oley Foundation Albany, NY TF 800-776-OLEY www.oley.org	S	Fee varies as applicable	Ongoing	Maintains contact lists of patients and caregivers to be contacted in person or through foundation's toll-free numbers	Anyone sustained on IV or tube feeding because of gastrointestinal disease
United Ostomy Association, Inc. United States, Canada, Puerto Rico, and Bermuda TF 800-826-0826 www.uoa.org	E, S	Fee varies as applicable	Ongoing	Hundreds of chapters throughout the United States, Canada, Puerto Rico, and Bermuda; online discussion forums for teens, young adults, and parents; social networks; conferences; visitation program	People with intestinal or urinary diversions
Head and Neck Cancer					
International Association of Laryngectomees (IAL) Stockton, CA TF 866-425-3678 www.larynxlink.com	S	Club dues; S10 for members at large	Ongoing	250 support clubs throughout the United States and 14 other countries; members visit new patients	People with laryngectomies and their family members

(Continued on next page)

Appendix. Psychosocial Support Programs and Resources for People Surviving Cancer and Their Families (Continued)

Program	Purpose	Fees[a]/Sponsor	Duration/ Frequency	Focus	Cancer Populations
Let's Face It Bellingham, WA 360-676-7325 www.faceit.org	S	Fee varies as applicable	Ongoing	Phone consultation and self-help network directory	People with facial disfigurement and their caregivers
Support for People with Oral and Head and Neck Cancer (SPOHNC) Locust Valley, NY TF 800-377-0928 www.spohnc.org	S	Fee varies as applicable	Ongoing	Survivor/family member matching with volunteers; newsletter	People surviving head and neck cancer and their families
Hematologic Cancers					
International Myeloma Foundation (IMF) U.S./Canada hot line TF 800-452-2873 Elsewhere 818-487-7455 www.myeloma.org	E, S	Fee varies as applicable	Ongoing	Maintains contact information for more than 100 support groups worldwide; retreats for support group leaders	People surviving multiple myeloma
Leukemia & Lymphoma Society White Plains, NY 914-949-5213 www.leukemia-lymphoma.org	E, S	Fee varies as applicable	Ongoing	Chapters throughout the United States; peer-to-peer telephone support program; 230 family support groups; annual financial stipend available for treatment or travel	All people affected by blood-related cancers

(Continued on next page)

Appendix. Psychosocial Support Programs and Resources for People Surviving Cancer and Their Families (Continued)

Program	Purpose	Fees[a]/Sponsor	Duration/ Frequency	Focus	Cancer Populations
Lymphoma Research Foundation New York, NY TF 800-235-6848 Los Angeles, CA TF 800-500-9976 www.lymphoma.org	E, S	Fee varies as applicable	Ongoing	Patient-to-patient telephone network; newsletter	People surviving lymphoma and their families
Lung Cancer					
Lung Cancer Alliance Washington, DC TF 800-298-2436 www.lungcanceralliance.org	E, S	Fee varies as applicable	Ongoing	Hot line; "phone buddies"; multiple types of support groups	People surviving lung cancer and their families and friends
Ovarian Cancer					
Gilda Radner Familial Ovarian Cancer Registry Buffalo, NY TF 800-682-7426 (OVARIAN) www.ovariancancer.com	E, S	Fee varies as applicable	Ongoing	Question help line for high-risk women; newsletter; online support forum under development	Women at risk for, with questions about, and/or surviving ovarian cancer
The International Ovarian Cancer Connection Amarillo, TX 806-355-2565 www.ovarian-news.org	S	Free; donations accepted	Ongoing	Support groups throughout the United States and Canada; newsletter, *Conversations!*	Women surviving ovarian cancer

(Continued on next page)

Appendix. Psychosocial Support Programs and Resources for People Surviving Cancer and Their Families *(Continued)*

Program	Purpose	Fees[a]/Sponsor	Duration/ Frequency	Focus	Cancer Populations
SHARE: Self-Help for Women With Breast or Ovarian Cancer New York, NY TF peer hot line 866-891-2392 www.sharecancersupport.org	E, S, W	Fee varies as applicable	Ongoing	Wellness workshops; support groups; educational programs	Women surviving breast and/or ovarian cancer and their families
Pain					
American Chronic Pain Association (ACPA) Rocklin, CA 916-632-0922 TF 800-533-3231 www.theacpa.org	E, S, W	$30 initial membership fee; $15 annual renewal to receive newsletter and workbook and participate in member discussion board	Contact to find a local group	Peer support groups, online forums, and information to assist people in living well with chronic pain	All people experiencing chronic pain
Vulvar Pain Foundation Graham, NC 336-226-0704 www.vulvarpainfoundation.org	E, S	$40 membership fee (installment plan or reduced fee available with approval)	Ongoing	Membership entitles women to newsletter, support group information, and other wellness opportunities	Women with chronic vulvar pain

(Continued on next page)

Appendix. Psychosocial Support Programs and Resources for People Surviving Cancer and Their Families (Continued)

Program	Purpose	Fees[a]/Sponsor	Duration/Frequency	Focus	Cancer Populations
Pancreatic Cancer					
National Organization for Rare Disorders (NORD) Danbury, CT TF 800-999-NORD (6673) www.rarediseases.org	E, S	Fee varies as applicable	Ongoing	Family counseling; information; newsletter	People with rare diseases (e.g., pancreatic islet cell)
Pancreatic Cancer Action Network El Segundo, CA TF 877-272-6226 www.pancan.org	E, S	Fee varies as applicable	Ongoing	Patient and Liaison Services (PALS) for information and support; link to support groups in several states	People experiencing pancreatic cancer and their caregivers
Prostate Cancer					
US TOO International TF 800-808-7865 www.ustoo.com	E, S	Free; donations accepted	Ongoing	Network of chapter meetings and support groups	Men surviving prostate cancer and their families
Sarcoma					
The Sarcoma Alliance Mill Valley, CA 415-381-7236 www.sarcomaalliance.com	S	Fee varies as applicable	Ongoing	Peer-to-peer connection; online discussion forums	People surviving sarcoma

(Continued on next page)

Appendix. Psychosocial Support Programs and Resources for People Surviving Cancer and Their Families (Continued)

Program	Purpose	Fees[a]/Sponsor	Duration/Frequency	Focus	Cancer Populations
Thyroid Cancer					
ThyCa: Thyroid Cancer Survivors' Association, Inc. New York, NY TF 877-588-7904 www.thyca.org	S	Free; donations accepted	Ongoing	Support groups in 34 states; person-to-person matching network; "Membership Messenger" newsletter	All thyroid cancer survivors
All Cancers					
AMC Cancer Research Center—cancer information and counseling line Denver, CO TF 800-525-3777 counseling line www.amc.org	E, S	Fee varies as applicable	Ongoing	Information and support	All people surviving cancer
American Cancer Society Atlanta, GA www.cancer.org TF 800-ACS-2345					
• Cancer Survivors Network	S	Free—must register to participate in discussions	Ongoing	Secure online support and discussion; create own Web site; share experiences	All people surviving cancer

(Continued on next page)

Appendix. Psychosocial Support Programs and Resources for People Surviving Cancer and Their Families (Continued)

Program	Purpose	Fees[a]/Sponsor	Duration/Frequency	Focus	Cancer Populations
• I Can Cope (classic) • I Can Cope (compact) • I Can Cope (stand alone)	E, S	Free	Two hours; eight consecutive classes	Increase knowledge; promote positive attitude, decision making, and coping	Adults with any type of cancer and their families from diagnosis through treatment
• Taking Charge of Money Matters			Four modules; two hours each		Financial and work issues arising during or after treatment; guest speakers
• Relieving Cancer Pain • Nutritional Well-Being			Two-hours; one-time seminars		
• Reach to Recovery	S	Free	One-on-one in-person or over phone support (ongoing program)	Volunteer breast cancer survivors provide support and education from diagnosis through treatment	Women and men undergoing breast cancer treatment
• Man to Man	E, S	Free	Monthly meetings	Volunteers and speakers educate men about prostate cancer, treatment, and side effects	Men surviving prostate cancer (some meetings permit spouses/partners)

(Continued on next page)

Appendix. Psychosocial Support Programs and Resources for People Surviving Cancer and Their Families (Continued)

Program	Purpose	Fees[a]/Sponsor	Duration/Frequency	Focus	Cancer Populations
• Look Good . . . Feel Better (group, one-on-one, self-help; Spanish and bilingual materials available)	E, S	Free	1–2 hours; frequency varies by facility; self-help materials	Makeup techniques, skin and nail care, and head-covering options	Women undergoing cancer treatment
• Look Good . . . Feel Better for Teens - TF 800-395-LOOK - www.2bMe.org	E, S	Free	1½ hours; frequency varies by facility	Skin care and makeup techniques; hair loss issues; nutrition, exercise, fitness, and teen issues; available in 13 states	Males and females 13–17 years old undergoing treatment
Cancer Care New York, NY TF 800-813-HOPE (4673) www.cancercare.org	E, S	Free; donations accepted	Support groups monthly; contact them for other schedules	Emotional support from social workers and support groups via telephone; in-person or online support groups in several eastern U.S. cities	All people surviving cancer
Cancer Care Services Fort Worth, TX 817-921-0653 www.cancercareservices.org	E, S, W	Fee varies as applicable	"Surviving with Cancer" seven-week series	Support groups; yoga; visits by social workers; play therapy for children	All people surviving cancer and their families and friends

(Continued on next page)

Appendix. Psychosocial Support Programs and Resources for People Surviving Cancer and Their Families (Continued)

Program	Purpose	Fees[a]/Sponsor	Duration/ Frequency	Focus	Cancer Populations
Cancer Hope Network Chester, NJ TF 877-467-3638 www.cancerhopenetwork.org	S	Free; donations accepted	Ongoing	One-on-one support from cancer survivors with same or similar cancers; matching people with similar cancer situations	All people with cancer and their family members
Cancer House of Hope Westfield, MA 413-562-0110, ext. 1191 www.center-of-hope.org	E, W	Free; donations accepted	Ongoing	Outdoor activities; lectures; newsletter; support groups; library	All cancer survivors and their friends and families
Cancervive Los Angeles, CA TF 800-4-TO-CURE www.cancervive.org	E, S	Fee varies as applicable	Ongoing	Sponsors support groups, conferences, and camps	All people surviving cancer (focus on life after cancer)
Cancer Wellness Center Northbrook, IL TF 866-292-9355 or Local 847-509-9595 www.cancerwellness.org	E, S, W	Free; donations accepted	Monthly networking and eight-week commitment support groups available; contact them for schedule	Emotional support; support groups; spirituality healing; education; complementary therapies; 24-hour support hot line	All people surviving cancer, their families, and others

(Continued on next page)

Appendix. Psychosocial Support Programs and Resources for People Surviving Cancer and Their Families (Continued)

Program	Purpose	Fees[a]/Sponsor	Duration/ Frequency	Focus	Cancer Populations
Caring Bridge Eagan, MN 651-452-7940 www.caringbridge.com	S	Free; donations accepted	Ongoing	Offers free Web pages to patients on which they can place health information for friends and family to review and reply with short notes	All people with cancer and their family and friends
Caring Connections Salt Lake City, UT 801-585-9522 www.nurs.utah.edu/caringconnections	S	University of Utah College of Nursing; $40; scholarships available	Eight weekly sessions held five times per year	Multiple facilitated grief support groups for adults, children, and adolescents	Anyone adjusting to the death of a family member or friend resulting from a variety of circumstances
DES Cancer Network Washington, DC TF 800-337-6384 www.descancer.org E-mail: desnetwrk@aol.com	S	Fee varies as applicable	Ongoing	Patient-to-patient support	All people (men and women) who were exposed to diethylstilbestrol and now have cancer
Dia de la Mujer Latina, Inc. Marietta, GA 678-494-8879 www.diadelamujerlatina.org	E, S	Fee varies as applicable	Ongoing	Promotes health in Latina community, including resource information and patient navigation for Latina women diagnosed with cancer	Primarily Latina women surviving cancer in Georgia
Dream Foundation Santa Barbara, CA 805-564-2131 www.dreamfoundation.org	S	Donations accepted	Ongoing	Attempts to fulfill the last wishes of adults with cancer	Adults with a life expectancy of less than one year

(Continued on next page)

Appendix. Psychosocial Support Programs and Resources for People Surviving Cancer and Their Families (Continued)

Program	Purpose	Fees[a]/Sponsor	Duration/ Frequency	Focus	Cancer Populations
Gillette Women's Cancer Connection www.gillettecancerconnect.org	S	Fee varies as applicable	Ongoing	Supportive reading materials; sponsors programs nationally; maintains list of U.S. support groups	Women cancer survivors and their families and friends
The Group Room Radio Talk Show Sherman Oaks, CA TF 800-GRP-ROOM (477-7666) www.vitaloptions.org	E, S	Fee to receive previously taped broadcasts	Weekly; listen online or see list of local radio stations carrying broadcast	Call-in radio talk show about cancer topics linking survivors with each other and healthcare professionals	All adults surviving cancer
Kathy's Group Wakefield, RI TF 888-5-Kathys	S	Free; donations accepted	Weekly	Support groups for lesbians and their families; bereavement support	Lesbians and their families/ friends affected by any type of cancer or life-threatening illness in New England
Lesbian Community Cancer Project Chicago, IL 773-561-4662 www.lccp.org	E, S	Fee varies as applicable	Weekly	Support, education, advocacy, services, stress management and buddy program for newly diagnosed women with cancer	Women surviving cancer regardless of sexual orientation; special focus on providing access to lesbian-sensitive care
Mautner Project for Lesbians with Cancer Washington, DC 202-332-5536 www.mautnerproject.org	E, S	Fee varies as applicable	Ongoing	Emotional and practical support to families; support and bereavement groups; phone peer support	Lesbians surviving cancer of any type and their partners and other family members

(Continued on next page)

Appendix. Psychosocial Support Programs and Resources for People Surviving Cancer and Their Families *(Continued)*

Program	Purpose	Fees[a]/Sponsor	Duration/ Frequency	Focus	Cancer Populations
National Association for Continence Charleston, SC TF 800-BLADDER www.nafc.org	E, S	Fee varies as applicable	Ongoing	Bladder Control Forum online discussion group	All people with urinary continence issues
Partnership for Caring Washington, DC 24-hour help line 800-989-9455 www.partnershipforcaring.org	E, S, W	Donations accepted	Ongoing	Guidance in completing living wills, pain management at end of life, and talking with family about dying; live online chat room and moderated discussion groups currently being developed	All people with questions about preparing for death
Pathways Minneapolis, MN 612-822-9061 www.pathwaysminneapolis.org	S, W	Free; donations accepted	Ongoing extensive calendar	Psychological, emotional, and spiritual healing	Adults with life-threatening illnesses
Patient Advocate Foundation Newport News, VA TF 800-532-5274 www.patientadvocate.org	E, S	Fee varies as applicable	Ongoing	Link to multiple resources to assist with resolution of legal, insurance, and workplace issues	All people surviving cancer
People Living Through Cancer Albuquerque, NM 505-242-3263 (support hot line) www.pltc.org	S	Fee varies as applicable	Ongoing	Peer support services throughout New Mexico; Native American training program	All people surviving cancer

(Continued on next page)

Appendix. Psychosocial Support Programs and Resources for People Surviving Cancer and Their Families *(Continued)*

Program	Purpose	Fees[a]/Sponsor	Duration/ Frequency	Focus	Cancer Populations
Planet Cancer Austin, TX 512-481-9010 www.planetcancer.org	S	Free; donations accepted	Ongoing	Online support and discussion forums; support groups throughout the United States	Family and friends of children and young adults surviving cancer
Pregnant With Cancer Network Buffalo, NY TF 800-743-4471 www.pregnantwithcancer.org	S	Fee varies as applicable	Ongoing	Matches pregnant patients with cancer via phone or e-mail with women postpartum surviving the same cancer; newsletter	Women diagnosed with any cancer during pregnancy
R.A. Bloch Cancer Foundation, Inc. Kansas City, MO 816-WE-BUILD www.blochcancer.org	S	Fee varies as applicable	Ongoing	Matches cancer survivors for support	All people surviving cancer
Renewing Life Nationwide www.renewinglife.org E-mail: pathways@mtn.org	E, S	Fee varies as applicable	Eight consecutive weeks or three-day intensive education and support program	Counseling, information, practical tools, support and encouragement to treat the person as a whole and see illness as a growth opportunity	Adults with cancer and healthcare professionals

(Continued on next page)

Appendix. Psychosocial Support Programs and Resources for People Surviving Cancer and Their Families (Continued)

Program	Purpose	Fees[a]/Sponsor	Duration/ Frequency	Focus	Cancer Populations
RESOLVE: The National Infertility Association Somerville, MA 617-623-0744 TF 888-623-0744 help line www.resolve.org	E, S	Fee varies as applicable	Ongoing	More than 50 local chapters throughout the United States; Internet chat on specific topics and bulletin board support postings; local newsletters and support groups	All people experiencing infertility issues for any reason
The Simon Foundation for Continence Wilmette, IL TF 800-23-SIMON www.simonfoundation.org	E, S	Fee varies as applicable	Ongoing	Online support and discussion forum	All people with urinary continence issues
Susie Q. Foundation and Cancer Telecall Survivor Update c/o Mark Kocsis 6112 S. 95th Street Omaha, NE 68127-4036 402-996-1818 (registration) www.cancertelecall.com	S	Free; service provided by StarTouch International	Service provided 24 hours a day; available nationally	Password-protected voicemail system where patients leave health-related information for family and friends to access by calling 877-469-8732	Anyone with cancer able to speak on the telephone and their family and friends
University of Arizona Program in Integrative Medicine Tucson, AZ 520-626-6417 http://integrativemedicine.arizona.edu	W	Contact regarding fees	Ongoing	Consultation with physicians specializing in integrative (mind, body, spirit) medicine	All people surviving cancer

(Continued on next page)

Appendix. Psychosocial Support Programs and Resources for People Surviving Cancer and Their Families (Continued)

Program	Purpose	Fees*/Sponsor	Duration/ Frequency	Focus	Cancer Populations
Well Spouse Association Freehold, NJ TF 800-838-0879 www.wellspouse.org	S	Fee varies as applicable	Ongoing	Support groups throughout the United States and Canada; quarterly newsletter	Spousal caregivers of people surviving cancer
The Wellness Community Washington, DC TF 888-793-WELL www.thewellnesscommunity.org	E, S, W	Free; donations accepted	Ongoing	Worldwide facilities that provide home-like setting for connecting with other cancer survivors; "virtual" online wellness community forums	All people with cancer and their loved ones
Children (Support and Retreats/Camps)					
Big Sky Kids Bozeman, MT 406-586-1781 www.eaglemount.org	S, W	Free; donations accepted	Various camps for differing age groups	Retreat at Yellowstone National Park and surrounding area; horseback riding, fly fishing, kayaking; opportunity to meet friends	Children and young adults (ages 5–23 years) surviving cancer
Brain Tumor Foundation for Children, Inc. Atlanta, GA 770-458-5554 www.btfcgainc.org	E, S	Fee varies as applicable	Ongoing	Family support, education, telephone support network, meetings and events	Children with brain tumors and their parents
Camp Good Grief Boca Raton, FL 561-395-5031, ext. 5059 www.hospicebytheseafl.org	S	Free; donations accepted	Weekend twice per year	Bereavement camp with cabins, arts, crafts, bonfires, and sports	Children ages 6–13 who have lost a loved one, in any location, from any cause in the past three years

(Continued on next page)

Appendix. Psychosocial Support Programs and Resources for People Surviving Cancer and Their Families (Continued)

Program	Purpose	Fees[a]/Sponsor	Duration/ Frequency	Focus	Cancer Populations
Camp Mak-A-Dream Missoula, MT 406-549-5987 www.campdream.org	E, S, W	Free (limited number of travel scholarships)	See Web site for programs.	Outdoor fishing, hiking, ropes course, and horseback riding	Children and young adults surviving cancer and their siblings
Camp Okizu Novato, CA 415-382-9058 (karmaforkids hot line) 415-382-9038 (main) www.okizu.org	S, W	Free; donations accepted	Week-long camps; weekend camps for families and teens	Outdoor adventures and experiences; medical care available	Children and teens surviving cancer
Camp Special Love Winchester, VA TF 888-930-2707 www.speciallove.org	S, W	Contact for information	Week-long camps; year-round activities; special weekends for 13–25-year-olds and 18–25-year-olds	Variety of outdoor and other activities to support and encourage children and young adults to experience wellness	Children and young adults surviving cancer and their families and friends
Camp Sunshine Decatur, GA 404-325-7979 www.mycampsunshine.com	S, W	Low to no cost (can be waived for those unable to pay); contact for information	Year-round programs	Encourages children to be children through a variety of activities	Children, teens, and young adults surviving cancer (primarily in Georgia area)

(Continued on next page)

Appendix. Psychosocial Support Programs and Resources for People Surviving Cancer and Their Families (Continued)

Program	Purpose	Fees[a]/Sponsor	Duration/ Frequency	Focus	Cancer Populations
Camp Sunshine Casco, ME 207-655-3800 www.campsunshine.org	S, W	Free; donations accepted	Week-long camps	Counseling; recreational and medical support	Children with life-threatening illness and their families
Camp Wapiyapi Denver, CO 303-315-8255 www.wapiyapi.com	W	Free; donations accepted	Annual, week-long summer camp	Encourages healing and allows children the freedom to be children	Children surviving cancer and their siblings
CancerCare Helping Children Cope Program New York, NY TF 800-813-HOPE www.cancercare.org	S	Fee varies as applicable	Ongoing	Support groups and phone counseling	Children of parents with cancer
Candlelighters Childhood Cancer Foundation Kensington, MD TF 800-366-2223 www.candlelighters.org	S	Fee varies as applicable	Ongoing	Programs and services; camps; e-mail support group for parents; bereavement services; chapters throughout the United States	Families of children with cancer of any type
Children's Brain Tumor Foundation New York, NY TF 866-228-HOPE (support line) 212-448-9494 www.cbtf.org	S, W	Fee varies as applicable	Ongoing	Parent-to-parent support network and hot line; summer camps	Families of children surviving brain tumors

(Continued on next page)

Appendix. Psychosocial Support Programs and Resources for People Surviving Cancer and Their Families (Continued)

Program	Purpose	Fees[a]/Sponsor	Duration/ Frequency	Focus	Cancer Populations
First Descents Vail, CO 970-328-1806 www.firstdescents.com	W	Free; donations accepted	Week-long camps	Kayaking camp; professional athlete speakers	Young adults (15–22 years) surviving cancer
Hole in the Wall Gang Camp Ashford, CT 860-429-3444 www.holeinthewallgang.org	S, W	Free; donations accepted	Year-round programs; camps; support groups	Variety of outdoor activities; includes a Western-style camp, barn, recreational center, Olympic-size pool, and medical staff to help children to gain a renewed sense of childhood	Children with cancer and hematologic diseases and their families
Kids Cancer Network Santa Barbara, CA www.kidscancernetwork.org E-mail: info@kidscancernetwork.org	S	Free	Ongoing	Online support through positive story sharing and prayer requests	Children and parents surviving cancer
Kids Konnected Laguna Hills, CA TF 800-899-2866 www.kidskonnected.org	S	Free	Ongoing	24-hour hot line for children; support through camps, grief workshops, online newsletter and chat room, and teddy bears	Children ages three through teens who have a parent diagnosed with cancer
KOA Care Camps Birmingham, AL 205-824-0022 www.koacarecamps.com	S, W	Free; donations accepted	Varies by state	Listing of 37 camps throughout the United States and Canada providing outdoor adventure and support	Children of all ages and young adults surviving cancer and their siblings

(Continued on next page)

Appendix. Psychosocial Support Programs and Resources for People Surviving Cancer and Their Families *(Continued)*

Program	Purpose	Fees[a]/Sponsor	Duration/ Frequency	Focus	Cancer Populations
Make-A-Wish Phoenix, AZ TF 800-722-WISH (9474) www.wish.org	S, W	Free to child and family as applicable; donations accepted	Ongoing	Grants wishes to children with life-threatening illness to enhance their lives	Children (from age 2½ to 18) with a life-threatening illness (a terminal diagnosis is not necessary although medical eligibility is required)
The National Children's Cancer Society St. Louis, MO TF 800-532-6459 www.children-cancer.com	E, S	Fee varies as applicable	Ongoing	Emotional support services and education	Children (birth to 18 years) with cancer and their parents
Starlight Starbright Children's Foundation Los Angeles, CA 310-479-1212 www.starlight.org	S, W	Fee varies as applicable; relies on sponsor; donations accepted	Ongoing	Programs in more than 1,000 hospitals in the United States to provide bedside entertainment to children; family outings; grants wishes	Children ages 4–18 years
SunKeeper Mentorship Program Calgary, Alberta, Canada 403-216-9210, ext. 231 www.kidscancercare.ab.ca	E, S, W	Free; sponsored by Kids Cancer Care Foundation of Alberta	Week-long and year-round camps and activities	Variety of outdoor experiential activities; leadership and mentorship camps for young adults	Children ages three to young adults surviving cancer
Sunshine Foundation Feasterville, PA TF 800-767-1976 www.sunshinefoundation.org	S, W	Free; however, financial and medical eligibility required; donations accepted	Ongoing	Grants wishes of seriously ill children	Children/young adults ages 3–21 years who are seriously ill, challenged, or abused and whose families are experiencing financial strain

(Continued on next page)

Appendix. Psychosocial Support Programs and Resources for People Surviving Cancer and Their Families *(Continued)*

Program	Purpose	Fees[a]/Sponsor	Duration/ Frequency	Focus	Cancer Populations
Teens Living with Cancer Henrietta, NY 585-334-0858 www.teenslivingwithcancer.com	E, S	Donations accepted	Ongoing	Online support for teens and families; patients send stories and pictures to share	Teens surviving cancer, their families, and friends
The Ulman Cancer Fund for Young Adults Ellicott City, MD TF 888-393-FUND www.ulmanfund.org	E, S	Fee varies as applicable	Ongoing	Networking service that matches patients for support; support groups throughout the United States	All young adults surviving cancer and their friends and family
The World's Greatest Camp Orange, CA 949-855-1972 www.ocf-ocf.org/camp.html	S, W	Free; donations accepted	Retreat twice a year	YMCA camp in Big Bear, CA that includes a variety of outdoor activities	Children and young adults with cancer and their families
Lodging and Travel					
Gilda's Club Worldwide International; 14 locations TF 888-GILDA-4-U www.gildasclub.org	S, W	Free	Non-residential home-like settings	Social and emotional support	Men, women, and children undergoing cancer treatment and their families
Hope Lodge 15 states and Puerto Rico TF 800-ACS-2345 www.cancer.org	S, W	Free; American Cancer Society program	Temporary lodging	Supportive, home-like atmosphere	Eligible people receiving cancer treatment and their families

(Continued on next page)

Appendix. Psychosocial Support Programs and Resources for People Surviving Cancer and Their Families (Continued)

Program	Purpose	Fees[a]/Sponsor	Duration/Frequency	Focus	Cancer Populations
National Association of Hospital Hospitality Houses, Inc. Asheville, NC TF 800-542-9730 www.nahhh.org	S	Free or low cost	Temporary lodging	Directory of member and non-member housing opportunities throughout the United States	Patients and families receiving treatment away from home
National Patient Travel Center Virginia Beach, VA TF 800-296-1217 (24-hour help line) 757-318-9145 (outside the United States) www.patienttravel.org	S	No cost; eligibility requirements apply	No limit on number of trips	Referral and information service to organizations providing travel	People of all ages with financial hardship needing to travel a long distance for specialized medical evaluation, diagnosis, or treatment
Ronald McDonald House Oak Brook, IL 212 houses in 20 countries 630-623-7048 www.rmhc.org	S	$5–$20/day; free if unable to pay	Temporary lodging near medical facilities	Support; convenience	Children with serious illness and their families
Adult Retreats and Wellness Centers—Southwest					
Cancer Wellness House Salt Lake City, UT 801-236-2294 www.cancer-wellness.org	E, S, W	Free services; fee varies as applicable for events	Weekly resource offerings	Home-like setting providing emotional support and educational resources	All people (including children and teens) with cancer and their families and friends
Commonweal Cancer Help Program Bolinas, CA 415-868-0970 www.commonweal.org	S, W	All-inclusive basic $1,880 fee (partial scholarships available)	Week-long retreats; approximately six per year	California plus several other states and Canada; provides support, relaxation, and complementary therapies	People surviving cancer and their spouses or close support person

(Continued on next page)

Appendix. Psychosocial Support Programs and Resources for People Surviving Cancer and Their Families *(Continued)*

Program	Purpose	Fees[a]/Sponsor	Duration/ Frequency	Focus	Cancer Populations
Healing Odyssey Irvine, CA 949-494-2447 www.healingodyssey.org	W	$250; includes lodging, meals, ropes course, and educational materials (scholarships available)	Weekends	Two- to three-day retreats; ropes course	All female cancer survivors
Image Reborn: Living Beyond Breast Cancer Park City, UT 435-649-4287 www.imagerebornfoundation.org	E, S, W	Image Reborn Foundation	Week-long and extended weekend	Renewal retreat with group counseling, music, art, journaling, and light exercise	Women surviving breast cancer
Life Beyond Cancer Tucson, AZ www.lifebeyondcancer.com E-mail: lifebeyondcancer@usoncology.com	E, S, W	Scholarships available; $100 non-refundable registration fee	Four days	Retreats for inspiration; wellness activities; educational speakers	Female survivors of all cancers Participants are highly encouraged to take learning back to community.
Scripps Clinic San Diego, CA 858-554-3300 www.scrippsclinic.com	W	Fee varies as applicable	Ongoing	Variety of complementary therapy courses to improve coping with stress, pain, and illness	All people wishing to improve their health and wellness
Spa for the Spirit Foundation Denver, CO 303-675-4709	W	Granted through the Susan G. Komen Denver Affiliate Contact for fee information	Four-day retreats	Mountain retreats that include music, art, massage, and movement	Women living with advanced breast cancer or recently diagnosed breast cancer

(Continued on next page)

Appendix. Psychosocial Support Programs and Resources for People Surviving Cancer and Their Families *(Continued)*

Program	Purpose	Fees[a]/Sponsor	Duration/ Frequency	Focus	Cancer Populations
Sunstone Cancer Retreats Tucson, AZ 520-749-1928 www.sunstonehealing.net	E, S, W	Sunstone Cancer Support Foundation $500–$750	Two to three nights; lodging, meals, program, and personal services such as massage	Refocusing physically and psychologically	Cancer survivors, healthcare professionals, support groups, and nonprofessional caregivers
Tutu's House Waimea, HI 808-885-6777 www.tutushouse.org	W	Free	Ongoing	Experiential programs; support; emphasis on mind, body, spirit wellness, and Hawaiian culture	People of all ages seeking wellness
Adult Retreats and Wellness Centers—Central					
A New Beginning Cancer Retreat Ellston, IA 641-722-4276 www.cancer-retreat.org	E, S, W	Free to survivors	Year-round; Monday through Wednesday or weekend retreats available	Individual and group counseling; nutrition; support groups for a variety of participants; Look Good . . . Feel Better wig and makeup assistance	All survivors (family may join in at designated times and may stay for a fee on weekends)

(Continued on next page)

Appendix. Psychosocial Support Programs and Resources for People Surviving Cancer and Their Families (Continued)

Program	Purpose	Fees[a]/Sponsor	Duration/ Frequency	Focus	Cancer Populations
Breast Cancer Recovery Foundation, Inc. Madison, WI 608-821-1140 www.bcrf.org	S, W	$100–$1,000 (approximately 1% of the woman's household income); covers food, lodging, activities, and supplies	One to several days of adventures/ seminars throughout year	"Infinite Boundaries" retreats (many on Madeline Island, Lake Superior) providing support and opportunity to challenge self	Women surviving breast cancer
Cancer Support Center Homewood, IL www.cancersupportcenter.org	E, S, W	Free	Ongoing	Nonprofit programs to support social, physical, and spiritual needs, exercise, relaxation, counseling	All people surviving cancer and their family and friends
North Memorial Medical Center Hubert H. Humphrey Cancer Center Minneapolis, MN 763-520-5158 (day long) 763-520-5211 (wilderness) www.northmemorial.com	S, W	Contact for rates	Day-long retreat	Wellness Retreat at Aveda Institute	All people surviving cancer and their support person
			Four-day winter or five-day fall retreat in northern Minnesota wilderness	Women in Nature confidence building, relaxation	Women surviving cancer

(Continued on next page)

Appendix. Psychosocial Support Programs and Resources for People Surviving Cancer and Their Families (*Continued*)

Program	Purpose	Fees/Sponsor	Duration/ Frequency	Focus	Cancer Populations
Recovery in the Wilderness Pinewood, MI 847-328-4130 www.wildernessbay.org	S, W	$275	Three days	Wilderness retreat with nature walks, ropes course, and canoeing to increase independence and confidence	Women surviving breast cancer
Wellness House Hinsdale, IL 630-323-5150 www.wellnesshouse.org	E, S, W	Fee varies as applicable	Ongoing (no lodging)	Home-like environment that provides education, support, exercise, and nutrition courses and groups	All cancer survivors, family, and friends
Wellness Weekend Retreat Oklahoma City, OK TF health line 888-951-2277 www.integris-health.com	E, S, W	Sponsored by several area cancer centers; $30–$45; scholarships available	Annual fall weekend	Workshops, hiking, and relaxation with focus on life enrichment	All adult cancer survivors and family members
Adult Retreats and Wellness Centers—Northwest					
The Center for Cancer Support Bozeman, MT 406-582-1600 www.bigskycancerresource.org	E, S, W	Contact for information	Ongoing programs	Supportive and educational care; buddy program; support groups; retreat	People surviving cancer, family, friends, and caregivers
Harmony Hill Cancer Care Retreat Union, WA 360-898-2363 www.harmonyhill.org	W	No fee	Three-day retreats throughout year	Healing, quality of life, group activity, imagery, stress reduction, complementary care techniques, and whole-food meals	All adult residents surviving cancer and their loved ones (some retreats designed for local residents or minority groups)

(Continued on next page)

Appendix. Psychosocial Support Programs and Resources for People Surviving Cancer and Their Families *(Continued)*

Program	Purpose	Fees[a]/Sponsor	Duration/ Frequency	Focus	Cancer Populations
Adult Retreats and Wellness Centers—South					
Surviving and Thriving San Antonio, TX 210-616-5570 www.ccc.saci.org/patientservices/wellness.htm E-mail: mjackson@saci.org	E, W	Contact regarding fee (negotiable based on needs); Cancer Therapy and Research Center Wellness Center	Three-day event in spring	Education, exercise, humor, relaxation, creativity, and stress reduction	Adult survivors and caregivers
Adult Retreats and Wellness Centers—East					
Adirondack Experience Lake Placid, NY TF 800-300-1718 www.adkexp.com	W	$350 (less if participant brings own tent); some scholarships available	Two-night retreat every other month	Personal growth and challenge, ropes course, reflection, and healing	Women surviving breast cancer
Exceptional Cancer Patients Meadville, PA 814-337-8192 www.ecap-online.org	E, S, W	Fee varies as applicable; associated with the Mind-Body Wellness Center and Bernie Siegel, MD	Varies	Wellness seminars	People surviving chronic illnesses and health professionals

(Continued on next page)

Appendix. Psychosocial Support Programs and Resources for People Surviving Cancer and Their Families (*Continued*)

Program	Purpose	Fees[a]/Sponsor	Duration/ Frequency	Focus	Cancer Populations
The Gathering Place Cleveland, OH 216-595-9546 www.touchedbycancer.org	E, S, W	Free; donations accepted	Ongoing	Emotional support; educational resources; healing touch, yoga, and camping for children whose parents or loved one is a participant; bereavement and other support groups	Adults surviving cancer and their loved ones
Smith Farm Cancer Help Program Washington, DC; retreats in Comus, MD 202-483-8600 www.smithfarm.com/cancer.html	E, S, W	Fee varies as applicable	Week-long retreats; ongoing	Physical, emotional, and spiritual healing; yoga, counseling, groups, relaxation	All cancer survivors and spouses
Two Roads Maine Freeport, ME 207-865-4517 www.tworoadsmaine.org	S, W	Fee varies by trip	Three- to four-day trips year-round	Outdoor adventure experiences in Maine with goal of reestablishing one's connection with nature	People surviving life-threatening illness or experiencing a major life change, their friends, and family
Retreats in Variable Locations					
Camp Bluebird Camps in 13 states TF 800-811-8925 www.campbluebird.com	S, W	Fee varies as applicable (St. Vincent's Foundation, Birmingham, AL—national sponsor)	Contact sites for details	Outdoors; focus on listening, learning, and sharing with cancer survivors	All adults surviving cancer whether in or completed with treatment

(Continued on next page)

Appendix. Psychosocial Support Programs and Resources for People Surviving Cancer and Their Families (Continued)

Program	Purpose	Fees[a]/Sponsor	Duration/ Frequency	Focus	Cancer Populations
Casting for Recovery Manchester, VT TF 888-553-3500 www.castingforrecovery.org	W	Free; donations accepted	Weekends (May through September)	Trips in 15 states; fly fishing; focus on emotional and physical wellness	Women surviving breast cancer
Expedition Inspiration Trips in various states 208-726-6456 www.expeditioninspiration.org	W	Contact for information	Five-day trips (approximately) February through October	Mountain climbing to promote physical and emotional wellness and raise funds for program expansion and breast cancer research	Women surviving breast cancer and others wishing to participate
Team Survivor Santa Monica, CA Teams in approximately 16 states www.teamsurvivor.org	W	Free; donations accepted	Ongoing training and events	Physical activity; health education; support to regain body confidence and feeling of accomplishment	Female cancer survivors
We Can Weekend TF 800-ACS-2345 www.cancer.org	E, S, W	$40/family including lodging and meals; American Cancer Society	Two-day annual program	Focus on communication, relaxation, stress management, spirituality, and nutrition	People undergoing treatment and their families
Periodicals					
Coping With Cancer www.copingmag.com/CopPages/CgHome. html	E, S	Available through most clinics or $19 annual subscription	Six times/ year	Enlightens and motivates readers	All people surviving cancer

(Continued on next page)

Appendix. Psychosocial Support Programs and Resources for People Surviving Cancer and Their Families *(Continued)*

Program	Purpose	Fees[a]/Sponsor	Duration/Frequency	Focus	Cancer Populations
CURE: Cancer Updates, Research & Education www.curetoday.com	E, S	Free to people with cancer; $20 annually for others	Quarterly	Provides support and information through science and personal stories	All people surviving cancer
OQ (Ostomy Quarterly magazine) www.uoa.org/publications_oq.htm	E, S	$25 annually	Quarterly	Is the only national periodical for ostomates	People with intestinal or urinary diversions
General					
National Alliance of Breast Cancer Organizations (NABCO) New York, NY TF 888-80-NABCO	E	Fee varies as applicable	Ongoing	Network of organizations in the United States dedicated to all aspects of breast cancer detection, care, and survivorship	Patients with and people affected by breast cancer; professionals
National Cancer Institute Bethesda, MD TF 800-4-CANCER www.cancer.gov	E	Fee varies as applicable	Ongoing	Education; resources; clinical research trial information	All people with cancer, families, friends, and professionals
National Coalition for Cancer Survivorship Silver Spring, MD TF 877-622-7937 www.canceradvocacy.org	E, S	Fee varies as applicable	Ongoing	Educational resources; news updates; events; "tool kit" audio tapes for coping with cancer	All people with cancer, families, friends, and professionals.
National Comprehensive Cancer Network Jenkintown, PA 215-690-0280 www.nccn.org	E	Fee varies as applicable	Ongoing	Education; treatment guidelines; decision-making assistance; clinical research trial information	All people experiencing a cancer diagnosis

E—education; S—support; TF—toll-free telephone number; W—wellness
[a] Fees indicated are those at the time of publication and are subject to change.

Index

INDEX

The letter f after a page number indicates that relevant content appears in a figure; the letter t, in a table.

A

abandonment, patient's fear of, 14, 33
action
   direct, 67, 81
   inhibition of, 68
active listening, 388–389, 409
acute fatigue, 170. *See also* fatigue
adaptation, 62–65, 79–80, 80f. *See also* coping
addiction, 567–571. *See also* substance abuse
   assessment for, 573f, 573–575
   definition of, 569t
   fear of, 146, 217, 579–582
   pain and, 579–580
   relapse in, 570–571, 575–577, 578t, 580
   treatment for, 575–579, 576f–577f, 578t
adjustment disorders, 208–209
adolescents. *See* children/adolescents
advance directives, 494, 534
affective denial, 263, 263t. *See also* denial
African American culture, 73–74, 103–105, 104t, 109t, 110–112, 149, 373, 505, 538, 559
after-death communication, 308–309
age. *See also* children/adolescents; developmental stages; older adults
   cancer development by, 89, 89t, 94t
   cognitive functioning and, 192–193
   influence on coping, 89t, 90, 92–95, 93t
Agency for Healthcare Research and Quality, 440
aggression, 223, 225, 235. *See also* anger
agoraphobia, 209
akathisia (motor restlessness), 210, 217, 361
ALARM model, for sexual functioning assessment, 336f
alcohol abuse. *See also* addiction; substance abuse
   and anxiety, 210–211, 214
   and cancer development/treatment, 571–573

and depression, 246
   epidemiology of, 565–567
   family history of, 570
alopecia
   and body image, 280
   from chemotherapy, 8–9
   effect on sexuality, 332
alpha interferon, side effects of, 175, 467
alprazolam, for anxiety, 216
alternative therapies. *See also* complementary and alternative medicine
   definition of, 531, 532t, 534f
   and denial, 265, 268
   and guilt, 319
Alzheimer disease, 193, 195, 356. *See also* dementia
amantadine (Symmetrel), 186
American Association of Sex Educators, Counselors, and Therapists, 347
American Geriatrics Society, Clinical Practice Committee, 361
American Medical Association
   Code of Ethics (1847), 4
   on physician-patient e-mail, 442
Americans with Disabilities Act (ADA), 36
amitriptyline, 217, 248t
amoxapine, 249t
amygdala, role in anger, 225
amyotrophic lateral sclerosis (ALS), 252
analgesics
   for pain management, 149, 185–186
   tolerance to, 580
anastrozole (Arimidex), 333
anemia
   cognitive impairment from, 195
   fatigue from, 173, 173f, 182f, 183
anger
   assessment of, 232–234, 233t, 236f
   in bereavement process, 230, 295, 309–310
   at cancer diagnosis, 229